AF118158

A Personalized Medicine Approach to the Diagnosis and Management of Autism Spectrum Disorder

A Personalized Medicine Approach to the Diagnosis and Management of Autism Spectrum Disorder

Editors

Richard E. Frye
Richard G. Boles
Shannon Rose
Daniel A. Rossignol

MDPI • Basel • Beijing • Wuhan • Barcelona • Belgrade • Manchester • Tokyo • Cluj • Tianjin

MDPI

Editors
Richard E. Frye
Director of Research
Rossignol Medical Center
Phoenix, AZ
United States

Richard G. Boles
Mitochondrial & Molecular
Medicine
Neurabilities Healthcare
Voorhees, NJ
United States

Shannon Rose
Department of Pediatrics
University of Arkansas for
Medical Sciences
Little Rock, AR
United States

Daniel A. Rossignol
Rossignol Clinic
Rossignol Medical Center
Aliso Viejo, CA
United States

Editorial Office
MDPI
St. Alban-Anlage 66
4052 Basel, Switzerland

This is a reprint of articles from the Special Issue published online in the open access journal *Journal of Personalized Medicine* (ISSN 2075-4426) (available at: https://www.mdpi.com/journal/jpm/special_issues/Personalized_Medicine_Approach_ASD).

For citation purposes, cite each article independently as indicated on the article page online and as indicated below:

LastName, A.A.; LastName, B.B.; LastName, C.C. Article Title. *Journal Name* **Year**, *Volume Number*, Page Range.

ISBN 978-3-0365-3221-9 (Hbk)
ISBN 978-3-0365-3220-2 (PDF)

© 2022 by the authors. Articles in this book are Open Access and distributed under the Creative Commons Attribution (CC BY) license, which allows users to download, copy and build upon published articles, as long as the author and publisher are properly credited, which ensures maximum dissemination and a wider impact of our publications.
The book as a whole is distributed by MDPI under the terms and conditions of the Creative Commons license CC BY-NC-ND.

Contents

About the Editors ix

Preface to "A Personalized Medicine Approach to the Diagnosis and Management of Autism Spectrum Disorder" xi

Richard E. Frye, Shannon Rose, Richard G. Boles and Daniel A. Rossignol
A Personalized Approach to Evaluating and Treating Autism Spectrum Disorder
Reprinted from: *J. Pers. Med.* **2022**, *12*, 147, doi:10.3390/jpm12020147 1

Harshit Bokadia, Richa Rai and Elizabeth Barbara Torres
Digitized ADOS: Social Interactions beyond the Limits of the Naked Eye
Reprinted from: *J. Pers. Med.* **2020**, *10*, 159, doi:10.3390/jpm10040159 7

Areej G. Mesleh, Sara A. Abdulla and Omar El-Agnaf
Paving the Way toward Personalized Medicine: Current Advances and Challenges in Multi-OMICS Approach in Autism Spectrum Disorder for Biomarkers Discovery and Patient Stratification
Reprinted from: *J. Pers. Med.* **2021**, *41*, , doi:10.3390/jpm11010041 33

María Luján Ferreira and Nicolás Loyacono
Rationale of an Advanced Integrative Approach Applied to Autism Spectrum Disorder: Review, Discussion and Proposal
Reprinted from: *J. Pers. Med.* **2021**, *11*, 514, doi:10.3390/jpm11060514 57

Genevieve Grivas, Richard Frye and Juergen Hahn
Pregnant Mothers' Medical Claims and Associated Risk of Their Children being Diagnosed with Autism Spectrum Disorder
Reprinted from: *J. Pers. Med.* **2021**, *11*, 950, doi:10.3390/jpm11100950 69

Heather Way, Grant Williams, Sharon Hausman-Cohen and Jordan Reeder
Genomics as a Clinical Decision Support Tool: Successful Proof of Concept for Improved ASD Outcomes
Reprinted from: *J. Pers. Med.* **2021**, *11*, 596, doi:10.3390/jpm11070596 93

Rena J. Vanzo, Aparna Prasad, Lauren Staunch, Charles H. Hensel, Moises A. Serrano, E. Robert Wassman, Alexander Kaplun, Temple Grandin and Richard G. Boles
The Temple Grandin Genome: Comprehensive Analysis in a Scientist with High-Functioning Autism
Reprinted from: *J. Pers. Med.* , *11*, 21, doi:10.3390/jpm11010021 107

Emily L. Casanova, Carolina Baeza-Velasco, Caroline B. Buchanan and Manuel F. Casanova
The Relationship between Autism and Ehlers-Danlos Syndromes/Hypermobility Spectrum Disorders
Reprinted from: *J. Pers. Med.* **2020**, *10*, 260, doi:10.3390/jpm10040260 119

Sara Calderoni, Ivana Ricca, Giulia Balboni, Romina Cagiano, Denise Cassandrini, Stefano Doccini, Angela Cosenza, Deborah Tolomeo, Raffaella Tancredi, Filippo Maria Santorelli and Filippo Muratori
Evaluation of Chromosome Microarray Analysis in a Large Cohort of Females with Autism Spectrum Disorders: A Single Center Italian Study
Reprinted from: *J. Pers. Med.* **2020**, *10*, 160, doi:10.3390/jpm10040160 141

Andrew R. Pines, Bethany Sussman, Sarah N. Wyckoff, Patrick J. McCarty, Raymond Bunch, Richard E. Frye and Varina L. Boerwinkle
Locked-in Intact Functional Networks in Children with Autism Spectrum Disorder: A Case-Control Study
Reprinted from: *J. Pers. Med.* **2021**, *11*, 854, doi:10.3390/jpm11090854 . . . . **159**

Patrick J. McCarty, Andrew R. Pines, Bethany L. Sussman, Sarah N. Wyckoff, Amanda Jensen, Raymond Bunch, Varina L. Boerwinkle and Richard E. Frye
Resting State Functional Magnetic Resonance Imaging Elucidates Neurotransmitter Deficiency in Autism Spectrum Disorder
Reprinted from: *J. Pers. Med.* **2021**, *11*, 969, doi:10.3390/jpm11100969 . . . . **171**

Fatir Qureshi, James Adams, Kathryn Hanagan, Dae-Wook Kang, Rosa Krajmalnik-Brown and Juergen Hahn
Multivariate Analysis of Fecal Metabolites from Children with Autism Spectrum Disorder and Gastrointestinal Symptoms before and after Microbiota Transfer Therapy
Reprinted from: *J. Pers. Med.* **2020**, *10*, 152, doi:10.3390/jpm10040152 . . . . **179**

Richard E Frye, Janet Cakir, Shannon Rose, Raymond F. Palmer, Christine Austin, Paul Curtin and Manish Arora
Mitochondria May Mediate Prenatal Environmental Influences in Autism Spectrum Disorder
Reprinted from: *J. Pers. Med.* **2021**, *11*, 218, doi:10.3390/jpm11030218 . . . . **205**

Rita Barone, Jean Bastin, Fatima Djouadi, Indrapal Singh, Mohammad Azharul Karim, Amrit Ammanamanchi, Patrick John McCarty, Leanna Delhey, Rose Shannon, Antonino Casabona, Renata Rizzo and Richard Eugene Frye
Mitochondrial Fatty Acid β-Oxidation and Resveratrol Effect in Fibroblasts from Patients with Autism Spectrum Disorder
Reprinted from: *J. Pers. Med.* **2021**, *11*, 510, doi:10.3390/jpm11060510 . . . . **221**

Natasha Bobrowski-Khoury, Vincent T. Ramaekers, Jeffrey M. Sequeira and Edward V. Quadros
Folate Receptor Alpha Autoantibodies in Autism Spectrum Disorders: Diagnosis, Treatment and Prevention
Reprinted from: *J. Pers. Med.* **2021**, *11*, 710, doi:10.3390/jpm11080710 . . . . **235**

Daniel A. Rossignol and Richard E. Frye
Cerebral Folate Deficiency, Folate Receptor Alpha Autoantibodies and Leucovorin (Folinic Acid) Treatment in Autism Spectrum Disorders: A Systematic Review and Meta-Analysis
Reprinted from: *J. Pers. Med.* **2021**, *11*, 1141, doi:10.3390/jpm11111141 . . . . **251**

Daniel A. Rossignol and Richard E. Frye
The Effectiveness of Cobalamin (B12) Treatment for Autism Spectrum Disorder: A Systematic Review and Meta-Analysis
Reprinted from: *J. Pers. Med.* **2021**, *11*, 784, doi:10.3390/jpm11080784 . . . . **275**

James B. Adams, Anisha Bhargava, Devon M. Coleman, Richard E. Frye and Daniel A. Rossignol
Ratings of the Effectiveness of Nutraceuticals for Autism Spectrum Disorders: Results of a National Survey
Reprinted from: *J. Pers. Med.* **2021**, *11*, 878, doi:10.3390/jpm11090878 . . . . **297**

Daniel A Rossignol and Richard E Frye
A Systematic Review and Meta-Analysis of Immunoglobulin G Abnormalities and the Therapeutic Use of Intravenous Immunoglobulins (IVIG) in Autism Spectrum Disorder
Reprinted from: *J. Pers. Med.* **2021**, *11*, 488, doi:10.3390/jpm11060488 . . . . **319**

Theoharis C. Theoharides
Ways to Address Perinatal Mast Cell Activation and Focal Brain Inflammation, including Response to SARS-CoV-2, in Autism Spectrum Disorder
Reprinted from: *J. Pers. Med.* **2021**, *11*, 860, doi:10.3390/jpm11090860 . . . . **339**

Stephen T. Foldes, Amanda R. Jensen, Austin Jacobson, Sarah Vassall, Emily Foldes, Ann Guthery, Danni Brown, Todd Levine, William James Tyler and Richard E. Frye
Transdermal Electrical Neuromodulation for Anxiety and Sleep Problems in High-Functioning Autism Spectrum Disorder: Feasibility and Preliminary Findings
Reprinted from: *J. Pers. Med.* **2021**, *11*, 1307, doi:10.3390/jpm11121307 . . . . **363**

Alessandro Musetti, Tommaso Manari, Barbara Dioni, Cinzia Raffin, Giulia Bravo, Rachele Mariani, Gianluca Esposito, Dagmara Dimitriou, Giuseppe Plazzi, Christian Franceschini and Paola Corsano
Parental Quality of Life and Involvement in Intervention for Children or Adolescents with Autism Spectrum Disorders: A Systematic Review
Reprinted from: *J. Pers. Med.* **2021**, *11*, 894, doi:10.3390/jpm11090894 . . . . **387**

About the Editors

Richard E. Frye

Dr. Richard Frye is a Child Neurologist with expertise in neurodevelopmental and neurometabolic disorders. He received an MD and PhD in Physiology and Biophysics from Georgetown University and a Masters in Biomedical Science and Biostatistics from Drexel University. He completed a residency in Pediatrics at the University of Miami, Residency in Child Neurology and Fellowship in Behavioral Neurology and Learning Disabilities at Children's Hospital Boston and Fellowship in Psychology at Boston University. He holds board certifications in Pediatrics and in Neurology with Special Competence in Child Neurology. He has authored over 200 peer-reviewed publications and book chapters and is currently the Editor-in-Chief for the Section on Mechanisms of Diseases of the *Journal of Personalized Medicine*. Dr. Frye is a national leader in autism spectrum disorder (ASD) research. His studies focus on defining the clinical, behavioral, cognitive, genetic and metabolic characteristics of children with ASD and metabolic disorders and clinical trials demonstrating the efficacy of safe and novel treatments that target underlying physiological abnormalities in children with ASD, including a recent double-blind placebo controlled trial on leucovorin.

Richard G. Boles

Dr. Richard Boles is the Director of NeuroGenomics at Neurabilities Healthcare. This innovative program uses telemedicine to assist families across the USA, and physicians worldwide, to order, interpret, and act on whole-genome (DNA) sequencing. Dr. Boles also has a private telemedicine practice under the name of Mitochondrial & Molecular Medicine. Additionally, he is a founder and Chief Medical & Scientific Officer of NeuroNeeds LLC, a company dedicated to making food supplement products for people with a variety of neurological, neurodevelopmental, and functional disorders. In the past, Dr. Boles was affiliated with four different clinical laboratories, including being a Medical Director of the genetic testing companies Courtagen and Lineagen. He became involved in genetic testing in order to facilitate the translation of the vast amounts of acquired genetic knowledge into applications that improve routine medical care. Genetic testing remains the focus of his current clinical practice. Dr. Boles is a Clinical Geneticist with expertise in mitochondrial/metabolic, functional (e.g., chronic pain, fatigue, nausea, etc.), and neurodevelopmental disorders. He completed medical school at UCLA, a pediatric residency at Harbor-UCLA, and a genetics fellowship at Yale. He has been board certified in Pediatrics, Clinical Genetics, and Clinical Biochemical Genetics (metabolic disorders). He has authored over 80 peer-reviewed publications, mostly in Mitochondrial Medicine.

Shannon Rose

Dr. Shannon Rose is an Assistant Professor in the Department of Pediatrics, Division of Allergy/Immunology at the University of Arkansas for Medical Sciences and Arkansas Children's Research Institute in Little Rock, AR, USA. Dr. Rose was trained as a cell biologist and now runs a research program utilizing a combination of novel cell biology and immunology techniques and metabolomics to study mitochondrial and redox biology in health and pediatric metabolic disorders, including autism, obesity and diabetes. She received her PhD in Interdisciplinary Biomedical

Sciences at the University of Arkansas for Medical Sciences, under the training of S. Jill James, PhD, and conducted her postdoctoral training at Arkansas Children's Research Institute in the laboratory of Richard E. Frye, MD, PhD. By applying state-of-the-art Seahorse extracellular flux technology to autism to understand the relationship between oxidative stress, environmental exposures, and mitochondrial dysfunction using immune cells, she distinguished subgroups of children with autism with atypical mitochondrial function and increased susceptibility to oxidant-induced dysfunction.

Daniel A. Rossignol

Dr. Rossignol, MD FAAFP, is a board-certified family physician. He received his Doctorate of Medicine at the Medical College of Virginia and completed his residency in family medicine at the University of Virginia. Coming from an academic background, Dr. Rossignol has a special interest in evidence-based medicine, especially concerning autism spectrum disorder and has published over 70 papers, abstracts, editorials, and book chapters (including those in press) concerning autism and related conditions. Dr. Rossignol has a special interest in autism spectrum disorders, PANS/PANDAS, cerebral palsy, and related neurological and developmental disorders as well as medically complex children and adults. Dr. Rossignol is a Fellow of the American Academy of Family Physicians (FAAFP).

Preface to "A Personalized Medicine Approach to the Diagnosis and Management of Autism Spectrum Disorder"

Autism spectrum disorder (ASD) is estimated to affect 1 in every 44 children (>2%) in the United States. Through the monitoring of ASD by the Center for Disease Control and Prevention, a 241% increase in prevalence has been seen over the last 20 years. More troublesome is the fact that there has been little progress in diagnosing ASD early in life when behavioral therapy may be most effective.

ASD is a difficult disorder to diagnose and treat, both because diagnosis is not based on objective biomarkers but rather behavioral observations and because there are many underlying causes which are difficult to identify. Additionally, response to treatment for individuals with ASD is extremely variable and unpredictable. Each individual with ASD is unique and, thus, could greatly benefit from a personalized approach to diagnosis, treatment and management.

This collection of articles starts to provide an overview of the current and future methods for applying a personalized medicine approach to the diagnosis, management, and treatment of ASD. These articles discuss innovative methods for understanding the individual components of ASD, with many of the articles outlining quantitative methods to subtype ASD to better understand the underlying etiology or select effective treatments. By understanding ASD using the framework of personalized medicine, it may be possible to improve the lives of individuals with ASD and their families by identifying ASD earlier and more accurately and by selecting effective treatments to achieve optimal outcomes.

This collection of articles spans many disciplines, from psychology to genetics to biochemistry to neuroimaging, demonstrating the wide number of specialties involved in ASD. Individuals from all areas should no doubt be enlightened and interested in this collection of works. Indeed, the editors hope that these articles demonstrate how different disciplines can be integrated together to understand ASD. We thank the authors of the individual manuscripts for their creativity and ingenuity and for paving the way forward in developing new tools and approaches to understanding a complex disorder.

Richard E. Frye, Richard G. Boles, Shannon Rose, and Daniel A. Rossignol
Editors

Journal of *Personalized Medicine*

MDPI

Editorial

A Personalized Approach to Evaluating and Treating Autism Spectrum Disorder

Richard E. Frye [1,2,*], Shannon Rose [3,4], Richard G. Boles [5] and Daniel A. Rossignol [6]

[1] Section on Neurodevelopmental Disorders, Barrow Neurological Institute at Phoenix Children's Hospital, Phoenix, AZ 85016, USA
[2] Department of Child Health, University of Arizona College of Medicine—Phoenix, Phoenix, AZ 85004, USA
[3] Arkansas Children's Research Institute, Little Rock, AR 72202, USA; SROSE@uams.edu
[4] Department of Pediatrics, University of Arkansas for Medical Sciences, Little Rock, AR 72205, USA
[5] NeurAbilities Healthcare, Voorhees, NJ 08043, USA; rboles@neurabilities.com
[6] Rossignol Medical Center, 24541 Pacific Park Drive, Suite 210, Aliso Viejo, CA 92656, USA; rossignolmd@gmail.com
* Correspondence: rfrye@phoenixchildrens.com; Tel.: +1-602-933-1100

Citation: Frye, R.E.; Rose, S.; Boles, R.G.; Rossignol, D.A. A Personalized Approach to Evaluating and Treating Autism Spectrum Disorder. *J. Pers. Med.* **2022**, *12*, 147. https://doi.org/10.3390/jpm12020147

Received: 11 January 2022
Accepted: 17 January 2022
Published: 24 January 2022

Publisher's Note: MDPI stays neutral with regard to jurisdictional claims in published maps and institutional affiliations.

Copyright: © 2022 by the authors. Licensee MDPI, Basel, Switzerland. This article is an open access article distributed under the terms and conditions of the Creative Commons Attribution (CC BY) license (https://creativecommons.org/licenses/by/4.0/).

The most recent Center for Disease Control and Prevention estimates suggest that 1 in every 44 children (>2%) in the United States (US) is affected by autism spectrum disorder (ASD). Despite decades of research, it is difficult to identify ASD early in infancy when treatments are likely to be most effective. Recent evidence suggests that optimal outcomes for individuals with ASD may be better achieved by substantially improving our understanding of the underlying biological mechanisms or causes of ASD and from identifying effective treatments. One of the limitations for understanding ASD in greater depth is the well-known heterogeneity in clinical presentation, genes and pathways involved, co-morbid medical conditions, and response to treatment. Many have suggested that ASD is best represented as a set of distinct subgroups known as 'Autisms' rather a spectrum with a hereunto undefined number of dimensions, but little evidence points to one or the other approach as being the most valid. Thus, a personalized medicine approach may be optimal for understanding and treating each individual with ASD based on their individual unique characteristics.

Regardless of whichever approach is best, the fact remains that patients with ASD are all unique in many ways and require a personalized approach to their care. In this sense, we developed this Special Issue in order to start to better understand ASD by using a personalized medicine approach so that an eventual plan for understanding and treating patients with ASD can be developed as we go forward into the future. The Special Issue published 21 articles with 8 research articles, 10 review articles and 3 case studies. Of these articles, 14 discussed different underlying phenotypes of ASD, 12 discussed evidence for potential promising treatments, two described prenatal factors that might influence the development of ASD, and one described an alternative approach to understanding social interactions to improve diagnosis.

One major limitation to identifying and treating children with ASD is the diagnostic tests used. One of the current gold-standard diagnostic tests, the Autism Diagnostic Observation Schedule (ADOS), uses a trained examiner to elicit social 'presses' designed to evoke social interactions in the patient. A paper from the group at Rutgers University uses the standard ADOS examination to expand on an analysis of social interactions [1]. The group advances the examination by postulating that social interactions are not one-sided but involve a social dyad of interacting nervous systems processing sensory-motor information. Using wearable devices to digitally monitor movements, this group analyzes behaviors at both micro and macro levels with non-linear dynamic equations to derive advanced metrics of social interaction such as strength, coherence and variability of the dyad interactions. As such, this paper provides an interesting conceptual advance by both uncovering an underlying limitation of current approaches of evaluating social interactions and expands the use of such instruments to improve diagnosis by integrating a more complex analysis of the underlying dynamics of the nervous system.

The etiology of ASD is unknown in many, perhaps the majority, of cases. An increasing number of studies have pointed to genetic vulnerabilities interacting with environmental factors to trigger the development of ASD. It is being increasingly recognized that one of the most influential environments that will shape an individual's life is the prenatal maternal environment. This research is particularly insightful as it not only points to potential pathophysiological factors that cause ASD but also provides insight into potential strategies for preventing ASD from developing in the first place. Using a large dataset of medical claims across 123,824 pregnancies, researchers from the Rensselaer Polytechnic Institute identified pregnancy factors, which both increased and decreased the risk of developing ASD [2]. A common shortfall of research on prenatal factors is that most studies are associational rather than mechanistic. In this Special Issue, a group of researchers who have recently linked specific prenatal environmental exposures, including air pollution and nutritional metals, to long-term changes in mitochondrial function provide a comprehensive review of evidence linking prenatal factors that have been previously epidemiologically linked to ASD with mitochondrial dysfunction, thus providing a potential mechanism for these prenatal influences [3]. Connections with oxidative stress and disruption of the immune system are also outlined.

One of the most rational methods of approaching the management of individuals with ASD is to define subgroups. Fourteen papers describe various potential subgroups. This set of papers illustrates multiple viewpoints and techniques that can be used to define subgroups. Two papers describe methods for stratifying subgroups. A group of leaders in the treatment of ASD in Argentina describe their approach for defining subgroups by concentrating on the diagnosis and treatment of common concomitant medical problems and propose a classification system based on responses to the treatment of these concomitant problems [4]. A nice overview from a group in Qatar outlines the potential for biomarker use in the stratification of ASD [5]. This paper provides nice illustrations of the various biomarkers and approaches as well as provides some limited examples of the biomarkers described.

One important subgroup of patients with ASD that can be rather rigorously defined consists of those with known genetic changes. One article reported females with potential causative copy number changes on the chromosomal microarray. Variants involved in synaptic structure and transmission were most prominent, although other pathways including ion channels, neuron projection, and mRNA/protein processing, all mechanisms previously linked to ASD, were also identified. An interesting exploratory analysis found significantly lower restrictive and repetitive behaviors in those with presumed disease causative copy number variations as compared to females without such genetic changes [6]. One of the mysteries of ASD is the high heritability index without a high rate of common causative inherited genetic mutations. This is potentially due to several phenomena and historically has often been attributed to extreme genetic heterogeneity with multiple rare variants in many genes being causal for ASD. Another potential explanation is the complex interaction of genetic variations which by themselves may not be severe enough to express the ASD phenotype but together may result in disease. By analyzing the genome of a well-known professor with high-functioning ASD, Dr Temple Grandin, insight into how interactions between a complexity of genetic variations may result in the ASD phenotype is discussed in one article [7]. In another article, a genomic clinical decision support tool that focuses on relatively common DNA variants in pathways that can be targeted for treatment to improve symptoms is described along with several cases successfully treated using this tool [8]. In many cases, the complexity of genetic changes (as well as potential environmental interactions) is not clear. In a nice article, the overlap between ASD and Ehlers-Danlos syndromes and hypermobility spectrum disorders (EDS/HSD) is discussed [9]. This latter set of disorders also is believed to have an inherited component, which, similarly to ASD, remains elusive in many cases. Hypermobility spectrum disorders are being increasing recognized in ASD, in addition to comorbidities associated with both disorders including autonomic and immune dysregulation.

Two articles discuss aspects of the immune phenotype related to ASD. By conducting a meta-analysis on the literature, evidence for two specific subtypes of immunoglobulin dysregulation, low total IgG, and elevations in IgG4 are found [10]. Other phenotypes such as those with immune deficiencies as well as those with autoimmune encephalopathies are also described. In another article, the importance of mast cell activation in activating microglia resulting in focal brain inflammation and disrupted synaptic pruning is discussed [11]. Similar to EDS/HSD, aberrant mast cell activation and related symptomatology are common in cohorts with ASD and may designate endophenotypes of diseases.

Metabolic subtypes of ASD are also being recognized. One article describes a potential important subtype of ASD with a unique type of mitochondrial dysfunction, which may be related to environmental exposures [3]. In another article, researchers from Italy and France demonstrate that children with ASD who had elevations in acyl-carnitines in their blood exhibit changes in fatty-acid oxidation and electron transport chain complex activity in their fibroblasts [12]. Another article describes neurotransmitter dysregulation associated with mitochondrial disease in a unique patient [13]. Most interestingly, these changes in central neurotransmitters were discovered non-invasively by using resting state functional magnetic resonance imaging (rsfMRI) and confirmed by examination of the cerebrospinal fluid. Another study examined fecal metabolites from individuals with ASD and gastrointestinal symptoms, demonstrating that a model with five metabolites provides excellent separation between the ASD and a typically developing control group [14].

Two articles describe an increasingly recognized subgroup of children with ASD who have a unique metabolic-immune disorder that may influence their brain development both prenatally and postnatally. Autoantibodies that bind the folate receptor alpha (FRα), the major transporter of folate into the brain and across the placenta, are found in children with ASD as well as their parents. One article discusses FRα autoantibodies in a broad context, discussing the overlap with cerebral folate deficiency (CFD) and neural tube defects and a subgroup of ASD patients who may be more severely affected due to both prenatal and postnatal autoantibody exposure [15]. Another article conducts a meta-analysis on the available data to provide more concrete prevalence values of FRα autoantibodies in children with ASD and their families [16]. Interestingly, the prevalence rates suggest that FRα autoantibodies have a familial component, although the mechanism of this is not well understood and may be polygenic with environmental influences. This latter article also provides a meta-analysis to better define the overlap between children with ASD and those with CFD.

Two papers discuss regressive-type ASD, which may constitute yet another endophenotype of ASD. One paper describes a unique type of mitochondrial dysfunction that might underlie metabolic disturbance in children with ASD and neurodevelopmental regression [3]. In the other article, researchers at Barrow Neurologic Institute at Phoenix Children's Hospital use rsfMRI to demonstrate that children with regressive-type ASD appear to have intact cognitive networks that potentially cannot be expressed because of aberrant interfering networks, essentially creating a locked-in network syndrome [17].

Eleven papers provide either original data of treatment effectiveness or review the current literature of potentially effective treatments. Five papers describe treatments addressing specific metabolic defects. Building on the subgroup of children with FRα autoantibodies, one paper provides insight into the potential prenatal and postnatal treatment to prevent and treat ASD [15], while a second paper uses meta-analysis to document evidence for effectiveness and efficiency of *d,l*-leucovorin, the major treatment for children with ASD and FRα autoantibodies, across published clinical trials [16]. In another systematic review and meta-analysis, the effectiveness of cobalamin, a treatment that targets dysfunctional methylation and redox pathways, is analyzed, along with an examination of its metabolic effects [18]. Researchers from Italy and France demonstrate that resveratrol may be effective in correcting metabolic defects in fibroblasts from children with ASD and fatty-acid oxidation defects [12]. Lastly, researchers from Arizona State University demonstrate that Microbiota Transfer Therapy appear to normalize abnormal fecal metabolites in a group of people with ASD [14].

Two papers discuss potential treatments for immune dysfunction in ASD. Using a systematic review and meta-analysis approach, evidence for the effectiveness of intravenous immunoglobulin (IVIG) in ASD is presented [10], while another study discusses approaches to treating mast cell disorders with an emphasis on luteolin [11].

Two papers examine general treatments for children with ASD. In a large national survey of 1286 participants across the US, several nutraceuticals, including folate and cobalamin, were found to be rated by families to have greater benefits than a similar survey of psychiatric and seizure medications [19]. Another study demonstrates how examining genetic variations can help consider targeting common nutraceutical treatments on a personalized basis [8].

Transdermal Electrical Neuromodulation (TEN) is an approved safe non-invasive treatment for several disorders including attention-deficit hyperactivity disorder and migraines. In the first study using TEN to treat individuals with ASD, researchers at the Barrow Neurologic Institute at Phoenix Children's Hospital demonstrate the feasibility and potential effectiveness of TEN treatment for anxiety as well as demonstrate how autonomic system biomarkers may be used to predict response to TEN treatment [20].

Lastly, in an important and enlightening systematic review, evidence is presented that parental involvement in therapy relates to improved parental quality of life [21].

We believe that this collection of articles provides insight into the current state of ASD diagnosis, evaluation, and treatment using a personalized medicine approach. While each of these articles individually advances this goal, we believe that this collection fits in with the current understanding of ASD and advances this understanding. Perhaps most apparent, these articles underline the primacy of mitochondria in ASD, including oxidative stress and redox regulation, which are themselves major functions of mitochondria. Although the connection between ASD and this important cellular organelle is hardly new, this collection of papers serves to demonstrate the ubiquitous nature of the connection, which ranges from mitochondrial aspects in the prenatal and environmental risk factors/exposures [2,3,8] to biomarkers/metabolites [5,8,12–16], enzymology [12], and the positive response to therapy, at least in part targeting the mitochondria [8,11,12,15,16,18,19].

Many papers also relate to another potential etiology of ASD, particularly the immune system, in which multiple interactive domains are highlighted, including innate immunity, immune deficiency, autoimmunity, inflammation, and mast cell activation [7,8,10,11,15,16]. However, similarly to neurons, leukocytes are highly dependent on energy metabolism, and the connections between energy and immunity are many and important. In one example, folate transport to brain is affected predominately by autoimmunity and mitochondrial function [16].

Is ASD itself a result of abnormal mitochondria, with effects on neurons and/or leukocytes—essentially a "Bad Trio" of mitochondrial dysfunction, oxidative stress and redox regulation, and immune system dysfunction [3]? Is there a room for a primary role in pathogenesis for other pathways, including synapses [6–8], methylation [8,18], autonomic nervous function [9,20], ion channels [6], hypermobility [9], and microbiome [14], at least in some cases? Or, perhaps, do these concepts work within the mitochondrial hypothesis? For example, synapses have high-energy requirements and have high densities of mitochondria. Folate and cobalamin, important cofactors in methylation, are also important cofactors in energy metabolism. Similar to all neurons, autonomic neurons have high energy requirements. Leaking ion channels require ATP-driven pumps to reestablish homeostasis placing additional pressure on energy metabolism. Joint mobility is dependent on muscle tone, which is yet another tissue with high-energy requirements. Additionally, the microbiome produces metabolites that cross over into the body and likely interact with mitochondrial metabolism of the host, especially if the blood–brain barrier is compromised.

In any event, each of these concepts, from synapses to microbiome, are important to include in further research and to consider in a personalized medicine approach for the diagnosis and treatment in the individual ASD patient.

If mitochondria are the key to ASD, why is it that the vast majority of ASD patients that have undergone whole genome sequencing (WGS) have yet to have identifiable pathogenic variants in genes involved in mitochondrial function? Certainly, people with mitochondrial disease (a primary genetic mutation affecting energy metabolism) often have ASD, and many people with ASD do have mitochondrial disease, but this is a minority per our present understanding. Perhaps the answer is in the combined effects of multiple genetic variants, each one benign in of itself and oftentimes common [7]. Perhaps the presence of primary mutations in many different pathways among people with ASD, in hundreds of different genes suggests that abnormal mitochondria are rarely the cause of ASD, but rather an important downstream mechanism in the common pathophysiology of ASD. Thus, mitochondrial dysfunction may be acquired in most people with ASD [3]. Perhaps the answer is a little of both as well as other mechanisms not considered herein or even not yet proposed. Further research is needed to examine these possibilities.

Effective treatment and management for individuals with ASD is only starting to be uncovered, but we believe the articles within this volume provide insight and a starting point for the evolution of rational and optimal treatments for individuals with ASD.

Author Contributions: Conceptualization, R.E.F., S.R., R.G.B. and D.A.R.; writing—original draft preparation, R.E.F.; writing—review and editing, R.E.F., S.R., R.G.B. and D.A.R. All authors have read and agreed to the published version of the manuscript.

Funding: This research received no external funding.

Institutional Review Board Statement: Not applicable.

Informed Consent Statement: Not applicable.

Data Availability Statement: Not applicable.

Acknowledgments: We thank all authors who contributed their work and in so doing made the Special Issue a success. We also thank the staff of *JPM* for their excellent support throughout the editorial process.

Conflicts of Interest: The authors declare no conflict of interest.

References

1. Bokadia, H.; Rai, R.; Torres, E.B. Digitized ADOS: Social Interactions beyond the Limits of the Naked Eye. *J. Pers. Med.* **2020**, *10*, 159. [CrossRef] [PubMed]
2. Grivas, G.; Frye, R.; Hahn, J. Pregnant Mothers' Medical Claims and Associated Risk of Their Children being Diagnosed with Autism Spectrum Disorder. *J. Pers. Med.* **2021**, *11*, 950. [CrossRef] [PubMed]
3. Frye, R.; Cakir, J.; Rose, S.; Palmer, R.; Austin, C.; Curtin, P.; Arora, M. Mitochondria May Mediate Prenatal Environmental Influences in Autism Spectrum Disorder. *J. Pers. Med.* **2021**, *11*, 218. [CrossRef] [PubMed]
4. Ferreira, M.; Loyacono, N. Rationale of an Advanced Integrative Approach Applied to Autism Spectrum Disorder: Review, Discussion and Proposal. *J. Pers. Med.* **2021**, *11*, 514. [CrossRef] [PubMed]
5. Mesleh, A.G.; Abdulla, S.A.; El-Agnaf, O. Paving the Way toward Personalized Medicine: Current Advances and Challenges in Multi-OMICS Approach in Autism Spectrum Disorder for Biomarkers Discovery and Patient Stratification. *J. Pers. Med.* **2021**, *11*, 41. [CrossRef]
6. Calderoni, S.; Ricca, I.; Balboni, G.; Cagiano, R.; Cassandrini, D.; Doccini, S.; Cosenza, A.; Tolomeo, D.; Tancredi, R.; Santorelli, F.M.; et al. Evaluation of Chromosome Microarray Analysis in a Large Cohort of Females with Autism Spectrum Disorders: A Single Center Italian Study. *J. Pers. Med.* **2020**, *10*, 160. [CrossRef]
7. Vanzo, R.J.; Prasad, A.; Staunch, L.; Hensel, C.H.; Serrano, M.A.; Wassman, E.R.; Kaplun, A.; Grandin, T.; Boles, R.G. The Temple Grandin Genome: Comprehensive Analysis in a Scientist with High-Functioning Autism. *J. Pers. Med.* **2021**, *11*, 21. [CrossRef]
8. Way, H.; Williams, G.; Hausman-Cohen, S.; Reeder, J. Genomics as a Clinical Decision Support Tool: Successful Proof of Concept for Improved ASD Outcomes. *J. Pers. Med.* **2021**, *11*, 596. [CrossRef]
9. Casanova, E.; Baeza-Velasco, C.; Buchanan, C.; Casanova, M. The Relationship between Autism and Ehlers-Danlos Syndromes/Hypermobility Spectrum Disorders. *J. Pers. Med.* **2020**, *10*, 260. [CrossRef]

10. Rossignol, D.; Frye, R. A Systematic Review and Meta-Analysis of Immunoglobulin G Abnormalities and the Therapeutic Use of Intravenous Immunoglobulins (IVIG) in Autism Spectrum Disorder. *J. Pers. Med.* **2021**, *11*, 488. [CrossRef]
11. Theoharides, T.C. Ways to Address Perinatal Mast Cell Activation and Focal Brain Inflammation, including Response to SARS-CoV-2, in Autism Spectrum Disorder. *J. Pers. Med.* **2021**, *11*, 860. [CrossRef] [PubMed]
12. Barone, R.; Bastin, J.; Djouadi, F.; Singh, I.; Karim, M.; Ammanamanchi, A.; McCarty, P.; Delhey, L.; Shannon, R.; Casabona, A.; et al. Mitochondrial Fatty Acid β-Oxidation and Resveratrol Effect in Fibroblasts from Patients with Autism Spectrum Disorder. *J. Pers. Med.* **2021**, *11*, 510. [CrossRef] [PubMed]
13. McCarty, P.J.; Pines, A.R.; Sussman, B.L.; Wyckoff, S.N.; Jensen, A.; Bunch, R.; Boerwinkle, V.L.; Frye, R.E. Resting State Functional Magnetic Resonance Imaging Elucidates Neurotransmitter Deficiency in Autism Spectrum Disorder. *J. Pers. Med.* **2021**, *11*, 969. [CrossRef] [PubMed]
14. Qureshi, F.; Adams, J.; Hanagan, K.; Kang, D.-W.; Krajmalnik-Brown, R.; Hahn, J. Multivariate Analysis of Fecal Metabolites from Children with Autism Spectrum Disorder and Gastrointestinal Symptoms before and after Microbiota Transfer Therapy. *J. Pers. Med.* **2020**, *10*, 152. [CrossRef] [PubMed]
15. Bobrowski-Khoury, N.; Ramaekers, V.; Sequeira, J.; Quadros, E. Folate Receptor Alpha Autoantibodies in Autism Spectrum Disorders: Diagnosis, Treatment and Prevention. *J. Pers. Med.* **2021**, *11*, 710. [CrossRef]
16. Rossignol, D.A.; Frye, R.E. Cerebral Folate Deficiency, Folate Receptor Alpha Autoantibodies and Leucovorin (Folinic Acid) Treatment in Autism Spectrum Disorders: A Systematic Review and Meta-Analysis. *J. Pers. Med.* **2021**, *11*, 1141. [CrossRef]
17. Pines, A.R.; Sussman, B.; Wyckoff, S.N.; McCarty, P.J.; Bunch, R.; Frye, R.E.; Boerwinkle, V.L. Locked-in Intact Functional Networks in Children with Autism Spectrum Disorder: A Case-Control Study. *J. Pers. Med.* **2021**, *11*, 854. [CrossRef]
18. Rossignol, D.A.; Frye, R.E. The Effectiveness of Cobalamin (B12) Treatment for Autism Spectrum Disorder: A Systematic Review and Meta-Analysis. *J. Pers. Med.* **2021**, *11*, 784. [CrossRef]
19. Adams, J.B.; Bhargava, A.; Coleman, D.M.; Frye, R.E.; Rossignol, D.A. Ratings of the Effectiveness of Nutraceuticals for Autism Spectrum Disorders: Results of a National Survey. *J. Pers. Med.* **2021**, *11*, 878. [CrossRef]
20. Foldes, S.T.; Jensen, A.R.; Jacobson, A.; Vassall, S.; Foldes, E.; Guthery, A.; Brown, D.; Levine, T.; Tyler, W.J.; Frye, R.E. Transdermal Electrical Neuromodulation for Anxiety and Sleep Problems in High-Functioning Autism Spectrum Disorder: Feasibility and Preliminary Findings. *J. Pers. Med.* **2021**, *11*, 1307. [CrossRef]
21. Musetti, A.; Manari, T.; Dioni, B.; Raffin, C.; Bravo, G.; Mariani, R.; Esposito, G.; Dimitriou, D.; Plazzi, G.; Franceschini, C.; et al. Parental Quality of Life and Involvement in Intervention for Children or Adolescents with Autism Spectrum Disorders: A Systematic Review. *J. Pers. Med.* **2021**, *11*, 894. [CrossRef] [PubMed]

Journal of *Personalized Medicine*

MDPI

Article

Digitized ADOS: Social Interactions beyond the Limits of the Naked Eye

Harshit Bokadia [1], Richa Rai [1] and Elizabeth Barbara Torres [1,2,*]

[1] Department of Psychology, Rutgers University Center for Cognitive Science, The State University of New Jersey, Rutgers, NJ 08854, USA; hb271@scarletmail.rutgers.edu (H.B.); rr708@psych.rutgers.edu (R.R.)

[2] Department of Computer Science, Computational Biomedicine Imaging and Modelling Centre, Rutgers, The State University of New Jersey, Rutgers, NJ 08854, USA

* Correspondence: ebtorres@psych.rutgers.edu; Tel.: +1-732-208-3158

Received: 14 September 2020; Accepted: 1 October 2020; Published: 8 October 2020

Abstract: The complexity and non-linear dynamics of socio-motor phenomena underlying social interactions are often missed by observation methods that attempt to capture, describe, and rate the exchange in real time. Unknowingly to the rater, socio-motor behaviors of a dyad exert mutual influence over each other through subliminal mirroring and shared cohesiveness that escape the naked eye. Implicit in these ratings nonetheless is the assumption that the other participant of the social dyad has an identical nervous system as that of the interlocutor, and that sensory-motor information is processed similarly by both agents' brains. What happens when this is not the case? We here use the Autism Diagnostic Observation Schedule (ADOS) to formally study social dyadic interactions, at the macro- and micro-level of behaviors, by combining observation with digital data from wearables. We find that integrating subjective and objective data reveals fundamentally new ways to improve standard clinical tools, even to differentiate females from males using the digital version of the test. More generally, this work offers a way to turn a traditional, gold-standard clinical instrument into an objective outcome measure of human social behaviors and treatment effectiveness.

Keywords: digital biomarkers; wearables; time series analysis; autism; social dyads; socio-motor parameters; network connectivity; non-linear complex dynamics; stochastic analysis

1. Introduction

The wearable sensors revolution has brought behavioral science to a new era of precision. Across many research areas in basic and translational sciences, it is now possible to monitor natural motions continuously, as they unfold between two people in a social dyad, or even as part of a social group. Indeed, the advent of new advances in digital technology opens many new avenues of inquiry in the social, clinical, and psychological sciences. It is now possible to track multi-layered activities generated by our nervous systems while our brain controls our bodies in motion. Such tracking affords various levels of discourse, including a macro- and a micro-level of description.

At a macro-level (Figure 1A), we can describe the overt motions of our body to some degree, i.e., the motions that we can unambiguously perceive and explicitly describe. However, it is at the micro-level of analysis where information that transpires largely beneath awareness can help us understand the patterns of socio-motor behaviors underlying social interactions (Figure 1B). From facial micro-expressions to voice micro-fluctuations to bodily micro-gestures, all these non-verbal forms of communication permeate everything that we share socially with others, ever since birth (and even in uterus as we interact with our mother's biorhythms [1,2]) in pre-cognitive stages of neurodevelopment. We are born with the capacity for social readiness and our perceptual systems help us make sense of the social world, whenever we receive appropriate support from an early age. Such support comes from our parents and from other social beings whose speech cadence and facial and bodily patterns we spontaneously imitate from an early age [3–5] through synchronous patterns and socio-motor entrainment.

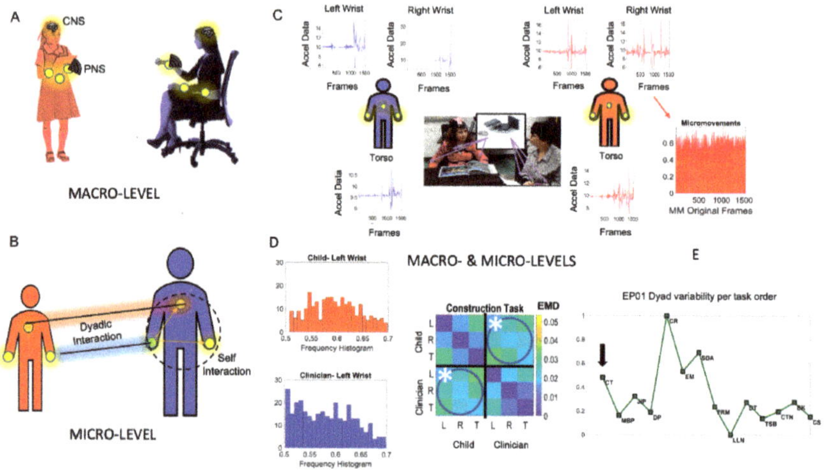

Figure 1. Leveraging the wearable sensors revolution to significantly augment traditional pencil and paper methods and advance the behavioral sciences. (**A**) The macro-level of behavioral description inevitably misses fast and subtle information in dyadic social interactions, as information flows between the Central and the Peripheral Nervous Systems (the CNS and the PNS). (**B**) Micro-level coherence information, automatic social mirroring, lead-lag patterns, and micro-gestures of the face and body, among other socio-motor behaviors, can only be captured with high grade instrumentation and proper analytics. (**C**) Macro- and micro-levels of inquiry can be integrated to advance social behavioral sciences, e.g., the Autism Diagnostic Observation Schedule (ADOS) is used as a backdrop experimental assay to probe dyadic social interactions, combined with wearables. to digitize standard clinical criteria. Light wearables embedded in the clothing unobtrusively and continuously co-register child and clinician (certified as rater) during the administration of the ADOS test to detect autism. Micro-fluctuations in the timeseries data from these wearables (e.g., acceleration waveforms) can be converted to standardized micro-movement spikes (MMS) to derive various socio-motor biometrics. (**D**) The Earth Mover's Distance (EMD) metric is used to ascertain the pairwise difference between frequency histograms of MMS and build a matrix with entries capturing the dyadic interactions (circled entries) and the self-interactions of body nodes. (**E**) The averaged sum across all dyadic interaction entries per unit time, obtained task by task, in the order in which they were administered, gives us a session profile of the dyadic variability, as one example of several metrics used here to objectively quantify socio-motor behavior simultaneously at the macro- and micro-levels of inquiry.

There is a form of autonomous mirroring that tends to occur in social interactions from birth, when within a few weeks human babies can entrain their bodily biorhythms to the rhythmic speech of their mother [6,7] and perceive changes in facial micro-gestures with emotional content [8–11]. From birth, babies can distinguish biological motions [12,13], and by eight months of age they can dissociate structural and dynamic information from non-biological vs. biological motions [14]. Between four and five years of age, their socio-motor kinematics, to communicate decisions and desires through pointing gestures, mature into fundamentally different statistical signatures [15,16]. Their statistics transition from random and noisy to predictive signals necessary for proper motor control in order to start schooling and formal instruction [17,18].

The body of work on human development and the capacity of human babies for social readiness has relied on high grade instruments, microfilm, wearables, and other means beyond human observation. This is so because several of these pre-cognitive socio-motor behaviors are much too complex, variable and subtle to be captured by the naked eye [19,20]. They require sensors with proper sampling resolutions, to register the micro-fluctuations in biorhythmic activities across the nervous systems of the two people engaged in the social exchange. Using such means, it is then possible to discern important aspects of the interaction and distinguish synchronous intent, mutual trust, joint goals and overall coordination that leads to good rapport, successful gestural communication and anticipatory control [21].

We know that people automatically sway together when they converse and when they joke [22,23], that their bodies entrain when they build social rapport and that they show disjointed patterns when communication fails [24]. When one of the parties prevails in excess over the other, and that person leads the interaction most of the time, there is no opportunity for the other party to communicate [24]. They then dance to a different beat [25]. What is supposed to be a social dyadic dialogue breaks into a dyadic monologue. One of the agents no longer participates as it should in a social exchange. How could we study such phenomena more systematically and help current research in autism, the disorder of the nervous system that leads to fundamental differences in socio-motor control [26] and social communication [27]?

One possible way to probe the social dyad in a systematic manner is by using as the backdrop of our experiment well-established and broadly adopted tests of social interaction that have already been standardized in some form (Figure 1C). One such a test is the gold standard to detect autism in clinical and in research settings: The Autism Diagnostic Observation Schedule (ADOS) [28]. This test was designed precisely to detect the extent to which a person fails to reach a set of criteria, rendering the interaction socially appropriate. The rater of the test provides a numeric score reflecting the severity of the inability to carry on an appropriate social exchange. The test is one sided in that the certified rater both poses social presses to evoke social overtures in response and actively participates in the exchange. Then, from the outcome of such interactions, the rater scores the responses of the other person. This is very taxing on the rater who is both interacting with and observing the person being scored. It is also taxing on the person being scored, because the test takes a long time (approximately one hour), while the information obtained is very discrete, necessarily missing key aspects of the exchange that escape the busy rater's eyes.

Social interactions naturally occur in a very different manner (i.e., no one is rating the other person as the interaction unfolds.) Natural interactions are extremely complex, dynamic, and flow organically in (at times) unpredictable manners. One of the advantages of using the ADOS as a backdrop of our study is precisely that it is conceived to allow for such fluidity using several tasks that can be administered in the order in which the situation affords, rather than in a fixed order. Yet, despite this fluidity, because of the standard ways in which each task is conceived, the overall test preserves a systematic manner of administration across different ages and different verbal capacities, ranging from minimally to fluidly verbal cases.

The ADOS test has not officially included neurotypical controls to build a normative scale [29]. It is a criterion-based rather than a norm-based test, yet this does not preclude us from using this test to probe neurotypicals while applying our micro-level inquiry, paired with wearables. Combining wearables which co-register simultaneously the bodily motions of both the rater and the participant with high sampling frequency and extract information both at the macro- and micro-levels of the social exchange, can give us a very rich picture of the highly non-linear complex dynamics taking place during the interactions. We hypothesize that the digital ADOS will reveal new aspects of the shared space spanned by the cohesive dyadic micro-movements of the child and clinician.

Integrating macro-and micro-levels of analysis will augment in unprecedented ways our knowledge about action execution and action observation in this closed loop of highly variable, transient, and sustained dyadic cohesiveness (e.g., Figure 1C–E). We may provide biometrics of a social dialogue through bodily activity. informing us not only about the person's capacity for social readiness, but more importantly instructing us on how-to best nurture that potential. We may even be able to broaden the potential to help the person's socio-motor tendencies to adapt and converge toward the desirable social norms of any given culture. Furthermore, because such bodily activities are sampled with high frequency, and because the micro-fluctuations derived from biorhythms shift with context and pick up subtle nuances otherwise hidden to the naked eye of the observer, we will be able to add significantly to the information that the macro-level ADOS test already provides. It may be also possible to detect differences between females and males in the cohort when examining the dyadic interactions, as social rapport emerges between the child and clinician, and does so differently for males than for females across the ADOS tasks. More generally, we may be able to transition such valuable clinical tests from a quasi-static discrete method of detection, to a highly dynamic, continuous tracking tool, one capable of providing an outcome measure for any treatment's effectiveness during the naturalistic activities of daily living.

In the social sciences in general, this approach could advance more than one line of inquiry into the non-linear, dynamic, and stochastic complexity of micro-level social exchange, making these important aspects of our social being no longer hidden to the naked eye.

2. Materials and Methods

2.1. Ethics Information

This study was approved by the Rutgers University Institutional Review Board. The study is compliant with the Helsinki Act.

2.2. Design

This study used the tasks from the research grade ADOS-2 [28], a standard clinical test to evoke social situations, rate the child's responses and detect autism in cases whereby social affect and repetitive restrictive behaviors impede proper social interactions with the rater. (The term Repetitive Restrictive Behaviors (RRB) is used here to be congruent with the clinical jargon of the ADOS test. According to our quantitative metrics, these motions reflect, rather, adaptation of the nervous systems in order to enhance kinesthetic reafferent feedback (i.e., feedback from intentional movements) which in autism shows highly random noisy patterns in relation to neurotypical controls [15]).

The experiment consisted of four visits. In the first visit, the neurotypical control participants were administered the tasks from the ADOS-2 module that were most appropriate in terms of age and verbal capacity. The first visit also examined autistic subjects under similar ADOS-2 module criteria, i.e., using the most appropriate module according to the child's age, verbal status, and cognitive capabilities (as determined by the rater clinician.) The autistic participants were familiar with one of the two raters but not the other. Controls only participated in visit one.

The second visit employed an ADOS-2 module that was compatible with the child's verbal ability, even if it was easier than the most appropriate module used in visit one. The idea was to vary the module while keeping the rater familiar to the children in both visits. The third visit switched to a new, unfamiliar rater but kept the most appropriate module. The fourth visit kept that rater but changed the module to an easier one, feasible but not the most appropriate (if one were to use the ADOS-2 to detect autism.) In our case, we used this test as an experimental assay to evoke dyadic social interactions. Table S2 shows the tasks' names (and initials used in Figures labels) along with the corresponding module numbers. The raters are certified clinicians naïve to the purpose of the study.

2.3. Sampling Plan and Inclusion/Exclusion Criteria

We tested a total of 29 participants, 10 females and 19 males (see Table S3). There were 11 control children of school age (mean age 9.9 years old) and 18 autistic children (mean age 8.3 years old). In this set 26/29 dyads (10 females and 16 males) had completed the digitized ADOS with six synchronous sensors, three on the child and three on the clinician co-registering their motions in tandem) and these were included in visit one. The 3/29 dyads not included in these analyses had grids with 12 sensors, and/or the child had a diagnosis of Fragile X. These will be the focus of a different publication, so we include only idiopathic autism in the present work. Furthermore, eight autistic children returned in visits one and two, six returned to the lab in visits one–three and one in visits one–four. The details of these participants, along with the module delivered and ADOS-2 score assigned across all the visits, are summarized in Tables S2 and S3 of the Supplementary Material. Autistic children were referred to our laboratory by local clinics and by the community, with help from the New Jersey Autism Center of Excellence (https://njace.us/), funded by the New Jersey Governor's Council for the Medical Research and Treatments of Autism.

Because of the data type and methods that we introduce for personalized behavioral analyses, this cohort was sufficient in size. We test the proposition that combining pencil-and-paper methods with digital means would reveal information about dyadic behaviors that we would miss using observation alone.

We built indexes that combined the rater's scores derived from observation with digital data collected using light wearable sensors. The sensors (APDM Opals, Portland, OR, USA) synchronously co-registered motions continuously at 128 Hz, thus providing big data for personalized analyses. We study here linear acceleration (for results using angular velocity, see Supplementary Material) co-registered synchronously across six sensors (Figure 1B.) The six sensors were positioned at the wrist and torso of the participants, conceptualized as an interconnected network. Sessions took place in a socially controlled environment, using the standard ADOS tasks and set up (Figure 1C). Tasks were administered by two clinicians, who were naïve to the experimental goals of the study. Both clinicians had ADOS certification for research reliability.

2.4. Analysis Plan

We developed new data types and analytics to simultaneously track the participating agents of the dyad within the context of the social interactions that the ADOS-2 test evokes. Importantly, our analytical methods consider the biorhythmic activities of each participant (individually) and of the shared spatio-temporal parameters of the dyad acting in concert (Figure 1A). We co-registered synchronously the upper body motions of both participants using a grid of unobtrusive wearable biosensors (Figure 1B) and examined each sensor's activity pairwise in relation to the other sensor's activity. The moment by moment fluctuations in the amplitude of the signals from each sensor are normalized to account for anatomical differences that impact motion parameters. A new standardized data type coined micro-movement spikes (MMS) is then obtained together with various indexes derived from the frequency and temporal domains of these data.

An index of Dyadic Strength is built as a ratio whereby the numerator is derived from the Dyadic Coherence, using analyses in the frequency domain (Figure 2A,B). The denominator uses the Dyadic Variability extracted from the MMS, providing information about the fluctuations in signal amplitude in the time domain. In both Dyadic Coherence and Dyadic Variability, we sum the dyadic-interaction entries of the 6×6 matrices that we build from pairwise sensors' computations. Figure 2C shows the parameterization of the MMS cross-coherence, phase, and frequency matrices. These were conceptualized as adjacency matrices and combined to represent dynamically evolving weight-directed graphs. We then adapted network connectivity analyses using the Brain Connectivity Toolbox of MATLAB [30,31] to uncover various relevant connectivity metrics across the six nodes. The shared activity in the dyadic interaction entries were then used to obtain the Dyadic Coherence quantity per unit time. As with Dyadic Variability, we obtained this for each task of the session in the order in which the tasks were administered. The Dyad Strength metric was thus built from the ratio of Dyad Coherence divided by Dyad Variability and normalized between 0 and 1.

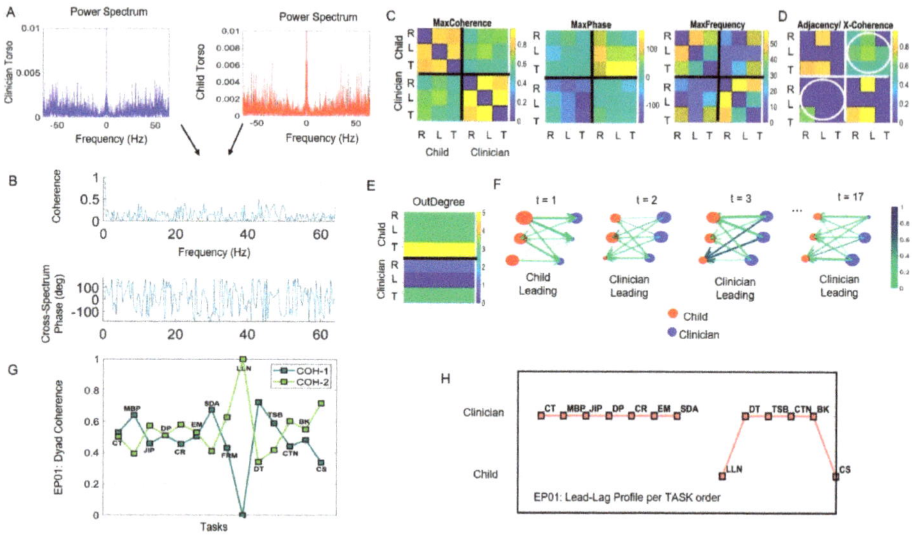

Figure 2. Analytical pipeline and visualization tools. (**A**) Frequency domain power spectrum analysis of pairwise sensor data provides input to obtain cross coherence spectrum phase across frequencies. (**B**,**C**) A parameterization of the data into three corresponding matrices: MaxCoherence, MaxPhase, MaxFrequency. Each entry contains the maximal cross coherence value obtained pairwise across all sensors. For example, row 1 contains the values for the child's right wrist (R) sensor in relation to all other sensors (child left wrist L, child torso T, clinician right wrist R, clinician left wrist L, and clinician torso T. Dyad entries of the matrix are at the right upper quadrant (child→clinician) and left lower quadrant (clinician→child). Self-interaction entries are at the left upper quadrant (child) and the right lower quadrant (clinician). Corresponding entries in the MaxPhase matrix reflect the phase value at which the pairwise coherence is maximal while the same entry in the MaxFrequency reflect the corresponding frequency value. (**D**) Adjacency matrix used to represent a dynamically changing weighted connected graph is obtained by retaining the entries at positive phase under convention i→j for the (i,j) entry. Dyadic interaction entries are circled. (**E**) Outdegree for each node denotes the number of links from that node to other nodes. (**F**–**H**) Visual tools and sample metrics to characterize socio-motor behaviors in social dyads. (**F**) Visualizing the network to track its states as they dynamically change in the Construction Task for a child-clinician dyad (EP01, with 17-unit times of 12 s time length for each sample under Independent Identically Distributed (IID) assumption, explained in Methods). The size of the node corresponds to the OutDegree value, the arrow's color is the maximum cross-coherence value, the thickness is the phase value and the direction comes from the computation involving Outdegree (see methods.) (**G**) Sample profile over tasks of Experimental Participant 01, EP01 showing the COH1 and COH2 unfolding within the session. These terms are used to obtain a socio-motor metric (see Methods.) (**H**) Lead profile for the dyad involving EP01 and revealing the clinician prevalent leadership for most tasks, but Loneliness (LLN) and Creating a Story (CS), where the child leads (please see Supplementary Material Table S2 for task description and acronyms).

We analyze data in the time and frequency domains and construct various socio-motor indexes. In the time domain, we examine the variability in MMS using in-home developed analyses of time series data. These include the characterization of the MMS as deviations from an empirically estimated mean, determined using maximum likelihood estimation (MLE) of the best continuous family of probability distributions fitting the data. Previous studies involving natural behaviors had revealed the continuous Gamma family as a good characterization of human digital data registered with these wearables [15,32,33]. The MMS trains were windowed according to an optimal time block yielding tight confidence intervals for the optimal parameters in an MLE sense. They were analyzed task by task, using the simultaneously co-registered data from the six sensors that the child and rater wore (Figure 1C). To that end, using the Earth Mover's Distance (EMD) metric [34], we examine the pairwise differences in frequency histograms derived from the MMS of the linear acceleration (see angular speed in Supplementary Material) and build a 6×6 matrix whereby entries provide information about variability in the micro-fluctuations of linear acceleration amplitude for dyadic- and for self-interactions (Figure 1D). The dyadic-interaction variability was obtained by summing all dyadic entries of one of the circled blocks of this symmetric matrix. This quantity was then used as the denominator of a ratio coined Dyadic Strength.

We derived several adjacency matrices to represent these activities using dynamically evolving weighted directed graphs. Furthermore, we adapted various network connectivity analyses from brain research and used them here to characterize a grid of sensors registering the continuous naturalistic social interactions of a dyad. We focus on the cohesiveness of the dyadic interactions from the spatio-temporal spaces shared. We also examine the kinematic synergies of self-interactions in each dyad participant.

Among the connectivity metrics that we used, we specifically assessed possible differences between males and females across the cohort. We used the clustering coefficient metric, a measure of the degree to which nodes in a graph tend to cluster together. We used the Betweenness Centrality metric, measuring the extent to which a vertex lies on paths between other vertices. Vertices with high betweenness may have considerable influence within a network by virtue of their control over information passing between other vertices. Related to this, we examined the characteristic path length, the average shortest distance path (geodesic), denoting he number of edges in the shortest paths between all vertex pairs. In all cases we gathered the data generated by the dyad across the tasks and used the same number of data points in males and in females, to ask if, given a scatter of similar size, the values distributed significantly differ. Since we had fewer females (10) than males (16), we relied on the minimum number of values in the females and cycled through all the values of the males (bootstrapping from the data) to ascertain the degree to which they differed when the number of elements were identical for each parameter and for each cohort. To compare the groups, we used the rank-sum test and visualized the histograms and the scatters across all connectivity parameters scaled to range between 0 and 1. This normalization allowed us to visually compare males and females across network connectivity metrics and stochastic parameters.

2.5. Data Types

We used Euclidean norm (Equation (1)) to obtain the scalar value of acceleration from the tri-axial acceleration time series, sampled $\vec{A}_c(t) = \left(A_c(t)_x, A_c(t)_y, A_c(t)_z\right)$ at the sampling frequency of 128 Hz.

$$A_c(t) = \sqrt{A_c(t)_x^2 + A_c(t)_y^2 + A_c(t)_z^2} \tag{1}$$

The resultant time series of peaks and valleys for an experiment's participant (EP01), during the ADOS "Construction task", and the rater are shown in Figure 1C. The sensors co-registered orientation data through a tri-axial gyroscope. Similarly, we computed the angular speed capturing rotational data (results shown in Supplementary Material).

These time series of linear acceleration and angular speed have peaks and valleys that fluctuate in amplitude and inter-peak interval times. We focused in this paper on the fluctuations in signal amplitude, taken as relative deviations from the empirically estimated Gamma mean. To estimate the mean, we fit the continuous Gamma family of probability distributions to the frequency histogram of the raw data peaks. The Gamma family fits the data in an MLE sense with 95% confidence intervals for the shape and the scale parameters, respectively [15]. Using these parameters, we estimated the Gamma moments and used the mean to obtain the absolute deviation of each point in the time series. We then construct our waveform of interest denoting micro-fluctuations in bodily biorhythms during social interactions, derived from the original raw data of linear acceleration (and angular speed).

The peak amplitude data mean, shifted and centered at the empirically estimated mean, was then scaled to the real valued interval (0,1) using Equation (2)

$$NormPeak = \frac{Peak}{Peak + Avrg_{\text{min to min}}} \tag{2}$$

These unitless waveforms are called micro-movement spikes (MMS) (see Figure 1C). The MMS are in reduced frames as they capture only the absolute deviations from the estimated mean. We zero-pad values below the deviations to reconstruct the original number of frames across all six sensors. This standardized waveform accounts for allometric effects [35] owing to anatomical differences impacting the motion data and allows us to combine data from multiple sensors with different physical units [19]. Here we focus on the linear acceleration and present the results in the main paper. The Supplementary Material presents the results for angular speed.

We chose 12 s time windows as our unit for the Gamma parameter estimation because this was the minimal task segment across the entire set and it provided tight confidence intervals at 128 Hz sampling rate.

2.6. Socio-Motor Metrics

Several metrics per unit time (12 s windows independently sampled without overlap) are derived to quantify socio-motor phenomena, inclusive of leading patterns within the dyad agents, cohesiveness and phase delays. Below we enumerate these metrics in the temporal and frequency domains. Furthermore, we explain our adaptation of network connectivity analyses commonly used in brain science [30,31] to the analyses of interacting nodes on a grid of synchronous sensors, sampling biorhythmic activities generated by bodies producing social motions and emotions.

Dyad Variability (temporal domain): To quantify the differences in frequency histograms derived from the MMS, we use the Earth Mover's Distance metric [36] commonly employed in machine learning [34]. The average pairwise EMD per unit time is taken across all time windows of each task, owing to variable task time lengths. We sample windows under the independent identically distributed (IID) assumption for each task and average across these uniform units of time. Thus, our results are reported as quantity per unit time, using our uniformly determined unit of time. For each child-clinician dyad, this information produces a 6×6 matrix with the first three rows representing the child data from the right wrist (R), left wrist (L) and the torso (T) sensors in that order. The following rows represent the clinician's sensors in the same order as the child's sensors. Likewise, the columns follow this convention such that entry [1,2] in row 1 and column 2 represents the pairwise $EMD_{1,2}$ quantity between the right wrist and the left wrist of the child, whereas entry in row 5 and column 2 represent the $EMD_{5,2}$ between the left wrist of the clinician and the left wrist of the child. $EMD_{1,2}$ captures variability in bodily nodes' self-interaction because these are from the child's own body. In contrast, $EMD_{5,2}$ captures variability in dyadic interactions because they are from a shared dyadic spatio-temporal pattern derived from pairwise activities between the clinician and the child. Figure 1D shows sample frequency histograms from the child and clinician right wrist MMS used to obtain the entry marked by an asterisk on the EMD matrix. The sum over the Child-Clinician (or the Clinician-Child) entries reflect Dyadic Variability (note this is a symmetric positive matrix as EMD is a proper distance metric.) This quantity is obtained for each task across the time length that the task may take, using 12 s long time windows under IID assumption. The average for each task is then plotted across the tasks (normalized by maximal value to plot it as (0,1) values). Figure 1E shows an example of this profile for EP01-clinician dyad.

Coherence-Phase-Frequency Parameterization (frequency domain): Power spectrum analyses (Figure 2A) of the MMS and pairwise cross-coherence analyses across the grid of sensors were used to build a parameterization of the data in the frequency domain. To that end, for each task we obtain the pairwise cross-coherence and cross-spectrum phase across frequencies, thus providing maximal cross-coherence with the corresponding phase and frequency, forming three matrices lined up in

Figure 2C. These matrices are used to derive several socio-motor parameters using network connectivity analyses (see below).

The first matrix comprises the maximal cross-coherence value at each entry. For example, entry $MaxCoherence_{2,3}$ represents the maximal cross-coherence value between the left wrist (L) of the child and the torso (T) of the child. This is the maximal level of synchronicity between these self-body parts. As with the EMD matrix before, here we focus on the self-interaction entries and on the dyadic entries, separately. Under this convention, entry $MaxCoherence_{2,3}$ represents a self-interaction entry. The corresponding entry in the MaxPhase matrix has 0 value, thus indicating that these two self-body parts are synchronized with 0 lag and this occurs at 30Hz, the corresponding entry in the MaxFrequency matrix.

The MaxCoherence is conceptualized as an adjacency matrix representing a weighted connected graph. We use it to derive an interconnected network of nodes (body parts) and links between nodes. The links represent the level of pairwise maximal coherence. We use network connectivity analyses and obtain OutDegree, InDegree, total degree, strength, modularity, clustering coefficient, etc., to capture different states of network connectivity across tasks representing states of the dyad whose biorhythmic activity dynamically evolves over time. For the corresponding MaxPhase matrix, we adopt the convention that node i leads node j in the (i, j) entry. Lastly, the frequency matrix provides information about the frequency range at which the cross-coherence is maximal at a phase lag. We can examine the activities for known physiological ranges up to 30 Hz, and/or beyond those ranges up to 64 Hz in this case, focusing on different frequency bands to examine different patterns of entrainment for different dyads, etc. (see other examples [24,37].) In this paper, we focus on the activities across all bands. Figure 2D shows the adjacency matrix that we use to represent the connected network, while focusing on the positive phase leads and zeroing out the entries corresponding to negative phase. The OutDegree vector for a construction task time window is shown in Figure 2E and used to represent network connectivity in the third row. There the color bar represents the maximal coherence values in a color gradient used to color the arrows linking the nodes, with direction according to the positive phase value captured by the arrow thickness. The size of the node is the OutDegree value capturing all the links that the node connects to all other nodes. Two states of the network are represented as an example of transitions, whereby the child leads on average in one and the clinician leads on average in the other. Figure 2F reveals other states where different network patterns evolve as the dyad performs the construction task.

Dyad Coherence Metric: The total dyad coherence is obtained by summing over the entries of the dyadic portions of the matrix (circled in Figure 2D). The lower left quadrant circled entries represent coherence from clinician-to-child (COH-1) and the upper right quadrant represents coherence from child-to-clinician (COH-2). COH-1 + COH-2 is tracked for all the tasks performed during the session in Figure 2G. Note here that the maximum cross coherence metric is symmetric, but the matrix derived using the phase-lags with positive values to build the adjacency matrix is not symmetric.

Dyad Strength Index: An index measuring the strength of the dyad (Equation (3)) combines the value from the Dyad Coherence metric in the numerator and the value from the Dyad Variability metric in the denominator. Higher value of the ratio indicates lower variability and higher cross-coherence during the interaction. This quantity was normalized between (0,1) using the maximal value across all tasks.

$$DyadStrength = \frac{DyadCoherence}{DyadVariability} \tag{3}$$

Delay in Cohesiveness: For maximal coherence values, we sum the lag values over the dyadic entries of the phase matrix to determine, under our (i, j) order convention which person lags behind the other person when the shared dyadic body parts are maximally coherent.

Social Readiness Metric: Using the combination of macro-level data (ADOS scores) and micro-level Dyad Strength quantity, we build a parameter space where we localize all controls and autistic participants to learn where in that parameter space the controls lie. The assumption here is that the control with the highest value of Dyad Strength and the lowest value of ADOS score has high social readiness potential. Then we build a relative metric of Social Readiness by taking the difference between this representative participant and every other participant in the cohort. This is a positive quantity spanning from 0 to the maximal value across the cohort. We normalize both the ADOS scores and the Social Readiness quantity using the corresponding maximal values, and we can then profile the full cohort simultaneously at the macro- and micro-level of inquiry. This can inform us about the potential of each child in the cohort for appropriate social interactions that the clinical test expects and that the body performs.

Leading Profile: To assess who leads, the child and clinician, during the dyadic interaction for each task, we use the OutDegree metric (Figure 2E) obtained from the weighted directed graph that the cross-coherence adjacency matrix produces for each task (e.g., in Figure 2D). Given two nodes, the node with the higher value of OutDegree is said to lead the interaction. There are nine possible cases of inter-body connections (3 (child) × 3 (clinician)) in the dyadic network shared by the child and clinician. As the interaction unfolds, these states change (e.g., Figure 2F). At each time unit where we update the state of the network, the maximal OutDegree represents the leading person. Since the total time for every task is different, we calculate the lead-lag dynamics across all the time units in the manner explained above (with 12s windows taken under IID assumption) and sum up the total for each child and clinician. The person leading a greater number of time units for each given task is said to lead the task. Figure 2H shows the lead-lag for every task performed by EP01 during the session.

As an example of lead-lag calculation for EP01, he spent 17 time units in the Construction Task (CT) with a 12 s time unit (128 Hz × 12 s gives 1536 frames and this is the minimum time length of a task across the entire cohort.) This number of frames provided enough information to empirically estimate statistical parameters with 95% confidence intervals. At time $t = 1$, the OutDegree patterns could be $(3\ (LW), 3\ (RW), 5\ (Torso))_{Child}$ and $(1\ (LW), 0\ (RW), 3\ (Torso))_{Clinician}$.

Each of the entries in the Child vector are compared to the entries in the Clinician vector, giving a total of nine possible dyadic interactions. For example, the first interaction, being LW_{Child} (OutDegree = 3), is compared to $LW_{Clinician}$ (OutDegree = 1). The Child leads this interaction as it has a higher value of OutDegree. Similarly, the Child leads seven to nine interactions, none are led by the Clinician and two are balanced (with equal OutDegree value). Consequently, at time $t = 1$, the Child leads.

The lead-lag patterns can be visualized as in Figure 2F, where the color of the lines depicts the coherence value, the line thickness represents the phase lag, and the size of the node is the OutDegree. Here the direction of the arrows represents who leads the interaction at time t. We can see that at $t = 1$, the child leads as explained above. The calculation for the other time units follows and a profile across tasks is shown in Figure 2F. Similar to the dyadic interaction portion of the matrix, we can also quantify the self-interaction for each child and clinician separately, to see which sensor (Left Wrist, Right Wrist or Torso) leads during each of the tasks.

3. Results

The combination of macro- and micro-level of inquiries can be appreciated in Figure 3A where we plot the ADOS sub-scores as a function of the Dyad Strength for each child in the cohort.

3.1. Potential for Social Readiness Revealed by Micro-Level Socio-Motor Biometrics Is Missed by Macro-Level Criteria

Figure 3A shows that neurotypical children have low ADOS scores (total, social affect, and repetitive restricted behaviors) and higher Dyad Strength than the autistic participants, according to linear acceleration data (angular speed data in Figure S1 is congruent.) However, several autistic subjects with high ADOS scores also have strong Dyad Strength, in the range of neurotypicals. Their bodily biorhythms synchronize with those of the rater as they socially interact. This shared level of cohesiveness suggests a potential for social readiness captured by the digital data but missed by the naked eye.

To further characterize that potential, we compute the difference between the neurotypical participant with the highest Dyad Strength value and that of every other participant in the cohort. We then normalize this quantity by dividing it by the maximal value of that difference across the group. The corresponding normalized ADOS score is plotted for each participant along with this relative measure of Social Readiness. The closer to 0 this quantity is, the higher the Social Readiness potential. This can be appreciated in Figure 3B inclusive of neurotypical controls and autistic subjects.

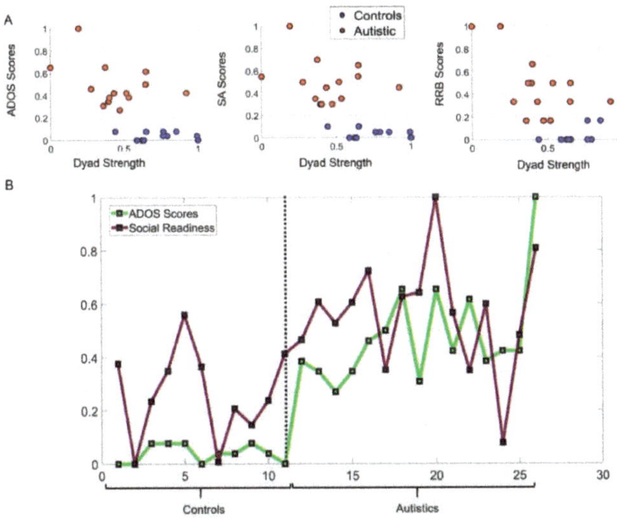

Figure 3. A measure of social readiness potential: Dyadic strength expressed in relation to ADOS sub-scores (Social Affect, (SA) and the so-called Repetitive Ritualistic Behaviors, (RRB)). (**A**) Dyad strength (see methods) tends to be higher in neurotypical controls, with a tendency towards lower (normalized) ADOS scores and some higher variations in the more ambiguous RRB sub-score. The trend in the autistic dyadic strength scores is towards lower values and higher ADOS score, yet 5/15, (33.3%) fall within the neurotypical lower range despite higher ADOS scores, thus signaling a hidden capacity for social dyadic exchange. (**B**) This information can be further unfolded for each participant, whereby a score of social readiness potential is obtained as a relative quantity measuring the absolute difference between each participant and the neurotypical with the highest dyad strength. Many of the autistic participants do have socio-motor strength in the dyadic interaction, despite high ADOS scores.

Notice that several of the autistic participants have social readiness potential in the range of controls, despite high ADOS scores.

3.2. Mirroring of Social Actions Inevitably Biases the Rater

Another metric that we can derive from the network connectivity analysis is the extent to which each node leads other nodes in the grid of six sensors, conceptualized as an interconnected network. To that end, we use the OutDegree metric (e.g., Figure 2E) which signals the number of links with high cross-coherence from each node to each other node (visualized in Figure 2F.) When examining self-interaction nodes, we focus on the person's nodes and obtain the OutDegree metric of each node, signaling the phase lead (in degrees per unit time) for each of the maximal cross-coherence values obtained pairwise. We do this for each child in the neurotypical and autistic subgroups and for the rater clinician interacting with these children. Figure 4A shows this profile as % of the neurotypical children's cohort leading with the highest positive phase at maximal cross-coherence (left panel in 4A). This quantity is plotted for each of the tasks that the children performed for a given module (along the x-axis) across all three sensors. The right-hand panel in 4A depicts the information for the clinician.

The neurotypical children and the rater clinician have comparable ranges of leading index values. In contrast, the same clinician shows a very different range of leading index values when the children are autistic. This mirroring effect of Figure 4A,B strongly suggest a socio-motor bias that inevitably occurs largely beneath awareness, but that nonetheless skews the performance of the task by the rater.

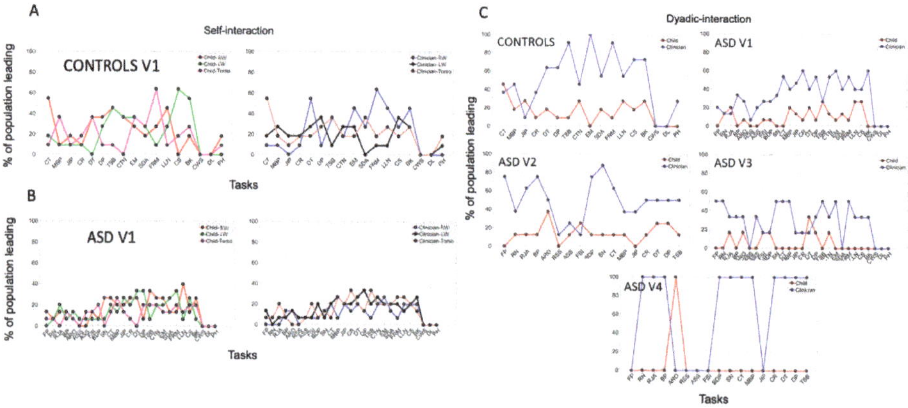

Figure 4. Mirroring Bias Effects. (**A**,**B**) Biased rating in the ADOS test quantified through mirroring metric of lead-lag social patterns of self-interactions (individual kinematic synergies) as percentage in leading patterns across the cohort. Neurotypical Controls and Clinician show broader range of values than Autistics the visit one, under the most appropriate module and same rater. (**C**) Mirroring effect and raters' leading bias persist in the shared dyadic cohesiveness as the module and rater change. Visit one and three (appropriate module) under two different raters show a reduction in parameter range for autistics relative to controls. Visit two and four (less appropriate module and by then familiar rater) show an increase in parameter range for autistics relative to visits one and three.

When the interlocutor is neurotypical, the rater's patterns mirror the range of neurotypical values, but when the interlocutor is autistic, this range shrinks. Since these are self-interactions (inter-node cross-coherence phase for each agent) and the dyad also shares the intra-node cross-coherence, we then obtained graphs in Figure 4C exploring similar a question for each visit. Controls only visit once, whereas autistics come back three more times. In each case, we now examine the OutDegree leading patterns of the dyadic nodes of the matrix. The angular speed data in Figure S2 shows consistent patterns with the linear acceleration data of Figure 4.

3.3. *Systematic Leading Bias of Rater Remains Across ADOS Modules and Familiarity with the Child*

We see that, as with the self-interaction nodes, the dyadic interaction nodes reveal a mirroring bias whereby, for the same clinician, same child and same module, the range of values in the leading parameter is on average much higher when the children are neurotypical (Figure 4C, left-panel) but shrinks when the children are autistic (Figure 4C, right-panel). Then, in visit two, when the module changes to an easier one, the range of values broadens across the autistic children. This effect on the person leading the interaction shows the mirroring effects of shared socio-motor parameters that raters inevitably miss when relying on observation alone.

The same cohort of children returns to visits three and four, but we change the rater. As in visit one, during visit three, the rater administers the most appropriate module for each child. In visit four (as in visit two), the module is the less language-appropriate one. In visit three, the children perform the appropriate module, as in visit one. Despite the familiarity with that module, the patterns of leadership ranges shrink with the new, unfamiliar rater. Here we see that the new rater's range becomes much broader when the children are familiar with her in visit four, and the module is already familiar to the child, from visit one. For both raters, there is an implicit mirroring effect with the autistic children that is inevitably bound to bias their scoring. The raters are interacting in a closed loop with the child and influencing the interaction that they evoke, respond to and rate. The cross-coherence network connectivity metrics capture the inherent biases in the leading patterns across the ADOS tasks. In all cases the rater dominates the interaction albeit with marked differences between controls and autistics in the full range of values across the cohort, susceptibility to familiarity with the rater and easiness of module.

3.4. *The ADOS Test Probing Appropriateness in Social Interactions Is Administered as a Monologue*

The network connectivity analyses invariably reveal for controls and autistics that the rater leads the interaction most of the time. This can be appreciated in Figure 5A, while Figure 5B shows the summary across all four visits for the autistic cohort and for visit one for the controls. Although natural social interactions of a dyad are supposed to unfold like a dialogue between two agents, the test administration switches the interaction to a monologue style. The rater is unaware of these socio-motor parameters, as they evolve implicitly, from the synchronous cross-cohesive patterns that self-emerge from the two bodies in micro-motion. At the macro-level of the social dyad, these aspects of the dynamically unfolding behavior occur much too quickly to be picked up by the rater, who is busy trying to evoke, react to and rate the child's social overtures. Figure S3 shows consistent results for angular speed data as Figure 5 does for linear acceleration data.

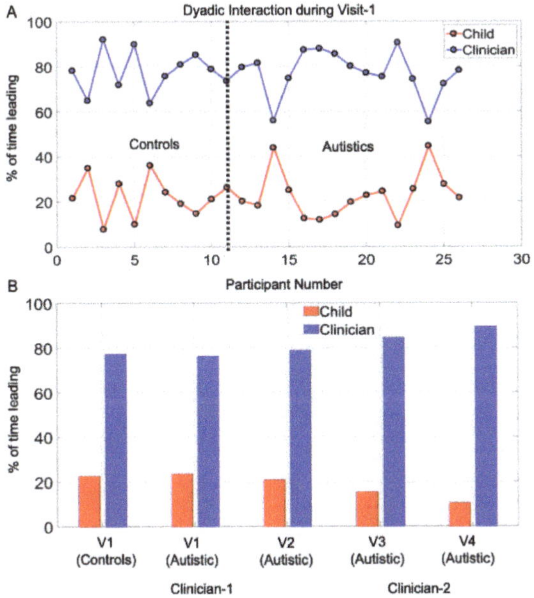

Figure 5. Monologue style of ADOS test. Rater leads social interaction a large percentage of the time for each child. (**A**) For all 26 children divided into neurotypical controls and autistics on the x-axis and on the y-axis, the % of time (taken across all ADOS tasks) that the rater or the child leads the interaction. Clinician rater leads on average for each child, across all tasks. (**B**) Group data per visit showing the summary of the % time that the person leads the social interaction.

3.5. *Micro-Level Analyses Capture Socio-Motor Changes Missed by Macro-Level Scores*

Figure 6 shows data from a representative autistic experiment participant who returned to the lab for a second visit and was rated by the same clinician during performance of the same

ADOS-appropriate module in both visits. We note that the child did not perform all tasks in each visit but performed a subset of them in both visits. While his ADOS scores remained unchanged, his socio-motor patterns markedly changed from visit to visit. Figure 6A shows the patterns of leadership for both visits, while Figure 6B shows the patterns of Dyad Variability. Figure 6C,D show the patterns of Dyad Coherence between child and clinician in the clinician→child and child→clinician directions, respectively. While neurodevelopment continued its complex micro-dynamic course in this autistic participant over two visits separated months apart, at the macro-level the ADOS scores remained deterministically static over time. Figure S4 shows consistent results for angular speed data as Figure 6 does for linear acceleration data.

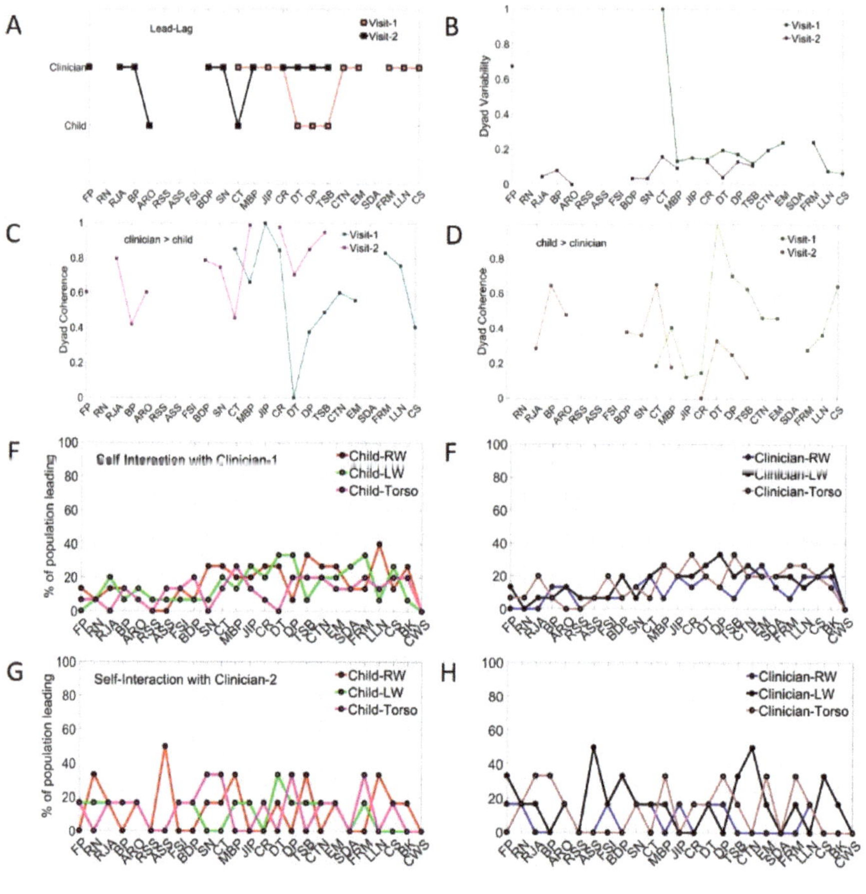

Figure 6. High sensitivity of micro-level metrics captures socio-motor changes over time and serves to measure rater's reliability-style. (**A–D**) ADOS scoring system does not capture change in developmental socio-motor physiology. Across visits, the macro-level scores remain static, but the micro-level socio-motor parameters change. These include leading profile, Dyadic Variability and Dyadic Coherence. (**E,F**) High sensitivity to changing clinician rater prevails across all children and tasks. The self-interaction parameters (individual kinematic synergies) of autistic participants are sensitive (at the micro-level) to changing the rater. (**G,H**) Leading profiles in the same autistic cohort shift as the raters differ.

3.6. High Sensitivity to Change in Clinician Across All Children of the Cohort

Two raters participated in the study, one in visits one and two, the other in visits three and four. As mentioned, the appropriate ADOS module was administered in visits one and three. Less appropriate modules were administered in visits two and four. This experimental assay allowed us to probe the responses of the dyad to the switch in raters (same ADOS module, different raters.) For the autistic children, the leading profile derived from the self-interaction entries of the matrix changes with the change in clinician, despite maintaining the same ADOS module, whether appropriate or not (Figure 6E,F). This suggests that the child's nervous system is sensitive to changes in the social environment, a desirable feature that could be further used to enhance social interactions across different situations.

3.7. Stratification of Sub-Types in Autism Is Not Possible Using Macro-Level Criteria Alone

Among the experimental participants, several had similar ADOS scores. This is not surprising, given the narrow numerical range of discrete values of these scores and the large heterogeneous population sample. Upon taking a random draw of participants from the population, it is not possible to cover all different subtypes using these discrete scores' range from macro-level criteria. To instantiate this point, we present the socio-motor data derived from the biosensors for two experiment participants with identical ADOS scores but fundamentally different socio-motor phenotype. We examined their ADOS activities using the same module and rater. Figure 7A shows the leadership profile across tasks for these two representative autistic participants with very different socio-motor activity. At the macro-level of ADOS description they are similar. At the micro-level of socio-motor behavior they differ. In an interventional therapy following this ADOS detection, these children would likely require different approaches that such discrete coarse clinical criteria could not differentiate. Panel 7B further shows the distinct profiles of Dyad Variability for these participants, while panels 7C and 7D show the profiles of Dyad Coherence across tasks, taken from the clinician→child and child→clinician dyadic entries of the cross-coherence matrix representing the interconnected network of sensors. Figure S5 shows consistent results for the angular speed data as Figure 7 does for linear acceleration data.

3.8. Two Different Clinicians Perceive the Same Child's Socio-Motor Patterns Highly Differently

Likewise, following up the sensitivity of the children's nervous system to changes in clinician, we here asked if the same autistic child interacting with the two clinicians in different visits would be differentially perceived by the clinicians. We tested this question using the micro-level socio-motor patterns from the clinicians and comparing them across the tasks that were common to the child. Figure 7E shows the differences in leadership patterns of the clinicians for the same child while Figure 7F shows the profile of Dyad Variability. Figure 7G,H show the pattern of Dyadic Coherence for the clinician→child and child→clinician directions, respectively.

3.9. Task Ranking and Target Treatment

Given the sensitivity of micro-level socio-motor patterns to changes in clinician, modules and the passage of time from visit to visit, we then ascertain the extent to which we could use the digital data derived using the ADOS test as an outcome measure and possibly turn this test into an intervention tool, beyond the static notion of a macro-level detection instrument. Adding the socio-motor micro-dynamics is amenable to further investigating this question, task by task. To that end, we probe the delay in attaining cohesiveness as a metric of natural social interactions. Delay in Cohesiveness (see methods) is obtained by summing over phase-lag values of the entries of the phase matrix for which maximal cross-coherence was attained between the child's and the clinician's biorhythmic activities. This is the socio-motor space cohesively shared by the two agents of the dyad when their bodily biorhythms synchronize with different phase lags. At 0 lag they are perfectly in sync, but that state is often transient. Lag patterns add up to out-of-phase synchronous patterns across child and clinician. We measure that

Delay in Cohesiveness and build a parameter space to learn about this as a function of Dyadic Strength (previously defined.) We find that controls span the full range of Delay in Cohesiveness while most lie on the higher values of Dyadic Strength (Figure 8A). In contrast, autistics are mostly on the upper left quadrant of the graph, with high values of Delay in Cohesiveness and, on average, lower values in Dyadic Strength than controls.

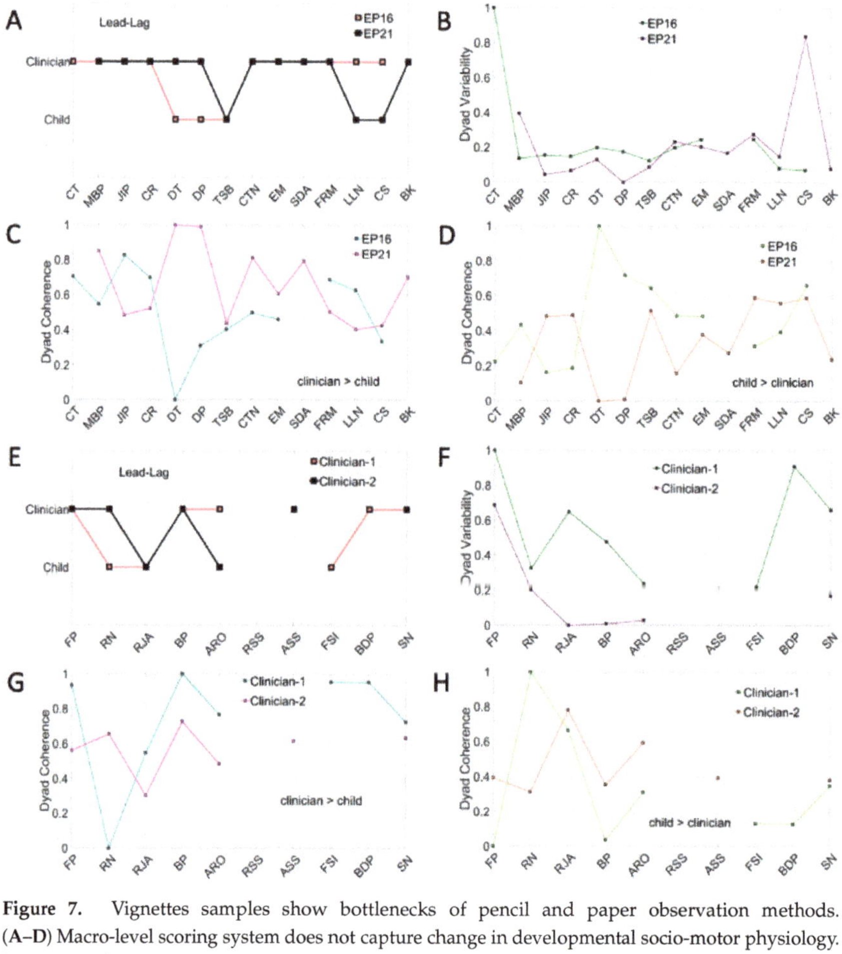

Figure 7. Vignettes samples show bottlenecks of pencil and paper observation methods. (**A–D**) Macro-level scoring system does not capture change in developmental socio-motor physiology. Experimental participants EP16 and EP21 are perceived very different by the same clinician in relation to leading patterns (**A**); Dyad Variability (**B**) and Dyad Coherence (**C**,**D**) in each of the clinician→child and child→clinician directions. (**E–H**) Ill-posed autism detection problem: Given the ADOS score, what is the most likely socio-motor phenotype? Each clinician perceives the same child differently across all micro-level socio-motor indexes.

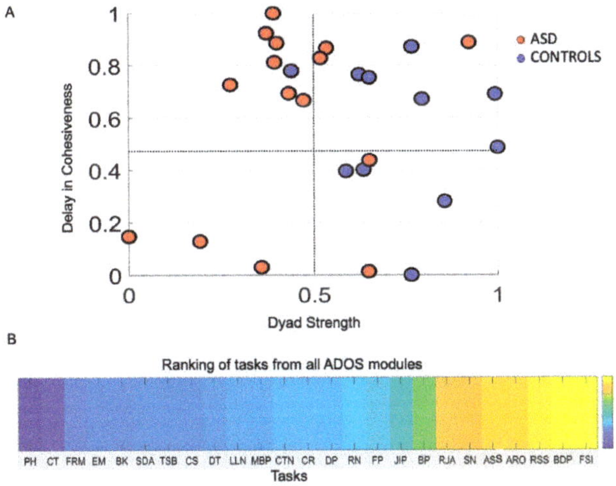

Figure 8. Digital biomarker for personalized design of adaptive targeted therapy. (**A**) Parameter space spanned by dyad strength on x-axis and delay in cohesiveness (see text for details) on the y-axis. Ideally within a social interaction one would desire high dyad strength and a broad range of response cohesiveness, spanning from fast to slow. Note that most controls have high dyad strength and their responses vary broadly from lower to higher cohesiveness delay, whereas autistics are primarily in the region of low dyad strength and delayed cohesiveness (i.e., they synchronize their body biorhythms with those of the rater, but there is a larger lag than desirable.) (**B**) Task ranking criteria based on dyad strength calculated for various tasks from participants in visit one. Functional and Symbolic Imitation, FSI is assigned the highest rank (easiest task to perform) as it depicts the best dyad strength while PH having the lowest dyad strength is assigned the lowest rank (most difficult task to perform).

This result motivated us to examine the tasks individually and propose a task training regime whereby, in a personalized manner, one could rank which tasks have highest Dyad strength, with variable delay in cohesiveness that converges toward the right lower quadrant of the graph. Then we can use those tasks to start gradually training the person while incorporating other tasks, as social learning improves in the precise sense that Dyad Strength increases, Delay in Coherence is variable and, at the macro-level, the rater begins to unambiguously perceive the positive changes. Figure 8B provides an example of the continuous digital scale derived from the tasks, ranging from lowest to highest Dyad Strength value. These scales encompass both macro- and micro-level of information but is dynamic, as it depends on the evolving socio-motor skills of the person interacting in a dyad. Table S1 shows the tasks that are significantly different at the alpha of 0.05 when comparing controls and autistics. Figure S6 shows consistent results for angular speed data as Figure 8 does for linear acceleration data.

3.10. The Digitazed ADOS Separates Males and Females Using Network Connectivity Metrics and Noise to Signal Ratio (NSR)

The network connectivity analyses revealed fundamental differences between males (16) and females (10) in the cohort. Figure 9 shows the distributions and scatters of several parameters used to assess dyadic socio-motor behavior. For each parameter we used the same number of points, 1730, which was the minimum set in the females derived from the 27 tasks. We cycled across all participants of the cohort and sampled multiple sets to systematically compare males vs. females. The sets represent a random draw of the population, inclusive of autistics and controls, whereby females revealed a very different connectivity and NSR profile than males. All parameters were statistically different with significance at the 0.01 level, $p << 0.01$ according to the non-parametric rank-sum test.

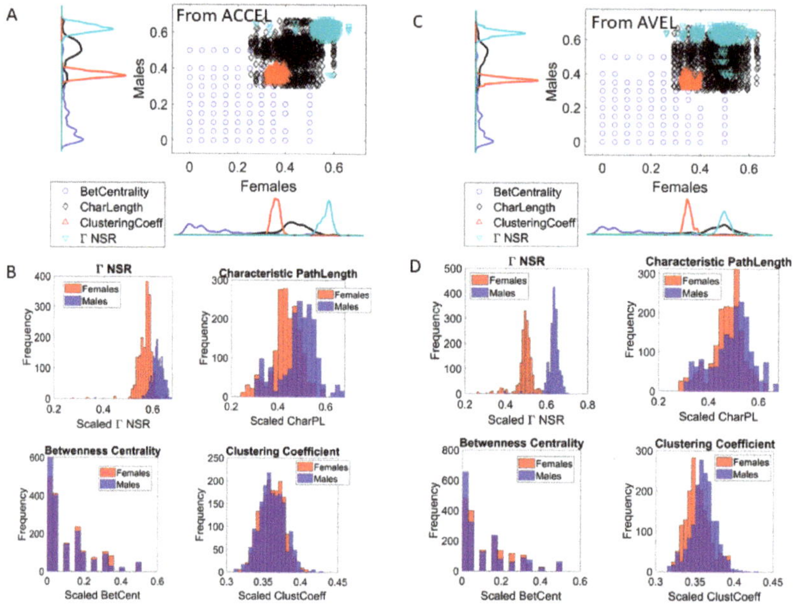

Figure 9. Digital ADOS automatically separates females from males in a random draw of the population. (**A**) Scatters and histograms of parameters derived from interconnected networks representing the dynamic dyad provide evidence for fundamental differences in connectivity across the nodes of the network composed by the child and clinician dyad. (**B**) The empirically estimated Gamma scale parameter (the noise to signal ratio, (NSR)) of the micro-movement spikes (MMS) derived from acceleration separate females from males with lower NSR in females and tighter distribution than males. The characteristic pathlength denoting average shortest distance path from each node to every other node of the network is significantly shorter in females than in males. The betweenness centrality is higher in females than males and the clustering coefficient is also higher in females. All differences are statistically significant with $p << 0.01$. (**C**) Summary graph for angular speed is consistent with the acceleration patterns. (**D**) Females show lower NSR, lower characteristic pathlength and higher betweenness centrality and lower clustering coefficient. All differences are statistically significant according to non-parametric rank-sum test $p << 0.01$.

The network connectivity parameters revealed better connectivity patterns in females than males. Since these patterns are derived from the dynamic dyad, they imply better social rapport with the clinician in females than males. The characteristic pathlength was significantly shorter in females than males, suggesting faster information transmission throughout the network, a feature that was accompanied by significantly lower NSR in females, lower clustering coefficient values denoting more distributed network in females, with more efficient (sparser) dyadic node information accompanied by higher betweenness centrality in the dyad nodes. These patterns turned out to be highly different when comparing males' and females' micro-movement data, as generated by the dyadic network from the digital ADOS. However, better connectivity patterns in females may make it harder for the clinician to visually recognize social difficulties in the female phenotype. All comparisons of these parameters yielded highly significant differences for the time series data from the accelerometer (Figure 9A,B) and from the gyroscope (Figure 9C,D).

4. Discussion

This study leveraged the digital data output by wearable sensors during the performance of a standard clinical test to significantly augment the information that we could gain during the assessment of dyadic social interactions. Turning the standard tasks of the research ADOS test into experimental assays and manipulating several parameters of the experiment, we were able to improve the characterization of socio-motor behaviors across the population, inclusive of neurotypical controls and autistic participants.

We digitized this test while neurotypical children interacted with the rater and uncovered new aspects of the test that helped reveal the potential for social readiness in autistic children. We also learned that the rater dominates the interaction, leading most of the time in both neurotypicals and autistics, with a mirroring effect that inevitably biases the shared cohesiveness of the interaction, channeling a broader range of variability in leadership patterns for neurotypicals and a much narrower range in autistics. The mirroring effects occur at the personal level of activity in what we coin self-interactions of the nodes (conceptualized as kinematic synergies across the bodily biorhythmic fluctuations of each interlocutor in the dyad.) It also occurs at the shared spatio-temporal patterns of cross-coherence between several body parts of the child and the rater. This shared cohesiveness that self-emerges and evolves across the tasks in a session contributes to the strength in dyadic interactions present in autistic children and is therefore revealing of their potential for social readiness. We would not have discovered this socio-motor parameter had we not included neurotypicals in our research-ADOS assessment. As social interactions depend on developmental socio-motor milestones, and these in turn depend on the maturation of the nervous system, our results underscore the need to include normative data from neurotypical participants in any study or assessment of autistic social behaviors. Furthermore, objectively quantifying the level of bias from the rater during the interactions enables us to curtail it or enhance it as needed, thus providing new means to causally induce a child's reaction in a much more controlled manner than has been traditionally done.

The use of the research ADOS standardized modules in our study allowed us to test the same child with the same rater under different social demands. When the module was appropriate, we saw a consistent reduction in the range of variability in the leading patterns across raters, in relation to their patterns for a less appropriate module under a context of more familiarity with the rater. This is important because, at the micro-level of socio-motor behaviors, the same child may demonstrate more social competence, given that s/he is more familiar with the person and/or the tasks. This is not something apparent to the naked eye of an observer and much less so when the observer may be also distracted when trying to rate the interaction. There is a bottleneck in information processing that inevitably prevents the rater from seeing this aspect of the interaction. Adding the micro-level of analysis thus presents us with the opportunity to harness this potential for social readiness and offer the child (autistic or otherwise) better social support. We can then utilize this standardized test as an avenue to train the child to be social without having to instruct how to do so, but rather by leveraging this micro-layer of information that we can extract from the shared spatio-temporal cohesiveness of the dyad under more relaxed conditions (e.g., more familiarity with the rater and the task.) Socio-motor phenomena are adaptable. We can use these biometrics to track the progression of adaptation at the micro-level of inquiry, underscoring once again how much more we gain by integrating them into the current behavioral assessments tools at the research and at the clinical levels.

Dyadic social interactions are typically a dialogue with balanced contributions from both parties involved. They succeed at communicating when there is appropriate turn taking, when joint attention is not sustained for too long or when it is not too brief, and when the entrainment between the bodily biorhythms lead to implicit agreement supporting non-verbal communication. There is a delicate balance at the micro-level activity that scaffolds social rapport of the interacting dyad at the macro-level. The results from our analyses reveal a prevalence of the rater leading the interaction with both neurotypicals and autistics. This rater dominance turned the test into a quasi-monologue style of interaction, perhaps an unintended consequence of having the same person evoke the social overture of the child, while responding to it, and rating the outcome. Inevitably, the leadership role of the rater skews the interaction. Although this is not discussed in the social behavioral sciences, here we reveal it using micro-level analyses of the shared spatio-temporal and frequency parameters, characterizing the fluctuations of the biorhythmic activity generated by the two bodies in motion during the dyadic exchange.

This strong skewing influence of the rater on the dyadic social behaviors changes the outcomes of the child's socio-motor patterns for the exact same task and module when different clinicians administer the research ADOS to that child. Consequently, not only at the micro-level of social responses, but also at the macro-level of observable responses, a given child could be perceived very differently by different clinicians. There are both positive and negative consequences here. The positive side is that we can precisely characterize the child–rater's reactions to each other and, in the context of therapy, use this digitized instrument to determine which therapist has by default more rapport with the child. This would be especially relevant in the early stages of the therapy. Likewise, we could use this test and biometrics in the context of a teacher-child relationship, to select the teacher that will most likely (by default) have the best rapport with the child. This is important for emotional social learning in general.

The negative aspect is that, for a test that aims at detecting something with high precision, there is no chance that it will do so. The detection problem becomes ill-posed: given a score, what is the most likely socio-motor phenotype? The map from score to socio-motor phenotype is many-to-one. This result bears implications for our (in)ability to define the autistic phenotype(s) and reliably uncover autistic subtypes in a random draw of the population. We could not use this test to stratify the broad spectrum of autism.

Since this test informs and largely steers the science of autism, and since given the ADOS score it is not possible to infer the most likely socio-motor phenotype, for detection purposes it may be beneficial to combine different levels of inquiry and produce a more reliable objective metric impervious to rating styles, personality or cultural nuances. This should be possible by providing a digital characterization of social interactions in general, as we have done here, with a clinical example that uses standard pre-specified tasks amenable to illustrate these various points.

We emphasize that there are many more possible biometrics that we can derive from these tasks and interactions [37–40]. The examples used here are merely illustrative of the broad variety of socio-motor parameters that digital data can offer. Wearable biosensors today sample at high frequency even when they are off-the-shelf, such as smart phones, smart watches, etc. [41] affording science and clinical areas a new level of granularity sensitive to the detection of change and its rate during neurodevelopment. This information is now at the tip or our fingers owing to the wearable sensors revolution, offering continuity to behavioral science even in times of physical (social) distancing.

One important aspect of the study was that some of the autistic children returned to the lab for a total of four visits. This passage of time was important to assess the extent to which the socio-motor phenomena assessed at different levels of inquiry would reflect the rate of change in neurodevelopment that the children underwent. We found that while the macro-level of description from observation (using in this case the research ADOS scoring criteria) remained static, the micro-level of description and statistical inference fluctuated over time, describing a stochastic trajectory that could reveal individual trends for each child and for the cohort.

Having the ability to assess developmental trajectories in tandem with changes in somatic-sensory-motor physiology is important to build the notion of a dynamic diagnosis chart that could reflect such changes in maturation and function. Underlying all these socio-motor biorhythmic phenomena is a growing, adapting and developing (coping) nervous system. Thus, relying exclusively on coarse observational metrics that fail to capture change will prevent the ability to provide proper support to nurture the growth of these systems and the social axes that they scaffold. Introducing these digital biometrics of socio-motor behaviors can help us bridge the gap between neurodevelopmental rates of change and coarse clinical behavioral criteria.

Another aspect of the study that is worthwhile underscoring is the fundamental differences in network connectivity patterns that we found between males and females. These differences in connectivity patterns relate to socio-motor parameters derived from the dynamically interacting dyad. Thus, unlike the paper-and-pencil version of the ADOS, which has failed to detect social differences in females (by observation), here the digital ADOS does so across all parameters under consideration. Furthermore, we also examined the Gamma NSR empirically derived using MLE and found fundamental differences between the MMS signatures of males and females across the cohort. This result is congruent with prior work involving person-centered analyses of involuntary head motions [32,42,43], decision making by pointing to targets [44] and gait analyses [45] from our laboratory. The new result separating sex in autism is more relevant than the previous results reported because it is derived from the dyadic social interaction taking place during the very tasks that define the scores to detect the condition. These results mean that, across numerous socio-motor axes, there is a high likelihood of automatically (and blindly) detecting such sex differences in a random draw of the population performing the ADOS test. This randomly chosen cohort of 26 children opens a new line of inquiry with the potential to finally address the disparate 4-5:1 male to female ratio in autism [46,47]. Most important yet, we will be able to do so using the test that researchers and clinicians use to detect autism, if we digitize it. Because of the wearable sensors revolution, we can easily digitize the ADOS using off-the-shelf technology such as smart watches and web-cameras, an important advantage also in remote testing and telemedicine approaches due to the pandemic. Under these new conditions, clinicians have limited visibility from the point of view of the child-caregiver dyad at the other end of the screen. The connectivity metrics and the empirically derived Gamma-NSR are hidden to the naked eye, but visible to the digital data and to the analytics that we offer here. It will be important to scale up this result and validate it across thousands of dyads performing the ADOS test while capturing the dynamic dyad digitally. We here note that our methods extend to more than two people, so remote model of telemedicine involving the clinician at one end and the parent-child dyad at the other end is also feasible.

Adopting standardized digital technology and integrating it with these gold-standard psychological tests may help us develop new outcome measures of treatments and provide parameter spaces where we can track the trajectories of interventions. A testable hypothesis is that, as participants repeat the ADOS performance, it may be possible to ascertain which tasks give higher dyad strength. If we were to focus on those tasks first to improve social interaction, then it would be possible to shift to the other tasks, thus aiming at broadening the repertoire of tasks that lead to appropriate social exchange, tailoring this to the child's inherent strengths in an individualized manner. Indeed, digitizing social behaviors could provide a guide to assess the changes in socio-motor parameters introduced here such as Dyad Strength and Delay in Cohesiveness, computed as relative metrics, obtained first in neurotypicals, and as such revealing of the expected course of socio-motor development, constructed along the path of least resistance. Our work offers more than one way to do this while leveraging the wearable sensors revolution and preserving the clinical gains already attained with observational means.

Caveats and Limitations of the Proposed Hybrid Methods

Although the digital characterization of the ADOS test may hold the promise of revealing new aspects of the ADOS interactions that may otherwise remain hidden to the naked eye, there are several caveats regarding the adoption and use of the present methods. The major limitation is the current lack of mechanisms that can scale up the results from this reduced cohort in the laboratory to thousands of participants in clinical settings. Future use of the analytics presented here can be extended to biorhythms registered with off-the-shelf wearables such as smart watches and web cameras outputting shareable digital data, even across remote settings. To that end, our laboratory has developed a new concept "The Lab in a Box". This remote kit for behavioral data acquisition and analyses offers continuity to the administration of behavioral tests such as the ADOS in times of social (physical) distancing. However, deploying such methods on a large scale would require a concerted effort across multiple disciplines, business models and entrepreneurship beyond academic settings. This exceeds the scope of this paper, but it is perhaps something to keep in mind in order to translate the present results to clinical and home settings, offering the possibility to scale up the use of this technology to tens of thousands of users.

Another limitation of the present analysis is that other pipelines could have been used to analyze the data. This begs the question of whether the general results would have dramatically changed in that case. In earlier preliminary analyses of these data sets using different analytical pipelines, larger number of sensors in the interconnected grid, different bodily locations for the additional sensors, different kinematic parameters, and different children, we observed similar trends [24]. As such, we are confident that the trends would remain invariant to such nuances. However, we do acknowledge that the interpretation and inference are to be discussed and validated across the community, to provide a consensus on the clinical interpretability of digital data in general. In other words, the characterization of the digital ADOS data that we provide here needs to be further validated across thousands of participants and clinicians. This is the case for any new scientific approach. In this sense, we invite the reader to reproduce the results using ours and other data sets provided in GitHub by our laboratory. Our analytics do not make theoretical assumptions about the likelihoods and probabilities of representing data features. Our new methods, rather, empirically estimate these from the micro-fluctuations inherently present in the signals that we register from natural behaviors. In this sense, we remain confident that cross-sectional and longitudinal data captured with various means will find trends similar to those found in this random draw of the population of autistics and neurotypical controls. This work extends an invitation to the clinical community, as well as to the scientific community, to collaborate and take steps toward combining different levels of inquiry in the study of general social behaviors beyond autism and other neurodevelopmental conditions.

5. Conclusions

We have shown that by integrating macro-level rubrics used to assess appropriateness of social exchange with micro-level biorhythmic activities co-registered synchronously in both agents of the social dyad, we can uncover much more than we would when using one level of inquiry alone. Our work underscores the need to combine pencil and paper methods with objective instruments that add a finer layer of granularity to the study of the complex dynamics of social phenomena. Without a doubt, this is a case where the overall sum amounts to much more than its individual parts.

6. Patents

EBT holds the US Patent "Methods and Systems for the Diagnoses and Treatments of Nervous Systems Disorders" combined in the paper as micro-movement spikes, MMS data type and Gamma process.

Supplementary Materials: The following are available online at http://www.mdpi.com/2075-4426/10/4/159/s1, Figure S1. A measure of social readiness potential: Dyadic strength expressed in relation to ADOS sub-scores (Social Affect, SA and the so-called Repetitive Ritualistic Behaviours, RRB), Figure S2: Mirroring Bias Effects, Figure S3: Monologue style of ADOS test, Figure S4: High sensitivity of micro-level metrics captures socio-motor changes over time and serves to measure rater reliability-style, Figure S5: Vignettes samples show bottlenecks of pencil and paper observation methods, Figure S6: Digital biomarker for personalized design of adaptive targeted therapy, Table S1: Wilcoxon RankSum test statistics (p-value) at 5% significance level for common tasks between Controls and Autistics, Table S2: Details of the tasks across all ADOS modules, Table S3: Details of participants (only whose data is available/ analyzed) across all the visits.

Author Contributions: Conceptualization, E.B.T.; methodology, E.B.T.; software, E.B.T. and H.B.; validation, E.B.T., H.B. and R.R.; formal analysis, H.B.; investigation, E.B.T., H.B. and R.R.; resources, E.B.T.; data curation, R.R.; writing—original draft preparation, E.B.T., H.B.; writing—review and editing, E.B.T., H.B. and R.R.; visualization, E.B.T., H.B.; supervision, E.B.T.; project administration, E.B.T.; funding acquisition, E.B.T. All authors have read and agreed to the published version of the manuscript.

Funding: This research was funded by the New Jersey Governor's Council for the Medical Research and Treatments of Autism CAUT14APL018 and by the Nancy Lurie Marks Family Foundation to E.B.T. Career Development Award.

Acknowledgments: We thank the children and the families who participated in the study. We thank Caroline P. Whyatt for her valuable contribution to the coordination and data acquisition during the early stages of the study. We thank Rutgers University Psychology undergraduates who helped curate the video and pencil and paper data.

Conflicts of Interest: The authors declare no conflict of interest.

References

1. Cowlyn, T. Maternal Voice and Communicative Musicality: Sharing the Meaning of Life Before Birth. In *Early Vocal Contact and Preterm Infant Brain Development: Bridging the Gap between Research and Practice*; Filippa, M., Kuhn, P., Westup, B., Eds.; Springer: Cham, Switzerland, 2017; pp. 3–24.
2. Moon, C. Prenatal Experience with the Maternal Voice. In *Early Vocal Contact and Preterm Infant Brain Development: Bridging the Gap between Research and Practice*; Filippa, M., Kuhn, P., Westrup, B., Eds.; Springer: Cham, Switzerland, 2017; pp. 25–38.
3. Trehub, S.E. The Maternal Voice as a Special Signal for Infants. In *Early Vocal Contact and Preterm Infant Brain Development: Bridging the Gap between Research and Practice*; Filippa, M., Kuhn, P., Westrup, B., Eds.; Springer: Cham, Switzerland, 2017; pp. 39–55.
4. Gratier, M.; Devouche, E. The Development of Infant Participation in Communication. In *Early Vocal Contact and Preterm Infant Brain Development: Bridging the Gap between Research and Practice*; Filippa, M., Kuhn, P., Westrup, B., Eds.; Springer: Cham, Switzerland, 2017; pp. 55–70.
5. Grandjean, D. Brain Mechanisms in Emotional Voice Production and Perception and Early Life Interactions. In *Early Vocal Contact and Preterm Infant Brain Development: Bridging the Gap between Research and Practice*; Filippa, M., Kuhn, P., Westrup, B., Eds.; Springer: Cham, Switzerland, 2017; pp. 71–91.
6. Condon, W.S.; Sander, L.W. Synchrony demonstrated between movements of the neonate and adult speech. *Child Dev.* **1974**, *45*, 456–462. [CrossRef]
7. Condon, W.S.; Sander, L.W. Neonate movement is synchronized with adult speech: Interactional participation and language acquisition. *Science* **1974**, *183*, 99–101. [CrossRef] [PubMed]
8. Brazelton, T.B.; Tronick, E.; Adamson, L.; Als, H.; Wise, S. Early mother-infant reciprocity. *Ciba Found. Symp.* **1975**, 137–154. [CrossRef]
9. Gusella, J.L.; Muir, D.; Tronick, E.Z. The effect of manipulating maternal behavior during an interaction on three- and six-month-olds' affect and attention. *Child Dev.* **1988**, *59*, 1111–1124. [CrossRef] [PubMed]
10. Weinberg, M.K.; Tronick, E.Z. Beyond the face: An empirical study of infant affective configurations of facial, vocal, gestural, and regulatory behaviors. *Child Dev.* **1994**, *65*, 1503–1515. [CrossRef]
11. Weinberg, M.K.; Tronick, E.Z. Infant affective reactions to the resumption of maternal interaction after the still-face. *Child Dev.* **1996**, *67*, 905–914. [CrossRef]
12. Bardi, L.; Regolin, L.; Simion, F. Biological motion preference in humans at birth: Role of dynamic and configural properties. *Dev. Sci.* **2011**, *14*, 353–359. [CrossRef]
13. Simion, F.; Regolin, L.; Bulf, H. A predisposition for biological motion in the newborn baby. *Proc. Natl. Acad. Sci. USA* **2008**, *105*, 809–813. [CrossRef]
14. Reid, V.M.; Hoehl, S.; Landt, J.; Striano, T. Human infants dissociate structural and dynamic information in biological motion: Evidence from neural systems. *Soc. Cogn. Affect. Neurosci.* **2008**, *3*, 161–167. [CrossRef]
15. Torres, E.B.; Brincker, M.; Isenhower, R.W.; Yanovich, P.; Stigler, K.A.; Nurnberger, J.I.; Metaxas, D.N.; Jose, J.V. Autism: The micro-movement perspective. *Front. Integr. Neurosci.* **2013**, *7*, 32. [CrossRef]
16. Torres, E.B.; Yanovich, P.; Metaxas, D.N. Give spontaneity and self-discovery a chance in ASD: Spontaneous peripheral limb variability as a proxy to evoke centrally driven intentional acts. *Front. Integr. Neurosci.* **2013**, *7*, 46. [CrossRef] [PubMed]
17. Konczak, J.; Borutta, M.; Topka, H.; Dichgans, J. The development of goal-directed reaching in infants: Hand trajectory formation and joint torque control. *Exp. Brain Res.* **1995**, *106*, 156–168. [CrossRef] [PubMed]
18. Thelen, E. Dynamic Mechanisms of Change in Early Perceptual-Motor Development. In *Mechanisms of Cognitive Development: Behavioral and Neural Perspectives*; McClelland, J., Siegler, R.S., Eds.; Lawrence Erlbaum Associates Inc.: Mahwah, NJ, USA; London, UK, 2001; pp. 161–184.
19. Torres, E.B.; Smith, B.; Mistry, S.; Brincker, M.; Whyatt, C. Neonatal Diagnostics: Toward Dynamic Growth Charts of Neuromotor Control. *Front. Pediatr.* **2016**, *4*, 121. [CrossRef] [PubMed]

20. Delafield-Butt, J.T.; Freer, Y.; Perkins, J.; Skulina, D.; Schogler, B.; Lee, D.N. Prospective organization of neonatal arm movements: A motor foundation of embodied agency, disrupted in premature birth. *Dev. Sci.* **2018**, *21*, e12693. [CrossRef] [PubMed]
21. Knoblich, G.; Jordan, J.S. Action coordination in groups and individuals: Learning anticipatory control. *J. Exp. Psychol. Learn Mem. Cogn.* **2003**, *29*, 1006–1016. [CrossRef] [PubMed]
22. Marsh, K.L.; Richardson, M.J.; Schmidt, R.C. Social connection through joint action and interpersonal coordination. *Top. Cogn. Sci.* **2009**, *1*, 320–339. [CrossRef] [PubMed]
23. Schmidt, R.C.; Nie, L.; Franco, A.; Richardson, M.J. Bodily synchronization underlying joke telling. *Front. Hum. Neurosci.* **2014**, *8*, 633. [CrossRef]
24. Whyatt, C.; Torres, E.B. The social-dance: Decomposing Naturalistic dyadic interaction dynamics to the micro-level. In Proceedings of the Movement and Computing, London, UK, 28–30 June 2017.
25. Amos, P. Rhythm and timing in autism: Learning to dance. *Front. Integr. Neurosci.* **2013**, *7*, 27. [CrossRef]
26. Torres, E.B.; Whyatt, C. *Autism: The Movement Sensing Perspective*; CRC Press/Taylor & Francis Group: Boca Raton, NJ, USA, 2018; p. xviii, 386p.
27. American Psychiatric Association. *Diagnostic and Statistical Manual of Mental Disorders*, 5th ed.; American Psychiatric Association: Arlington, VA, USA, 2013. [CrossRef]
28. Lord, C.; Risi, S.; Lambrecht, L.; Cook, E.H., Jr.; Leventhal, B.L.; DiLavore, P.C.; Pickles, A.; Rutter, M. The autism diagnostic observation schedule-generic: A standard measure of social and communication deficits associated with the spectrum of autism. *J. Autism Dev. Disord.* **2000**, *30*, 205–223. [CrossRef]
29. Torres, E.B.; Rai, R.; Mistry, S.; Gupta, B. Hidden Aspects of the Research ADOS Are Bound to Affect Autism Science. *Neural Comput.* **2020**, *32*, 515–561. [CrossRef]
30. Sporns, O. *Networks of the Brain*; MIT Press: Cambridge, MA, USA, 2011; p. xi. 412p, 418p.
31. Sporns, O. *Discovering the Human Connectome*; MIT Press: Cambridge, MA, USA, 2012; p. xii. 232p.
32. Torres, E.B.; Denisova, K. Motor noise is rich signal in autism research and pharmacological treatments. *Sci. Rep.* **2016**, *6*, 37422. [CrossRef] [PubMed]
33. Wu, D.; Jose, J.V.; Nurnberger, J.I.; Torres, E.B. A Biomarker Characterizing Neurodevelopment with applications in Autism. *Sci. Rep.* **2018**, *8*, 614. [CrossRef] [PubMed]
34. McClelland, J.; Koslicki, D. EMDUniFrac: Exact linear time computation of the UniFrac metric and identification of differentially abundant organisms. *J. Math Biol.* **2018**, *77*, 935–949. [CrossRef]
35. Lleonart, J.; Salat, J.; Torres, G.J. Removing allometric effects of body size in morphological analysis. *J. Theor. Biol.* **2000**, *205*, 85–93. [CrossRef] [PubMed]
36. Monge, G. Memoire sur la theorie des deblais et des remblais. In *Histoire de l' Academie Royale des Science, avec les Memoired de Mathematique et de Physique*; De L'imprimerie Royale: Paris, France, 1781.
37. Kalampratsidou, V.; Torres, E.B. Peripheral Network Connectivity Analyses for the Real-Time Tracking of Coupled Bodies in Motion. *Sensors* **2018**, *18*, 3117. [CrossRef] [PubMed]
38. Ryu, J.; Torres, E.B. The Autonomic Nervous System Differentiates Between Levels of Motor Intent and Hand Dominance. *bioRxvi* **2020**. [CrossRef]
39. Ryu, J.; Vero, J.; Dobkin, R.D.; Torres, E.B. Dynamic Digital Biomarkers of Motor and Cognitive Function in Parkinson's Disease. *J. Vis. Exp.* **2019**. [CrossRef]
40. Ryu, J.; Vero, J.; Torres, E.B. Methods for Tracking Dynamically Coupled Brain-Body Activities during Natural Movement. In Proceedings of the MOCO '17: 4th International Conference on Movement Computing, London, UK, 28–30 June 2017; pp. 1–8.
41. Torres, E.B.; Vero, J.; Rai, R. Statistical Platform for Individualized Behavioral Analyses Using Biophysical Micro-Movement Spikes. *Sensors* **2018**, *18*, 1025. [CrossRef]
42. Torres, E.B.; Mistry, S.; Caballero, C.; Whyatt, C.P. Stochastic Signatures of Involuntary Head Micro-movements Can Be Used to Classify Females of ABIDE into Different Subtypes of Neurodevelopmental Disorders. *Front. Integr. Neurosci.* **2017**, *11*, 10. [CrossRef]
43. Caballero, C.; Mistry, S.; Vero, J.; Torres, E.B. Characterization of Noise Signatures of Involuntary Head Motion in the Autism Brain Imaging Data Exchange Repository. *Front. Integr. Neurosci.* **2018**, *12*, 7. [CrossRef]
44. Torres, E.B.; Isenhower, R.W.; Yanovich, P.; Rehrig, G.; Stigler, K.; Nurnberger, J.; Jose, J.V. Strategies to develop putative biomarkers to characterize the female phenotype with autism spectrum disorders. *J. Neurophysiol.* **2013**, *110*, 1646–1662. [CrossRef] [PubMed]

45. Torres, E.B.; Nguyen, J.; Mistry, S.; Whyatt, C.; Kalampratsidou, V.; Kolevzon, A. Characterization of the Statistical Signatures of Micro-Movements Underlying Natural Gait Patterns in Children with Phelan McDermid Syndrome: Towards Precision-Phenotyping of Behavior in ASD. *Front. Integr. Neurosci.* **2016**, *10*, 22. [CrossRef] [PubMed]
46. Loomes, R.; Hull, L.; Mandy, W.P.L. What Is the Male-to-Female Ratio in Autism Spectrum Disorder? A Systematic Review and Meta-Analysis. *J. Am. Acad. Child Adolesc. Psychiatry* **2017**, *56*, 466–474. [CrossRef] [PubMed]
47. Lundstrom, S.; Marland, C.; Kuja-Halkola, R.; Anckarsater, H.; Lichtenstein, P.; Gillberg, C.; Nilsson, T. Assessing autism in females: The importance of a sex-specific comparison. *Psychiatry Res.* **2019**, *282*, 112566. [CrossRef] [PubMed]

© 2020 by the authors. Licensee MDPI, Basel, Switzerland. This article is an open access article distributed under the terms and conditions of the Creative Commons Attribution (CC BY) license (http://creativecommons.org/licenses/by/4.0/).

Journal of
Personalized
Medicine

Review

Paving the Way toward Personalized Medicine: Current Advances and Challenges in Multi-OMICS Approach in Autism Spectrum Disorder for Biomarkers Discovery and Patient Stratification

Areej G. Mesleh [1], Sara A. Abdulla [2,*] and Omar El-Agnaf [1,2,*]

1 Division of Genomics and Precision Medicine (GPM), College of Health & Life Sciences (CHLS), Hamad Bin Khalifa University (HBKU), Doha 34110, Qatar; Armesleh@hbku.edu.qa
2 Neurological Disorder Center, Qatar Biomedical Research Institute (QBRI), HBKU, Doha 34110, Qatar
* Correspondence: saabdulla@hbku.edu.qa (S.A.A.); oelagnaf@hbku.edu.qa (O.E.-A.)

Abstract: Autism spectrum disorder (ASD) is a multifactorial neurodevelopmental disorder characterized by impairments in two main areas: social/communication skills and repetitive behavioral patterns. The prevalence of ASD has increased in the past two decades, however, it is not known whether the evident rise in ASD prevalence is due to changes in diagnostic criteria or an actual increase in ASD cases. Due to the complexity and heterogeneity of ASD, symptoms vary in severity and may be accompanied by comorbidities such as epilepsy, attention deficit hyperactivity disorder (ADHD), and gastrointestinal (GI) disorders. Identifying biomarkers of ASD is not only crucial to understanding the biological characteristics of the disorder, but also as a detection tool for its early screening. Hence, this review gives an insight into the main areas of ASD biomarker research that show promising findings. Finally, it covers success stories that highlight the importance of precision medicine and the current challenges in ASD biomarker discovery studies.

Keywords: autism spectrum disorder; biomarker; omics; precision medicine; proteomics; transcriptomics; epigenetics; metabolomics; patient stratification

Citation: Mesleh, A.G.; Abdulla, S.A.; El-Agnaf, O. Paving the Way toward Personalized Medicine: Current Advances and Challenges in Multi-OMICS Approach in Autism Spectrum Disorder for Biomarkers Discovery and Patient Stratification. *J. Pers. Med.* **2021**, *11*, 41. https://doi.org/10.3390/jpm11010041

Received: 9 November 2020
Accepted: 8 January 2021
Published: 13 January 2021

Publisher's Note: MDPI stays neutral with regard to jurisdictional clai-ms in published maps and institutio-nal affiliations.

Copyright: © 2021 by the authors. Licensee MDPI, Basel, Switzerland. This article is an open access article distributed under the terms and conditions of the Creative Commons Attribution (CC BY) license (https://creativecommons.org/licenses/by/4.0/).

1. Introduction

Autism spectrum disorder (ASD) is a multifactorial neurodevelopmental disorder characterized by impairments in two main areas: social communication, which includes poor eye contact, difficulty understanding facial expressions, and delayed speaking skills; and repetitive and restricted behavior patterns such as hands flapping, headbanging, and complex body movements. ASD can also include individuals with intact language but impaired social and communication skills. The prevalence of ASD has increased in the past two decades [1]. However, it is not known whether the evident escalation in ASD prevalence is due to changes in diagnostic criteria or an actual increase in ASD cases. The prevalence of ASD varies. It accounts for 1–2.5% of the total population; also, males are more likely to be affected by ASD compared to females at approximately a 4:1 ratio [1,2]. Autistic disorder, Asperger's syndrome (AS), childhood disintegrative disorder, and pervasive developmental disorder not otherwise specified (PDD-NOS) are classified under the umbrella of ASD. These sub-classifications are diagnosed using the criteria of the diagnostic and statistical manual of mental disorders (DSM-5) that was released by the American Psychiatric Association (www.dsm5.org) and the International Classification of Disease 10 (ICD-10). Other diagnostic tools such as Autism Diagnostic Observation Schedule (ADOS) and Childhood Autism Rating Scale (CARS) have further been used to diagnose ASD. In the majority of cases, ASD is diagnosed at school age [3], with a mean age of 6 years old [4], although it should be diagnosed earlier. Additionally, late positive diagnosis of ASD after an initial negative diagnosis is not uncommon, which may imply flaws in diagnostic methods [5,6]. Furthermore, due to the complexity and heterogeneity of ASD, symptoms vary in severity and may be accompanied by comorbidities such as epilepsy, attention deficit hyperactivity disorder (ADHD), and gastrointestinal (GI) disorders [7]. Moreover, given the lack of effective drugs to alleviate or reduce the core symptoms of ASD, early behavioral interventions are key for better outcomes, as it improves cognitive performance as well as behavioral and language skills [8]. Consequently, identifying biomarkers of ASD is not only crucial towards understanding the biological characteristics of the disorder, but also as a detection tool for its early screening. Additionally, it supports the currently available diagnostic methods and paves a platform for a more robust and objective methodology.

This review provides insight into the main areas of ASD biomarker research that show promising findings, especially in genomics, transcriptomics, proteomics, metabolomics, microbiome, brain imaging, and eye-tracking. Furthermore, this review discusses some success stories that show the importance of precision medicine and the current challenges in ASD biomarker discovery studies and patient stratification.

2. Genetics of ASD: Understanding the Etiology and the Heritability

Genetics studies account for the majority of research published on ASD [9]. The recurrence rate of ASD is 2–8% higher between the siblings of a diagnosed child compared to the general population. Moreover, the concordance of ASD in monozygotic twins (MZ) ranges between 60–92% and from 0–10% in dizygotic twins (DZ) [10]. These observations highlight the importance of genetic factors for diagnosing and understanding ASD pathogenesis. While identifying ASD causal genes may not change current intervention protocols, it would, however, help in understanding the etiology behind ASD and it may help in developing genetic biomarker diagnostic tools. In some cases, ASD manifestations have been linked to a variety of well-known single-gene (monogenic) conditions. Common examples are fragile X syndrome (FXS) caused by a mutation in the *FMR1* gene and tuberous sclerosis complex (TSC) caused by a mutation in *TSC1* and *TSC2* genes. The notion that ASD is not caused by a single gene can be deduced from the fact that the aforementioned conditions are caused by different genes and patients with these different conditions can develop ASD. Epidemiological studies found that 25–40% of individuals with the abovementioned conditions tend to develop autistic traits [11,12]. Interestingly, even though ASD is known to be highly heritable, the diagnostic yield of ASD in terms of genetic evaluation varies, as it reached 40% [13], and as low as 8–10% in other studies [14,15]. However, much of these findings depend on the diagnostic tiers and techniques implemented by the clinical laboratory. Moreover, only 5–15% of total ASD cases are attributed to the abovementioned monogenic conditions (i.e., FXS and TSC) [16]. Consequently, the majority of the cases are classified as idiopathic (iASD).

ASD can be caused by rare or de novo single nucleotide variants (SNV), structural variants (SV), or copy number variants (CNV) that may affect multiple genes [16,17]. Large SVs are linked to ASD along with other comorbidities such as epilepsy, hyperactivity, behavioral problems, schizophrenia, and dysmorphic features [18]. SVs are usually detected using cytogenetic and comprehensive genomic hybridization (CGH) techniques in addition to next-generation sequencing (NGS). The CGH technique enhanced the detection of SVs such as large and small/submicroscopic duplications deletions and inversions in non-syndromic autism and mental retardation conditions [14]. A genome-wide CNV study done on ASD patients and healthy controls showed that SVs tend to encompass *NLGN1, ASTN2, UBE3A, PARK2, RFWD2*, and *FBXO40* in ASD patients [19]. These genes are known to be involved in cell-adhesion and ubiquitin pathways, as these pathways are important for synaptic formation, neuronal connection, and proper neuronal cell functions as shown in Table 1.

Table 1. Genes associated with autism spectrum disorder (ASD).

Gene Name	Function	Reference
Astrotactin- 2 (*ASTN2*)	Neuronal adhesion molecule has a role in glial migration.	[19]
Contactin 4 (*CNTN4*)	Neuronal maintenance and plasticity.	[20]
F-Box Protein- 40 (*FBXO40*)	Ubiquitin-protein transferase activity.	[19]
FMRP translational regulator-1 (FMR1)	mRNA trafficking from the nucleus to the cytoplasm. Synaptic plasticity.	[21]
Potassium voltage-gated channel subfamily Q member 2 (*KCNQ2*)	Transports potassium ions inside and outside the cells.	[22]
lysine methyltransferase 2E (KMT2E)	Regulates gene transcription.	[22]
Mono-ADP-Ribosylhydrolase (MACROD2)	Remove ADP-ribose from mono-ADP-ribosylated proteins.	[22]
Methyl CpG binding protein- 2 (MeCP2)	Chromosomal protein that binds to methylated DNA, it binds to single methy-CpG pairs.	[21]
Neuronal growth regulator- 1 (*NEGR1*)	Regulates synapses formation in the hippocampus.	[22]
Neuroligin-1 (*NLGN1*)	Synaptic functions and transmission.	[19]
Neurexin- 1 (*NRXN1*)	Binds neuroligins and formation of synaptic contacts.	[23]
Parkin (PARK2)	Part of protease complex multiprotein that guides to proteasomal degradation.	[19]
Polypyrimidine tract binding protein-2 (*PTBP2*)	Control assembly of splicing- regulatory proteins and important for alternative splicing in early development.	[22]
Ring finger and WD domain 2 (*RFWD2*) Also, known as *COP1*	Mediates ubiquitination and substrate protein degradation.	[19]
SH3 and multiple ankyrin repeat domains protein-3 (*SHANK3*)	Scaffold protein of the postsynaptic density.	[24]
Tuberous sclerosis complex (*TSC1* and *TSC2*)	Tumor suppressor gene that activate GTPase activating protein tuberin.	[25]
ubiquitin protein ligase E3A (UBE3A)	E3 ubiquitin-protein ligase.	[19]

On the contrary, common SNVs were also investigated in the context of ASD. As it is suggested that the majority of ASD cases are caused by common variants. These variants and their corresponding genes have different levels of penetrance that are known to impact chronic and complex diseases such as type 2 diabetes mellitus (T2DM) and cardiovascular diseases (CVD), as reported in many genome-wide association studies (GWAS). Furthermore, these diseases are similar to ASD in the sense that they all share a complex interplay between genetic and environmental factors, as incomplete penetrance of common SNVs in different genes contributes to the burden of these diseases/disorders along with lifestyle and other environmental factors. Similarly, GWAS and other genomic studies resulted in unwinding the complexity of ASD by identifying common variants associated with ASD. For instance, one GWAS study showed that certain SNVs that encompass genes such as *NEGRI, PTBP2, CADP2, KCNQ2, KMT2E,* and *MACROD2* significantly present in ASD subjects [22]. Nevertheless, according to the SFARI (Simon Foundation Autism Research Initiative), 913 genes are implicated in autism in humans (https://www.sfari.org/resource/sfari-gene/); some of these genes (Table 1) are important for brain development, synapses formation, and gene expression.

Overall, genetic and genomic studies are essential in understanding ASD etiology and pattern of ASD heritability, as well as family counseling, although there are some cases where the counseling recommendations are already fairly clear, such as for FXS. However, they may not be suitable as biomarker screening tools because of their complexity in terms of incomplete penetrance, high variability, polygenicity, and pleiotropic effect associated with ASD-related genes. Nevertheless, the implementation of sequencing technologies such as targeted sequencing, whole-genome sequencing (WGS), and whole-exome sequencing (WES) is expected to enhance the clinical diagnostic yield. Although NGS is still difficult to implement in clinical settings, a workflow that considers clinical manifestations and incorporates a variety of molecular techniques is suggested to reduce the cost and enhance the efficiency of ASD diagnosis.

3. Non-Coding RNA's as Biomarkers for ASD

MicroRNAs (miRNAs) are a group of non-coding RNAs (ncRNA) family. Other forms of non-coding RNA include long non-coding RNAs (lncRNA), small nuclear RNA (snRNA), small nucleolar RNA (snoRNA), ribosomal RNA (rRNA), and pseudogenes. The main function of miRNA is to regulate gene expression at the posttranscriptional level. Since the discovery of ncRNA in blood and other body fluids, miRNAs in particular have gained considerable interest as potential biomarkers for diseases such as cancer [26]. A study examining the serum of ASD patients and matched controls, through the use of a miRNA PCR array specific for neurological miRNAs, identified five potential microRNAs that were capable of differentiating healthy subjects from ASD subjects; these miRNAs are miR-19b-3p, miR-130a-3p, miR-181b-5p, miR-320a, and miR-572 [27]. Additionally, others have shown that miR-140-3p was upregulated in both serum and saliva [28,29]. Interestingly, in these studies, miR-140-3p was detected in different techniques, RNA-Seq in saliva and TaqMan low-density array (TLDA) in serum which suggests that miR-140-3p might have a particular role in ASD. In line with the aforementioned studies, one study used a multiplex reverse transcriptase-polymerase chain reaction (RT-PCR) on ASD postpartum samples and found that miR-140-3p and other miRNAs' expression were dysregulated in ASD cerebral cortex [30]. Furthermore, a large-scale study done on ASD patients used salivary miRNA to differentiate between ASD and other neurodevelopmental disorders such as developmental delay (DD) from typically developed children (TD). In this study, they found that the salivary miRNAs were able to differentiate ASD subjects with moderate accuracy [31]. Salloum-Asfar, Satheesh, and Abdulla have extensively reviewed ASD miRNA studies; these studies are summarized in Table 1 in their paper [32].

miRNA biomarker studies need further validation using in vivo and in vitro studies as the majority of existing studies used in silico prediction as a way to investigate the function and the validity of miRNAs discovered. Furthermore, inconsistencies between the studies in terms of findings do not necessarily mean that miRNAs fail as biomarkers, but rather, it may suggest two main issues: variation in protocols and the need for a better approach for ASD sub-classification. Although miRNA biomarkers have been the most popular in the ncRNA family, other ncRNAs have shown considerable potential as biomarkers. For instance, a study utilizing peripheral blood identified a signature set of 20 ncRNA, which includes some pseudogenes, lncRNA, snRNA, snoRNA, and rRNA. In their study, they discovered ncRNAs markers that showed an excellent robustness assessed by ROC curve analysis when tested on different ages, genders, and ASD sub-classifications [33]. Some of these ncRNA, such as POLR2KP2, TUBB2BP1, RNU1-16P, and RNVU1-15, are moderately to highly expressed in the neurons, which may suggest a possible association of these ncRNA to ASD pathogenesis in the brain. However, these findings need to be validated on a larger scale, because this study used a total of 186 samples divided into a training set and a validation set followed by 23 ASD patients and 23 controls samples to further validate these markers. Furthermore, the abovementioned studies underline the importance of utilizing panels that contain a group of a validated set of ncRNAs that could serve a purpose in discriminating ASD from normal children.

4. Evidence of Epigenetics Modifications in ASD

Epigenetic modifications, such as changes in DNA methylation patterns, are also elements that may potentially serve as biomarkers. As mentioned above, ASD widely overlaps with some monogenic conditions such as FXS and Rett syndrome. The pathophysiology of these conditions is known to be linked to dysregulation in DNA methylation [34,35]. A recent epigenome-wide DNA methylation study (EWAS), done on 223 postpartum brain sections of the prefrontal cortex, temporal cortex, and cerebellum, taken from 43 ASD patients and 38 non-psychiatric controls, showed significant differences in CpG methylation patterns; mainly in the cortical regions compared to the cerebellum in ASD brain tissue [36]. They inferred from their findings that there is a convergence in molecular signature between different forms of ASD [36]. Indeed, brain tissue is not accessible for biomarker discovery purposes; however, replication of these finds can be very powerful in validating the authenticity of the identified biomarker, as brain tissue is the main site of ASD's pathophysiology. As a consequence, a study that was done on ASD peripheral blood showed that there is an overlap in methylation patterns between ASD and other mendelian neurodevelopmental diseases that display mutation in epigenetic machinery genes [37]. Although the overlap was minimal, it did suggest similarities in the initial events of these disorders. Moreover, their machine-learning tools were able to differentiate the unique epi-signature of each disorder, which is crucial for diagnosing diseases with overlapping clinical manifestations [37].

A study done on ASD discordant twins using lymphoblastoid cells derived from blood lymphocytes showed that 2 CpG islands were hypermethylated. These CpG islands belong to B-cell lymphoma 2 (*BCL2*) and RAR-related orphan receptor A(*RORA*) genes, their findings were confirmed using bisulfite sequencing and methylation-PCR, and these genes were found to be downregulated in the brain [38]. Moreover, a study done on ASD MZ pairs using whole-peripheral blood revealed differences in methylation levels at many CpG sites. Moreover, they found that these changes in DNA methylation surround genes that have been previously linked to ASD, such as AF4/FMR2 family member 2 (*AFF2*), *NRXN1, NLGN3,* and *UBE3A* [39]. On the other hand, a large-scale case-control EWAS used DNA from blood failed to attribute any CpG site to ASD because they did not achieve the Bonferroni discovery threshold ($p < 1.12 \times 10^{-7}$) [40].

The contradictions between these findings suggest that the sample of choice, and maybe the cell type/matrix used may affect the final results. Unlike genetic mutations, epigenetic modification such as methylation is tissue-specific, and using different cell types/matrix or even a mix of a heterogeneous population of cells may influence the findings. Another essential point is the selection of the studied subjects. For instance, as mentioned above, Nguyen et al. [38] and C. C. Wong et al. [39] studies used ASD twins, as these subjects share genetics, age, and the maternal environment in utero. However, in the Andrews et al. study [40], although they used a considerably large sample size, the heterogeneity of their ASD subjects may have hindered possible CpG methylated sites; unlike the abovementioned studies that used twins, who are more likely to share many of the genetic and environmental exposures.

5. Proteomics: A Fundamental Tool That Helps in Biomarker Discovery

Proteins are the final products that carry function. Protein abnormalities reflect upstream molecular problems that occur at the DNA and the RNA levels and these problems can be mirrored by a change in protein activity, structure, and abundance. Similarly, proteins can also be modified by external stimuli. For example, high sugar intake will increase glycated hemoglobin 1c (HbA 1c), and this biomarker is important for long-term monitoring of a diabetic's diet [41]. There are many different methods of using proteomics for biomarker discovery studies. Common, unbiased approaches include a bottom-up approach, where the proteins are digested into peptide fragments and then run into mass spectrometry (MS) [42], and a top-down approach, where the intact proteins are separated and run through MS. Both strategies allow for gel and gel-free separation of the proteins/peptides [43]. Moreover, the top-down approach is better at identifying post-translational modifications (PTM) [43]. Applying the MS-based proteomics approach for biomarker discovery has opened the door for neurodevelopmental and neuropsychiatric disorders providing an unbiased method for a better understanding of these complex conditions. Other methods of proteomic biomarker investigation are immunoassays. These methods require prior knowledge of the protein's function and their expression in a particular tissue/body fluid. Consequently, this allows for the generation of immunoassays to capture proteins and evaluate possible upregulation/downregulation as well as PTM on a set of proteins. These techniques are used mostly in the validation phase after biomarker discovery phase and they are easy to implement in a clinical setting [44].

Proteomic investigations on the gray matter of the frontal lobe of ASD individuals, identified single amino acid substitutions from alanine to glutamic acid in a protein called glyoxalase I (Glo1). This noticeable change has a higher frequency in ASD postpartum brain tissue compared to healthy controls [45]. This substitution caused a reduction in the enzymatic activity of Glo1 which, as a consequence, resulted in the accumulation of advanced glycation end products (AGE). Therefore, Glo1 substitution may affect certain crucial functions during neural development in early life [45]. Furthermore, a study exploring the Brodmann area 10 (BA10) and the cerebellum region (CB) of postpartum tissues showed differential expression of proteins related to synaptic connectivity, axon myelination, glial cells function, and metabolic activities in both regions [46]. Some of these proteins are glial fibrillary acidic protein (GFAP), creatine kinase B (CKB), myelin basic protein (MBP), and synapsin II (SYN2).

Many studies tried to identify biomarkers in accessible body fluids such as cerebrospinal fluid (CSF), serum/plasma, saliva, and urine, Figure 1. For instance, a quasi-prospective study was done on neonatal CSF samples, that were formerly collected from mildly febrile neonates (0–3 months old) that later developed ASD, to check whether biochemical differences exist before ASD is phenotypically manifested. They showed that arginine vasopressin (AVP) is significantly decreased in 11 ASD neonates compared to 22 controls [47]. This study was based on a pre-determined knowledge about the role of AVP and preliminary results published earlier [48]. The same group had found reduced CSF AVP levels in ASD's samples and lower levels were associated with severe ASD symptoms. Unlike the former study, this study focused on older 1.5–9 years old ASD subjects [49]. Both studies imply a persistent and robust link between AVP and ASD even at an early age, as early as a few days. Interestingly, no significant difference was found on oxytocin (OXT) between the groups [47]. These findings may underline a possible subtype of ASD with a dysregulation in certain peptide hormones such as AVP. However, these findings need further validation using a larger cohort.

Unfortunately, the risk associated with drawing CSF samples at an early age is also present, thus, using a less invasive body fluid is needed as a source for ASD biomarker discovery. For instance, one study tried to investigate whether there is a correlation between AVP concentration in plasma and the CSF. They showed that the blood concentration of AVP positively correlated with the corresponding CSF sample [50]. Many proteomic studies were done using the unbiased MS approach, listed in Table 2. In these studies, serum and plasma were amongst the most common matrix utilized due to their mild invasiveness. The majority of these studies found a differential expression in proteins that are linked to the immune system, lipid metabolism, and platelet function pathways [51–53]. Paradoxically, one study failed to confirm the identity of the 8 peaks that were detected in MS and were found to be differentially expressed in ASD subjects [54].

Table 2. Proteomics studies on ASD.

Sample Type	Detection Method	Proteins Identified	Function	Reference
Serum	Tricine-PAGE LC-MS/MS	ApoA1, ApoA4, PON1.	Cholesterol metabolism Oxidative damage	[55]
Serum	multiplex immunoassay LC-MS	Immune assays Females: ADIPO, APOA1, IgA Males: IL-12p70, IL-16, TF, TNF-alpha, BMP6, CTGF, ICAM1. Both: CHGA, EPO, IL-3, TENA, PAP, SHBG. LC-MS Females: APOC2, APOE, ARMC3, CLC4K, FETUB, GLCE, MRRP1, PTPA, RN149, TLE1, TRIPB, ZC3HE. Males: RGPD4.	Cholesterol metabolism and transport Inflammation Androgens	[56]
Serum	MALDI-TOF MS	SERPINA5, PF4, FABP1, APOC1, AFP, CPB2, TAAR6, FGA.	Platelets and coagulation functions Cholesterol metabolism	[53]

It is important to note that biomarker discoveries are not limited to the brain, CSF, serum, and plasma; other body fluids such as saliva and urine can also be utilized. Two studies utilized saliva samples from ASD patients and age-matched controls [51,58]. Although there were some subtle differences in their methodology, both studies were able to show significant differential expression of proteins related to the immune system pathway. Interestingly, one protein called prolactin-induced protein (PIP) was replicated in both studies mentioned above. The function of PIP is not well-understood; however, it is a promising biomarker for breast cancer [61]. Moreover, PIP is known to bind to CD4+ on T cells; therefore, it may have some immunomodulatory function [62]. In one study, the proteome of urine, first-morning void, was used to search for biomarkers in ASD subjects. They found three proteins were significantly more abundant in ASD compared to controls; these proteins are kininogen 1(KNG1), immunoglobulin heavy constant gamma 1 (IGHG1), and mannan binding lectin serine peptidase (MASP2). Their findings were validated using ELISA, and showed a significant increase in KNG1 in all ASD patients compared to controls [60].

Many studies have used multiplex immunoassays for proteomics biomarker discovery. For instance, a study done on AS, a subtype of ASD wherein individuals present without delays in language development and normal or superior IQ, yet exhibit difficulties in social and communication skills, showed a difference in the plasma proteome of the AS group in comparison to healthy controls in a sex-specific manner [63]. They found an increase in inflammatory cytokines molecules such as interleukin-3 (IL-3), tumor necrosis factor-alpha (TNF-α), and epithelial-derived neutrophil-activating protein (ENA-78) in males, while in females, they observed an increase in androgens, growth, and metabolic pathways such as luteinizing hormone (LH) and insulin [63].

Altered immune response was also evident in ASD, as some studies have shown that cytokines such as TNF-α is significantly expressed in the brain, CSF, and peripheral blood mononuclear cells (PBMCs) of individuals with ASD [64–66]. TNF-α is mainly produced by M1 macrophages and it is important for NF-kB activation, which is a transcription factor and an essential regulator of inflammatory genes [67]. The evident increase in TNF-α may suggest a dysregulation in the inflammatory response in ASD. Furthermore, a study found an increased NF-kB binding activity to DNA in the PBMCs of ASD patients [68]. Another essential cytokine is interferon-gamma (IFN-γ), which was found to be elevated in the brain and whole blood of ASD compared to controls [64,69]. Moreover, mothers of individuals who were later diagnosed with autism showed an elevated level of serum IFN-γ, as well as interleukins (IL-4 and IL-5) during mid-gestation [70]. IFN-γ is a pro-inflammatory cytokine that activates CD4+ T-helper 1 (Th1) response [71]. Another pro-inflammatory cytokine interleukin-6 (IL-6) showed a significant production in monocytes of ASD compared to controls when their PBMCs were stimulated with lipopolysaccharide (LPS) in vitro [72]; IL-6 is known to induce T-helper 17 (Th17). Interestingly, when IL-17a was induced in pregnant dam mothers, the offspring exhibited an abnormal cortical development and autistic-phenotypes; even when IL-17a was administrated directly into the fetal brain [73]. Conversely, the administration of anti-IL-17a antibodies in dam mothers during the pregnancy resulted in a reduction in the abnormal behavioral phenotype [73]. These findings highlight the importance of cytokines in discriminating ASD from controls. In addition, they point toward a possible link between immune dysfunction and ASD subtype.

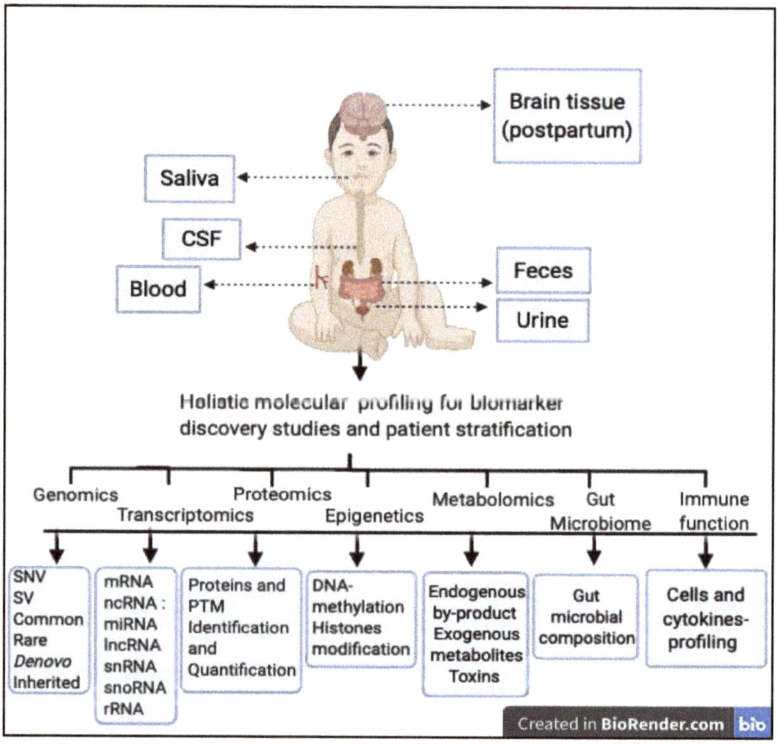

Figure 1. Schematic showing possible body fluids and tissues that may be essential for biomarker discovery in ASD patients. Blood is the most common site for biomarker discovery. However, saliva, urine, and feces are easily accessible and have been used recently for biomarker discovery studies. Although CSF and brain tissues could also be used for biomarker discovery in ASD, their accessibility is very difficult or even impossible (in the case of the brain, unless it is postpartum) for such purposes. Collecting huge biological data from a range of body fluids may help in performing holistic molecular profiling in the area of genomics, transcriptomics, proteomics, epigenetics, metabolomics, gut microbiome, and immune system, which may enhance biomarker discovery and patient stratification.

Synucleins have also been studied in the context of ASD. Synucleins are a family of proteins that are abundantly expressed in the presynaptic terminals of the neocortex, cerebellum, thalamus, and striatum [74]. The synuclein family includes α, β, and γ-synucleins (syn). Of a particular interest, the function of α-syn is not well understood. However, α-syn is thought to be involved in vesicle stabilization, synaptic plasticity, and regulates dopamine release [75,76]. α-syn is known to be involved in Parkinson's disease pathology through an intracellular aggregation process that results in Lewy body formation inside the neurons and eventually, cell death. Although α-syn may play a role in synaptic function, which is thought to be impaired in ASD, there are a limited number of studies on α-syn in the context of ASD. Two studies showed a consistent decrease in α-syn concentration in serum and plasma, respectively [77,78]. However, the latter study was done only on males. On the other hand, β-syn was shown to be higher in ASD patient's plasma compared to the age-matched controls [78]. Interestingly, autoantibodies against α-syn and other brain proteins were shown to increase in serum of ASD children and their corresponding mothers [79]. This finding may explain the reduced concentration of α-syn in serum/plasma that was evident in the aforementioned studies. Those autoantibodies may mask α-syn epitopes, which could result in α-syn being under-detected.

Furthermore, Tau, which is a major microtubule-associated protein in mature neurons and was known to be hyperphosphorylated in Alzheimer's disease patients. This hyperphosphorylation causes neurofibrillary tangles and neuronal death [80]. A study showed that Tau concentration decreases in the serum of ASD males [77]. More studies need to be done to elucidate the role of synucleins and Tau in ASD. Moreover, more research needs to be done on more pathogenic forms such as oligomeric and fibril forms of synuclein and Tau.

It is important to note that since ASD risk is traced to around 1000 genetic factors and many environmental factors, it is impractical to assume that individual proteins could be used as a universal biomarker for ASD. Thus, utilizing unbiased methods for proteomics profiling, as discussed in the metabolomic section [81,82], could be more beneficial for patient stratification and biomarker discovery.

6. Autoantibodies Biomarkers Suggest a Potential Molecular Sub-Class of ASD

There is growing evidence that supports the involvement of maternal immunity in developing ASD. The notion that maternal autoimmunity may be a cause of ASD in children has been around since the 1970s, as they observed that maternal IgG was present in children's CSF [83]. A second piece of supporting evidence was by a study cohort that included a large number of subjects (689,196 children). Out of these subjects, 3325 were diagnosed with ASD. The study showed that the risk of ASD increased if the mother had one on the following autoimmune diseases: rheumatoid arthritis, celiac disease, or a family history of diabetes mellitus (DM) type 1 [84]. Comparatively, another systematic review meta-analysis found similar findings, in addition to increased risk of ASD in mothers with hypothyroidism and psoriasis as well [85]. Additionally, when polyclonal antibodies from mothers with children that have ASD were administrated to pregnant mice, the offspring exhibited autistic-like features [86]. Furthermore, monoclonal antibodies against contactin-associated protein-like 2 (Caspr2), which is a membrane protein expressed in the CNS and essential for voltage-gated potassium channels localization in myelinated axons, were generated. Those monoclonal antibodies were successfully able to induce autistic-phenotypes in mouse offspring when exposed to anti-Caspr2 in utero [87]. These early studies laid the groundwork for other studies that aimed to elucidate the link between ASD and autoimmune impairment in the maternal system. Thus, this link could provide a potential biomarker for risk assessment, early intervention, screening, and monitoring for a sub-classification of ASD patients. To understand the role of maternal IgG antibodies in fetal development, some groups tested maternal serum against fetal brain proteins, and they found that maternal IgG antibodies exhibit reactivity against bands at the following molecular weights: 37 kDa, 73 kDa, and 39 kDa [88–90], listed in Table 3. Furthermore, the Heuer, Braunschweig, Ashwood, Van de Water, and Campbell study [91], was able to identify the proteins for 37 kDa, 73 kDa, and 39 kDa bands using 2D gel electrophoresis followed by MS. They showed that these bands correspond to lactate dehydrogenase 1 and 2 (LDH1, LDH2), stress-induced phosphoprotein 1 (STIP1), collapsing response mediator protein 1 and 2 (CRMP1, CRMP2), and Y-box binding protein 1 (YBX1); as listed in Table 3. Interestingly, one study tried to investigate the link of promoter allele C (rs1858830) of

MET gene with ASD-class that is categorized based on maternal autoantibodies positivity against fetal proteins [92]. The study observed a higher incidence of homozygote MET allele C/C in mothers with a positive fetal protein reactivity and ASD children compared to mothers with typically developed children. Additionally, the homozygote form of MET (rs1858830) C/C alleles were associated with reduced IL-10 concentration, thus it may cause prolonged inflammation [92]. Nevertheless, it is still vague whether the link between maternal autoimmunity to ASD is due to an overlap in susceptibility genes between some autoimmune diseases and ASD or simply a product of IgG infiltration into the fetus's CNS, hence, interfering with brain development. Solving this dilemma may help in the accurate subclassification of ASD, early diagnosis, and intervention.

Table 3. Autoantibodies studies on ASD.

Observed Autoantibodies Reactivities	Molecular Weight	Samples Used	Reference
Human fetal brain proteins Human adult brain proteins	73 kDa and 37 kD -	Mother's serum of: ASD vs. non-ASD (DD) * vs. TD *	[90]
Human fetal brain proteins	39 kDa, 39 kDa and 73 kDa	Mother's plasma of: AU * vs. ASD vs. DD * vs. TD *	[88]
Human fetal brain proteins Human adult brain proteins Rodent embryo brain proteins Rodent adult brain proteins	36 kDa, 39 kDa and 61 kDa caudate at 155 kDa and BA9 at 63 kDa 36 kDa and 73 kDa 27 kDa	Mother's serum of: ASD vs. controls	[93]
LDH 1, LDH2, STIP, CRMP1, CRMP2, and YBX1	37 kDa, 39 kDa, 48 kDa, 62 kDa and 68 kDa	Mother's plasma of: ASD vs. controls	[91]

* AU: full autism; DD: developmental delay; TD: typically developed child.

7. Metabolomics and Gut Microbiome's Biomarkers in ASD

Metabolic abnormalities are known to be multidimensional in the sense that they cross many pathways such as mitochondrial, oxidative, cholesterol, fatty acid, and neurotransmitters metabolism. Studies suggest a level of dysfunction in these metabolic pathways in ASD patients [94]. Moreover, metabolic pathways are influenced by internal factors such as gene mutations as seen in inborn error of metabolism diseases, and external factors, such as diet, gut microbiome, and exposure to toxins [94]. Some of these metabolites are highlighted in Table 4. The most relevant metabolites to ASD are endocannabinoids, namely anandamide, a fatty acid neurotransmitter and a cannabinoid receptor-1 ligand. The level of anandamide was associated with autism-like features in preclinical animal models including monogenic, fragile-X, and neuroligin 3 models; polygenic, BTBR15, and environmental, valproic acid-induced [95–98]. As a consequence, two studies found that children with ASD exhibited a significant decrease in plasma and serum anandamide concentration compared to healthy age-matched children [99,100]. Furthermore, another study on rodents showed an alleviation of rodent autism-like traits after rescuing the anandamide pathway by inhibiting its degradation [101]. These findings on the endocannabinoid system do not only help in searching for a biomarker for ASD but also may represent a potential therapeutic system to target. Endocannabinoids are being tested in clinical trials for reducing behavioral problems in ASD subjects (NCT02956226). On the other hand, more studies are shifting toward unbiased methods for metabolite discovery aiming at stratifying patients and looking for sets of biomarkers as therapeutic targets. For instance, a study tried to cluster ASD individuals based on their metabotype focusing on plasma amino acids (AA) profile. They were able to identify a subtype of ASD with an imbalance in AA: branched-chain amino acids (BCAAs). In addition, some amines such as glutamine and ornithine were able to discriminate ASD females in a sex-specific manner [81]. In line with those findings, a clinical trial (NCT02548442) is being tested on

ASD subjects aiming to identify biomarkers and stratify ASD based on the metabolomic profile of plasma and urine.

Other interesting metabolomes to be considered are gamma-aminobutyric acid (GABA) and glutamate. These metabolites are important neurotransmitters in the brain. A notable disturbance of the glutamatergic and GABAergic balance in individuals with ASD in comparison to controls has been identified, with a decreased glutamate to GABA ratio, making it a potential area of biomarker exploration for ASD [102]. Although the vast majority of these neurotransmitters are synthesized by the neurons in the brain [103], it is still unclear why their concentration in the peripheral blood is affected. Moreover, short-chain fatty acids (SCFA), produced by intestinal microbiota, was reported to be lower in ASD fecal samples [104]. SCFA act as histone deacetylase inhibitor (HDAC), which is important for glial cell function, and regulate tryptophan 5-hydroxylase 1, which is important for serotonin and tyrosine hydroxylase, a rate-limiting enzyme for the synthesis of dopamine, noradrenaline, and adrenaline [105].

Gut metabolomic studies further point toward a disruption of the normal gut flora and studying the metabolome of body fluids helps in identifying the composition of the gut microbiome. Gut microbiota is known to impact many neurological processes such as blood-brain barrier formation, myelination, and synthesis of neurotransmitters including GABA, dopamine, and others [106]. Those processes are mediated through the microbiota-gut-brain axis, which is a path of bidirectional communication between the CNS and the gut. The link between the gut microbiome and ASD was made because GI disturbances have been frequently detected in ASD [107,108]. One study showed that ASD patients with GI disturbances tend to be more anxious in social situations compared to those with no GI symptoms [109]. The autonomic nervous system that controls gut function is called the enteric nervous system (ENS) and this system shares many structural and functional characteristics with the CNS [110]. Furthermore, a study showed that individuals with ASD that exhibit mutations in the chromodomain helicase DNA binding protein 8 (*CHD8*) gene were reported to have constipation. Furthermore, GI abnormalities were also observed in the zebrafish model with *CHD8* mutations [111]. In addition, germ-free mice that received microbiota transfer from ASD donors showed autistic-like behaviors compared to mice that received a transfer from typically-developed donors [112]. Those mice displayed differences in their metabolome and microbiome profiles evaluated using metagenomic analysis [112]. The evidence that links ASD core symptoms to GI disturbances is strong, and it is being explored in clinical trials. For instance, one clinical trial is trying to test fecal transfer therapy from healthy participants to ASD individuals with GI disorders (NCT03408886).

Gut microbiome diversity is essential for maintaining redundancy and robustness of gut-biochemistry against environmental changes. A study showed that fecal samples taken from ASD subjects showed less gut microbiome diversity and quantity compared to healthy neurotypical controls [113]. In addition, it showed a significant reduction in a genus called *Prevotella* in ASD compared to controls [113]. *Prevotella* is known to colonize the large intestine, and it plays a major role in carbohydrate digestion, which was shown to be disrupted in ASD individuals with GI problems [114]. It has been suggested that clostridium species may exacerbate the symptoms of ASD via exposures to their toxic spores [115]. Another interesting finding is the presence of amino acid phenylaniline metabolites, 3-(3-hydroxyphenyl)-3-hydroxy propionic acid (HPHPA) which is a product of *clostridia* species, in the urine of ASD children [116]. Furthermore, a decrease in the plasma metabolite p-hydroxyphenyllactat, which acts as an antioxidant and is a by-product of *bifidobacteria* and *lactobacillus* [82], has been identified in individuals with ASD. A product called Para-cresol (p-cresol) was shown to be increased in urine [117,118] and feces [119] of ASD patients. p-cresol is produced by *Clostridium difficile* (*C. difficile*) which is a spore-producing anaerobic bacteria, and it has a negative influence on other gut microbiomes especially Gram-negative bacteria [120]. In addition, the severity of ASD symptoms correlated with p-cresol concentration in urine [117]; p-cresol is known to compete with neurotransmitters on the sulfonation process [121]. Moreover, other types of gut microbiome are also affected in ASD, as evidence points toward an elevation in *Firmicutes* to *Bacteroidetes* ratio in feces of ASD patients due to the relative reduction in *Bacteroidetes* [119,122]. Interestingly, a specific species of *Bacteroidetes* called *Bacteroidetes fragilis (B. fragilis)* was shown to improve gut integrity and reduce ASD behavioral symptoms such as anxiety and repetitive behavior when it was administrated in ASD induced mice [123]. The administration of probiotics seems to be beneficial for ASD patients, as it has been explored in clinical trials (NCT02708901), and it showed a positive impact on ASD core symptoms in a subset of ASD patients [124].

Although this field is still in its infancy, it may help in biomarker discovery, and it may add another dimension to the understanding of ASD pathogenesis. These findings suggest that gut-microbiome composition and its metabolome may be used as a clue to understanding how external factors may affect ASD pathogenesis and severity. However, more studies need to be done to delineate the exact mechanisms of how microbiome imbalance contributes to ASD core symptoms.

Table 4. Metabolomic biomarkers in ASD.

Metabolite	Sample Type	Method of Detection	Effect/Function	Reference
Anandamide (decrease)	Serum/Plasma	LC-MS/MS	Endocannabinoid signaling	[99,100]
HPHPA (increase)	Urine	GC-MS	A by-product of *clostridium* species and a probable tyrosine analog of m-tyrosine (3-hydroxyphenylalanine), that may depletes brain catecholamines.	[116]
p-hydroxyphenyllactat (decrease)	Plasma	LC-HRMS	A by-product of *bifidobacteria* and *lactobacillus,* act as an anti-oxidant	[82]
p-cresol (increase)	Urine Feces	HPLC-UV GC-MS/SPME	Competes with neurotransmitters on the sulfonation process and disturbs gut microbiome	[117–119]
GABA (increase)	Plasma	ELISA	Neurotransmitter	[102,125]
Glutamic acid (increase)	Plasma	LC-HRMS	Amino acid	[82]
SCFA (decrease)	Feces	FID-GC	Regulate tryptophan 5-hydroxylase 1 which is important for serotonin, dopamine, adrenaline and nor adrenaline production.	[104]
Lactate (increase)	Serum	ELISA and colorimetric assays	Energy metabolism	[125]
Pyruvate (increase)	Serum	ELISA and colorimetric assays	Energy metabolism	[125]
5-Aminovaleric acid (increase)	Plasma	LC-HRMS	Lysine degradation product and week inhibitor of coagulation	[82]
DHEA-sulfate (increase)	Plasma	LC-HRMS	Sex-hormone	[82]

8. Mitochondria Dysfunction in ASD

Mitochondrial dysfunction is linked to ASD. A systematic meta-analysis study showed that the prevalence of mitochondrial diseases in ASD was 4–5%, which is markedly higher than the general population (around 0.01%) [126,127]. Lactate was the first biomarker that was found to be elevated in ASD children's serum [126,127]. Other mitochondrial biomarkers that were shown to be elevated in children with ASD are AST, pyruvate, and creatine kinase [126,128]. On the other hand, carnitine was shown to decline [126]. Mitochondrial abnormalities such as increased hydrogen peroxide, reduced NADH, as well as mitochondrial DNA (mDNA) over-replication, were observed in lymphocytes isolated from ASD subjects [128]. Using an MS approach for mitochondria biomarker discovery, one study constructed a signature metabolomic pattern that is highly sensitive and specific in predicting ASD patients using plasma samples [82]. Most of these signature molecules identified have been previously reported such as creatinine, fatty acids, 3-aminoisobutyric acid, tricarboxylic acid, and BCAAs [82]. More evidence is pointing towards an association between neurodevelopmental regression (NDR) ASD with mitochondrial dysfunction [129,130]. A recent study has shown that the mitochondrial respiratory rate is elevated in ASD with NDR compared to ASD with no NDR, suggesting a potential subtype of ASD [127].

9. Brain Imaging, ERPs, and Eye-Tracking

Biomarker discovery is not confined by the boundaries of molecular investigations. Multiple studies have tried to investigate changes in brain structure and function using brain imaging tools such as magnetic resonance imaging (MRI), computerized tomography (CT) scan, and positron emission tomography (PET) scan. These scanning tools are commonly used to identify different brain features between ASD and typically developed individuals in a hope of improving early diagnosis of ASD. In general, an increase in brain volume was consistently observed in ASD patients compared to healthy controls [131,132]. In addition, the volume of the temporal, frontal lobe, as well as the CSF and lateral ventricles, were found to be increased in ASD subjects [133–135]. On the other hand, the corpus callosum, cerebellum, and cerebellar vermin volumes were reduced in ASD subjects [134,136,137]. Paradoxically, despite the fact that the amygdala is known to have a role in fear, social, and communicative activities, which are the core issues in ASD, it was shown to be enlarged only in ASD children not in adults. However, abnormal hippocampus size was noted even during adolescence [138,139].

Shen et al. performed a prospective study that was the first to investigate the extra-axial fluid accumulation in the brain [140]. In their study, they observed fifty-five infants that were divided into two groups. The first group was a high-risk group, which included infants with a family history of ASD (siblings with ASD). The second group was a low-risk group, which included infants with no family history of ASD. They recorded the infant's brains at different time points between 6–24 months old using MRI. Their results showed that infants who developed ASD later in life had a significant accumulation of extra-axial fluid mainly in the frontal lobes, and larger cerebral volume compared to typically-developed and developmental delay infants [140]. Similarly, another study that used functional connectivity-MRI (fcMRI) imaging on 6-month-old infants with a high risk of ASD showed an accurate prediction of ASD diagnosis by 24 months old, when ASD is known to manifest. They incorporated a machine-learning algorithm to capture the differences in fcMRI images between ASD and non-ASD infants [141].

Utilizing electroencephalographic recordings has been used to explore the ability of ASD individuals to recognize faces and objects by measuring high-density brain event-related potentials (ERPs) by measuring negative central (Nc) and P400 waves as parameters. A study found that ASD individuals failed to show amplitude differences in ERPs of familiar versus unfamiliar faces, while they did show amplitude differences in Nc and P400 in familiar versus unfamiliar objects. In contrast to controls that showed differences in both familiar versus unfamiliar faces and familiar versus unfamiliar objects. This finding suggests impairment in face recognition in ASD individuals [142].

Furthermore, robust findings in ASD brain imaging were noted at an early age (<6 years of age) [143], which may suggest that brain imaging could be a potential tool for early ASD risk assessment. Although MRI imaging is relatively safe, the use of dyes, sedative, or even distress during the procedure may pose a minimal risk to ASD children at that age [144]. As a consequence of that, guardians may be skeptical. Thus, these circumstances call for an urgent need for more age-friendly tools for ASD biomarkers studies or diagnosis.

A new emerging technique for ASD diagnosis is eye-tracking. It is a non-invasive, objective technique in which the subjects are presented with a picture of a human that they need to look at; the device will measure eye gazing time and location [145]. ASD children are known to avoid gazing into the eyes or the center of the face [146]. Likewise, studies done using eye-tracking showed that ASD subjects have significantly lower gazing time at the eyes and the face [146–148], and would rather gaze at irrelevant subjects. Interestingly, a preliminary study showed an even more significant difference when ASD subjects (from 4–6 years of age) were asked to look at a speaking face. Their findings suggest that ASD subjects had reduced fixation time at the speaking face compared to the typically developed children. The reduced gazing time was mainly prominent in the areas of eyes, mouth, body, person, face, and outer-person [149]; however, increased gazing time to the mouth was observed in another study [150].

10. Lessons from Other Diseases in Precision Medicine

To date, there is a lack of approved biomarkers for ASD screening and diagnosis. Despite the fact that many studies showed promising results in many areas, most of the studies are still in their infancy and lack consistency. This further includes studies that have reached the first and second phase of clinical trials, which later failed to proceed [151]. The causes of these issues are most likely due to the extreme heterogeneity of ASD and the fact that it overlaps with other comorbidities. Hence, models of ASD biomarker discovery, may need to consider its multidimensional complexity. Indeed, after the tremendous improvement in biomedical science technology and sequencing of the human genome, it became possible to use big data to enhance our understanding of ASD by incorporating OMICS into both research and clinics, as illustrated in Figure 2. The ultimate goal of biomarker discovery is implementing biomarkers within clinical settings to provide ASD risk assessment, screening, diagnosis, monitoring, and stratifications for better therapeutic strategies. Biomarkers for early diagnosis and stratification are desperately needed for ASD, especially for early diagnosis, hence, early intervention, an essential key for better outcomes.

Likewise, it is important to develop biomarkers to stratify patients for therapeutic purposes so that trials could be more effective. For instance, if a particular drug seems to show a potential link to a biomarker, biomarker-targeted trials can be initiated using that drug (i.e., GABAergic biomarkers are used to monitor drugs that target the GABAergic system, and clinical trials are trying to target the GABAergic system as a therapeutic strategy for ASD, such as NCT03678129 clinical trial). Stratification of biomarkers in therapeutics is reviewed in [152].

A well-known example of utilizing precision medicine in patient stratification is cystic fibrosis (CF). CF is an autosomal recessive disease that is caused by mutations in the cystic fibrosis transmembrane conductance regulator (CFTR) gene. This gene can carry more than 1000 mutations and more than 100 are known to be pathogenic [153]. Understanding the effect of these mutations helped in stratifying individuals into six classes based on mutations and the defects they cause. Moreover, this classification helped in devising an optimal therapy plan for the patients. Additionally, although CF is a monogenetic disease, symptoms vary in severity even if patients bear the same genetic mutation, this phenomenon can be explained by exposure to environmental factors and modifier genes that contribute to the severity of CF [153]. Even though ASD and CF differ in many ways, applying a similar concept that utilizes multi-modal molecular stratification may help in tailoring the intervention strategies in such a way that is more suitable to the patients.

Another worthy example of the importance of patient stratification is anemia. Anemia is a blood disease caused by low hemoglobin concentration, with a prevalence of 24.8% worldwide as estimated by the World Health Organization (WHO) [154]. Hemoglobin is a characteristic protein expressed in red blood cells (RBC) and is important for gas exchange. There are many subtypes of anemia that are sub-classified based on multiple parameters, such as RBC microscopic morphology, mean corpuscular volume (MCV), and hemoglobin concentration (MCHC), iron levels, protein electrophoresis, sequencing as well as vitamin B12 and folate concentrations, and other parameters [155]. Different sub-classes of anemia may share many clinical symptoms; however, they differ at multiple cellular and molecular levels, and they have different treatment strategies. Similar examples of using biomarkers for stratification and targeted therapy were seen in cancer such as non-small cell lung cancer (NSCLC), breast cancer, colorectal cancer [156,157]. Genomics testing such as testing for *CYP2C9* and *VKORC1* variants are used for warfarin dosage determination for patients with cardiovascular diseases [158]. With regard to the CNS, neurons are structurally complicated compared to blood and other tissues, and the brain tissue is inaccessible, which makes it hard to study during human development. Nevertheless, those abovementioned examples show that heterogeneity exists in many diseases, and patient stratification is the solution for understanding pathogenesis and optimizing therapies.

With respect to precision medicine in ASD, a recent study highlighted the possibility of using a multi-modal approach for patient stratification. In this study, large WES data along with spatiotemporal expression of genes during brain development was used to identify variants that are deleterious, ASD-segregated, developmentally co-regulated, and sex-specific. They found dyslipidemia as a common theme in a subset of non-syndromic ASD individuals and their findings were validated using massive electrical health records (EHR) and medical claims [159].

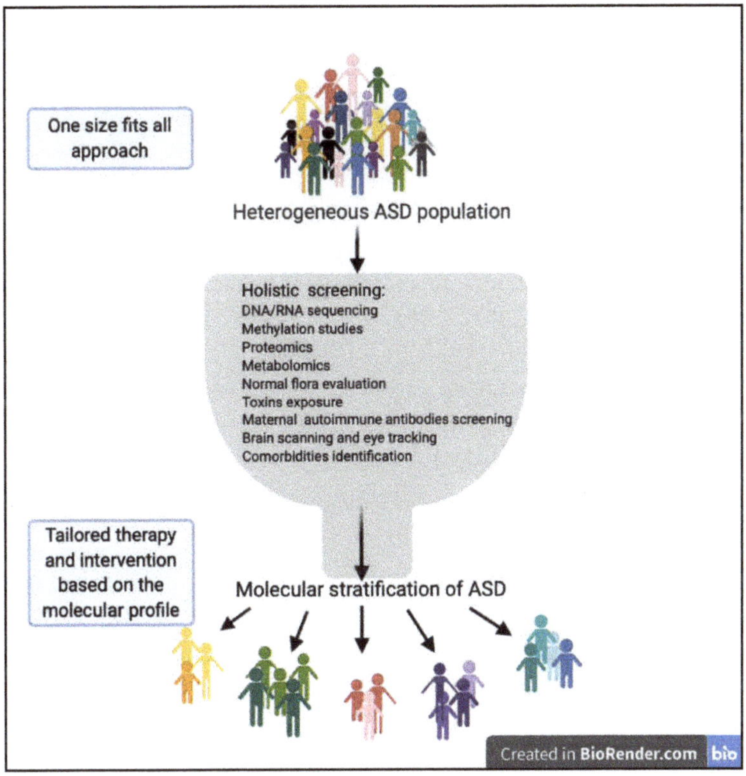

Figure 2. The extreme heterogeneity and complexity of ASD in terms of clinical manifestations, genetic background, and biological changes makes it hard for ASD to fit into a one size fits all treatment and diagnostic approach model; thus, applying a multi-modal approach utilizing modern technologies is a key for proper stratification and achieving tailored therapy that is most fitted to an individual's condition.

11. Contemporary Challenges and Future Directions

As the pathogenesis and the etiology of ASD are still not well-understood, OMICS multi-modal approaches could pave the way towards elucidating the etiology of ASD. Given the urgent need for an early diagnostic biomarker, researchers have been investigating all body fluids such as CSF, blood, saliva, urine, and stool looking for a possible set of biomarkers. Although there are many promising findings, it is still early to implement these findings for the early diagnosis of ASD. Alternatively, using these findings to thoroughly stratify ASD individuals based on their molecular profile could be a possible approach. Additionally, there are factors that need further consideration, these factors may contribute to the inconsistencies and the lack of replication between biomarker discovery studies. First, the definition of ASD and the method of diagnosis varied between studies. Additionally, comorbidities are not uncommon among ASD individuals. Subsequently, including these subjects could affect the accuracy of the findings, especially at the transcriptomic, proteomic, and metabolomic levels. The second important point is the consideration of therapies and medications that may have been undergone by ASD individuals while being involved in studies; these interventions may hinder or modify possible findings. Thirdly, the age range of the groups that participate in ASD biomarker studies is crucial, as reviewed above, mainly because the brain continues to change dramatically during childhood and adolescence. Furthermore, gender should also be considered during biomarker discovery studies. Finally, at the technical level, the method of sample processing is important because it is one of the main factors that contribute to the variability between the studies, not to mention the importance of selecting proper tissues/matrices mainly for proteomics, transcriptomics, and metabolomic studies.

Biomarker discovery has the potential to tailor therapeutic interventions to fit individualized conditions in order to receive maximum benefits. However, the question is why has it not been the case for ASD? Why have we not identified a robust set of ASD biomarkers that can be implemented in a clinical setting? Nevertheless, as biomedical technologies evolve and more discoveries on ASD pathogenesis surface, the more likely we are to utilize this knowledge for one's benefit. Furthermore, at this stage, having a tunneled vision at a specific aspect for biomarker discovery may not give the best answers, but rather, a thorough study on case-by-case bases and collecting data as much as possible at multiple levels on ASD may help unravel the answer.

Author Contributions: Original draft writing, A.G.M.; review and editing, S.A.A.; review and supervision O.E.-A. All authors have read and agreed to the published version of the manuscript.

Funding: This research received no external funding.

Institutional Review Board Statement: Not applicable.

Informed Consent Statement: Not applicable.

Data Availability Statement: Not applicable.

Acknowledgments: We would like to thank everyone who participated in building this review. We would also like to thank all the scientists who contributed in enriching the field. We hope that our work will add to the pile of knowledge and it will be a useful source for future work. The author is grateful for the scholarship provided by Qatar National Research Fund (QNRF). All the figures in this review were created by www.Biorender.com.

Conflicts of Interest: The authors declare no conflict of interest.

Abbreviations

ADHD	Attention deficit hyperactivity disorder
ADOS	Autism Diagnostic Observation Schedule
AGE	Glycation end products
ASD	Autism spectrum disorder
BA10	Brodmann area 10
CARS	Childhood Autism Rating Scale
CGH	Comprehensive genomic hybridization
CNV	Copy number variant
CSF	Cerebrospinal fluid
CVD	Cardiovascular diseases
DD	Developmental delay
ERP	Event-related potentials
GI	Gastrointestinal
T2DM	Diabetes mellitus type 2
DSM-5	Diagnostic and statistical manual of mental disorders- 5
DZ	Dizygotic
fcMRI	Functional connectivity magnetic resonance imaging
FXS	Fragile X syndrome
GC	Gas chromatography
GWAS	Genome wide association studies
iASD	Idiopathic Autism spectrum disorder
ICD-10	International Classification of Disease 10
LC	Liquid chromatography
MALDI-TOF	Matrix-Assisted Laser Desorption Ionization Time-of-Flight
miRNA	microRNA
MS	Mass spectrometry
mtDNA	mitochondrial DNA
MZ	Monozygotic
ncRNA	non-coding RNA
NGS	Next generation sequencing
NDR	Neurodevelopmental regression
PDD-NOS	Pervasive developmental disorder not otherwise specified
PTM	Post-translational modifications
rRNA	Ribosomal RNA
RT-PCR	Reverse transcriptase-polymerase chain reaction
snoRNA	Small nucleolar RNA
snRNA	Small nuclear RNA
SNV	Single nucleotide variant
SV	Structural variants
TD	Typically developed
TLDA	TaqMan low-density array
TSC	Tuberous sclerosis complex
WES	Whole-exome sequencing
WGS	Whole-genome sequencing

References

1. Sharma, S.R.; Gonda, X.; Tarazi, F.I. Autism Spectrum Disorder: Classification, diagnosis and therapy. *J. Pharmacol. Ther.* **2018**, *190*, 91–104. [CrossRef]
2. Hodges, H.; Fealko, C.; Soares, N. Autism spectrum disorder: Definition, epidemiology, causes, and clinical evaluation. *Transl. Pediatr.* **2020**, *9*, S55–S65. [CrossRef] [PubMed]
3. Mandell, D.S.; Novak, M.M.; Zubritsky, C.D. Factors Associated with Age of Diagnosis among Children with Autism Spectrum Disorders. *Pediatrics* **2005**, *116*, 1480–1486. [CrossRef] [PubMed]
4. Hrdlicka, M.; Vacova, M.; Oslejskova, H.; Gondžová, V.; Vadlejchova, I.; Kocourkova, J.; Koutek, J.; Dudova, I. Age at diagnosis of autism spectrum disorders: Is there an association with socioeconomic status and family self-education about autism? *Neuropsychiatr. Dis. Treat.* **2016**, *12*, 1639–1644. [CrossRef] [PubMed]

5. Davidovitch, M.; Levit-Binnun, N.; Golan, D.; Manning-Courtney, P. Late Diagnosis of Autism Spectrum Disorder after Initial Negative Assessment by a Multidisciplinary Team. *J. Dev. Behav. Pediatr.* **2015**, *36*, 227–234. [CrossRef] [PubMed]
6. Fusar-Poli, L.; Brondino, N.; Rocchetti, M.; Panisi, C.; Provenzani, U.; Damiani, S.; Politi, P. Diagnosing ASD in Adults without ID: Accuracy of the ADOS-2 and the ADI-R. *J. Autism Dev. Disord.* **2017**, *47*, 3370–3379. [CrossRef]
7. Brondino, N.; Fusar-Poli, L.; Miceli, E.; Di Stefano, M.; Damiani, S.; Rocchetti, M.; Politi, P. Prevalence of Medical Comorbidities in Adults with Autism Spectrum Disorder. *J. Gen. Intern. Med.* **2019**, *34*, 1992–1994. [CrossRef]
8. Warren, Z.; McPheeters, M.L.; Sathe, N.; Foss-Feig, J.H.; Glasser, A.; Veenstra-VanderWeele, J. A systematic review of early intensive intervention for autism spectrum disorders. *Pediatrics* **2011**, *127*, e1303–e1311. [CrossRef]
9. Rossignol, D.A.; Frye, R.E. A review of research trends in physiological abnormalities in autism spectrum disorders: Immune dysregulation, inflammation, oxidative stress, mitochondrial dysfunction and environmental toxicant exposures. *Mol. Psychiatry* **2012**, *17*, 389–401. [CrossRef]
10. Muhle, R.; Trentacoste, S.V.; Rapin, I. The Genetics of Autism. *Pediatrics* **2004**, *113*, e472–e486. [CrossRef]
11. Smalley, S.L. Autism and tuberous sclerosis. *J. Autism Dev. Disord.* **1998**, *28*, 407–414. [CrossRef] [PubMed]
12. Bailey, D.B., Jr.; Raspa, M.; Olmsted, M.; Holiday, D.B. Co-occurring conditions associated with FMR1 gene variations: Findings from a national parent survey. *Am. J. Med. Genet. A* **2008**, *146a*, 2060–2069. [CrossRef] [PubMed]
13. Schaefer, G.B.; Lutz, R.E. Diagnostic yield in the clinical genetic evaluation of autism spectrum disorders. *Genet. Med.* **2006**, *8*, 549–556. [CrossRef] [PubMed]
14. Herman, G.E.; Henninger, N.; Ratliff-Schaub, K.; Pastore, M.; Fitzgerald, S.; McBride, K.L. Genetic testing in autism: How much is enough? *Genet. Med.* **2007**, *9*, 268–274. [CrossRef] [PubMed]
15. Abdul-Rahman, O.A.; Hudgins, L. The diagnostic utility of a genetics evaluation in children with pervasive developmental disorders. *Genet. Med.* **2006**, *8*, 50–54. [CrossRef] [PubMed]
16. Devlin, B.; Scherer, S.W. Genetic architecture in autism spectrum disorder. *Curr. Opin. Genet. Dev.* **2012**, *22*, 229–237. [CrossRef] [PubMed]
17. Acuna-Hidalgo, R.; Veltman, J.A.; Hoischen, A. New insights into the generation and role of de novo mutations in health and disease. *Genome Biol.* **2016**, *17*, 241. [CrossRef]
18. Persico, A.M.; Napolioni, V. Autism genetics. *Behav. Brain Res.* **2013**, *251*, 95–112. [CrossRef]
19. Glessner, J.T.; Wang, K.; Cai, G.; Korvatska, O.; Kim, C.E.; Wood, S.; Zhang, H.; Estes, A.; Brune, C.W.; Bradfield, J.P.; et al. Autism genome-wide copy number variation reveals ubiquitin and neuronal genes. *Nature* **2009**, *459*, 569–573. [CrossRef]
20. Roohi, J.; Montagna, C.; Tegay, D.H.; Palmer, L.E.; DeVincent, C.; Pomeroy, J.C.; Christian, S.L.; Nowak, N.; Hatchwell, E. Disruption of contactin 4 in three subjects with autism spectrum disorder. *J. Med. Genet.* **2008**, *46*, 176–182. [CrossRef]
21. Farzin, F.; Perry, H.; Hessl, D.; Loesch, D.; Cohen, J.; Bacalman, S.; Gane, L.; Tassone, F.; Hagerman, P.; Hagerman, R. Autism Spectrum Disorders and Attention-Deficit/Hyperactivity Disorder in Boys with the Fragile X Premutation. *J. Dev. Behav. Pediatr.* **2006**, *27* (Suppl. 2), S137–S144. [CrossRef] [PubMed]
22. Grove, J.; Ripke, S.; Als, T.D.; Mattheisen, M.; Walters, R.K.; Won, H.; Pallesen, J.; Agerbo, E.; Andreassen, O.A.; Anney, R.; et al. Identification of common genetic risk variants for autism spectrum disorder. *Nat. Genet.* **2019**, *51*, 431–444. [CrossRef] [PubMed]
23. Onay, H.; Kacamak, D.; Kavasoglu, A.N.; Akgün, B.; Yalcinli, M.; Kose, S.; Ozbaran, B. Mutation analysis of the NRXN1 gene in autism spectrum disorders. *Balk. J. Med. Genet.* **2016**, *19*, 17–22. [CrossRef] [PubMed]
24. Durand, C.M.; Betancur, C.; Boeckers, T.M.; Bockmann, J.; Chaste, P.; Fauchereau, F.; Nygren, G.; Rastam, M.; Gillberg, I.C.; Anckarsäter, H.; et al. Mutations in the gene encoding the synaptic scaffolding protein SHANK3 are associated with autism spectrum disorders. *Nat. Genet.* **2006**, *39*, 25–27. [CrossRef] [PubMed]
25. Vignoli, A.; La Briola, F.; Peron, A.; Turner, K.; Vannicola, C.; Saccani, M.; Magnaghi, E.; Scornavacca, G.F.; Canevini, M.P. Autism spectrum disorder in tuberous sclerosis complex: Searching for risk markers. *Orphanet J. Rare Dis.* **2015**, *10*, 154. [CrossRef] [PubMed]
26. Beermann, J.; Piccoli, M.-T.; Viereck, J.; Thum, T. Non-coding RNAs in Development and Disease: Background, Mechanisms, and Therapeutic Approaches. *Physiol. Rev.* **2016**, *96*, 1297–1325. [CrossRef]
27. Vasu, M.M.; Anitha, A.; Thanseem, I.; Suzuki, K.; Yamada, K.; Takahashi, T.; Wakuda, T.; Iwata, K.; Tsujii, M.; Sugiyama, T.; et al. Serum microRNA profiles in children with autism. *Mol. Autism* **2014**, *5*, 40. [CrossRef]
28. Cirnigliaro, M.; Barbagallo, C.; Gulisano, M.; Domini, C.N.; Barone, R.; Barbagallo, D.; Ragusa, M.; Di Pietro, C.; Rizzo, R.; Purrello, M. Expression and Regulatory Network Analysis of miR-140-3p, a New Potential Serum Biomarker for Autism Spectrum Disorder. *Front. Mol. Neurosci.* **2017**, *10*, 250. [CrossRef]
29. Hicks, S.D.; Ignacio, C.; Gentile, K.; Middleton, F.A. Salivary miRNA profiles identify children with autism spectrum disorder, correlate with adaptive behavior, and implicate ASD candidate genes involved in neurodevelopment. *BMC Pediatr.* **2016**, *16*, 52. [CrossRef]
30. Abu-Elneel, K.; Liu, T.; Gazzaniga, F.S.; Nishimura, Y.; Wall, D.P.; Geschwind, D.H.; Lao, K.; Kosik, K.S. Heterogeneous dysregulation of microRNAs across the autism spectrum. *Neurogenetics* **2008**, *9*, 153–161. [CrossRef]
31. Hicks, S.D.; Carpenter, R.L.; Wagner, K.E.; Pauley, R.; Barros, M.; Tierney-Aves, C.; Barns, S.; Greene, C.D.; Middleton, F.A. Saliva MicroRNA Differentiates Children with Autism From Peers with Typical and Atypical Development. *J. Am. Acad. Child. Adolesc. Psychiatry* **2020**, *59*, 296–308. [CrossRef] [PubMed]

32. Salloum-Asfar, S.; Satheesh, N.J.; Abdulla, S.A. Circulating miRNAs, Small but Promising Biomarkers for Autism Spectrum Disorder. *Front. Mol. Neurosci.* **2019**, *12*, 253. [CrossRef] [PubMed]
33. Cheng, W.; Zhou, S.; Zhou, J.; Wang, X. Identification of a robust non-coding RNA signature in diagnosing autism spectrum disorder by cross-validation of microarray data from peripheral blood samples. *Medicine* **2020**, *99*, e19484. [CrossRef]
34. Persico, A.M.; Bourgeron, T. Searching for ways out of the autism maze: Genetic, epigenetic and environmental clues. *Trends Neurosci.* **2006**, *29*, 349–358. [CrossRef] [PubMed]
35. Loke, Y.J.; Hannan, A.J.; Craig, J. The Role of Epigenetic Change in Autism Spectrum Disorders. *Front. Neurol.* **2015**, *6*, 107. [CrossRef] [PubMed]
36. Wong, C.C.Y.; Smith, R.G.; Hannon, E.J.; Ramaswami, G.; Parikshak, N.N.; Assary, E.; Troakes, C.; Poschmann, J.; Schalkwyk, L.C.; Sun, W.; et al. Genome-wide DNA methylation profiling identifies convergent molecular signatures associated with idiopathic and syndromic autism in post-mortem human brain tissue. *Hum. Mol. Genet.* **2019**, *28*, 2201–2211. [CrossRef]
37. Aref-Eshghi, E.; Rodenhiser, D.I.; Schenkel, L.C.; Lin, H.; Skinner, C.; Ainsworth, P.; Paré, G.; Hood, R.L.; Bulman, D.E.; Kernohan, K.D.; et al. Genomic DNA Methylation Signatures Enable Concurrent Diagnosis and Clinical Genetic Variant Classification in Neurodevelopmental Syndromes. *Am. J. Hum. Genet.* **2018**, *102*, 156–174. [CrossRef]
38. Nguyen, A.; Rauch, T.A.; Pfeifer, G.P.; Hu, V.W. Global methylation profiling of lymphoblastoid cell lines reveals epigenetic contributions to autism spectrum disorders and a novel autism candidate gene, RORA, whose protein product is reduced in autistic brain. *FASEB J.* **2010**, *24*, 3036–3051. [CrossRef]
39. Wong, C.C.Y.; Meaburn, E.L.; Ronald, A.R.; Price, T.S.; Jeffries, A.R.; Schalkwyk, L.C.; Plomin, R.; Mill, J. Methylomic analysis of monozygotic twins discordant for autism spectrum disorder and related behavioural traits. *Mol. Psychiatry* **2014**, *19*, 495–503. [CrossRef]
40. Andrews, S.V.; Sheppard, B.; Windham, G.; Schieve, L.A.; Schendel, D.; Croen, L.A.; Chopra, P.; Alisch, R.S.; Newschaffer, C.J.; Warren, S.T.; et al. Case-control meta-analysis of blood DNA methylation and autism spectrum disorder. *Mol. Autism* **2018**, *9*, 40. [CrossRef]
41. Lyons, T.J.; Basu, A. Biomarkers in diabetes: Hemoglobin A1c, vascular and tissue markers. *Transl. Res.* **2012**, *159*, 303–312. [CrossRef] [PubMed]
42. Amunugama, R.; Jones, R.; Ford, M.; Allen, D. Bottom-Up Mass Spectrometry–Based Proteomics as an Investigative Analytical Tool for Discovery and Quantification of Proteins in Biological Samples. *Adv. Wound Care* **2013**, *2*, 549–557. [CrossRef] [PubMed]
43. Catherman, A.D.; Skinner, O.S.; Kelleher, N.L. Top Down proteomics: Facts and perspectives. *Biochem. Biophys. Res. Commun.* **2014**, *445*, 683–693. [CrossRef] [PubMed]
44. Del Campo, M.; Jongbloed, W.; Twaalfhoven, H.A.M.; Veerhuis, R.; Blankenstein, M.; Teunissen, C.E. Facilitating the Validation of Novel Protein Biomarkers for Dementia: An Optimal Workflow for the Development of Sandwich Immunoassays. *Front. Neurol.* **2015**, *6*, 202. [CrossRef]
45. Junaid, M.A.; Kowal, D.; Barua, M.; Pullarkat, P.S.; Brooks, S.S.; Pullarkat, R.K. Proteomic studies identified a single nucleotide polymorphism in glyoxalase I as autism susceptibility factor. *Am. J. Med. Genet.* **2004**, *131*, 11–17. [CrossRef]
46. Broek, J.A.; Guest, P.C.; Rahmoune, H.; Bahn, S. Proteomic analysis of post mortem brain tissue from autism patients: Evidence for opposite changes in prefrontal cortex and cerebellum in synaptic connectivity-related proteins. *Mol. Autism* **2014**, *5*, 41. [CrossRef]
47. Oztan, O.; Garner, J.P.; Constantino, J.N.; Parker, K.J. Neonatal CSF vasopressin concentration predicts later medical record diagnoses of autism spectrum disorder. *Proc. Natl. Acad. Sci. USA* **2020**, *117*, 10609–10613. [CrossRef]
48. Caldwell, H.K. Oxytocin and Vasopressin: Powerful Regulators of Social Behavior. *Neuroscientist* **2017**, *23*, 517–528. [CrossRef]
49. Oztan, O.; Garner, J.P.; Partap, S.; Sherr, E.H.; Hardan, A.Y.; Farmer, C.; Thurm, A.; Swedo, S.E.; Parker, K.J. Cerebrospinal fluid vasopressin and symptom severity in children with autism. *Ann. Neurol.* **2018**, *84*, 611–615. [CrossRef]
50. Carson, D.S.; Howerton, C.L.; Garner, J.P.; Hyde, S.A.; Clark, C.L.; Hardan, A.Y.; Penn, A.A.; Parker, K.J. Plasma vasopressin concentrations positively predict cerebrospinal fluid vasopressin concentrations in human neonates. *Peptides* **2014**, *61*, 12–16. [CrossRef]
51. Wetie, A.G.N.; Wormwood, K.L.; Russell, S.; Ryan, J.P.; Darie, C.C.; Woods, A.G. A Pilot Proteomic Analysis of Salivary Biomarkers in Autism Spectrum Disorder. *Autism Res.* **2015**, *8*, 338–350. [CrossRef] [PubMed]
52. Feng, C.; Chen, Y.; Pan, J.; Yang, A.; Niu, L.; Min, J.; Meng, X.; Liao, L.; Zhang, K.; Shen, L. Redox proteomic identification of carbonylated proteins in autism plasma: Insight into oxidative stress and its related biomarkers in autism. *Clin. Proteom.* **2017**, *14*, 2. [CrossRef] [PubMed]
53. Yang, J.; Chen, Y.; Xiong, X.; Zhou, X.; Han, L.; Ni, L.; Wang, W.; Wang, X.; Zhao, L.; Shao, D.; et al. Peptidome Analysis Reveals Novel Serum Biomarkers for Children with Autism Spectrum Disorder in China. *Proteom. Clin. Appl.* **2018**, *12*, e1700164. [CrossRef] [PubMed]
54. Chen, Y.; Du, H.-Y.; Shi, Z.-Y.; He, L.; He, Y.-Y.; Wang, D. Serum proteomic profiling for autism using magnetic bead-assisted matrix-assisted laser desorption ionization time-of-flight mass spectrometry: A pilot study. *World J. Pediatr.* **2018**, *14*, 233–237. [CrossRef] [PubMed]
55. Wetie, A.G.N.; Wormwood, K.; Thome, J.; Dudley, E.; Taurines, R.; Gerlach, M.; Woods, A.G.; Darie, C.C. A pilot proteomic study of protein markers in autism spectrum disorder. *Electrophoresis* **2014**, *35*, 2046–2054. [CrossRef] [PubMed]

56. Steeb, H.; Ramsey, J.M.; Guest, P.C.; Stocki, P.; Cooper, J.D.; Rahmoune, H.; Ingudomnukul, E.; Auyeung, B.; Ruta, L.; Baron-Cohen, S.; et al. Serum proteomic analysis identifies sex-specific differences in lipid metabolism and inflammation profiles in adults diagnosed with Asperger syndrome. *Mol. Autism* **2014**, *5*, 4. [CrossRef] [PubMed]
57. Corbett, B.A.; Kantor, A.B.; Schulman, H.; Walker, W.L.; Lit, L.; Ashwood, P.; Rocke, D.M.; Sharp, F.R. A proteomic study of serum from children with autism showing differential expression of apolipoproteins and complement proteins. *Mol. Psychiatry* **2006**, *12*, 292–306. [CrossRef]
58. Wetie, A.G.N.; Wormwood, K.L.; Charette, L.; Ryan, J.P.; Woods, A.G.; Darie, C.C. Comparative two-dimensional polyacrylamide gel electrophoresis of the salivary proteome of children with autism spectrum disorder. *J. Cell. Mol. Med.* **2015**, *19*, 2664–2678. [CrossRef]
59. Castagnola, M.; Messana, I.; Inzitari, R.; Fanali, C.; Cabras, T.; Morelli, A.; Pecoraro, A.M.; Neri, G.; Torrioli, M.G.; Gurrieri, F. Hypo-Phosphorylation of Salivary Peptidome as a Clue to the Molecular Pathogenesis of Autism Spectrum Disorders. *J. Proteome Res.* **2008**, *7*, 5327–5332. [CrossRef]
60. Suganya, V.; Geetha, A.; Sujatha, S. Urine proteome analysis to evaluate protein biomarkers in children with autism. *Clin. Chim. Acta* **2015**, *450*, 210–219. [CrossRef]
61. Gangadharan, A.; Nyirenda, T.; Patel, K.; Jaimes-Delgadillo, N.; Coletta, D.; Tanaka, T.; Walland, A.C.; Jameel, Z.; Vedantam, S.; Tang, S.; et al. Prolactin Induced Protein (PIP) is a potential biomarker for early stage and malignant breast cancer. *Breast* **2018**, *39*, 101–109. [CrossRef] [PubMed]
62. Urbaniak, A.; Jablonska, K.; Podhorska-Okolow, M.; Ugorski, M.; Dziegiel, P. Prolactin-induced protein (PIP)-characterization and role in breast cancer progression. *Am. J. Cancer Res.* **2018**, *8*, 2150–2164. [PubMed]
63. Schwarz, E.; Guest, P.C.; Rahmoune, H.; Wang, L.; Levin, Y.; Ingudomnukul, E.; Ruta, L.; Kent, L.; Spain, M.; Baron-Cohen, S.; et al. Sex-specific serum biomarker patterns in adults with Asperger's syndrome. *Mol. Psychiatry* **2011**, *16*, 1213–1220. [CrossRef] [PubMed]
64. Li, X.; Chauhan, A.; Sheikh, A.M.; Patil, S.; Chauhan, V.; Li, X.M.; Ji, L.; Brown, T.; Malik, M. Elevated immune response in the brain of autistic patients. *J. Neuroimmunol.* **2009**, *207*, 111–116. [CrossRef] [PubMed]
65. Chez, M.; Dowling, T.; Patel, P.B.; Khanna, P.; Kominsky, M. Elevation of Tumor Necrosis Factor-Alpha in Cerebrospinal Fluid of Autistic Children. *Pediatric Neurol.* **2007**, *36*, 361–365. [CrossRef] [PubMed]
66. Ashwood, P.; Krakowiak, P.; Hertz-Picciotto, I.; Hansen, R.; Pessah, I.N.; Van De Water, J. Altered T cell responses in children with autism. *Brain Behav. Immun.* **2011**, *25*, 840–849. [CrossRef]
67. Chu, W.M. Tumor necrosis factor. *Cancer Lett.* **2013**, *328*, 222–225. [CrossRef]
68. Naik, U.S.; Gangadharan, C.; Abbagani, K.; Nagalla, B.; Dasari, N.; Manna, S.K. A Study of Nuclear Transcription Factor-Kappa B in Childhood Autism. *PLoS ONE* **2011**, *6*, e19488. [CrossRef]
69. Croonenberghs, J.; Bosmans, E.; Deboutte, D.; Kenis, G.; Maes, M. Activation of the Inflammatory Response System in Autism. *Neuropsychobiology* **2002**, *45*, 1–6. [CrossRef]
70. Goines, P.E.; Croen, L.A.; Braunschweig, D.; Yoshida, C.K.; Grether, J.; Hansen, R.; Kharrazi, M.; Ashwood, P.; Van De Water, J.A. Increased midgestational IFN-γ, IL-4 and IL-5 in women bearing a child with autism: A case-control study. *Mol. Autism* **2011**, *2*, 13. [CrossRef]
71. Tau, G.; Rothman, P. Biologic functions of the IFN-gamma receptors. *Allergy* **1999**, *54*, 1233–1251. [CrossRef] [PubMed]
72. Jyonouchi, H.; Sun, S.; Le, H. Proinflammatory and regulatory cytokine production associated with innate and adaptive immune responses in children with autism spectrum disorders and developmental regression. *J. Neuroimmunol.* **2001**, *120*, 170–179. [CrossRef]
73. Choi, G.B.; Yim, Y.S.; Wong, H.; Kim, S.; Kim, H.; Hoeffer, C.A.; Littman, D.R.; Huh, J.R. The maternal interleukin-17a pathway in mice promotes autism-like phenotypes in offspring. *Science* **2016**, *351*, 933–939. [CrossRef] [PubMed]
74. Burré, J. The Synaptic Function of α-Synuclein. *J. Parkinsons Dis.* **2015**, *5*, 699–713. [CrossRef] [PubMed]
75. Bellani, S.; Sousa, V.L.; Ronzitti, G.; Valtorta, F.; Meldolesi, J.; Chieregatti, E. The regulation of synaptic function by α-synuclein. *Commun. Integr. Biol.* **2010**, *3*, 106–109. [CrossRef]
76. Cheng, F.; Vivacqua, G.; Yu, S. The role of α-synuclein in neurotransmission and synaptic plasticity. *J. Chem. Neuroanat.* **2011**, *42*, 242–248. [CrossRef]
77. Cetin, I.; Tarakçıoğlu, M.C.; Özer, Ö.F.; Kaçar, S.; Çimen, B.; Kadak, M.T. Low Serum Level α-Synuclein and Tau Protein in Autism Spectrum Disorder Compared to Controls. *Neuropediatrics* **2015**, *46*, 410–415. [CrossRef]
78. Sriwimol, W.; Limprasert, P. Significant Changes in Plasma Alpha-Synuclein and Beta-Synuclein Levels in Male Children with Autism Spectrum Disorder. *BioMed Res. Int.* **2018**, *2018*, 4503871. [CrossRef]
79. Abou-Donia, M.B.; Suliman, H.B.; Siniscalco, D.; Antonucci, N.; Elkafrawy, P. De novo Blood Biomarkers in Autism: Autoantibodies against Neuronal and Glial Proteins. *Behav. Sci.* **2019**, *9*, 47. [CrossRef]
80. Iqbal, K.; Liu, F.; Gong, C.-X.; Grundke-Iqbal, I. Tau in Alzheimer Disease and Related Tauopathies. *Curr. Alzheimer Res.* **2010**, *7*, 656–664. [CrossRef]
81. Smith, A.M.; King, J.J.; West, P.R.; Ludwig, M.A.; Donley, E.L.; Burrier, R.E.; Amaral, D.G. Amino Acid Dysregulation Metabotypes: Potential Biomarkers for Diagnosis and Individualized Treatment for Subtypes of Autism Spectrum Disorder. *Biol. Psychiatry* **2019**, *85*, 345–354. [CrossRef] [PubMed]

82. West, P.R.; Amaral, D.G.; Bais, P.; Smith, A.M.; Egnash, L.A.; Ross, M.E.; Palmer, J.A.; Fontaine, B.R.; Conard, K.R.; Corbett, B.A.; et al. Metabolomics as a Tool for Discovery of Biomarkers of Autism Spectrum Disorder in the Blood Plasma of Children. *PLoS ONE* **2014**, *9*, e112445. [CrossRef] [PubMed]
83. Adinolfi, M.; Beck, S.E.; Haddad, S.A.; Seller, M.J. Permeability of the blood-cerebrospinal fluid barrier to plasma proteins during foetal and perinatal life. *Nature* **1976**, *259*, 140–141. [CrossRef] [PubMed]
84. Atladóttir, H.Ó.; Pedersen, M.G.; Thorsen, P.; Mortensen, P.B.; Deleuran, B.; Eaton, W.W.; Parner, E.T.; Sutton, R.M.; Niles, D.; Nysaether, J.; et al. Association of Family History of Autoimmune Diseases and Autism Spectrum Disorders. *Pediatrics* **2009**, *124*, 687–694. [CrossRef] [PubMed]
85. Wu, S.; Ding, Y.; Wu, F.; Li, R.; Xie, G.; Hou, J.; Mao, P. Family history of autoimmune diseases is associated with an increased risk of autism in children: A systematic review and meta-analysis. *Neurosci. Biobehav. Rev.* **2015**, *55*, 322–332. [CrossRef]
86. Singer, H.S.; Morris, C.; Gause, C.; Pollard, M.; Zimmerman, A.W.; Pletnikov, M. Prenatal exposure to antibodies from mothers of children with autism produces neurobehavioral alterations: A pregnant dam mouse model. *J. Neuroimmunol.* **2009**, *211*, 39–48. [CrossRef]
87. Brimberg, L.; Mader, S.; Jeganathan, V.; Berlin, R.; Coleman, T.R.; Gregersen, P.K.; Huerta, P.T.; Volpe, B.T.; Diamond, B. Caspr2-reactive antibody cloned from a mother of an ASD child mediates an ASD-like phenotype in mice. *Mol. Psychiatry* **2016**, *21*, 1663–1671. [CrossRef]
88. Braunschweig, D.; Duncanson, P.; Boyce, R.; Hansen, R.; Ashwood, P.; Pessah, I.N.; Hertz-Picciotto, I.; Van De Water, J.A. Behavioral Correlates of Maternal Antibody Status Among Children with Autism. *J. Autism Dev. Disord.* **2011**, *42*, 1435–1445. [CrossRef]
89. Croen, L.A.; Braunschweig, D.; Haapanen, L.; Yoshida, C.K.; Fireman, B.; Grether, J.K.; Kharrazi, M.; Hansen, R.L.; Ashwood, P.; Van De Water, J. Maternal Mid-Pregnancy Autoantibodies to Fetal Brain Protein: The Early Markers for Autism Study. *Biol. Psychiatry* **2008**, *64*, 583–588. [CrossRef]
90. Braunschweig, D.; Ashwood, P.; Krakowiak, P.; Hertz-Picciotto, I.; Hansen, R.; Croen, L.A.; Pessah, I.N.; Van De Water, J.A. Autism: Maternally derived antibodies specific for fetal brain proteins. *NeuroToxicology* **2007**, *29*, 226–231. [CrossRef]
91. Braunschweig, D.; Krakowiak, P.; Duncanson, P.; Boyce, R.; Hansen, R.L.; Ashwood, P.; Hertz-Picciotto, I.; Pessah, I.N.; Van De Water, J.A. Autism-specific maternal autoantibodies recognize critical proteins in developing brain. *Transl. Psychiatry* **2013**, *3*, e277. [CrossRef] [PubMed]
92. Heuer, L.; Braunschweig, D.; Ashwood, P.; Van De Water, J.A.; Campbell, D.B. Association of a MET genetic variant with autism-associated maternal autoantibodies to fetal brain proteins and cytokine expression. *Transl. Psychiatry* **2011**, *1*, e48. [CrossRef] [PubMed]
93. Singer, H.S.; Morris, C.M.; Gause, C.D.; Gillin, P.K.; Crawford, S.; Zimmerman, A.W. Antibodies against fetal brain in sera of mothers with autistic children. *J. Neuroimmunol.* **2008**, *194*, 165–172. [CrossRef]
94. Shen, L.; Liu, X.; Zhang, H.; Lin, J.; Feng, C.; Iqbal, J. Biomarkers in autism spectrum disorders: Current progress. *Clin. Chim. Acta* **2020**, *502*, 41–54. [CrossRef] [PubMed]
95. Jung, K.-M.; Sepers, M.; Henstridge, C.M.; Lassalle, O.; Neuhofer, D.; Martin, H.; Ginger, M.; Frick, A.; DiPatrizio, N.V.; Mackie, K.; et al. Uncoupling of the endocannabinoid signalling complex in a mouse model of fragile X syndrome. *Nat. Commun.* **2012**, *3*, 1080. [CrossRef]
96. Földy, C.; Malenka, R.C.; Südhof, T.C. Autism-Associated Neuroligin-3 Mutations Commonly Disrupt Tonic Endocannabinoid Signaling. *Neuron* **2013**, *78*, 498–509. [CrossRef]
97. Wei, D.; Dinh, D.; Lee, D.; Allison, A.; Anguren, A.; Moreno-Sanz, G.; Gall, C.M.; Piomelli, D. Enhancement of Anandamide-Mediated Endocannabinoid Signaling Corrects Autism-Related Social Impairment. *Cannabis Cannabinoid Res.* **2016**, *1*, 81–89. [CrossRef]
98. Kerr, D.; Downey, L.; Conboy, M.; Finn, D.; Roche, M. Alterations in the endocannabinoid system in the rat valproic acid model of autism. *Behav. Brain Res.* **2013**, *249*, 124–132. [CrossRef]
99. Karhson, D.S.; Krasinska, K.M.; Ahloy-Dallaire, J.; Libove, R.A.; Phillips, J.M.; Chien, A.S.; Garner, J.P.; Hardan, A.Y.; Parker, K.J. Plasma anandamide concentrations are lower in children with autism spectrum disorder. *Mol. Autism* **2018**, *9*, 18. [CrossRef]
100. Aran, A.; Eylon, M.; Harel, M.; Polianski, L.; Nemirovski, A.; Tepper, S.; Schnapp, A.; Ecassuto, H.; Wattad, N.; Tam, J. Lower circulating endocannabinoid levels in children with autism spectrum disorder. *Mol. Autism* **2019**, *10*, 2. [CrossRef]
101. Servadio, M.; Melancia, F.; Manduca, A.; Di Masi, A.; Schiavi, S.; Cartocci, V.; Pallottini, V.; Campolongo, P.; Ascenzi, P.; Trezza, V. Targeting anandamide metabolism rescues core and associated autistic-like symptoms in rats prenatally exposed to valproic acid. *Transl. Psychiatry* **2016**, *6*, e902. [CrossRef] [PubMed]
102. Al-Otaish, H.; Al-Ayadhi, L.Y.; Bjørklund, G.; Chirumbolo, S.; Urbina, M.A.; El-Ansary, A. Relationship between absolute and relative ratios of glutamate, glutamine and GABA and severity of autism spectrum disorder. *Metab. Brain Dis.* **2018**, *33*, 843–854. [CrossRef] [PubMed]
103. Valenzuela, C.F.; Puglia, M.P.; Zucca, S. Focus On: Neurotransmitter Systems. *Alcohol Res. Health J. Natl. Inst. Alcohol Abus. Alcohol.* **2011**, *34*, 106–120.
104. Adams, J.B.; Johansen, L.J.; Powell, L.D.; Quig, D.W.; Rubin, R.A. Gastrointestinal flora and gastrointestinal status in children with autism—Comparisons to typical children and correlation with autism severity. *BMC Gastroenterol.* **2011**, *11*, 22. [CrossRef]

105. Silva, Y.P.; Bernardi, A.; Frozza, R.L. The Role of Short-Chain Fatty Acids from Gut Microbiota in Gut-Brain Communication. *Front. Endocrinol.* **2020**, *11*, 25. [CrossRef]
106. Oh, D.; Cheon, K.-A. Alteration of Gut Microbiota in Autism Spectrum Disorder: An Overview. *J. Korean Acad. Child. Adolesc. Psychiatry* **2020**, *31*, 131–145. [CrossRef]
107. Fulceri, F.; Morelli, M.; Santocchi, E.; Cena, H.; Del Bianco, T.; Narzisi, A.; Calderoni, S.; Muratori, F. Gastrointestinal symptoms and behavioral problems in preschoolers with Autism Spectrum Disorder. *Dig. Liver Dis.* **2016**, *48*, 248–254. [CrossRef]
108. McElhanon, B.O.; McCracken, C.; Karpen, S.; Sharp, W.G. Gastrointestinal Symptoms in Autism Spectrum Disorder: A Meta-analysis. *Pediatrics* **2014**, *133*, 872–883. [CrossRef]
109. Chaidez, V.; Hansen, R.L.; Hertz-Picciotto, I. Gastrointestinal Problems in Children with Autism, Developmental Delays or Typical Development. *J. Autism Dev. Disord.* **2014**, *44*, 1117–1127. [CrossRef]
110. Rao, M.; Gershon, M.D. The bowel and beyond: The enteric nervous system in neurological disorders. *Nat. Rev. Gastroenterol. Hepatol.* **2016**, *13*, 517–528. [CrossRef]
111. Bernier, R.; Golzio, C.; Xiong, B.; Stessman, H.A.; Coe, B.P.; Penn, O.; Witherspoon, K.; Gerdts, J.; Baker, C.; Vulto-van Silfhout, A.T.; et al. Disruptive CHD8 Mutations Define a Subtype of Autism Early in Development. *Cell* **2014**, *158*, 263–276. [CrossRef] [PubMed]
112. Sharon, G.; Cruz, N.J.; Kang, D.-W.; Gandal, M.J.; Wang, B.; Kim, Y.-M.; Zink, E.M.; Casey, C.P.; Taylor, B.C.; Lane, C.J.; et al. Human Gut Microbiota from Autism Spectrum Disorder Promote Behavioral Symptoms in Mice. *Cell* **2019**, *177*, 1600–1618.e17. [CrossRef] [PubMed]
113. Kang, D.-W.; Park, J.G.; Ilhan, Z.E.; Wallstrom, G.; LaBaer, J.; Adams, J.B.; Krajmalnik-Brown, R. Reduced Incidence of Prevotella and Other Fermenters in Intestinal Microflora of Autistic Children. *PLoS ONE* **2013**, *8*, e68322. [CrossRef] [PubMed]
114. Williams, B.L.; Hornig, M.; Buie, T.; Bauman, M.L.; Paik, M.C.; Wick, I.; Bennett, A.; Jabado, O.; Hirschberg, D.L.; Lipkin, W.I. Impaired Carbohydrate Digestion and Transport and Mucosal Dysbiosis in the Intestines of Children with Autism and Gastrointestinal Disturbances. *PLoS ONE* **2011**, *6*, e24585. [CrossRef] [PubMed]
115. Parracho, H.M.R.T.; Bingham, M.O.; Gibson, G.R.; McCartney, A.L. Differences between the gut microflora of children with autistic spectrum disorders and that of healthy children. *J. Med. Microbiol.* **2005**, *54*, 987–991. [CrossRef] [PubMed]
116. Shaw, W. Increased urinary excretion of a 3-(3-hydroxyphenyl)-3-hydroxypropionic acid (HPHPA), an abnormal phenylalanine metabolite ofClostridiaspp. in the gastrointestinal tract, in urine samples from patients with autism and schizophrenia. *Nutr. Neurosci.* **2010**, *13*, 135–143. [CrossRef]
117. Altieri, L.; Neri, C.; Sacco, R.; Curatolo, P.; Benvenuto, A.; Muratori, F.; Santocchi, E.; Bravaccio, C.; Lenti, C.; Saccani, M.; et al. Urinary p cresol is elevated in small children with severe autism spectrum disorder. *Biomarkers* **2011**, *16*, 252–260. [CrossRef]
118. Gabriele, S.; Sacco, R.; Cerullo, S.; Neri, C.; Urbani, A.; Tripi, G.; Malvy, J.; Barthelemy, C.; Bonnet-Brihault, F.; Persico, A.M. Urinary p-cresol is elevated in young French children with autism spectrum disorder: A replication study. *Biomarkers* **2014**, *19*, 463–470. [CrossRef]
119. De Angelis, M.; Piccolo, M.; Vannini, L.; Siragusa, S.; De Giacomo, A.; Serrazzanetti, D.I.; Cristofori, F.; Guerzoni, M.E.; Gobbetti, M.; Francavilla, R. Fecal microbiota and metabolome of children with autism and pervasive developmental disorder not otherwise specified. *PLoS ONE* **2013**, *8*, e76993. [CrossRef]
120. Passmore, I.J.; Letertre, M.P.; Preston, M.D.; Bianconi, I.; Harrison, M.A.; Nasher, F.; Kaur, H.; Hong, H.A.; Baines, S.D.; Cutting, S.M.; et al. Para-cresol production by Clostridium difficile affects microbial diversity and membrane integrity of Gram-negative bacteria. *PLOS Pathog.* **2018**, *14*, e1007191. [CrossRef]
121. Clayton, T.A.; Baker, D.; Lindon, J.C.; Everett, J.R.; Nicholson, J.K. Pharmacometabonomic identification of a significant host-microbiome metabolic interaction affecting human drug metabolism. *Proc. Natl. Acad. Sci. USA* **2009**, *106*, 14728–14733. [CrossRef] [PubMed]
122. Strati, F.; Cavalieri, D.; Albanese, D.; De Felice, C.; Donati, C.; Hayek, J.; Jousson, O.; Leoncini, S.; Renzi, D.; Calabrò, A.; et al. New evidences on the altered gut microbiota in autism spectrum disorders. *Microbiome* **2017**, *5*, 24. [CrossRef] [PubMed]
123. Hsiao, E.Y.; McBride, S.W.; Hsien, S.; Sharon, G.; Hyde, E.R.; McCue, T.; Codelli, J.A.; Chow, J.; Reisman, S.E.; Petrosino, J.F.; et al. Microbiota Modulate Behavioral and Physiological Abnormalities Associated with Neurodevelopmental Disorders. *Cell* **2013**, *155*, 1451–1463. [CrossRef] [PubMed]
124. Santocchi, E.; Guiducci, L.; Prosperi, M.; Calderoni, S.; Gaggini, M.; Apicella, F.; Tancredi, R.; Billeci, L.; Mastromarino, P.; Grossi, E.; et al. Effects of Probiotic Supplementation on Gastrointestinal, Sensory and Core Symptoms in Autism Spectrum Disorders: A Randomized Controlled Trial. *Front. Psychiatry* **2020**, *11*, 550593. [CrossRef] [PubMed]
125. Hassan, W.M.; Al-Ayadhi, L.Y.; Bjørklund, G.; Alabdali, A.; Chirumbolo, S.; El-Ansary, A. The Use of Multi-parametric Biomarker Profiles May Increase the Accuracy of ASD Prediction. *J. Mol. Neurosci.* **2018**, *66*, 85–101. [CrossRef] [PubMed]
126. Rossignol, D.; Frye, R.E. Mitochondrial dysfunction in autism spectrum disorders: A systematic review and meta-analysis. *Mol. Psychiatry* **2011**, *17*, 290–314. [CrossRef]
127. Singh, K.; Singh, I.N.; Diggins, E.; Connors, S.L.; Karim, M.A.; Lee, D.; Zimmerman, A.W.; Frye, R.E. Developmental regression and mitochondrial function in children with autism. *Ann. Clin. Transl. Neurol.* **2020**, *7*, 683–694. [CrossRef]
128. Giulivi, C.; Zhang, Y.-F.; Omanska-Klusek, A.; Ross-Inta, C.; Wong, S.; Hertz-Picciotto, I.; Tassone, F.; Pessah, I.N. Mitochondrial Dysfunction in Autism. *JAMA* **2010**, *304*, 2389–2396. [CrossRef]

129. Shoffner, J.; Hyams, L.; Langley, G.N.; Cossette, S.; Mylacraine, L.; Dale, J.; Ollis, L.; Kuoch, S.; Bennett, K.; Aliberti, A.; et al. Fever Plus Mitochondrial Disease Could Be Risk Factors for Autistic Regression. *J. Child. Neurol.* **2009**, *25*, 429–434. [CrossRef]
130. Chaudhari, N.; Talwar, P.; Parimisetty, A.; Lefebvre d'Hellencourt, C.; Ravanan, P. A molecular web: Endoplasmic reticulum stress, inflammation, and oxidative stress. *Front. Cell. Neurosci.* **2014**, *8*, 213. [CrossRef]
131. Libero, L.E.; Nordahl, C.W.; Li, D.D.; Ferrer, E.; Rogers, S.J.; Amaral, D.G. Persistence of megalencephaly in a subgroup of young boys with autism spectrum disorder. *Autism Res.* **2016**, *9*, 1169–1182. [CrossRef] [PubMed]
132. Nordahl, C.W.; Braunschweig, D.; Iosif, A.-M.; Lee, A.; Rogers, S.; Ashwood, P.; Amaral, D.G.; Van De Water, J. Maternal autoantibodies are associated with abnormal brain enlargement in a subgroup of children with autism spectrum disorder. *Brain Behav. Immun.* **2013**, *30*, 61–65. [CrossRef] [PubMed]
133. Lai, M.; Lombardo, M.V.; Auyeung, B.; Chakrabarti, B.; Baron-Cohen, S. Sex/Gender Differences and Autism: Setting the Scene for Future Research. *J. Am. Acad. Child. Adolesc. Psychiatry* **2015**, *54*, 11–24. [CrossRef]
134. Foster, N.E.; Doyle-Thomas, K.A.; Tryfon, A.; Ouimet, T.; Anagnostou, E.; Evans, A.C.; Zwaigenbaum, L.; Lerch, J.P.; Lewis, J.D.; Hyde, K.L. Structural Gray Matter Differences During Childhood Development in Autism Spectrum Disorder: A Multimetric Approach. *Pediatric Neurol.* **2015**, *53*, 350–359. [CrossRef] [PubMed]
135. Haar, S.; Berman, S.; Behrmann, M.; Dinstein, I. Anatomical Abnormalities in Autism? *Cereb. Cortex* **2014**, *26*, 1440–1452. [CrossRef] [PubMed]
136. Ure, A.M.; Treyvaud, K.; Thompson, D.K.; Pascoe, L.; Roberts, G.; Lee, K.J.; Seal, M.L.; Northam, E.; Cheong, J.L.; Hunt, R.W.; et al. Neonatal brain abnormalities associated with autism spectrum disorder in children born very preterm. *Autism Res.* **2015**, *9*, 543–552. [CrossRef]
137. Brun, C.C.; Nicolson, R.; Leporé, N.; Chou, Y.-Y.; Vidal, C.N.; DeVito, T.J.; Drost, D.J.; Williamson, P.C.; Rajakumar, N.; Toga, A.W.; et al. Mapping brain abnormalities in boys with autism. *Hum. Brain Mapp.* **2009**, *30*, 3887–3900. [CrossRef]
138. Schumann, C.M.; Barnes, C.C.; Lord, C.; Courchesne, E. Amygdala Enlargement in Toddlers with Autism Related to Severity of Social and Communication Impairments. *Biol. Psychiatry* **2009**, *66*, 942–949. [CrossRef]
139. Schumann, C.M.; Hamstra, J.; Goodlin-Jones, B.L.; Lotspeich, L.J.; Kwon, H.; Buonocore, M.H.; Lammers, C.R.; Reiss, A.L.; Amaral, D.G. The Amygdala Is Enlarged in Children but Not Adolescents with Autism; the Hippocampus Is Enlarged at All Ages. *J. Neurosci.* **2004**, *24*, 6392–6401. [CrossRef]
140. Shen, M.D.; Nordahl, C.W.; Young, G.S.; Wootton-Gorges, S.L.; Lee, A.; Liston, S.E.; Harrington, K.R.; Ozonoff, S.; Amaral, D.G. Early brain enlargement and elevated extra-axial fluid in infants who develop autism spectrum disorder. *Brain* **2013**, *136*, 2825–2835. [CrossRef]
141. Emerson, R.W.; Adams, C.; Nishino, T.; Hazlett, H.C.; Wolff, J.J.; Zwaigenbaum, L.; Constantino, J.N.; Shen, M.D.; Swanson, M.R.; Elison, J.T.; et al. Functional neuroimaging of high-risk 6-month-old infants predicts a diagnosis of autism at 24 months of age. *Sci. Transl. Med.* **2017**, *9*, eaag2882. [CrossRef] [PubMed]
142. Dawson, G.; Carver, L.; Meltzoff, A.N.; Panagiotides, H.; McPartland, J.; Webb, S.J. Neural Correlates of Face and Object Recognition in Young Children with Autism Spectrum Disorder, Developmental Delay, and Typical Development. *Child. Dev.* **2002**, *73*, 700–717. [CrossRef] [PubMed]
143. Pagnozzi, A.M.; Conti, E.; Calderoni, S.; Fripp, J.; Rose, S.E. A systematic review of structural MRI biomarkers in autism spectrum disorder: A machine learning perspective. *Int. J. Dev. Neurosci.* **2018**, *71*, 68–82. [CrossRef] [PubMed]
144. Marshall, J.; Martin, T.; Downie, J.; Malisza, K. A Comprehensive Analysis of MRI Research Risks: In Support of Full Disclosure. *Can. J. Neurol. Sci.* **2007**, *34*, 11–17. [CrossRef] [PubMed]
145. Falck-Ytter, T.; Bölte, S.; Gredebäck, G. Eye tracking in early autism research. *J. Neurodev. Disord.* **2013**, *5*, 28. [CrossRef] [PubMed]
146. Falck-Ytter, T.; Fernell, E.; Hedvall, Å.L.; Von Hofsten, C.; Gillberg, C. Gaze Performance in Children with Autism Spectrum Disorder when Observing Communicative Actions. *J. Autism Dev. Disord.* **2012**, *42*, 2236–2245. [CrossRef] [PubMed]
147. Dalton, K.M.; Nacewicz, B.M.; Johnstone, T.; Schaefer, H.S.; Gernsbacher, M.A.; Goldsmith, H.H.; Alexander, A.L.; Davidson, R.J. Gaze fixation and the neural circuitry of face processing in autism. *Nat. Neurosci.* **2005**, *8*, 519–526. [CrossRef]
148. Klin, A.; Jones, W.; Schultz, R.; Volkmar, F.; Cohen, D. Visual Fixation Patterns during Viewing of Naturalistic Social Situations as Predictors of Social Competence in Individuals with Autism. *Arch. Gen. Psychiatry* **2002**, *59*, 809–816. [CrossRef]
149. Wan, G.; Kong, X.; Sun, B.; Yu, S.; Tu, Y.; Park, J.; Lang, C.; Koh, M.; Wei, Z.; Feng, Z.; et al. Applying Eye Tracking to Identify Autism Spectrum Disorder in Children. *J. Autism Dev. Disord.* **2019**, *49*, 209–215. [CrossRef]
150. Jones, W.; Carr, K.; Klin, A. Absence of Preferential Looking to the Eyes of Approaching Adults Predicts Level of Social Disability in 2-Year-Old Toddlers with Autism Spectrum Disorder. *Arch. Gen. Psychiatry* **2008**, *65*, 946–954. [CrossRef]
151. Loth, E.; Murphy, D.G.; Spooren, W. Defining Precision Medicine Approaches to Autism Spectrum Disorders: Concepts and Challenges. *Front. Psychiatry* **2016**, *7*, 188. [CrossRef] [PubMed]
152. Beversdorf, D.Q. Phenotyping, Etiological Factors, and Biomarkers: Toward Precision Medicine in Autism Spectrum Disorders. *J. Dev. Behav. Pediatrics* **2016**, *37*, 659–673. [CrossRef] [PubMed]
153. Chang, E.H.; Zabner, J. Precision Genomic Medicine in Cystic Fibrosis. *Clin. Transl. Sci.* **2015**, *8*, 606–610. [CrossRef] [PubMed]
154. McLean, E.; Cogswell, M.; Egli, I.; Wojdyla, D.; De Benoist, B. Worldwide prevalence of anaemia, WHO Vitamin and Mineral Nutrition Information System, 1993–2005. *Public Health Nutr.* **2008**, *12*, 444–454. [CrossRef] [PubMed]
155. Northrop-Clewes, C.A.; Thurnham, D.I. Biomarkers for the differentiation of anemia and their clinical usefulness. *J. Blood Med.* **2013**, *4*, 11–22.

156. Mitsudomi, T.; Suda, K.; Yatabe, Y. Surgery for NSCLC in the era of personalized medicine. *Nat. Rev. Clin. Oncol.* **2013**, *10*, 235–244. [CrossRef]
157. Ginsburg, G.S.; Phillips, K.A. Precision Medicine: From Science to Value. *Health Aff.* **2018**, *37*, 694–701. [CrossRef]
158. Dainis, A.M.; Ashley, E. Cardiovascular Precision Medicine in the Genomics Era. *JACC Basic Transl. Sci.* **2018**, *3*, 313–326. [CrossRef]
159. Luo, Y.; Eran, A.; Palmer, N.; Avillach, P.; Levy-Moonshine, A.; Szolovits, P.; Kohane, I.S. A multidimensional precision medicine approach identifies an autism subtype characterized by dyslipidemia. *Nat. Med.* **2020**, *26*, 1375–1379. [CrossRef]

Journal of
Personalized
Medicine

MDPI

Review

Rationale of an Advanced Integrative Approach Applied to Autism Spectrum Disorder: Review, Discussion and Proposal

María Luján Ferreira [1] and Nicolás Loyacono [1,2,*]

[1] TEA-Enfoque Integrador Group, Bahía Blanca 8000, Argentina; ferreiramaralujn@yahoo.com
[2] SANyTA (Sociedad Argentina de Neurodesarrollo y Trastornos Asociados), Migueletes 681, Piso 2, Departamento 2, BUE-Ciudad Autónoma de Buenos Aires C1426, Argentina
* Correspondence: nicoloya@hotmail.com; Tel.: +54-911-5825-5209

Abstract: The rationale of an Advanced Integrative Model and an Advanced Integrative Approach is presented. In the context of Allopathic Medicine, this model introduces the evaluation, clinical exploration, diagnosis, and treatment of concomitant medical problems to the diagnosis of Autism Spectrum Disorder. These may be outside or inside the brain. The concepts of static or chronic, dynamic encephalopathy and condition for Autism Spectrum Disorder are defined in this model, which looks at the response to the treatments of concomitant medical problemsto the diagnosis of Autism Spectrum Disorder. (1) Background: Antecedents and rationale of an Advanced Integrative Model and of an Advanced Integrative Approach are presented; (2) Methods: Concomitant medical problems to the diagnosis of Autism Spectrum Disorder and a discussion of the known responses of their treatments are presented; (3) Results: Groups in Autism are defined and explained, related to the responses of the treatments of the concomitant medical problems to ASD and (4) Conclusions: The analysis in the framework of an Advanced Integrative Model of three groups including the concepts of static encephalopathy; chronic, dynamic encephalopathy and condition for Autism Spectrum Disorder explains findings in the field, previously not understood.

Keywords: integrative; model; ASD; concomitant; condition; disorder

Citation: Ferreira, M.L.; Loyacono, N. Rationale of an Advanced Integrative Approach Applied to Autism Spectrum Disorder: Review, Discussion and Proposal. *J. Pers. Med.* **2021**, *11*, 514. https://doi.org/10.3390/jpm11060514

Academic Editors: Daniel Rossignol and Richard E. Frye

Received: 6 February 2021
Accepted: 27 May 2021
Published: 4 June 2021

Publisher's Note: MDPI stays neutral with regard to jurisdictional claims in published maps and institutional affiliations.

Copyright: © 2021 by the authors. Licensee MDPI, Basel, Switzerland. This article is an open access article distributed under the terms and conditions of the Creative Commons Attribution (CC BY) license (https://creativecommons.org/licenses/by/4.0/).

1. Introduction—The Background

This manuscript presents the rationale of a new model of approach to Autism Spectrum Disorder. There are several acronyms that will be used throughout this work:

Autism Spectrum Disorder = ASD
Advanced Integrative Model = AIM, a new model of approach to ASD
Advanced Integrative Approach = AIA. The AIA is the application of the AIM.
Concomitant medical problems to diagnosis = CMPD. The CMPD are the medical problems outside the brain (mainly competence of the General Practitioner in adulthood and Pediatricians in childhood) and inside the brain (competence of the fields of Neurology and Psychiatry).
Neuro-Developmental Disorders = NDDs
Diagnostic and Statistical Manual of Mental Disorders, fourth version = DSM-IV
Diagnostic and Statistical Manual of Mental Disorders, fifth version = DSM-5
Genetic Model = GM
Intellectual disability = ID
Attention deficit hyperactivity disorder = ADHD
Obsessive-compulsive disorder = OCD

1.1. One Finding, One Treatment—The Old Era of Simplification as the Goal

Most recent manuscripts introduce Autism Spectrum Disorder or ASD as "Autism spectrum disorder defines a broad group of NDDs characterized by (i) young age of onset, (ii) impairment in communication and social abilities, (iii) restricted interests and repetitive behaviors, and (iv) symptoms that affect patients' function in various areas of their life". Many of today's manuscripts about Autism Spectrum Disorder (ASD) begin with the phrase: "The complex pathophysiology of autism spectrum disorder encompasses interactions between genetic and environmental factors" or similar [1]. The diagnosis of ASD is given considering the Diagnostic and Statistical Manual of Mental Disorders (DSM) in 2021, with its fifth version or DSM-5. A recent review summarized the history of the DSM from Kanner to DSM-5 [2]. In precision medicine, the gap between bodily behaviors and genomics is being addressed, including the study of gene expression on tissues beyond the brain, in organs for vital functions. This approach is proposed to reframe Psychiatry [3].

Recent manuscripts reviewed the so-called comorbidities in ASD [4,5]. Comorbidities may be psychiatric [6], neurological [7], or related to medical conditions beyond the brain in the field of Pediatrics or General Medicine [8]. Recent literature has demonstrated that people with ASD diagnosis may have multiple comorbidities in different combinations and severity [9] and even temporal, transient hyper-multimorbidity. Multimorbidity is present when multiple medical issues (called comorbidities) are diagnosed in the same person. The present manuscript will call the medical issues that are frequently present in people with ASD as "concomitant medical problems to diagnosis" (of ASD) or CMPD. These CMPD are outside the brain or related to the brain (neurological and psychiatric CMPD of ASD). Previous attempts proposed potentially different roles for CMPD [10].

1.2. *Trans-Discipline for the Analysis of the So Called "Comorbidities"*

Complexity science forces us to see the dynamic properties of systems and the varying properties that are related to social roots [11,12]. ASD may be considered a complex diagnosis that resists the finding of new approaches via traditional models. It would be better tackled through interdisciplinary, systems-level approaches, considering implementation science [13,14].

Somatic health is a key point to move forward [15]. Several important reports have alerted about the need for the serious consideration of the CMPD of ASD [3,4,16–18] with transdisciplinary and interdisciplinary collaboration in the context of the multimorbidity [19]. As reference [17] cites, ASD is defined behaviorally. It includes the consideration of impairments in social behavior, stereotypic movements, and communication issues with impact on social skills, called "core symptoms of ASD". All these symptoms significantly impair the quality of life of people diagnosed with ASD [20,21].

Medical conditions such as gut dysbiosis [22], non-celiac gluten sensitivity [23], cerebral folate deficiency [24], food allergies and intolerances [25], gastrointestinal [26], metabolic [27] and biochemical issues [28], immune dysfunction [29], autoimmune problems [30], mitochondrial dysfunction [31], barrier permeabilities [32], oxidative stress [33], endocrine issues [34] and more are not explored (sometimes for years) in ASD patients. The most advanced approaches have shifted the focus of the "causation search" original framework to the study of the (epi) genetic susceptibility for ASD, from the brain to the whole body [1,35], and to the importance of humanism in medicine [36] as well as to the study of genes expressed in tissues outside of the brain [37]. As Constantino recently reported, the so-called "co-morbidities" of ASD are inappropriately named if they actually contribute to (or exacerbate) the severity of autism itself [38]. Multimorbidity affects the generation of evidence [39] and a new Evidence Pyramid in Evidence Based Medicine was recently proposed [40]. Multimorbidity and hyper-multimorbidity should be taken into account in the case of ASD. The field of ASD needs personalized medicine as the norm.

1.3. *What This Manuscript Is*

This manuscript is not a narrative or scoping review in a traditional sense [41]. It is not a systematic review, meta-analysis or meta-synthesis. Furthermore, it does not propose a medical hypothesis.

This manuscript presents a New Model, the Advanced Integrative Model (AIM) and its application, the Advanced Integrative Approach (AIA). AIA is the application of the AIM. Evaluation, diagnosis, and treatment of CMP to ASD diagnosis are very important in this model, considering those in the brain and beyond the brain. Mainly reviews and systematic reviews in CMPD were included in the revision. The selected language was English. These manuscripts were selected using PubMed, Scopus, and Medline, with keywords such as "ASD" and "health comorbidities", "health children", "physical health teen-adolescents", "physical health adults", "quality of life", "outcomes", "gastrointestinal", "immune", "autoimmune", "mitochondria", "symptoms", "physical conditions" and combinations of them with systematic review/review or general articles. Published manuscripts about prevalence, advocacy, neurodiversity, and genetics in ASD were also included. The publication dates of the 73 references are from 2011 to 2021, with nearly 24 published in 2020–2021 and only 4 before 2010.

The design and answer of three main questions relating to a person (child/teen/adult) diagnosed with ASD (but presented for a child) are discussed in this manuscript. These main questions are:

What does ASD mean?

How CMPD can be evaluated, diagnosed and treated rigorously and adequately today in this child with ASD?

Which would be the best combination of medical and non-medical tools for this child, considering the whole-body status at this moment in the Advanced Integrative Approach (AIA) thinking in multimorbidity?

2. When the Conclusion Should Not Be the Presumption

Looking at the published research in ASD, there is plenty of information about neurological [42], psychiatric [43] and biological (outside the brain) CMPD of ASD [3]. These are almost always called comorbidities. However, comorbidities mean that medical conditions present are not related to a main diagnosis, in this case ASD. The design of the research studies in ASD is performed considering OFAT (one factor at a time) instead of the context of multimorbidity. ASD is a model psychiatric disorder following the DSM-5 for the analysis of multimorbidity and personalized medicine.

In this case, multimorbidity is present in the brain (psychiatric and neurological issues) and outside the brain (biological problems in body systems outside the brain) with behavioral, emotional, motor, sensorial and communicational symptoms. The physicians related to these areas are from Psychiatry, Neurology and Pediatrics. The Pediatrician detects ASD and refers to other areas. However, in the Advanced Integrative Model the Pediatrician (or General Practitioner) by training, experience, and competence, is of paramount importance in the Advanced Integrative Approach.

2.1. *The Response to Treatment of CMPD in ASD*

When a family receives a diagnosis, CMPD are considered comorbid, not related to ASD and of little or no impact on core symptoms or trajectory of ASD. The recommended practice, if it includes exploration of CMPD, is only the limited exploration of gastrointestinal issues, beyond the neurological or psychiatric co-occurring medical problems. In a recent manuscript the recommendations were educational practices, developmental therapies, and behavioral interventions, but CMPD (in particular the out-of-the-brain biological issues) were not properly considered in the state-of-the art knowledge [44]. It has not been considered, historically, that the results of all the behavioral, relational, developmental or psychoeducative methods to approach ASD are strongly related to the biological status of the person with the ASD diagnosis.

The question is how could the treatment(s) of CMPD affect the ASD symptoms?

There are several possible outcomes to the treatments of CMPD of ASD outside the brain.

There are people diagnosed with ASD (mainly children) whose core ASD symptoms disappear after the adequate treatment of CMPD outside the brain. ASD symptoms seem to be only symptoms of a few CMPD outside the brain with a causal relation [45].

There are people diagnosed with ASD (all ages) whose core ASD symptoms ameliorate after the adequate treatment of CMPD outside the brain. Many times, several CMPD need to be considered and properly treated to show an impact in the core symptoms. ASD symptoms appear to be related to CMPD in ASD [46].

There are people diagnosed with ASD (all ages) whose core ASD symptoms do not change after the adequate treatment of CMPD outside the brain, even when several CMPD are considered and properly treated. ASD symptoms are not related to CMPD in ASD. In this case, they could be called "comorbid".

The individual response to the most rigorous, controlled, and serious allopathic treatments of CMPD in ASD, taking into account multimorbidity and complexity, gives clues to their roles. Therefore, the role of CMPD in ASD would be shown or concluded after and not before the treatment of them.

As Dr. Frye's group has reported, in ASD many neurological issues have links to biological problems not related to the brain [47]. Dr. Frye has published several important manuscripts about CMPD in ASD and from the design the work is presented differently than other manuscripts. The titles of these manuscripts generally are "XXX as treatment of YYY in ASD". This kind of approach to the problem takes into account, since the design, the multiple CMPD in ASD. Historically the presentation of the treatment of CMPD was "XXX as treatment of ASD". Many recent manuscripts detect, count, and report the so called "comorbidities" instead of considering new models for the role of these CMPD [4,48,49]. Not all children with gut dysbiosis have ASD, not all children with mitochondrial dysfunction or with some immune deficiency have ASD. There should be another component to take into account and address this complexity and this other component is the brain status in ASD.

2.2. The Controversy about Whether a Static or Dynamic Encephalopathy Contributes to ASD

Encephalopathy is a term used here for a diffuse disorder (or disease) that alters brain function or structure. An encephalopathy is dynamic when it responds to treatments of CMPD outside the brain. An encephalopathy is static when it does not change; it does not respond to treatments of CMPD. A central point is if the encephalopathy in ASD is static or dynamic and how. The dynamic encephalopathy in ASD is considered at first to be chronic and difficult to change, once present. The dynamism of the encephalopathy would also be related to the plastic nature of the brain and the number, combination, and severity of the CMPD. The development of the encephalopathy and the path to chronicity of it is then considered a process, not a genes-mediated fact for all people diagnosed with ASD. This process may begin prenatally (as vulnerability and/or through a genetic mutation/s or polymorphism/s and combinations of them with environmental impact) and/or postnatally. The mechanisms for the encephalopathy to develop involve the genetic susceptibility to CMPD in the brain and outside the brain and the individual response to in-series and in-parallel exposures in the second decade of the XXI century. From processed food to antibiotics, from contaminated water and air to mitochondrial impact, from dysbiosis to whole-body dysfunction and more the many pathways to gut barrier permeability and brain–blood barrier permeability in vulnerable people are explained looking at the model of ASD as symptoms of a dynamic (but chronic) encephalopathy.

Since the presentation of the genetic model (GM) with the manuscript of Folstein and Rutter [50], 44 years has shown the exploration of the genetic basis of ASD. Meanwhile, the prevalence has grown up to 1 in 54 from the CDC data [51], that is more related to 1 in 36 [52] and near 1 in 20 males in children up to 17 years or even higher [53]. The main point of the GM is the consideration of the root of ASD as a static encephalopathy of prenatal origin [54]. In the neurodiversity model, ASD is a way of being [55]. These two points of view do not explain many findings, do not give tools or resources to professionals, non-professionals and families to address the individual complex medical, non-medical, and educational needs of many children, teens and adults diagnosed with ASD. There are several recent reports about these unmet needs [56–58].

The Advanced Integrative Model (AIM) is a new model of ASD. In this model the CMPD outside the brain should be properly diagnosed and treated. These CMPD may be related to a chronic encephalopathy through the barrier's permeability. Gut and brain blood barrier permeabilities are important to understand in this proposal. The gut dysbiosis involves pathogenic bacteria, parasites, and fungus that may translocate and/or produce metabolites and correlates with inflammation in the presence of a permeable gut barrier. This abnormal situation produces an immune response. The immune system components and metabolites from gut dysbiosis reach the bloodstream due to the permeable gut barrier and finally the brain due to brain blood barrier permeability [15]. The idea of a chronic, dynamic encephalopathy as a model of ASD was presented by Dr. Herbert in 2005 [59] but unfortunately was not explored adequately up until the last 10 years and much more in the last 5 years.

In the framework of a model based on the explanation of ASD as a static encephalopathy of prenatal origin, the plausibility of a role of postnatal development disturbance is not taken into account and dismissed. CMPD have been labeled as "comorbid": medical issues that have no link to ASD. Coincidence or simply better health has been the explanation for the reported improvements after treatments of CMPD, which are sometimes very dramatic. Regression (loss of speech and/or abilities and/or skills) continues to happen today without explanation in these models. No other proposals have been presented, even when no genetic link in brain to regression can be clearly shown in ASD [60]. Today, regression has been reported to be present in prospective studies in up to 88% of people with ASD [61], although the consensus in retrospective studies is lower and nearer 30% [62]. Regression is understood in AIM as the final point of a pre-encephalopathy process. The pathway to chronicity is considered to be an individual process and not a single event [63] and the final point could be considered to be the regression. The chronic status of the encephalopathy would be related to chronic pathophysiological processes in the brain in ASD (see reference [52] for further explanation).

3. AIM Classification System

Core symptoms of ASD include impairments in social interaction and communication, and restricted and repetitive behaviors. There are no known efficacious treatments for the core social symptoms, although effects on repetitive behaviors have been reported [64].

The main groups in ASD following the AIM would now be:

Main Group 1—Core ASD symptoms disappear after the adequate treatment of CMPD outside the brain. In this case the encephalopathy is dynamic and completely reversible with loss of the ASD diagnosis.

Main Group 2—Core ASD symptoms ameliorate after the adequate treatment of CMPD outside the brain. In this case the encephalopathy is dynamic but chronic, partially reversible, with improvements in ASD symptoms from mild to huge, even without loss of the ASD diagnosis.

Main Group 3—Core ASD symptoms do not change after the adequate treatment of CMPD outside the brain, even when several CMPD are considered and properly treated. Some people diagnosed with ASD without intellectual disability (ID) and Asperger's syndrome following DSM-IV would be a subgroup where ASD is related to a condition as a way of being. Other subgroups would have strong links to genetics, with ID besides the ASD diagnosis, and the ASD symptoms would be related to a static encephalopathy in the subgroup called "syndromic autism" [65]. These subgroups are very different.

In these three main groups, many different subgroups may be defined, considering ID or not, speech problems, sex, age and more. Figure 1 shows the comparison between the Genetic Model (GM) and the Advanced Integrative Model (AIM) in their answer to the first of the three important questions this manuscript presents: What does ASD mean?

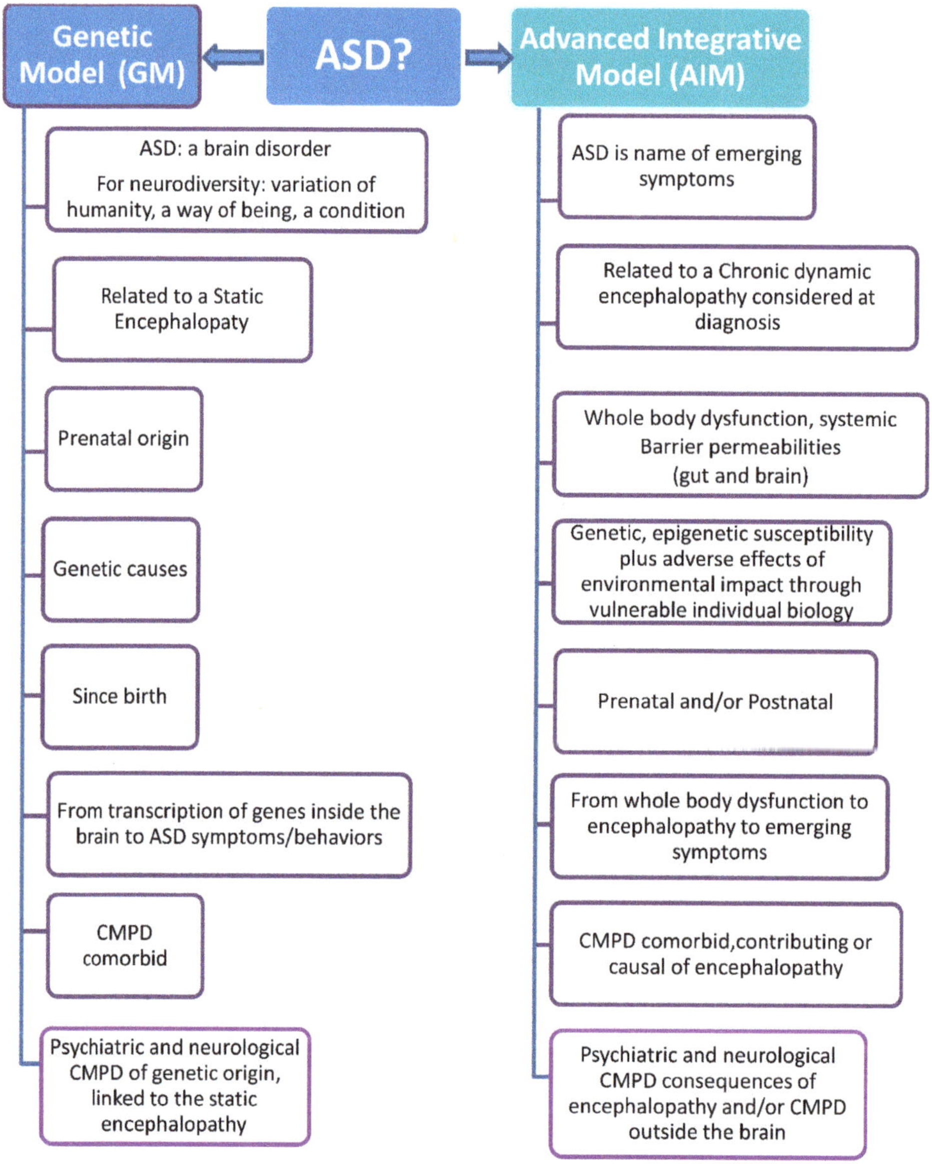

Figure 1. Genetic Model versus Advanced Integrative Model.

4. The Advanced Integrative Approach (AIA)

The second key question is what causes ASD? For the GM, the answer is genes or genes plus environment at the prenatal step or genes and epigenetics plus environment at the prenatal step. The manuscripts dealing with an important number of CMP generally obtain the information from medical records and report statistics. It is known that medical records in ASD are very incomplete because, many times, the extensive biological exploration outside the brain in ASD does not exist. The experience and the research show that many times, a person (child, teen or adult) with ASD diagnosis have CMPD in ASD outside the brain and neurological (seizures/epilepsy, movement disorders, sleep disorders), psychiatric diagnosis (from attention deficit hyperactivity disorder or ADHD to bipolar disorder, from anxiety to OCD/tics and more), language/speech problems (all the spectra of them), learning challenges, a spectra of intellectual disability and behavioral, emotional and psychological issues.

The question "What causes ASD in all children?" has shifted following the last 10 years of research to "What causes ASD in this child?"

The Advanced Integrative Approach (AIA) is the AIM in practice. The AIA is personalized and the answer to the question presented above is not straightforward. The model gives tools and resources to help and explore in different ways if medical problems outside the brain and at systemic level are at least part of the answer to that question for the person diagnosed with ASD.

Therefore, in an AIA, the second question is How CMPD can be evaluated, diagnosed and treated rigorously and adequately today in this child with ASD?

Medical and non-medical professionals do not receive the information about CMPD in ASD. If they receive it, it is incomplete or it is presented as hypothetical or "alternative" (when it is not). Discussion about models has been focused on neurodiversity versus the so called "medical model". This "medical model" includes the treatment of ASD in the context of the GM (with behavioral approaches, psychoeducative methods, and psychopharmacology). The individual symptoms of a person with an ASD diagnosis give the trained physician clues about what to explore. Many times symptoms of CMPD in ASD are only behavioral, emotional, or related to aggression/auto-aggression and more [66]. Disruptive behavior should be analyzed first, as a request for help due to potential pain, discomfort or an altered brain state [67].

The third question would be which would be the best combination of medical and non-medical tools for this child, considering the whole-body status at this moment in the Advanced Integrative Approach (AIA) thinking in multimorbidity? Figure 2 shows the hierarchy of the questions discussed in this section, expanded. The arrow shows the increasing difficulty of the questions to be answered. The last question is the most difficult to answer.

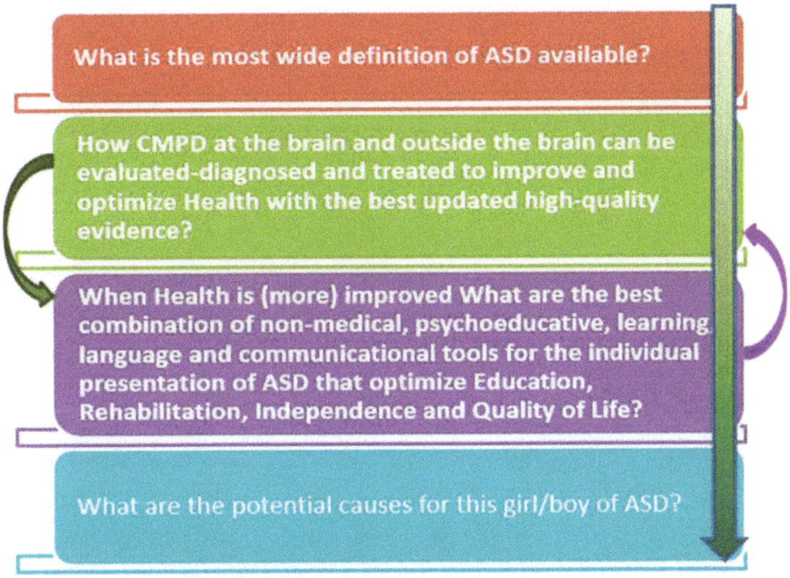

Figure 2. Main questions to present and to take into account.

5. When Genetics Is an Important Part in Building Individual Vulnerability

The genetics in ASD is of paramount importance. Genetic susceptibility in ASD is being presented more and more as increased vulnerability for the CMPD to develop. This analysis gives support to the genetics and epigenetic links in ASD but at a whole-body level, not only the brain [2].

Here, we present a new model called AIM that aims to represent a more comprehensive model for ASD:

From Genetic Susceptibility to Mutated Genes-Whole Body (including brain)-CMPD (in and outside the brain)-Permeable barriers-Chronic, Dynamic, Systemic (to Static) Encephalopathy or Condition-ASD Behavior.

In the AIM the role of genetics is different but no less important than in the GM.

6. Beyond the Brain and the System's Biology Updated to 2021

For many years, there has been a long discussion about if what is needed is health or education in the field of ASD. From the application of the AIM to an AIA, the answer is one or the other or both, depending on the individual ASD age, sex and individual presentation.

Main groups one to three include people diagnosed with ASD of all ages and presentations whose core ASD symptoms respond (or not) to treatment of CMPD, including people with Asperger's syndrome (following the DSM-IV), today included in ASD (following DSM-5). The needs are different in each main group in terms of education and/or health and other services. When core symptoms of ASD respond to treatment of CMPD, they are not a way of being or a condition, they are emerging symptoms. When core symptoms of ASD do not respond to the treatment of all the CMPD when properly and exhaustively considered, then the diagnosis of ASD could be related to a way of being for that particular person or to a static encephalopathy.

With adequate training, many symptoms historically assigned to "autism" may guide the clinician to the diagnosis and treatment of CMPD in ASD [3,4]. The treatments of CMPD are only that, they are not "ASD treatments". Even if core ASD symptoms do not respond, the treatment of adequately diagnosed CMPD in the main group three would improve the quality of life. The AIM involves the application in practice of the system´s biology updated to 2021, with the consideration of ASD as a whole-body disorder.

6.1. *Why Is the Progress So Slow in Practice When So Much Is Known from Published Research?*

Published research has been increasing regarding CMPD in ASD. The main groups one and two have not been properly studied from CMPD point of view. One of the most cited problems has been the confounding role of the intellectual disability (ID). This group also has increased the number of CMPD in ASD [3,8]. A selection bias to study people with ASD without ID was shown [68,69].

Even when it is clear that there are different subgroups of people diagnosed with ASD that respond positively, and sometimes spectacularly, to the treatment of CMPD; even when the information about these subgroups are data, not anecdotal; even when the optimal outcome was reported by several groups around the world [70,71]; even when the individual improvements after proper treatments were reported in many properly presented reports [24,39,72]; even when there are several manuscripts that show the importance of the individual response to CMPD [2], the research funding in CMPD has not been enough and in general only 9% was assigned to services research in ASD [73]. The updated information is not reaching the local sources of trusted information for doctors in practice.

The response to the treatment of CMPD gives clues to the nature of the underlying encephalopathy: static o dynamic, reversible or irreversible. The AIM allows and explains the possibility of a partial reversibility of the encephalopathy and (less reported as yet, possible) total reversibility and loss of an ASD diagnosis.

6.2. Advanced Integrative Approach (AIA): A New Model Taking Science into Medical Practice with Permanent Review

The application of an AIM requires Implementation Science, a careful design of the optimization of translational research. The higher the severity of ASD, the higher the number, combination and complexity of the CMPD. In physician practice (Pediatrician or General Practitioner), the AIA involves the careful consideration of the CMPD in ASD from the beginning. Figure 3 shows the sequence of learning about CMPD. First, the hypothesis in the AIA is that a chronic dynamic encephalopathy is underlying with the ASD diagnosis. Later, after a careful clinical exploration (also involving professionals from Neurology, Psychiatry and Genetics, if needed), CMPD are diagnosed and treated, sequentially or in parallel as needed. Finally, with the response to treatments of the CMPD in ASD the conclusion for the individual with ASD can be obtained: static encephalopathy, dynamic encephalopathy (partially or completely reversible), or condition. The complexity of the ASD presentation, the behavioral, emotional, sensorial, motor and speech/communication symptoms, and the CMPD from Pediatrics, Neurology, and Psychiatry plus their treatments require permanent review and updates.

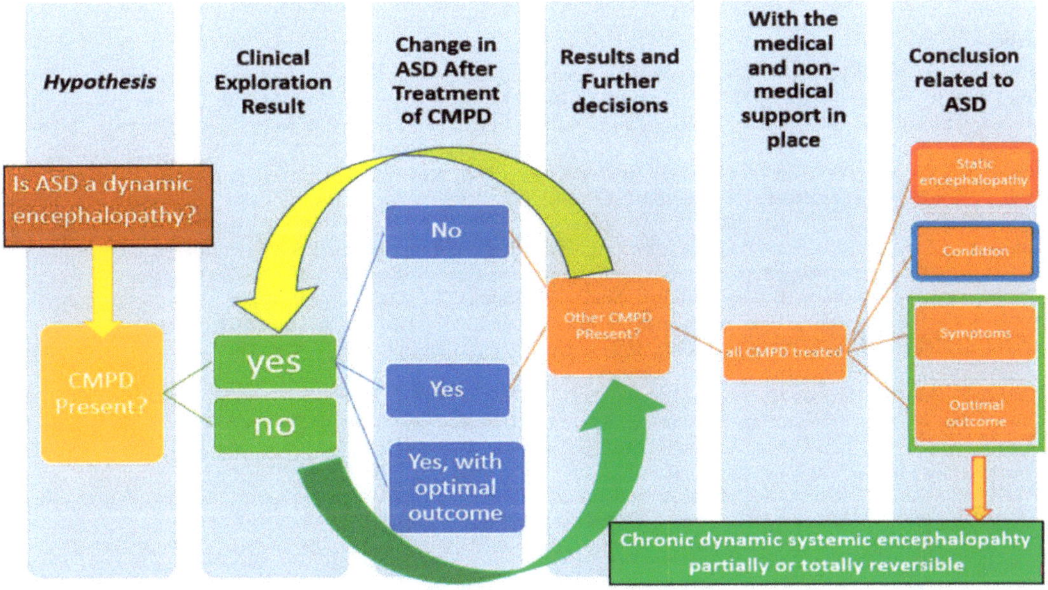

Figure 3. A path for the physician from hypothesis to conclusion in an Advanced Integrative Approach (AIA) of ASD.

7. Conclusions

The Advanced Integrative Model (AIM) and the Advanced Integrative Approach (AIA) are presented and explained in this manuscript. The consideration of the CMPD to ASD from an individual point-of-view and the analysis of the response to the proper treatment of all of them are the key to present the three different main groups. Considering the response to treatments of the CMPD of ASD, the conclusion for the individual ASD may be related to a static encephalopathy, to a chronic dynamic encephalopathy (partially or completely reversible) or to a condition. The Advanced Integrative Model for ASD includes the GM and also the idea of ASD as a condition for a subgroup of people diagnosed with ASD.

Author Contributions: Conceptualization; methodology, formal analysis, investigation, resources, M.L.F., N.L.; writing—original draft preparation, M.L.F.; writing—review and editing, N.L. and M.L.F.; visualization and supervision, N.L. All authors have read and agreed to the published version of the manuscript.

Funding: This research received no external funding.

Acknowledgments: The authors acknowledge the University of Buenos Aires (UBA, Argentina) and the Hospital de Clínicas José de San Martín (UBA, Argentina) for the support for and during the Consulting of M.L.F. (Researcher CONICET) from 2015 to 2019. N.L. and M.L.F. acknowledge Roberto Héctor Iermoli for his support of the project and the team of "ASD-Integrative Approach" (TEA-Enfoque Integrador).

Conflicts of Interest: María Luján Ferreira (Principal Res. CONICET) is the mother of a young man of 20 years, diagnosed in 2003 with Autism. From 06/2015 to 06/2019 she was an ad-honorem Consultor in ASD to the Hospital de Clínicas José de San Martín (Buenos Aires Argentina), directed by N. Loyacono and R. Iermoli (Res. Directorio CONICET 3070/2015). A presentation for a potential Agreement SANyTA (Director:N. Loyacono)-CONICET (Consejo Nacional de Investigaciones Científicas y Técnicas) -Argentina- is under development and will be presented for consideration to CONICET next months/year 2021. N. Loyacono declares no conflicts of interest.

References

1. Cheroni, C.; Caporale, N.; Testa, G. Autism spectrum disorder at the crossroad between genes and environment: Contributions, convergences, and interactions in ASD developmental pathophysiology. *Mol. Autism* **2020**, *11*, 1–18. [CrossRef]
2. Rosen, N.E.; Lord, C.; Volkmar, F.R. The Diagnosis of Autism: From Kanner to DSM-III to DSM-5 and Beyond. *J. Autism Dev. Disord.* **2021**. [CrossRef]
3. Torres, E.B. Reframing Psychiatry for Precision Medicine. *J. Pers. Med.* **2020**, *10*, 144. [CrossRef] [PubMed]
4. Sala, R.; Amet, L.; Blagojevic-Stokic, N.; Shattock, P.; Whiteley, P. Bridging the Gap Between Physical Health and Autism Spectrum Disorder. *Neuropsychiatr. Dis. Treat.* **2020**, *16*, 1605–1618.
5. Muskens, J.B.; Velders, F.P.; Staal, W.G. Medical comorbidities in children and adolescents with autism spectrum disorders and attention deficit hyperactivity disorders: A systematic review. *Eur. Child. Adolesc.* **2017**, *26*, 1093–1103. [CrossRef]
6. Lai, M.; Kassee, C.; Besney, R.; Bonato, S.; Hull, L.; Mandy, W.; Szatmari, P.; Ameis, S.H. Prevalence of co-occurring mental health diagnoses in the autism population: A systematic review and meta-analysis. *Lancet Psychiatry* **2019**, *6*, 819–829. [CrossRef]
7. Pan, P.Y.; Bölte, S.; Kaur, P.; Jamil, S.; Jonsson, U. Neurological disorders in autism: A systematic review and, meta-analysis. *Autism* **2020**. [CrossRef]
8. Dizitzer, Y.; Meiri, G.; Flusser, H.; Michaelovski, A.; Dinstein, I.; Menashe, I. Comorbidity and health services' usage in children with autism spectrum disorder: A nested case-control study. *Epidemiol. Psychiatr. Sci.* **2020**, *29*, e95. [CrossRef]
9. Cawthorpe, D. A 16-Year Cohort Analysis of Autism Spectrum Disorder-Associated Morbidity in a Pediatric Population. *FrontPsychiatry* **2018**, *9*, 635. [CrossRef] [PubMed]
10. Tye, C.; Runicles, A.K.; Whitehouse, A.J.O.; Alvares, G.A. Characterizing the Interplay Between Autism Spectrum Disorder and Comorbid Medical Conditions: An Integrative Review. *Front. Psychiatry* **2019**, *9*, 751. [CrossRef]
11. Miles, A. Complexity in medicine and healthcare: People and systems, theory and practice. *J. Eval. Clin. Pract.* **2009**, *15*, 409–410. [CrossRef]
12. Braithwaite, J.; Churruca, K.; Long, J.C.; Ellis, L.A.; Herkes, J. When complexity science meets implementation science: A theoretical and empirical analysis of systems change. *BMC Med.* **2018**, *16*, 63. [CrossRef]
13. Nilsen, P. Making sense of implementation theories, models and frameworks. *Implement. Sci.* **2015**, *10*, 53. [CrossRef]
14. Witteman, H.O.; Stahl, J.E. Facilitating interdisciplinary collaboration to tackle complex problems in health care: Report from an exploratory workshop. *Health Syst.* **2013**, *2*, 162–170. [CrossRef]
15. Pei-Yin, P.; Tammimies, G.; Bölte, S. The Association Between Somatic Health, Autism Spectrum Disorder, and Autistic. *Traits Behav. Genet.* **2020**, *50*, 233–246.
16. Panisi, C.; Guerini, F.R.; Abruzzo, P.M.; Balzola, F.; Biava, P.M.; Bolotta, A.; Brunero, M.; Burgio, E.; Chiara, A.; Clerici, M.; et al. Autism Spectrum Disorder from the Womb to Adulthood: Suggestions for a Paradigm Shift. *J. Pers. Med.* **2021**, *11*, 70. [CrossRef] [PubMed]
17. Vargason, T.; Frye, R.E.; McGuinness, D.L.; Hahn, J. Clustering of co-occurring conditions in autism spectrum disorder during early childhood: A retrospective analysis of medical claims data. *Autism Res.* **2019**, *12*, 1272–1285. [CrossRef] [PubMed]
18. Randolph-Gips, M.; Srinivasan, P. Modeling autism: A systems biology approach. *J. Clin. Bioinform.* **2012**, *2*, 17. [CrossRef] [PubMed]
19. Rohleder, N. Translating biobehavioral research advances into improvements in health care-a "network of networks" approach to multimorbidity. *J. Eval. Clin. Pract.* **2017**, *23*, 230–232. [CrossRef]

20. Happè, F.; Frith, U. Annual research review: Towards a developmental neuroscience of atypical social cognition. *J. Child. Psychol. Psych.* **2014**, *3*, 553–577. [CrossRef]
21. Pino, M.C.; Mariano, M.; Peretti, S.; D'Amico, S.; Masedu, F.; Valenti, M.; Mazza, M. When do children with autism develop adequate social behaviour? Cross-sectional analysis of developmental trajectories. *Eur. J. Develop. Psychol.* **2018**, *17*, 71–87. [CrossRef]
22. Zou, R.; Xu, F.; Wang, F.; Duan, M.; Guo, M.; Zhang, Q.; Zhao, H.; Zheng, H. Changes in the Gut Microbiota of Children with Autism Spectrum Disorder. *Autism Res.* **2020**, *13*, 1614–1625. [CrossRef] [PubMed]
23. Catassi, C.; Bai, J.C.; Bonaz, B.; Bouma, G.; Calabrò, A.; Carroccio, A.; Castillejo, G.; Ciacci, C.; Cristofori, F.; Dolinsek, J.; et al. Non-Celiac Gluten sensitivity: The new frontier of gluten related disorders. *Nutrients* **2013**, *5*, 3839–3853. [CrossRef]
24. Quadros, E.V.; Sequeira, J.M.; Brown, T.; Mevs, C.; Marchi, E.; Flory, M.; Jenkins Velinov, M.T.; Cohen, I.L. Folate receptor autoantibodies are prevalent in children diagnosed with autism spectrum disorder, their normal siblings and parents. *Autism Res.* **2018**, *11*, 707–712. [CrossRef] [PubMed]
25. Xu, G.; Snetselaar, L.G.; Jing, J.; Liu, B.; Strathearn, L.; Bao, W. Association of Food Allergy and Other Allergic Conditions with Autism Spectrum Disorder in Children. *JAMA Netw. Open* **2018**, *1*, e180279. [CrossRef]
26. Chakraborty, P.; Carpenter, K.L.; Major, S.; Deaver, M.; Vermeer, S.; Herold, B.; Franz, L.; Howard, J.; Dawson, G. Gastrointestinal problems are associated with increased repetitive behaviors but not social communication difficulties in young children with autism spectrum disorders. *Autism* **2020**. [CrossRef]
27. Frye, R.E.; Rossignol, D.A.; Scahill, L.; McDougle, C.J.; Huberman, H.; Quadros, E.V. Treatment of Folate Metabolism Abnormalities in Autism Spectrum Disorder. *Semin. Pediatr. Neurol.* **2020**, *35*, 100835. [CrossRef]
28. Delhey, L.M.; Tippett, M.; Rose, S.; Bennuri, S.C. Comparison of Treatment for Metabolic Disorders Associated with Autism: Reanalysis of Three Clinical Trials. *Front. Neurosci.* **2018**, *12*, 19. [CrossRef]
29. Pangrazzi, L.; Balasco, L.; Bozzi, Y. Oxidative Stress and Immune System Dysfunction in Autism Spectrum Disorders. *Int. J. Mol. Sci.* **2020**, *21*, 3293. [CrossRef]
30. Hughes, H.K.; Ko, E.M.; Rose, D.; Ashwood, P. Immune Dysfunction and Autoimmunity as Pathological Mechanisms in Autism Spectrum Disorders. *Front. Cell Neurosci.* **2018**, *12*, 405. [CrossRef]
31. Frye, R.E. Mitochondrial Dysfunction in Autism Spectrum Disorder: Unique Abnormalities and Targeted Treatments. *Semin. Pediatr. Neurol.* **2020**, *35*, 100829. [CrossRef] [PubMed]
32. Fiorentino, M.; Sapone, A.; Senger, S.; Camhi, S.S.; Kadzielski, S.M.; Buie, T.M.; Kelly, D.L.; Cascella, N.; Fasano, A. Blood-brain barrier and intestinal epithelial barrier alterations in autism spectrum disorders. *Mol. Autism* **2016**, *7*, 49. [CrossRef]
33. Hu, T.; Dong, Y.; He, C.; Zhao, M.; He, Q. The Gut Microbiota and Oxidative Stress in Autism Spectrum Disorders (ASD). *Oxid. Med. Cell. Longev.* **2020**, *2020*, 8396708. [CrossRef]
34. Wilson, H.A.; Creighton, C.; Scharfman, H.; Choleris, E.; MacLusky, N.J. Endocrine Insights into the Pathophysiology of Autism Spectrum Disorder. *Neuroscientist* **2020**. [CrossRef]
35. Nudel, R.; Appadurai, V.; Schork, A.J.; Buil, A.; Bybjerg-Grauholm, J.; Børglum, A.D.; Daly, M.J.; Mors, O.; Hougaard, D.M.; Mortensen, P.B.; et al. A large population-based investigation into the genetics of susceptibility to gastrointestinal infections and the link between gastrointestinal infections and mental illness. *Hum. Genet.* **2020**, *139*, 593–604. [CrossRef]
36. Loyacono, N.; Ferreira, M.L.; Iermoli, R. Humanism in medicine: The critical role of pediatricians in autism spectrum disorder. *Arch. Argent. Pediatr.* **2019**, *117*, 195–197.
37. Plummer, J.T.; Gordon, A.J.; Levitt, P. The Genetic Intersection of Neurodevelopmental Disorders and Shared Medical Comorbidities—Relations that Translate from Bench to Bedside. *Front. Psychiatry* **2016**, *7*, 142. [CrossRef] [PubMed]
38. Constantino, J.N. Deconstructing autism: From unitary syndrome to contributory developmental endophenotypes. *Int. Rev. Psychiatry* **2018**, *30*, 18–24. [CrossRef]
39. Weiss, C.O.; Varadhan, R.; Puhan, M.A.; Vickers, A.; Bandeen-Roche, K.; Boyd, C.M.; Kent, D.M. Multimorbidity and evidence generation. *J. Gen. Intern. Med.* **2014**, *29*, 653–660. [CrossRef]
40. Murad, M.H.; Asi, N.; Alsawas, M.; Alahdab, F. New evidence pyramid. *BMJ Evid. Based Med.* **2016**, *21*, 125–127. [CrossRef] [PubMed]
41. Grant, M.J.; Booth, A. A typology of reviews: An analysis of 14 review types and associated methodologies. *Health Inf. Libr. J.* **2009**, *26*, 91–108. [CrossRef]
42. Jeste, S.S. The neurology of autism spectrum disorders. *Curr. Opin. Neurol.* **2011**, *24*, 132–139. [CrossRef]
43. Hossain, M.; Khan, N.; Sultana, A.; Ma, P.; McKyer, E.L.J.; Ahmed, H.U.; Purohit, N. Prevalence of comorbid psychiatric disorders among people with autism spectrum disorder: An umbrella review of systematic reviews and meta-analyses. *Psychiatry Res.* **2020**, *287*, 112922. [CrossRef] [PubMed]
44. Hyman, S.L.; Levy, S.E.; Myers, S. Identification, Evaluation, and Management of Children with Autism Spectrum Disorder. *Pediatrics* **2020**, *145*, e20193447. [CrossRef] [PubMed]
45. Genuis, S.J.; Bouchard, T.P. Celiac disease presenting as autism. *J. Child. Neurol.* **2010**, *25*, 114–119. [CrossRef] [PubMed]
46. Adams, J.B.; Audhya, T.; Geis, E.; Gehn, E.; Fimbres, V.; Pollard, E.L.; Mitchell, J.; Ingram, J.; Hellmers, R.; Laake, D.; et al. Comprehensive Nutritional and Dietary Intervention for Autism Spectrum Disorder-A Randomized, Controlled 12-Month Trial. *Nutrients* **2018**, *10*, 369. [CrossRef]

47. Frye, R.E. Metabolic and mitochondrial disorders associated with epilepsy in children with autism spectrum disorder. *Epilepsy Behav.* **2015**, *47*, 147–157. [CrossRef]
48. Li, X.; Liu, G.; Chen, W.; Bi, Z.; Liang, H. Network analysis of autistic disease comorbidities in Chinese children based on ICD-10 codes. *BMC Med. Inform. Decis. Mak.* **2020**, *20*, 268. [CrossRef] [PubMed]
49. Brooks, J.D.; Bronskill, S.E.; Fu, L.; Saxena, F.E.; Arneja, J.; Pinzaru, V.B.; Anagnostou, E.; Nylen, K.; McLaughlin, J.; Tu, K. Identifying Children and Youth with Autism Spectrum Disorder in Electronic Medical Records: Examining Health System Utilization and Comorbidities. *Autism Res.* **2020**. [CrossRef] [PubMed]
50. Folstein, S.; Rutter, M. Infantile autism: A genetic study of 21 twin pairs. *J. Child. Psychol. Psychiatry* **1977**, *18*, 297–321. [CrossRef]
51. Maenner, M.J.; Shaw, K.A.; Baio, J.; Washington, A.; Patrick, M.; DiRienzo, M.; Christensen, D.L.; Wiggins, L.D.; Pettygrove, S.; Andrews, J.G.; et al. Prevalence of Autism Spectrum Disorder Among Children Aged 8 Years—Autism and Developmental Disabilities Monitoring Network, 11 Sites, United States, 2016. *MMWR Surveill. Summ.* **2020**, *69*, 1–12. [CrossRef] [PubMed]
52. Zablotsky, B.; Black, L.I.; Blumberg, S.J. *Estimated Prevalence of Children with Diagnosed Developmental Disabilities in the United States, 2014–2016*; NCHS Data Brief, No 291; National Center for Health Statistics: Hyattsville, MD, USA, 2017.
53. Chiarotti, F.; Venerosi, A. Epidemiology of Autism Spectrum Disorders: A Review of Worldwide Prevalence Estimates Since 2014. *Brain Sci.* **2020**, *10*, 274–284. [CrossRef]
54. Amaral, D.G.; Anderson, G.M.; Bailey, A.; Bernier, R.; Bishop, S.; Blatt, G.; Canal-Bedia, R.; Charman, T.; Dawson, G.; de Vries, P.J.; et al. Gaps in Current Autism Research: The Thoughts of the Autism Research Editorial Board and Associate Editors. *Autism Res.* **2019**, *12*, 700–714. [CrossRef] [PubMed]
55. Masataka, N. Implications of the idea of neurodiversity for understanding the origins of developmental disorders. *Phys. Life Rev.* **2017**, *20*, 85–108. [CrossRef]
56. Wills, J.; Evans, S. *Health and Service Provision for People with Autism Spectrum Disorders: A Survey of Parents in the United Kingdom, 2014*; Queen Mary University of London: London, UK, 2016.
57. Report from Autistica UK Personal Tragedies, Public Crisis, 2016, 12 Pages. Available online: https://www.autistica.org.uk/downloads/files/Personal-tragedies-public-crisis-ONLINE.pdf (accessed on 14 January 2020).
58. Drexler University Life Course Outcomes. Available online: https://drexel.edu/autismoutcomes/publications-and-reports/nat-autism-indicators-report/ (accessed on 2 June 2021).
59. Herbert, M. Autism a brain disorder or a disorder that affects the brain? *Clin. Neurol.* **2005**, *6*, 354–379.
60. Tammimies, K. Genetic mechanisms of regression in autism spectrum disorder. *Neurosci. Biobehav. Rev.* **2019**, *102*, 208–220. [CrossRef]
61. Ozonoff, S.; Gangi, D.; Hanzel, E.P.; Hill, A.; Hill, M.M.; Miller, M.; Schwichtenberg, A.J.; Steinfeld, M.B.; Parikh, C.; Iosif, A.M. Onset patterns in autism: Variation across informants, methods, and timing. *Autism Res.* **2018**, *11*, 788–797. [CrossRef]
62. Tan, C.; Frewer, V.; Cox, G.; Williams, K.; Ure, A. Prevalence and Age of Onset of Regression in Children with Autism Spectrum Disorder: A Systematic Review and Meta-analytical Update. *Autism Res.* **2021**. [CrossRef] [PubMed]
63. Tanner, A.; Dounavi, K. The Emergence of Autism Symptoms Prior to 18 Months of Age: A Systematic Literature Review. *J. Autism Dev. Disord.* **2020**. [CrossRef]
64. Farmer, C.; Thurm, A.; Grant, P. Pharmacotherapy for the Core Symptoms in Autistic Disorder: Current Status of the Research. *Drugs* **2013**, *73*, 303–314. [CrossRef] [PubMed]
65. Fernandez, B.A.; Scherer, S.W. Syndromic autism spectrum disorders: Moving from a clinically defined to a molecularly defined approach. *Dialogues Clin. Neurosci.* **2017**, *19*, 353–371. [CrossRef]
66. Buie, T.; Campbell, D.B.; Fuchs, G.J., 3rd; Furuta, G.T.; Levy, J.; VandeWater, J.; Whitaker, A.H.; Atkins, D.; Bauman, M.L.; Beaudet, A.L.; et al. Evaluation, diagnosis, and treatment of gastrointestinal disorders in individuals with ASDs: A consensus report. *Pediatrics* **2010**, *125* (Suppl. S1), S1–S18. [CrossRef]
67. Edelson, S.; Bostford Johnson, J. *Understanding and Treating Self-Injurious Behavior*; Jessica Kingsley Publishers: London, UK, 2016; Philadelphia (EEUU).
68. Russell, G.; Mandy, W.; Elliott, D.; White, R.; Pittwood, T.; Ford, T. Selection bias on intellectual ability in autism research: A cross-sectional review and meta-analysis. *Mol. Autism.* **2019**, *10*, 9. [CrossRef]
69. Jack, A.; Pelphrey, K.A. Annual Research Review: Understudied populations within the autism spectrum—Current trends and future directions in neuroimaging research. *J. Child. Psychol. Psychiatry* **2017**, *58*, 411–435. [CrossRef]
70. Fein, D.; Barton, M.; Eigsti, I.M.; Kelley, E.; Naigles, L.; Schultz, R.T.; Stevens, M.; Helt, M.; Orinstein, A.; Rosenthal, M.; et al. Optimal outcome in individuals with a history of autism. *J. Child. Psychol. Psychiatry* **2013**, *54*, 195–205. [CrossRef]
71. Herbert, M.R.; Buckley, J.A. Autism and dietary therapy: Case report and review of the literature. *J. Child. Neurol.* **2013**, *28*, 975–982. [CrossRef]
72. Yang, J.; Fu, X.; Liao, X.; Li, Y. Effects of gut microbial-based treatments on gut microbiota, behavioral symptoms, and gastrointestinal symptoms in children with autism spectrum disorder: A systematic review. *Psychiatry Res.* **2020**, *293*, 113471. [CrossRef]
73. Cervantes, P.E.; Matheis, M.; Estabillo, J.; Seag, D.E.M.; Nelson, K.L.; Peth-Pierce, R.; Hoagwood, K.E.; Horwitz, S.M. Trends Over a Decade in NIH Funding for Autism Spectrum Disorder Services Research. *J. Autism Dev. Disord.* **2020**. [CrossRef] [PubMed]

Journal of *Personalized Medicine*

Article

Pregnant Mothers' Medical Claims and Associated Risk of Their Children being Diagnosed with Autism Spectrum Disorder

Genevieve Grivas [1,2,3], Richard Frye [4,5] and Juergen Hahn [1,2,6,*]

1 Department of Biomedical Engineering, Rensselaer Polytechnic Institute, Troy, New York, NY 12180, USA; grivag@rpi.edu
2 Center for Biotechnology and Interdisciplinary Studies, Rensselaer Polytechnic Institute, Troy, New York, NY 12180, USA
3 OptumLabs Visiting Fellow, OptumLabs, Eden Prairie, MN 55344, USA
4 Department of Child Health, University of Arizona College of Medicine, Phoenix, AZ 85004, USA; rfrye@phoenixchildrens.com
5 Phoenix Children's Hospital, Phoenix, AZ 85016, USA
6 Department of Chemical and Biological Engineering, Rensselaer Polytechnic Institute, Troy, New York, NY 12180, USA
* Correspondence: hahnj@rpi.edu

Abstract: A retrospective analysis of administrative claims containing a diverse mixture of ages, ethnicities, and geographical regions across the United States was conducted in order to identify medical events that occur during pregnancy and are associated with autism spectrum disorder (ASD). The dataset used in this study is comprised of 123,824 pregnancies of which 1265 resulted in the child being diagnosed with ASD during the first five years of life. Logistic regression analysis revealed significant relationships between several maternal medical claims, made during her pregnancy and segmented by trimester, and the child's diagnosis of ASD. Having a biological sibling with ASD, maternal use of antidepressant medication and psychiatry services as well as non-pregnancy related claims such hospital visits, surgical procedures, and radiology exposure were related to an increased risk of ASD regardless of trimester. Urinary tract infections during the first trimester and preterm delivery during the second trimester were also related to an increased risk of ASD. Preventative and obstetrical care were associated with a decreased risk for ASD. A better understanding of the medical factors that increase the risk of having a child with ASD can lead to strategies to decrease risk or identify those children who require increased surveillance for the development of ASD to promote early diagnosis and intervention.

Keywords: autism spectrum disorder; medical claims; logistic regression analysis; retrospective analysis; associated risk

Citation: Grivas, G.; Frye, R.; Hahn, J. Pregnant Mothers' Medical Claims and Associated Risk of Their Children being Diagnosed with Autism Spectrum Disorder. *J. Pers. Med.* **2021**, *11*, 950. https://doi.org/10.3390/jpm11100950

Academic Editor: Farah R. Zahir

Received: 12 June 2021
Accepted: 21 September 2021
Published: 24 September 2021

Publisher's Note: MDPI stays neutral with regard to jurisdictional claims in published maps and institutional affiliations.

Copyright: © 2021 by the authors. Licensee MDPI, Basel, Switzerland. This article is an open access article distributed under the terms and conditions of the Creative Commons Attribution (CC BY) license (https://creativecommons.org/licenses/by/4.0/).

1. Introduction

Autism spectrum disorder (ASD) is an early onset neurodevelopmental disorder characterized by difficulties in social communication/interactions and by the presence of restricted and repetitive behaviors [1]. The prevalence of ASD has significantly increased over the last three decades [2] with the most recent estimate being 1 in every 54 eight-year-old children in the United States has been diagnosed with ASD with a 4.3 times higher occurrence in males than females [3]. The etiological understanding of ASD has also changed over the years, with current research suggesting a combination of genetic and environmental factors [4]. It is now generally acknowledged that investigation of environmental risk factors for ASD should not only be limited to the life of the child, but also include the prenatal and preconception period [5].

Numerous maternal body systems have been hypothesized to contribute to ASD including the gastrointestinal, immune, metabolic, and endocrine systems [6–10]. It is not surprising that research has extended these investigations to include the influence of maternal systems disorders. Maternal endocrine or hormonal disorders, such as polycystic ovary syndrome, show an increased risk of offspring developing ASD [11]. Maternal autoimmune disorders are notable ASD risk factors [12–15] with emphasis on hypothyroidism [16], psoriasis [17], and rheumatoid arthritis [18]. The presence of maternal infection during pregnancy significantly increases the risk of ASD in the offspring [19], with studies suggest this effect is specific for bacterial [20], viral [21], severe [22,23] or febrile [24,25] infections. In fact, the maternal immune activation (MIA) mouse model, a major animal model of ASD, induced ASD-like behavior in the offspring by activating the material immune system but also highlights the variability of this effect [26]. Though it may provide difficult to distinguish the confounding effects of the infection itself from the treatment for the infection, as some studies have shown antibiotic consumption is a risk factor, though there are discrepancies regarding the significance for antibiotics taken during the second or third trimester [21] or when taken for longer than 14 days [27].

It is well known that ASD is commonly linked to other cognitive or mental health disorders such as epilepsy, ADHD, and anxiety [28–31], and the role of brain development cannot be understated. Similarly, the influence of maternal mental disorders is crucial to understand and has been widely studied, with a heavy focus on maternal depression and antidepressant usage during pregnancy. Recent literature suggests the risk factor for ASD may be associated with prior antidepressant treatment or maternal psychological conditions rather than antidepressant consumption [5,32]. Another widely studied maternal pharmaceutical is prenatal vitamin supplementation, particularly folate (vitamin B9), which has been found to reduce the risk of offspring developing ASD by almost half [33–35].

Lastly, risk factors have also been found for delivery-related events such as preterm delivery [36,37] and cesarean delivery [38,39]. Though, these factors may be influenced by abnormal child development stemming from previously mentioned risk factors.

Given the large number of studies that have presented contradicting results, this work focuses on identifying ASD risk factors from a very large cohort of mothers in the United States. Specifically, this study is a retrospective analysis of maternal medical events that occurred during pregnancy and their effect on the risk of ASD in the child. These maternal events are reflected by diagnostic, procedural, and pharmaceutical claims from a private United States health plan.

2. Materials and Methods

2.1. Mother and Child Cohort Identification

This retrospective analysis used de-identified claims data with a family identifier and socioeconomic status information from the OptumLabs® Data Warehouse (OLDW), which included medical and pharmacy claims, laboratory results, and enrollment records for commercial and Medicare Advantage (MA) enrollees. The database contained longitudinal health information on enrollees and patients, representing a diverse mixture of ages, ethnicities and geographical regions across the United States [40]. As this study uses deidentified data, approval is exempt from the Institutional Review Board.

Children diagnosed with and without ASD, born between 1 January 2000 and 31 December 2010, were previously identified using the OLDW [10]. Vargason et al. (2019) used the children's diagnostic claims from their date of birth until five years of age to identify children diagnosed with ASD. This study identified the mother of these children through the use of family identifiers, policy holder relationship codes, and delivery claims within 10 days of the child's earliest enrollment date (assumed to be the child's date of birth) [41,42]. Diagnostic, pharmacy, and procedural claims (Table S1) were identified for each mother ten months prior to the birth of each child.

The processing steps used to identify children and their mothers, as well as the resulting number of women and children identified from the OLDW, are outlined in Table 1. Women were identified between the ages of 14 and 49 with commercial health coverage that included medical, pharmaceutical, and mental health coverage; this medical plan matched that of the children cohort. Step 4 outlined in Table 1 required that all children be labeled as "child" in relation to the policy holder. In Step 6, women were linked to children by having a delivery claim within 10 days of the child's first enrollment date. During this process, some children were found to be linked to multiple mothers, most likely due to different women under the same policy having birth claims at similar times; these mothers and children were excluded in Step 7. The final cohort sizes, shown in Step 8, identified various pairs of siblings (different children having the same mother) during the investigated time frame, resulting in a greater total number of children than women. This included siblings (single and multiple births) with different ASD outcomes, i.e., with and without an ASD diagnosis. For this study, each child was associated with the events that occurred during his or her gestational period, which were unique for siblings but identical for multiple births (i.e., twins and triplets). The final data set was comprised of 123,824 pregnancies identified using the OLDW data base; 1265 pregnancies resulted in children with ASD (ASD cohort), and 122,559 pregnancies resulted in children with no ASD diagnosis (population or POP cohort) during the investigated time frame. The ASD prevalence determined in this study agrees with the prevalence estimation performed by the Center for Disease Control during the same time period [43]. Within the dataset, 37,775 (30.5%) of all children had a sibling and of this 5616 (4.5%) were a part of multiple births.

Table 1. Data Attrition Steps for Identifying Mother Cohorts and Associated Children.

Data Attrition Step	Number of Women	Number of Children
1. Women who have delivery claim between 2000 and 2010	1,241,757	-
2. Women between the ages of 15 and 49, correct medical coverage, and known relationship ID	1,023,631	-
3. Children cohort identified by protocol in Vargason et al. 2019	-	283,644
4. Children with relationship ID as "child" and have a single OLDW family ID	-	234,366
5. Women and children with the same OLDW family ID	133,490	170,480
6. Women who have delivery claim within 10 days of child's first enrollment date	115,092	136,200
7. Women and children who have single linkage, and women who are continuously enrolled for one year prior to delivery claim	115,069	136,178
8. Women who have sociodemographic information on file	104,051	123,824

2.2. Medical Claims Identification

Medical claims were split up into the following three categories of variables: diagnostic claims identified by the International Classification of Diseases coding, version 9 (ICD-9), filled prescription claims determined by the National Drug Code (NDC) identifiers, and medical procedures claims denoted by their Current Procedural Terminology (CPT) coding. Total claims investigated included 478 ICD-9 diagnostic codes as variables, 10,810 NDC codes segmented into 132 pharmacy variables, and 3,808 CPT codes segmented into 122 procedural variables (Table S1). Pharmacy variables were created based on code descriptions embedded into the database. Procedural variables were based on CPT code descriptions. Table 2 shows the progression of variable selection from these categories, further outlined below.

Table 2. Progression of the Number of Variables for Diagnostic, Pharmacy, and Procedural Categories.

	Number of Variables		
	Diagnostic	Pharmacy	Procedural
Initially investigated with a claim within 10 months of delivery	478	132	122
Contained claims for greater than 2% of women within 10 months of delivery	82	27	45
Contained claims for greater than 2% of women within identified gestational days	77	25	44
Contained claims that were not highly correlated (r [1] < 0.7)	76	23	42

[1] Pearson correlation coefficient.

All variables had relatively similar percentages of claims between both cohorts (Table S1). A heuristic threshold was used to exclude variables due to uncommon claims, thereby eliminating small cell sizes and ensuring that all variables were present for both cohorts. If the number of claims fell below 2% for both cohorts combined (2476 of 123,824) or 2% for the ASD cohort only (25 of 1265) then the claim was excluded from further analysis. An example can be found in Figure S1, depicting the number of pregnancies that had a claim for the first 100 diagnostic variables (Table S1). Only variables with claims greater than 2% for the combined and ASD cohorts were further investigated (noted by the dashed lines in Figure S1, top and bottom, respectively). Thus, of the first 100 diagnostic variables, only 3 diagnostic variables were kept. Due to OptumLabs Data Policy, all cell values less than 11 are censored for de-identification purposes as noted by the y-axis starting at 11 for all figures.

Of the original 732 variables investigated, 156 remained after thresholding: 82 ICD-9 diagnostic codes, 27 pharmacy variables, and 45 procedural variables, see Table 2. These claims were then used to identify the mothers' gestational ages, as well as associated trimesters, using the same protocol presented in Li et al. [44]. Claims that fell outside of the identified gestational days were then removed and the remaining variables with claims above the threshold were kept. In addition, the following 6 maternal sociodemographic variables were included: race, home ownership, education level, income level, age, and a binary indicator for women who have had previous children with ASD. The latter variable, denoted as 'Previous ASD', refers to all subsequent children whose mother had a previous child diagnosed with ASD during the time frame of this study. This variable was included because women who have had previous children with ASD are at an increased risk of having another child with ASD [45].

For comparison, the sociodemographic data were analyzed based on individual women (referred to as "women cohorts") instead of pregnancies or resulting children (referred to as "pregnancy cohorts") to better represent the population. For this case, cohort separation is defined as women who have never had a child with ASD (population or POP) and women who have had one or more children with ASD (ASD). For ASD cohort women, age range refers to the age at which each woman had her first child with ASD, for POP cohort women it refers to the age at which she had her first child.

2.3. Statistical Analysis

A chi-square analysis was used to determine a statistically significant difference in proportions between the women's ASD and POP cohorts for the sociodemographic variables. For small cell sizes, a Fisher's exact test was used. For each age category, a Welch's t-test was used to determine statistically significant differences between mean age of the ASD and POP cohorts.

An F-test, with 5% significance level, was used to determine a statistically significant difference in variance between the ASD and POP cohort for total number of medical claims (diagnostic, pharmacy, and procedural combined), as well as each variable category individually. For categories that showed a statistically significant difference in variance, a

Welch two-sample *t*-test was used to determine a statistically significant difference between the mean number of claims for the ASD and POP cohorts, at a 5% significance level. For equal variance, a standard t-test was used at a 5% significance level. Histograms were normalized in order to better compare the two cohorts.

Logistic regression was used to estimate the relationship between the presence of ASD in the child over the investigated time frame and the maternal medical claim (diagnostic, pharmacy, or procedural) made during pregnancy [46]. Pearson correlation analysis was conducted to identify claims that were highly correlated with any other claim, $r >= 0.7$, of which those of lower significance (denoted using *p*-values calculated from the unadjusted logistic regression) were removed from the analysis (see Table 2) [47,48]. Adjusted odds ratios (ORs) were used to quantify the effect of the medical claim and the associated risk of the child being diagnosed with ASD later, using a 95% confidence interval [49]. An initial logistic regression model showed the previous ASD variable was highly skewed towards the ASD cohort due to bias associated with multiple births; to correct for this, two adjusted logistic regression models were used, one with all variables and one with all variables except previous ASD. The statistically significant variables determined from these two models were then used for a third adjusted logistic regression model, which allowed for correction of multiple comparisons by reducing the number of variables included in the model as well as identifying false significance from the latter models. A schematic of the model development can be found in Figure 1. Due to computational restrictions, all logistic regression models were built using 10% of the POP cohort data, resulting in a ratio of approximately 10:1 POP to ASD, stratified based on sociodemographic variables. This analysis was then repeated for each trimester excluding sociodemographic variables since these are constant throughout the entire pregnancy. For brevity, all statistically significant findings as defined in this section and reported in this study are referred to as significant.

Some diagnostic variables were further specified based on their ICD-9 coding. ICD-9 codes are structured through a numeric system where a whole value code can also contain decimal values to elaborate on a diagnosis. For example, ICD-9 code 649 corresponds to the variable Other Conditions Complicating Pregnancy and can be broken down as follows: 649.0 tobacco use disorder complicating pregnancy, 649.1 obesity complicating pregnancy, 649.2 bariatric surgery complicating pregnancy, etc. Claims are made using either whole values or decimal points, at the discretion of the medical professional. All statistically significant final diagnostic variables are further evaluated by their whole and single digit ICD-9 coding in a separate logistic regression analysis, shown in Figure 1. Variables were only included in this analysis if they contain claims greater than 11, and due to this smaller threshold were evaluated with both unadjusted and adjusted ORs.

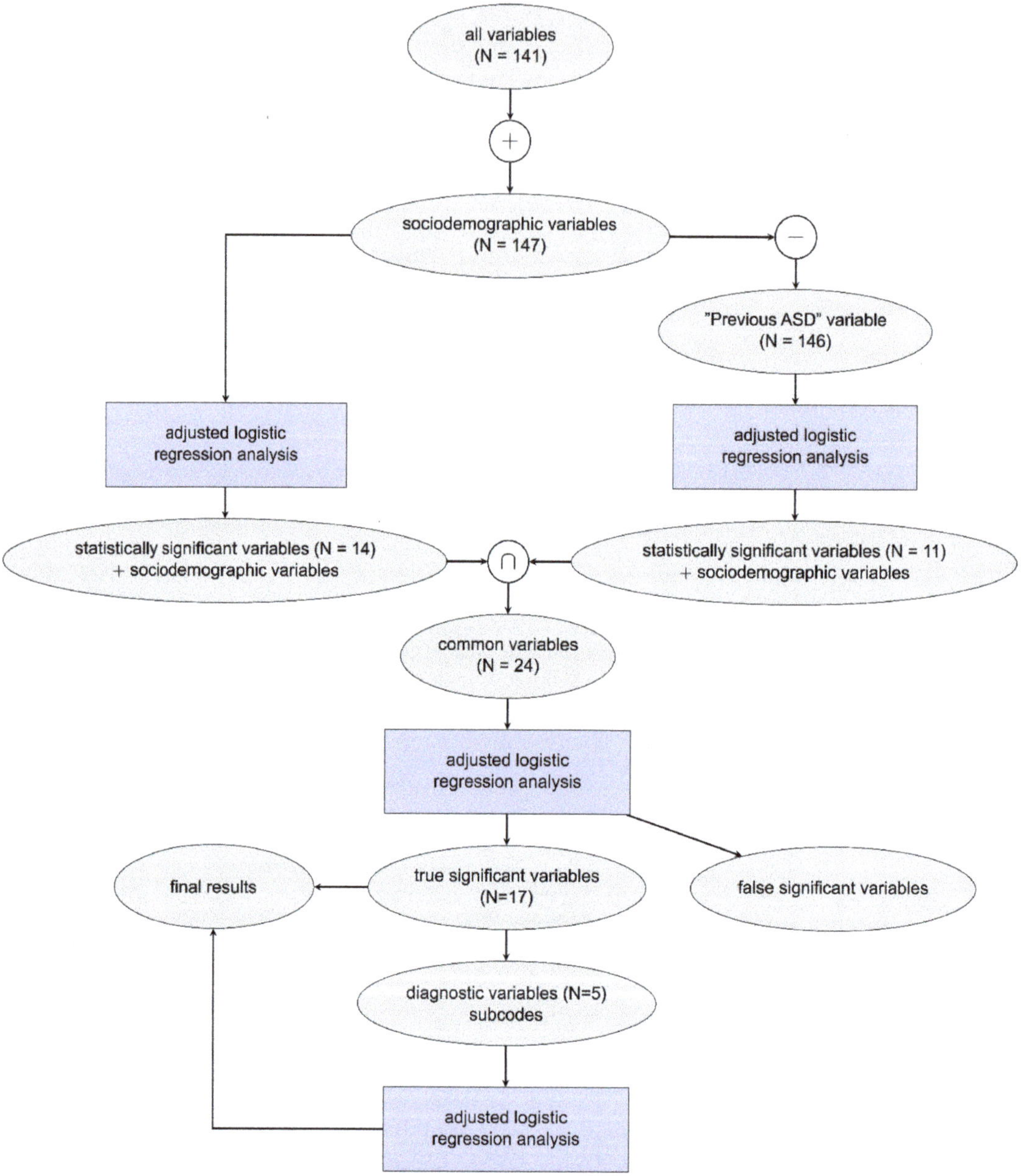

Figure 1. Schematic of model development where N represents the number of variables included for each analysis on claims data obtained throughout the entire pregnancy. This procedure was also repeated for each trimester individually (not shown).

3. Results

There were some key differences in sociodemographic data for the two women cohorts (Table 3). The percentages for race were for the most part comparable, with the majority being White, however, a significantly larger percentage of Asian pregnancies in the ASD cohort (10.4%) was found compared to the POP cohort (7.7%). In addition, the ASD cohort, as compared to the POP cohort, was significantly more educated (i.e., attained a degree higher than a Bachelor's degree), had higher income (i.e., income greater than USD 125,000) and was older (i.e., age 30 years or older), see Tables 3 and 4. Furthermore, the ASD cohort had a significantly smaller percentage of women having only a high school diploma, an income between USD 40,000–74,999, and being of age between 20–29 years old. The ASD cohort had a significantly higher percentage of previous ASD children, 245 (20.1%), compared to the 0 (0.0%) from the POP cohort. This was obviously expected since the women POP cohort is defined as women who have never had a child with ASD and thus will not have a previous ASD indicator.

Table 3. Sociodemographic Data on Women Cohorts.

		ASD Women		POP Women		
		1218 *n* [1]	%	102,833 *n* [1]	%	*p*-Value [2]
Race	Asian	127	10.4	7949	7.7	**<0.001**
	Black	91	7.5	8275	8.0	0.50
	Hispanic	119	9.8	11,088	10.8	0.28
	White	881	72.3	75,521	73.4	0.40
Home Owner-ship	Unknown	>118	>9.6	10,304	10.0	0.61
	Probable Owner	1089	89.4	92,117	89.6	0.88
	Probable Renter [3]	<11	<1.0	412	0.4	0.10
Education Level	Less than 12th Grade [3]	<11	<1.0	305	0.3	0.79
	High School Diploma	>153	>12.4	19,160	18.6	**<0.001**
	Less than a Bachelor's Degree	666	54.7	54,339	52.8	0.21
	Bachelor's Degree Plus	388	31.9	29,029	28.2	**0.006**
Income Range	<USD 40,000	79	6.5	7841	7.6	0.15
	USD 40,000–74,999	206	16.9	19,776	19.2	**0.045**
	USD 75,000–124,999	347	28.5	31,837	31.0	0.07
	USD 125,000–199,999	316	25.9	23,786	23.1	**0.023**
	>USD 200,000	270	22.2	19,593	19.1	**0.007**
Age Range	<20 [3]	<11	<1.0	290	0.3	0.27
	20–29	312	25.6	32,587	31.7	**<0.001**
	30–39	805	66.1	63,991	62.2	**0.006**
	40–49	>90	>7.3	5965	5.8	**<0.001**
Previous ASD	Yes	245	20.1	0	0.0	**<0.001**
	No	973	79.9	102,833	100.0	**<0.001**

[1] Number of women. [2] *p*-values are calculated using chi-squared analysis or Fisher's exact test for small cell values, significant *p*-values are shown in bold. [3] Values < 11 are censored for anonymity and *p*-values are calculated using Fisher's exact test.

Table 4. Age Statistics on Women Cohorts.

		ASD Women	POP Women	
		Mean (Median)		*p*-Value [1]
Age Range	<20 [2]			
	20–29	26.8 (27)	26.6 (27)	0.36
	30–39	34.1 (34)	33.8 (34)	**<0.001**
	40–49	42.3 (42)	42.3 (42)	0.80

[1] *p*-values are calculated using chi-squared analysis or Fisher's exact test for small cell values, significant *p*-values are shown in bold. [2] values < 11 are censored for anonymity and *p*-values are calculated using Fisher's exact test.

Correlation analysis for all variables during the entire pregnancy depicted six pairs of variables containing correlations of 0.7 or higher. These variables and their associated unadjusted p-values are shown in Table S2. The variable with the larger p-value in each pairwise correlation was discarded from the adjusted logistic regression analysis; variables that remain in the analysis are bolded in Table S2. Three pairs of highly correlated variables all related to the same medical event of receiving a vaccination (variables: Vaccinations, Need for Prophylactic Vaccination against Viral Diseases, and Immunization Administration for Vaccinations). The remaining three pairs of variables were associated with a cardiovascular procedure, diabetic-related materials (such as test strips), and a thyroid disorder.

Normalized histograms for claims from both the ASD and POP cohort can be found in Figure 2 with associated descriptive statistics in Table 5. These data were generated by summing claims made throughout each entire pregnancy. Histograms for all medical claims (diagnostic, pharmacy, and procedural) and only diagnostic claims (Figure 2A,B, respectively) closely followed a normal distribution as shown by the similar mean, median, and mode values listed in Table 5. Pharmacy claims and procedural claims (Figure 2C,D) were right- and left-skewed, respectively, where most women had few (1–2) prescriptions and many (14–16) procedural claims. For all categories of variables (including total combination), the ASD cohort had a statistically significantly higher mean number of claims than the POP cohort.

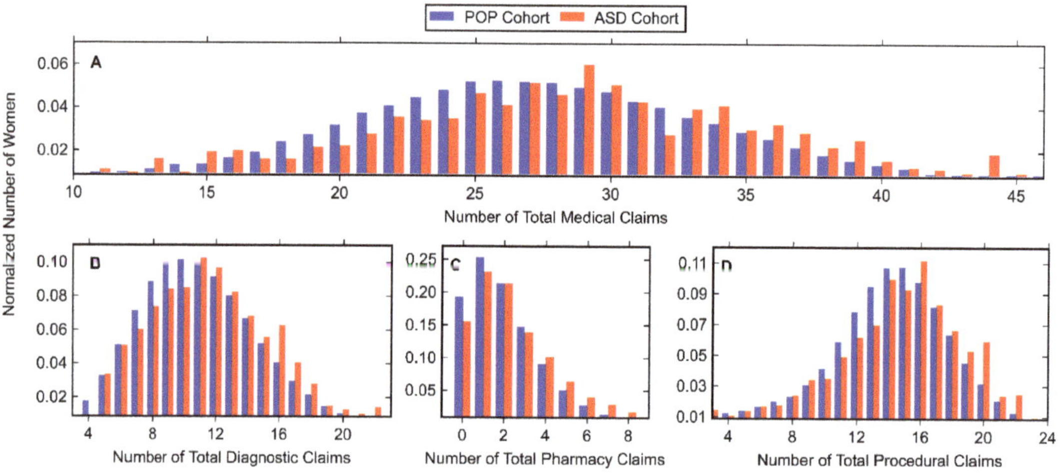

Figure 2. Histogram data of normalized number of women belonging to the POP and ASD cohorts (shown in blue and red, respectively) with (**A**) any medical claim, (**B**) diagnostic claim, (**C**) pharmacy claim, or (**D**) procedural claim. Values associated with small cell sizes are not shown in order to be compliant with OptumLabs' de-identification policy.

Table 5. Statistics on Number of Medical Claims during Entire Pregnancy.

							Difference in Distribution	
	Cohort	Max	Mean	Median	Mode	Stdev [2]	Variance p-Value [1] (95% CI [3])	Mean p-Value [1] (95% CI [3])
All Medical Claims	POP	73	27.1	27	26	8.6	**<0.001**	**<0.001** [4]
	ASD	59	28.6	29	29	9.4	(1.10, 1.40)	(1.13, 2.74)
Diagnostic Claims	POP	34	11.1	11	10	4.0	**<0.001**	**<0.001** [4]
	ASD	29	11.7	11	11	4.2	(1.09, 1.40)	(0.34, 1.06)
Pharmacy Claims	POP	15	2.1	2	1	1.8	**<0.001**	**<0.001** [4]
	ASD	15	2.5	2	1	2.1	(1.20, 1.54)	(0.29, 0.65)
Procedural Claims	POP	31	13.9	14	15	4.4	0.102	**<0.001** [5]
	ASD	26	14.4	15	16	4.7	(0.98, 1.26)	(0.36, 1.18)

[1] All p-values are calculated using random samples of 1000, significant p-values are shown in bold. [2] Standard deviation. [3] Confidence intervals. [4] Calculated using Welch two-sample t-test. [5] Calculated using two-sample t-test.

Normalized histograms for claims made in each trimester, along with descriptive statistics, can be found in Figures 3 and 4, as well as Table 6. The largest number of total medical claims was made in the third trimester with similar values for the first and second trimester. While the mean and median number of claims was greater in the first trimester compared to the second, the first trimester had a greater amount of zero-claims. In all trimesters, the majority of claims were made for procedures, followed by diagnostics and pharmacy. For all trimesters, the ASD cohort had a significantly higher mean number of diagnostics, pharmacy and procedural claims with one exception: diagnostic claims made in the first trimester showed no significant difference.

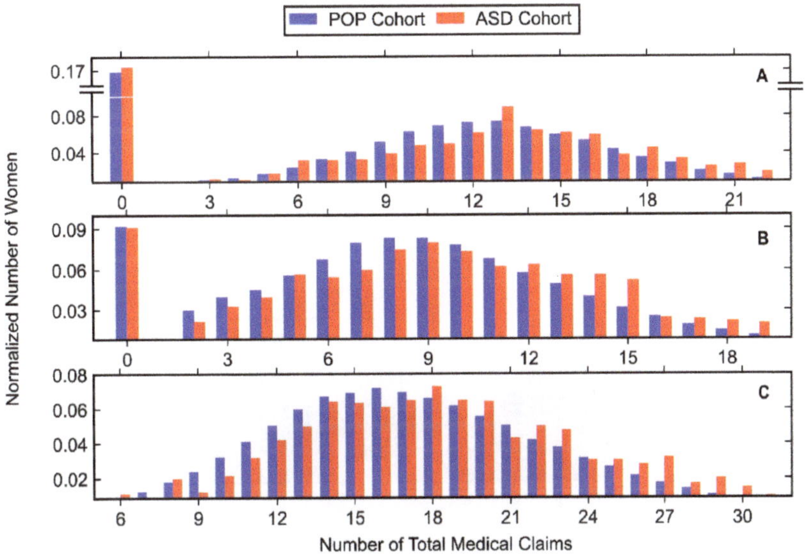

Figure 3. Histogram data of normalized number of women belonging to the POP and ASD cohorts (shown in blue and red, respectively) with any medical claim during the (**A**) first trimester, (**B**) second trimester, and (**C**) third trimester. Values associated with small cell sizes are not shown in order to be compliant with OptumLabs' de-identification policy.

Table 6. Statistics of Number of Medical Claims during Each Trimester.

	Cohort	Max	Mean	Median	Mode	Stdev [2]	Difference in Distribution: Variance p-Value [1] (95% CI [3])	Difference in Distribution: Mean p-Value [1] (95% CI [3])
Trimester 1 All Medical Claims	POP	38	10.6	11	0	6.5	**0.040**	**0.011** [4]
	ASD	33	11.2	12	0	7.0	(1.01, 1.29)	(0.18, 1.38)
Diagnostic Claims	POP	15	2.7	3	2	2.1	0.080	0.077 [5]
	ASD	11	2.8	3	0	2.2	(0.99, 1.26)	(−0.01,0.36)
Pharmacy Claims	POP	10	0.9	1	0	1.1	**<0.001**	**<0.001** [4]
	ASD	8	1.1	1	0	1.3	(1.19, 1.52)	(0.10, 0.30)
Procedural Claims	POP	21	7.0	8	0	4.2	0.076	**0.038** [5]
	ASD	18	7.2	8	0	4.5	(0.99, 1.27)	(0.02, 0.79)
Trimester 2 All Medical Claims	POP	36	8.7	9	0	5.2	**<0.001**	**<0.001** [4]
	ASD	36	9.5	9	0	5.7	(1.13, 1.44)	(0.53, 1.47)
Diagnostic Claims	POP	14	2.7	2	2	1.9	**<0.001**	**<0.001** [4]
	ASD	12	3.0	3	2	2.1	(1.20, 1.54)	(0.21, 0.56)

Table 6. *Cont.*

	Cohort	Max	Mean	Median	Mode	Stdev [2]	Difference in Distribution Variance p-Value [1] (95% CI [3])	Mean p-Value [1] (95% CI [3])
Pharmacy Claims	POP ASD	8 8	0.8 0.9	1 1	0 1	0.9 1.0	**0.022** (1.02, 1.31)	**<0.001** [4] (0.06, 0.23)
Procedural Claims	POP ASD	20 16	5.1 5.5	5 6	6 6	3.3 3.5	**0.019** (1.02, 1.31)	**0.002** [4] (0.17, 0.77)
Trimester 3 All Medical Claims	POP ASD	47 42	17.4 18.5	17 18	16 18	5.9 6.1	0.105 (0.98, 1.25)	**<0.001** [5] (0.75, 1.82)
Diagnostic Claims	POP ASD	21 17	7.7 8.1	7 8	7 8	2.6 2.6	0.420 (0.93, 1.19)	**0.002** [5] (0.13, 0.59)
Pharmacy Claims	POP ASD	9 8	1.1 1.3	1 1	0 1	1.1 1.3	**<0.001** (1.25, 1.60)	**<0.001** [4] (0.18, 0.40)
Procedural Claims	POP ASD	25 21	8.6 9.1	8 9	8 7	3.6 3.8	0.537 (0.92, 1.18)	**<0.001** [5] (0.31, 0.97)

[1] All p-values are calculated using random samples of 1000, significant p-values are shown in bold. [2] Standard deviation. [3] Confidence intervals. [4] Calculated using Welch two-sample t-test. [5] Calculated using two-sample t-test.

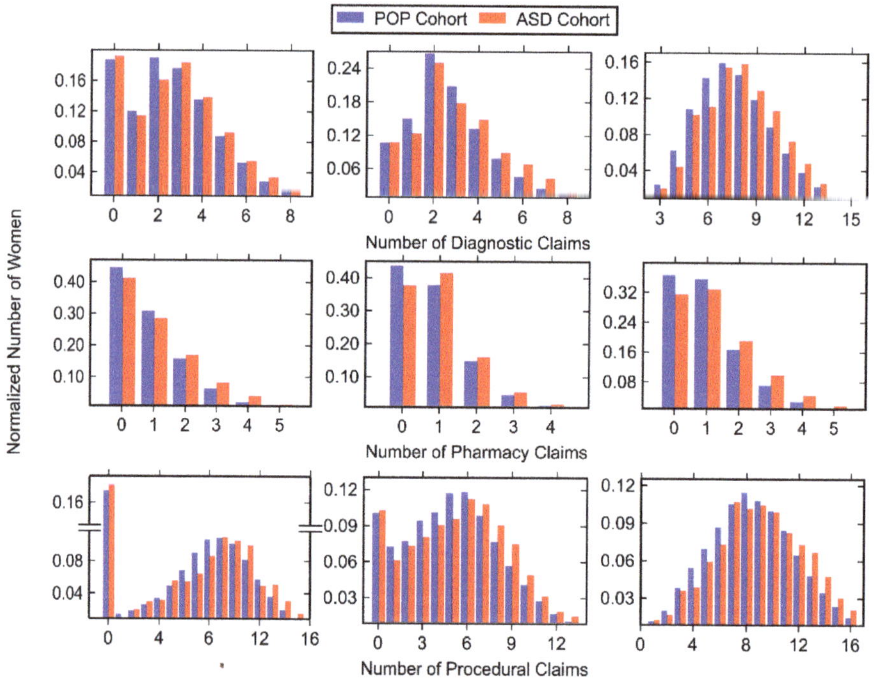

Figure 4. Histogram data of normalized number of women belonging to the POP and ASD cohorts (shown in blue and red, respectively) with any diagnostic (top row), pharmacy (middle row), and procedural (bottom row) claim during the first trimester (left column), second trimester (middle column), and third trimester (right column). Values associated with small cell sizes are not shown in order to be compliant with OptumLabs' de-identification policy.

The adjusted logistic regression models (with and without previous ASD) show a total of 20 significant variables (Table S3): 2 sociodemographic variables, 7 diagnostic variables, 3 pharmacy variables, and 8 procedural variables. When modeled by themselves, only 17 of these significant variables retained their significance (Table 7, full model results can be found in Table S3). A majority of the variables (13 of 17) were associated with an increased risk of having a child diagnosed with ASD. While both sociodemographic variables showed an increased risk, having a child previously diagnosed with ASD was associated with the largest increased risk of all variables, OR 16.09 (8.27, 32.12). Three diagnostic, all three pharmacy, and five procedural variables were also associated with an increased risk. The remaining four variables (two diagnostic and two procedural) were associated with a significantly decreased risk. Results for the subcode logistic regression analysis on diagnostic variables from the entire pregnancy can be found in Table S4.

Table 7. Logistic Regression Analysis Results of Variables Identified as Highly Significant during the Entire Pregnancy.

	Odds Ratio [1] (95% CI [2])	*p*-Value [1]
Sociodemographic Variables		
Previous ASD	16.1 (8.27, 32.1)	<0.001
Race—Asian	1.36 (1.11, 1.66)	0.003
Diagnostic Variables		
Special Screening for Blood Disorders	1.39 (1.06, 1.80)	0.015
Other Indications Related to Labor	1.28 (1.13, 1.45)	<0.001
Other Complications of Labor	1.27 (1.09, 1.47)	0.002
Other Conditions Complicating Pregnancy	0.70 (0.54, 0.88)	0.003
Special Screening for Malignant Neoplasms	0.79 (0.66, 1.00)	0.005
Pharmacy Variables		
Antidepressants	1.44 (1.15, 1.79)	0.001
Durable Medical Equipment Diabetic	1.27 (1.00, 1.59)	0.043
Nutritional Vitamins	1.18 (1.04, 1.33)	0.008
Procedural Variables		
Anesthesia Procedures Lower Abdomen	1.81 (1.30, 2.46)	<0.001
Procedures Pulmonary	1.66 (1.24, 2.19)	<0.001
Procedures Services Psychiatry	1.44 (1.17, 1.76)	<0.001
Services Consultation	1.37 (1.21, 1.56)	<0.001
Procedures Diagnostic Radiology	1.15 (1.02, 1.30)	0.025
Vaccinations	0.58 (0.46, 0.71)	<0.001
Evaluations Physical Medicine and Rehabilitation	0.77 (0.62, 0.94)	0.015

[1] *p*-value and odds ratios are calculated using adjusted logistic regression analysis. [2] Confidence intervals.

Results from the adjusted logistic regression analyses for all trimester variables can be found in Table S3. The final significant variables identified for each trimester can be found in Table 8; some of these variables differed from the entire pregnancy analysis due to the different number of claims that occur in each trimester. A larger number of significant variables occurred for the first and third trimesters (15) compared to the second trimester (13). While all trimesters had a majority of variables associated with increased risk, the third trimester had the most variables associated with increased risk (11) while the first trimester had the most variables that were associated with decreased risk (5). Multiple Gestation, Antidepressants, and Procedure Services Psychiatry variables were consistently associated with increased risk for all three trimesters.

The variable Other Conditions Complicating Pregnancy was associated with a significantly increased risk during the third trimester, however further analysis showed that no subcode was significant for this occurrence and thus this study is not able to determine what event influenced this diagnosis (see Table S4). Similarly, Services Office or Other Outpatient was associated with a significantly increased risk during the second trimester. This variable corresponds to a new patient visit; however, this study is unable to determine if this visit was related to pregnancy or another maternal health-related event.

Table 8. Logistic Regression Analysis Results of Variables Identified as Highly Significant during each Trimester.

	Trimester 1	Trimester 2	Trimester 3
	Odds Ratio [1] **(95% CI** [2]**)** ***p*-Value** [1]	**Odds Ratio** [1] **(95% CI** [2]**)** ***p*-Value** [1]	**Odds Ratio** [1] **(95% CI** [2]**)** ***p*-Value** [1]
Diagnostic Variables			
Multiple Gestation	1.49 (1.10, 1.98) 0.009	1.69 (1.33, 2.12) <0.001	1.56 (1.25, 1.94) <0.001
Other Disorders of Urethra and Urinary Tract	1.49 (1.19, 1.86) <0.001	–	–
Other Symptoms Involving Abdomen and Pelvis	1.42 (1.08, 1.83) 0.010	1.42 (1.09, 1.82) 0.007	–
Special Screening for Endocrine Nutritional Metabolic and Immunity Disorders	1.36 (1.05, 1.73) 0.016	–	–
Normal Pregnancy	–	1.33 (1.16, 1.54) <0.001	–
Acquired Hypothyroidism	–	–	1.31 (0.99, 1.70) <0.050
Other Indications Related to Labor	–	1.33 (1.14, 1.54) <0.001	1.27 (1.13, 1.43) <0.001
Other Complications of Labor	–	–	1.22 (1.05, 1.42) 0.010
Need for Prophylactic Vaccination against Certain Viral Diseases	–	0.60 (0.41, 0.83) 0.004	–
Antepartum Hemorrhage and Placenta Previa	–	–	0.71 (0.55, 0.92) 0.010
Other Conditions Complicating Pregnancy	–	–	0.74 (0.55, 0.97) 0.036
Abnormality of Pelvis	0.64 (0.44, 0.92) 0.019	–	0.86 (0.75, 0.99) 0.044
Special Screening for Malignant Neoplasms	0.76 (0.63, 0.91) 0.004	–	–
Antenatal Screening	0.82 (0.71, 0.95) 0.007	–	–
Special Investigations and Examinations	0.83 (0.73, 0.95) 0.006	–	–
Pharmacy			
Anti-inflammatory Glucocorticoids	1.44 (1.08, 1.89) 0.011	–	–
Antidepressants	1.40 (1.08, 1.81) 0.010	1.45 (1.08, 1.93) 0.011	1.55 (1.18, 2.00) 0.001
Respiratory Antihistamines	–	1.39 (1.03, 1.83) 0.026	1.62 (1.20, 2.15) 0.001
Nutritional Vitamins	–	1.19 (1.05, 1.34) 0.005	1.19 (1.06, 1.34) 0.004

Table 8. *Cont.*

	Trimester 1	Trimester 2	Trimester 3
	Odds Ratio [1] (95% CI [2]) *p*-Value [1]	Odds Ratio [1] (95% CI [2]) *p*-Value [1]	Odds Ratio [1] (95% CI [2]) *p*-Value [1]
Procedural Variables			
Consultations Clinical Pathology	1.76 (1.25, 2.45) 0.001	-	-
Procedures Services Psychiatry	1.66 (1.24, 2.19) <0.001	1.64 (1.20, 2.20) 0.001	1.46 (1.13, 1.85) 0.003
Surgical Procedures Female Genital System	1.65 (1.26, 2.15) <0.001	-	-
Services Consultation	1.56 (1.30, 1.87) <0.001	-	1.48 (1.25, 1.75) <0.001
Surgical Procedures Nervous System	-	-	1.32 (1.00, 1.72) 0.045
Surgical Procedures Maternity Care and Delivery	-	1.31 (1.09, 1.57) 0.004	-
Services Office or Other Outpatient	-	1.23 (1.08, 1.40) 0.002	-
Procedures Urinalysis	-	-	1.18 (1.04, 1.33) 0.012
Procedures Diagnostic Ultrasound	-	0.61 (0.51, 0.73) <0.001	-
Evaluations Physical Medicine and Rehabilitation	-	0.67 (0.48, 0.92) 0.016	-
Vaccinations	-	-	0.68 (0.47, 0.96) 0.037
Procedures Other Pathology and Laboratory	0.79 (0.65, 0.96) 0.022	-	-

[1] *p*-value and odds ratios are calculated using adjusted logistic regression analysis. [2] Confidence intervals.

4. Discussion

The majority of this study's significant findings were associated with an increased risk of having a child with ASD. Many of these correspond to a single variable in the model such as having a previous child with ASD (Table 7, Previous ASD), first pregnancy over the age of 35 (Table 7, Other Indications Related to Labor), current cesarean delivery (Tables 7 and 8, Other Complications of Labor), prescription for antidepressants (Tables 7 and 8), psychiatric services (Tables 7 and 8), pre-existing diabetes (Table 7, Durable Medical Equipment Diabetic), urinary tract infection during the first trimester (Table 8, Other Disorders of Urethra and Urinary Tract), and premature pregnancy (Table 8, variables Normal Pregnancy and Surgical Procedures Maternity Care and Delivery). Some of these variables were grouped in order to identify a common theme associated with ASD such as variables corresponding to standard obstetrical procedures, non-pregnancy related procedures, or maternal immune dysfunction and allergens. Lastly, a few variables and their associations with ASD disagreed with current literature, such as being of Asian race, having a prescription for pre-natal vitamins, and having multiple gestations. These findings, and others, have all been further discussed below and a summary can be found in Table 9, listed as they appear in this section.

Table 9. Summary of Study Findings.

Finding	Associated Risk of ASD
Being of Asian race	Increase
Having previous children diagnosed with ASD	Increase
First pregnancy over the age of 35	Increase
Current cesarean delivery	Increase
Prescription for antidepressants and procedure of psychiatric services	Increase
Pre-existing diabetes	Increase
Pre-natal vitamins	Increase
Vaccinations	Decrease
Standard obstetrical procedures	Decrease
Non-pregnancy related procedures	Increase
Urinary tract infection during the first trimester	Increase
Premature pregnancy	Increase
Maternal immune dysfunction or allergens	Increase
Multiple gestation	Increase

The data cohorts identified in this study found the highest percentage of ASD pregnancies among White children, followed by Asian, Hispanic, and Black children. This trend agrees with that reported in a CDC surveillance completed within the same time period as this study [43] except for those of Asian race, which was found to vary widely depending on location and where our study shows a significantly larger proportion in the ASD women's cohort (p-value < 0.001, Table 3). Asian race was associated with a 40% increased risk of having a child diagnosed with ASD (Table 7). The most recent CDC surveillance summary showed similar prevalence between Asian and White children within the United States [3]. Therefore, it is most likely that the increase in risk associated with Asian race found in this study was a result of sample bias as noted by the significantly greater percentage of Asian ASD women identified in Table 3.

It is well known that the recurrence risk for ASD in families is much greater than the risk for the general population, therefore, women who have a child with ASD are considered high-risk for having subsequent children diagnosed with ASD [45]. Our study confirmed and clarified this finding, suggesting a 16-fold increased risk associated with having another child with ASD when a previous child was diagnosed with ASD (Table 7). There was also evidence to suggest that this elevated risk increased with each additional child diagnosed with ASD [50,51]. However, having a child diagnosed with ASD may influence the parental decision of having subsequent children, known as reproductive stoppage, which is a confounding factor [51–53].

Sociodemographic trends for ASD noted a higher prevalence of the disorder among higher levels of education and income [54,55], similar to what was found in this study (see Table 3). While advanced maternal age was not reflected in the sociodemographic variables of the logistic regression analysis, it was reflected in the diagnostic subcode Elderly Primigravida (ICD-9 659.5, Table S4) of the variable Other Indications Related to Labor, ICD-9 659, which demonstrated an overall adjusted OR 1.28 (1.13, 1.45; Table 7). This subcode corresponds to women with their first pregnancy over the age of 35. Advanced maternal age has been associated with an increased risk of ASD, with studies showing the association for the highest age category [56], age greater than 35 [5,57], or age greater than 40 [58].

Our analysis showed that cesarean delivery (ICD-9 669.7, Table S4) was the significant contributing factor to the diagnostic variable Other Complications of Labor, ICD-9 669, OR 1.27 (1.09, 1.47), Table 7, overall as well as during the third trimester, OR 1.22 (1.05, 1.42), Table S4. Previous studies reported inconclusive results for associating ASD with cesarean delivery. Some studies showed a weak or no association [15,59,60] while others showed a significantly increased risk [39,61] though this may be correlated with the risk factors associated with the cause for cesarean delivery instead of the delivery itself [62,63]. Some studies find cesarean delivery with general anesthesia significantly increased the risk of ASD compared to cesarean delivery with regional anesthesia or other indications [38,64]. While some women elect to have a cesarean delivery, more commonly they occur due to complications that arise during pregnancy or delivery, which vary depending on maternal age [65]. Cesarean deliveries change the risk profiles for both the mother and newborn [66] and may directly affect the environment of newborns and possibly even their microbiome [67,68]. There are even long-term health risks associated with the delivery following a cesarean [69]. However, our study found that having a previous cesarean delivery (before the current pregnancy), code ICD-9 654.2, was associated with a decreased risk of ASD during the third trimester (Table S4), with an overall OR 0.86 (0.75, 0.99) denoted by Abnormality of Pelvis, ICD-9 654, Table 8. While currently there is little research on the effect of previous cesarean delivery or even vaginal birth after cesarean (VBAC) and having a child diagnosed with ASD, women with previous cesarean deliveries are more carefully managed, especially during labor [70,71]. It is possible that these extra precautions are a confounding factor as this finding contradicts other literature that associate prior cesarean delivery with an increased risk of adverse reproductive outcomes for subsequent pregnancies [72–75].

A prescription for antidepressants was significantly associated with an increased risk for ASD, with an overall risk greater than 40% and increased per trimester. Maternal antidepressant usage is a highly researched area as a potential risk factor for ASD. Many studies have shown that antidepressants, including the use of selective serotonin reuptake inhibitors (SSRIs), are associated with a significantly increased risk of the child developing ASD [5,76,77]. Contrary to this, other reviews find conflicting results [78,79] or no significant association [80]. However, recent investigations also examined the underlying mental illness, as many studies have shown that adjusting for depression attenuates the significant association of antidepressants while the association of mental illness remains strong [81–86]. Our analysis found a greater than 40% significantly increased risk associated with psychiatric services (Table 7), that increased to greater than 60% during the first trimester and decreased with each trimester (Table 8). We did not find a sufficient number of claims for Major Depression Disorder (ICD-9 311) to include in this analysis. As antidepressant medications are widely used for multiple psychiatric conditions, including anxiety, bipolar disorder and others, the data may suggest that an increased risk of ASD may be associated with a wider array of psychiatric conditions in the family, as have been documented in other studies [87]. However, it is clear that the risk associated with maternal antidepressant usage is heavily influenced based on study design [88], and that it is of great importance to acknowledge the underlying confounding effects of mental health disorders.

Our study did not have a sufficient number of claims to include the diagnosis of diabetes (ICD-9 250) and did not find a diagnosis for gestational diabetes (ICD-9 648) significant, but found that a prescription for Diabetic Durable Medical Equipment (DME, such as insulin needles) was associated with a significantly increased risk of ASD, OR 1.27 (1.00, 1.59), Table 7. This finding suggests a significant association with diabetes that may have been diagnosed before the time of our study. The risk of maternal diabetes associated with ASD remains unclear, with reviews suggesting a strong [89,90], moderate [15], or no [91] relationship. While some studies combine the effects of any type of diabetes, others suggest that familiar type 1 diabetes [13], gestational diabetes [92,93], or only diabetes in conjunction with obesity [94] are associated with an increased risk. Though, individuals who are predisposed to diabetes may act as a confounding factor. Extensive reviews have been conducted on how diabetes may relate to biological mechanisms involved in the development of ASD, specifically through the oxidative stress pathways [95].

Many studies show a significantly decreased risk associated with pre-natal vitamins [33,96], such as folic-acid supplements [34,97] or fatty acids [98]. However, our study showed an increased risk, overall OR 1.18 (1.04, 1.33), shown in Table 7, as well as a similar increased risk in the second and third trimesters, Table 8. This finding may not truly reflect the relationship between pre-natal vitamins and ASD as most vitamins are provided over the counter and therefore do not appear within an insurance claim and are not represented in this study. It is also possible that there are unknown reasons associated with receiving a prescription for nutritional vitamins that may be acting as a confounding factor such as economic concerns or medical conditions. For example, individuals with a previous child with ASD may specifically request a prescription for vitamins. The fact that a large well-done study demonstrated that higher folate supplementation was associated with a decreased risk of ASD would suggest other confounding factors are possible [35]. In addition, our study did not quantify the type of vitamins prescribed, (i.e., vitamin D, vitamin B, multivitamin, dietary supplements, etc.). For example, prescribing folic acid, an oxidized folate that is poorly metabolized and poorly transported across the placenta in some women, as opposed to a reduced folate which has much higher bioavailability, can result in high levels of unmetabolized folate in the blood in those with poor folate metabolism [99]. This can lead some to make the wrong conclusions that too much folate supplementation during pregnancy can be associated with an increased risk for ASD [100], whereas the problem lies with providing the correct type of bioavailable folate [101].

One finding that did show a significantly decreased risk of having a child with ASD, was a procedure claim for receiving a vaccination, OR 0.58 (0.46, 0.71), Table 7. This was also significant in the third trimester, OR 0.68 (0.47, 0.96), as well as the second trimester (diagnosis claim Need for Prophylactic Vaccination against Certain Viral Diseases), OR 0.60 (0.41, 0.83), Table 8. This study was unable to determine the type of vaccination, however. There is a limitation of relating this paper's findings to influenza vaccination as many instances of this vaccination can occur within the community, outside of a doctor's office, and thus would not appear within the claim's data. Vaccinations have been recommended during pregnancy in order to prevent infections [102].

Other standard obstetrical procedures showed a decreased risk, specifically Uterine Size and Date Discrepancy (Table S4, ICD-9 649.6), Special Screening of Malignant Neoplasms (of Cervix) overall and during the first trimester (Tables 7 and 8, respectively), Cervical Incompetence (ICD-9 654.5 Table S4) during the first trimester, Antenatal Screening and Pregnancy Evaluation (ICD-9 V28.5-6 and V72.4, respectively, see Table S4) during the first trimester, Diagnostic Ultrasound Procedures during the second trimester (Table 8), physical therapy (Evaluations Physical Medicine and Rehabilitation) overall and during the second trimester (Tables 7 and 8, respectively), and Procedures Other Pathology and Laboratory during the first trimester (Table 8). It is well documented that obstetric complications increase the risk of having a child with ASD [103–105] and it is clinically recommended that women who are at high risk should be closely monitored throughout their pregnancy [102]. Thus, these findings suggest that women with earlier and more aggressive obstetrical care have a decreased risk of ASD.

Various hospital procedures showed an increased risk such as an in-hospital consultation (Services Consultation) overall and during the first and third trimester (Tables 7 and 9, respectively), surgical procedures that may require anesthesia (Anesthesia Procedures Lower Abdomen shown in Table 7, Surgical Procedures Female Genital System during the first trimester and Surgical Procedures Nervous System during the third trimester shown in Table 8), ventilation or breathing tests (Procedures Pulmonary, Table 7), and Procedures Diagnostic Radiology (Table 7). While the following claims may not have required hospitalization they also show an increased risk: Special Screening for Blood Disorders (Table 7), Special Screening for Endocrine Nutritional Metabolic and Immunity Disorders during the first trimester, Abdominal Pain (Other Symptoms Involving Abdomen and Pelvis) during the first trimester, Acquired Hypothyroidism during the third trimester, Consultations Clinical Pathology during the first trimester, and Services Office or Other Outpatient during the second trimester (all of which can be found in Table 8). These findings suggest that claims not relating to the pregnancy nor delivery are associated with an increased risk of ASD regardless of trimester.

Our study showed an increased risk of UTI (Other Disorder of Urethra and Urinary Tract) but only during the first trimester, OR 1.49 (1.19, 1.86), shown in Table 8. UTIs have been shown to be common during pregnancy but have inconclusive associations with ASD [19–22,24,25,60,106]. Urinalysis procedures showed an increased ASD risk during the third trimester, OR 1.18 (1.04, 1.33), Table 8. However, urinalysis procedures refer to any urine examination and is not only associated with diagnosing UTI but may include other tests such as testing for pre-eclampsia. Pre-eclampsia has been shown to have an increased risk for ASD [5,107], but a diagnosis (ICD-9 642) was not found to be significant in this study. Maternal Antepartum Hemorrhage and Placenta Previa showed a decreased risk of ASD during the third trimester, OR 0.71 (0.55, 0.92), Table 8. Antepartum hemorrhage has been shown to be associated with intellectual disability but not ASD [60], while placenta previa is associated with a decreased incidence of pre-eclampsia [108].

Premature (pre-term) children, identified by the diagnostic variable Normal Pregnancy (ICD-9 V22) and the procedural variable Surgical Procedures Maternity Care and Delivery during the second trimester (Table 8), were associated with a 30% increased risk, consistent with Talmi et al. as well as other previous studies that found preterm to be a significant factor associated with ASD [37,109,110]. There is a higher prevalence of ASD among children born pre-term [111–116]. Though the risk has been shown to change depending on preterm gestational week cutoff [117]. Though, our study did not find any association with a diagnosis for Early or Threatened labor (ICD-9 642), a common diagnosis made at the discretion of medical personnel.

Other maternal prescriptions resulted in an increased risk of ASD, specifically Anti-inflammatory Glucocorticoids during the first trimester, OR 1.44 (1.08, 1.89), and Respiratory Antihistamines during the second and third trimester, OR 1.39 (1.03, 1.83) and 1.62 (1.20, 2.15), respectively, shown in Table 8. These prescriptions were common treatments for maternal immune dysfunctions and allergens, respectively. However, this study is limited to antihistamine prescriptions that were prescribed and cannot take into account any over-the-counter remedies. Many reviews have shown that maternal inflammatory events in conjunction with maternal immune activation or autoimmune diseases are associated with ASD [8,12,102,118]. Specifically, anti-inflammatory glucocorticoids are a common treatment for psoriasis, which was found to be significantly associated with ASD in one case-control study [17], although a diagnosis for psoriasis (ICD-9 696) was not included in this study due to lack of claims.

Multiple Gestation was found to have a significant increased risk on ASD in all three trimesters (Table 8). However, the study was unable to determine if the twins identified are monozygotic or dizygotic. Previous studies have shown that multiple births have not been associated with ASD, instead the association can be explained by the higher rate of ASD in monozygotic twins compared to their siblings [119,120].

This study does have limitations; the diagnostic codes inputted into each claim were made at the discretion of the medical personnel and were subject to potential bias and all pharmacy claims represented prescription being filled. All variables investigated originate from maternal claims received through insurance and thus does not provide a full representation of all environmental factors that occur outside of insurance claims such as over-the-counter medicines or supplements. Paternal claims were not able to be identified and therefore their influence is unknown. The claims investigated occurred during each woman's pregnancy and thus do not consider pre-existing conditions that may have been diagnosed or treated prior. Lastly, being limited to claims during pregnancy also ignores the possibility of attenuating these factors through consistent proper treatment during or even after pregnancy.

5. Conclusions

Some environmental effects that influence the development of ASD might be identifiable as early as the gestational period. This study identified maternal medical claims made throughout women's pregnancies and determined risk factors associated with having a child diagnosed with ASD. Identifying these factors that either increase or decrease risk is essential especially for women who are at high risk of having children diagnosed with ASD. It is also beneficially for the child by allowing for early screening, leading to earlier diagnosis and the start of interventions. Early intervention is crucial in children with ASD and has been shown to save costs in the long-term [121,122]. Future research would benefit from exploring medical claims made throughout an individual's lifetime to truly evaluate health trends and their influence on the risk of having a child with ASD. It would also be of interest to investigate paternal medical claims to emphasize the genetic influence in the development of ASD.

Supplementary Materials: The following are available online at https://www.mdpi.com/article/10.3390/jpm11100950/s1, Figure S1: Example of Variable Thresholding, Table S1: All Investigated Variables and Claims, Table S2: Highly Correlated Variables, Table S3: Logistic Regression Analyses Full Models, Table S4: Logistic Regression Analyses Subcodes.

Author Contributions: Conceptualization, J.H.; methodology, G.G.; software, G.G.; validation, G.G.; formal analysis, G.G.; investigation, G.G.; resources, J.H.; data curation, G.G.; writing—original draft preparation, G.G.; writing—eview and editing, G.G., R.F. and J.H.; visualization, G.G.; supervision, J.H.; project administration, J.H.; funding acquisition, J.H. All authors have read and agreed to the published version of the manuscript.

Funding: The authors gratefully acknowledge partial financial support from the National Institute of Health (Grant R01AI110642). Support for this research was also received from the Rensselaer Institute for Data Exploration and Applications. The authors express their gratitude to John Rodakis of the N of One: Autism Research Foundation for financially supporting the interactions with OptumLabs.

Institutional Review Board Statement: Ethical review and approval were waived for this study, due to use of de-identified data.

Informed Consent Statement: Patient consent was waived due to the use of de-identified data.

Data Availability Statement: Restrictions apply to the availability of these data. OptumLabs carefully manages access to its data to ensure appropriate use in accordance with its mission and values, policies and procedures, and prevention of re-identification. Users may, therefore, only access OLDW under an agreement with OptumLabs, and compliance with this policy.

Acknowledgments: The authors express their gratitude to the staff at OptumLabs for supporting the study design.

Conflicts of Interest: The authors declare no conflict of interest. The funders had no role in the design of the study; in the collection, analyses, or interpretation of data; in the writing of the manuscript, or in the decision to publish the results.

References

1. American Psychiatric Association (Ed.) Neurodevelopmental Disorders: Autism Spectrum Disorder. In *Diagnostic and Statistical Manual of Mental Disorders: DSM-5*; American Psychiatric Association: Washington, DC, USA, 2013; pp. 50–59, ISBN 978-0-89042-554-1.
2. Van Naarden Braun, K.; Christensen, D.; Doernberg, N.; Schieve, L.; Rice, C.; Wiggins, L.; Schendel, D.; Yeargin-Allsopp, M. Trends in the Prevalence of Autism Spectrum Disorder, Cerebral Palsy, Hearing Loss, Intellectual Disability, and Vision Impairment, Metropolitan Atlanta, 1991–2010. *PLoS ONE* **2015**, *10*, e0124120. [CrossRef]
3. Maenner, M.J.; Shaw, K.A.; Baio, J.; Washington, A.; Patrick, M.; DiRienzo, M.; Christensen, D.L.; Wiggins, L.D.; Pettygrove, S.; Andrews, J.G.; et al. Prevalence of Autism Spectrum Disorder Among Children Aged 8 Years—Autism and Developmental Disabilities Monitoring Network, 11 Sites, United States, 2016. *MMWR Surveill. Summ.* **2020**, *69*, 1–12. [CrossRef]
4. Gaugler, T.; Klei, L.; Sanders, S.J.; Bodea, C.A.; Goldberg, A.P.; Lee, A.B.; Mahajan, M.; Manaa, D.; Pawitan, Y.; Reichert, J.; et al. Most Genetic Risk for Autism Resides with Common Variation. *Nat. Genet.* **2014**, *46*, 881–885. [CrossRef]
5. Kim, J.Y.; Son, M.J.; Son, C.Y.; Radua, J.; Eisenhut, M.; Gressier, F.; Koyanagi, A.; Carvalho, A.F.; Stubbs, B.; Solmi, M.; et al. Environmental Risk Factors and Biomarkers for Autism Spectrum Disorder: An Umbrella Review of the Evidence. *Lancet Psychiatry* **2019**, *6*, 590–600. [CrossRef]
6. Adams, J.B.; Vargason, T.; Kang, D.-W.; Krajmalnik-Brown, R.; Hahn, J. Multivariate Analysis of Plasma Metabolites in Children with Autism Spectrum Disorder and Gastrointestinal Symptoms Before and After Microbiota Transfer Therapy. *Processes* **2019**, *7*, 806. [CrossRef]
7. Lyall, K.; Croen, L.; Daniels, J.; Fallin, M.D.; Ladd-Acosta, C.; Lee, B.K.; Park, B.Y.; Snyder, N.W.; Schendel, D.; Volk, H.; et al. The Changing Epidemiology of Autism Spectrum Disorders. *Annu. Rev. Public Health* **2017**, *38*, 81–102. [CrossRef]
8. Meltzer, A.; Van de Water, J. The Role of the Immune System in Autism Spectrum Disorder. *Neuropsychopharmacology* **2017**, *42*, 284–298. [CrossRef]
9. Qureshi, F.; Adams, J.; Hanagan, K.; Kang, D.-W.; Krajmalnik-Brown, R.; Hahn, J. Multivariate Analysis of Fecal Metabolites from Children with Autism Spectrum Disorder and Gastrointestinal Symptoms before and after Microbiota Transfer Therapy. *J. Pers. Med.* **2020**, *10*, 152. [CrossRef]

10. Vargason, T.; McGuinness, D.L.; Hahn, J. Gastrointestinal Symptoms and Oral Antibiotic Use in Children with Autism Spectrum Disorder: Retrospective Analysis of a Privately Insured U.S. Population. *J. Autism Dev. Disord.* **2019**, *49*, 647–659. [CrossRef]
11. Katsigianni, M.; Karageorgiou, V.; Lambrinoudaki, I.; Siristatidis, C. Maternal Polycystic Ovarian Syndrome in Autism Spectrum Disorder: A Systematic Review and Meta-Analysis. *Mol. Psychiatry* **2019**. [CrossRef]
12. Chen, S.; Zhong, X.; Jiang, L.; Zheng, X.; Xiong, Y.; Ma, S.; Qiu, M.; Huo, S.; Ge, J.; Chen, Q. Maternal Autoimmune Diseases and the Risk of Autism Spectrum Disorders in Offspring: A Systematic Review and Meta-Analysis. *Behav. Brain Res.* **2016**, *296*, 61–69. [CrossRef] [PubMed]
13. Hughes, H.K.; Mills Ko, E.; Rose, D.; Ashwood, P. Immune Dysfunction and Autoimmunity as Pathological Mechanisms in Autism Spectrum Disorders. *Front. Cell. Neurosci.* **2018**, *12*. [CrossRef] [PubMed]
14. Keil, A.; Daniels, J.L.; Forssen, U.; Hultman, C.; Cnattingius, S.; Söderberg, K.C.; Feychting, M.; Sparen, P. Parental Autoimmune Diseases Associated with Autism Spectrum Disorders in Offspring. *Epidemiology* **2010**, *21*, 805–808. [CrossRef]
15. Modabbernia, A.; Velthorst, E.; Reichenberg, A. Environmental Risk Factors for Autism: An Evidence-Based Review of Systematic Reviews and Meta-Analyses. *Mol. Autism* **2017**, *8*. [CrossRef] [PubMed]
16. Andersen, S.; Laurberg, P.; Wu, C.; Olsen, J. Attention Deficit Hyperactivity Disorder and Autism Spectrum Disorder in Children Born to Mothers with Thyroid Dysfunction: A Danish Nationwide Cohort Study. *BJOG Int. J. Obstet. Gynaecol.* **2014**, *121*, 1365–1374. [CrossRef]
17. Croen, L.A.; Grether, J.K.; Yoshida, C.K.; Odouli, R.; Van de Water, J. Maternal Autoimmune Diseases, Asthma and Allergies, and Childhood Autism Spectrum Disorders: A Case-Control Study. *Arch. Pediatr. Adolesc. Med.* **2005**, *159*. [CrossRef]
18. Rom, A.L.; Wu, C.S.; Olsen, J.; Jawaheer, D.; Hetland, M.L.; Mørch, L.S. Parental Rheumatoid Arthritis and Autism Spectrum Disorders in Offspring: A Danish Nationwide Cohort Study. *J. Am. Acad. Child Adolesc. Psychiatry* **2018**, *57*, 28–32.e1. [CrossRef]
19. Jiang, H.; Xu, L.; Shao, L.; Xia, R.; Yu, Z.; Ling, Z.; Yang, F.; Deng, M.; Ruan, B. Maternal Infection during Pregnancy and Risk of Autism Spectrum Disorders: A Systematic Review and Meta-Analysis. *Brain Behav. Immun.* **2016**, *58*, 165–172. [CrossRef]
20. Zerbo, O.; Qian, Y.; Yoshida, C.; Grether, J.K.; Van de Water, J.; Croen, L.A. Maternal Infection during Pregnancy and Autism Spectrum Disorders. *J. Autism Dev. Disord.* **2015**, *45*, 4015–4025. [CrossRef]
21. Atladottir, H.O.; Henriksen, T.B.; Schendel, D.E.; Parner, E.T. Autism after Infection, Febrile Episodes, and Antibiotic Use during Pregnancy: An Exploratory Study. *Pediatrics* **2012**, *130*, e1447–e1454. [CrossRef]
22. Al-Haddad, B.J.S.; Jacobsson, B.; Chabra, S.; Modzelewska, D.; Olson, E.M.; Bernier, R.; Enquobahrie, D.A.; Hagberg, H.; Östling, S.; Rajagopal, L.; et al. Long-Term Risk of Neuropsychiatric Disease after Exposure to Infection in Utero. *JAMA Psychiatry* **2019**, *76*, 594. [CrossRef]
23. Lee, B.K.; Magnusson, C.; Gardner, R.M.; Blomström, Å.; Newschaffer, C.J.; Burstyn, I.; Karlsson, H.; Dalman, C. Maternal Hospitalization with Infection during Pregnancy and Risk of Autism Spectrum Disorders. *Brain Behav. Immun.* **2015**, *44*, 100–105. [CrossRef]
24. Brucato, M.; Ladd-Acosta, C.; Li, M.; Caruso, D.; Hong, X.; Kaczaniuk, J.; Stuart, E.A.; Fallin, M.D.; Wang, X. Prenatal Exposure to Fever Is Associated with Autism Spectrum Disorder in the Boston Birth Cohort: Prenatal Fever Exposure and Autism Risk. *Autism Res.* **2017**, *10*, 1878–1890. [CrossRef] [PubMed]
25. Croen, L.A.; Qian, Y.; Ashwood, P.; Zerbo, O.; Schendel, D.; Pinto-Martin, J.; Daniele Fallin, M.; Levy, S.; Schieve, L.A.; Yeargin-Allsopp, M.; et al. Infection and Fever in Pregnancy and Autism Spectrum Disorders: Findings from the Study to Explore Early Development. *Autism Res.* **2019**. [CrossRef]
26. Ji-Xu, A.; Vincent, A. Maternal Immunity in Autism Spectrum Disorders: Questions of Causality, Validity, and Specificity. *J. Clin. Med.* **2020**, *9*, 2590. [CrossRef] [PubMed]
27. Hamad, A.F.; Alessi-Severini, S.; Mahmud, S.M.; Brownell, M.; Kuo, I.F. Prenatal Antibiotics Exposure and the Risk of Autism Spectrum Disorders: A Population-Based Cohort Study. *PLoS ONE* **2019**, *14*, e0221921. [CrossRef]
28. Kohane, I.S.; McMurry, A.; Weber, G.; MacFadden, D.; Rappaport, L.; Kunkel, L.; Bickel, J.; Wattanasin, N.; Spence, S.; Murphy, S.; et al. The Co-Morbidity Burden of Children and Young Adults with Autism Spectrum Disorders. *PLoS ONE* **2012**, *7*, e33224. [CrossRef] [PubMed]
29. Mannion, A.; Leader, G.; Healy, O. An Investigation of Comorbid Psychological Disorders, Sleep Problems, Gastrointestinal Symptoms and Epilepsy in Children and Adolescents with Autism Spectrum Disorder. *Res. Autism Spectr. Disord.* **2013**, *7*, 35–42. [CrossRef]
30. Muskens, J.B.; Velders, F.P.; Staal, W.G. Medical Comorbidities in Children and Adolescents with Autism Spectrum Disorders and Attention Deficit Hyperactivity Disorders: A Systematic Review. *Eur. Child Adolesc. Psychiatry* **2017**, *26*, 1093–1103. [CrossRef] [PubMed]
31. Rydzewska, E.; Hughes-McCormack, L.A.; Gillberg, C.; Henderson, A.; MacIntyre, C.; Rintoul, J.; Cooper, S.-A. Prevalence of Sensory Impairments, Physical and Intellectual Disabilities, and Mental Health in Children and Young People with Self/Proxy-Reported Autism: Observational Study of a Whole Country Population. *Autism* **2019**, *23*, 1201–1209. [CrossRef]
32. Ornoy, A.; Koren, G. SSRIs and SNRIs (SRI) in Pregnancy: Effects on the Course of Pregnancy and the Offspring: How Far Are We from Having All the Answers? *Int. J. Mol. Sci.* **2019**, *20*, 2370. [CrossRef]
33. Guo, B.-Q.; Li, H.-B.; Zhai, D.-S.; Ding, S.-B. Maternal Multivitamin Supplementation Is Associated with a Reduced Risk of Autism Spectrum Disorder in Children: A Systematic Review and Meta-Analysis. *Nutr. Res.* **2019**, *65*, 4–16. [CrossRef] [PubMed]

34. Iglesias Vázquez, L.; Canals, J.; Arija, V. Review and Meta-analysis Found That Prenatal Folic Acid Was Associated with a 58% Reduction in Autism but Had No Effect on Mental and Motor Development. *Acta Paediatr.* **2018**. [CrossRef]
35. Schmidt, R.J.; Iosif, A.-M.; Guerrero Angel, E.; Ozonoff, S. Association of Maternal Prenatal Vitamin Use with Risk for Autism Spectrum Disorder Recurrence in Young Siblings. *JAMA Psychiatry* **2019**, *76*, 391. [CrossRef] [PubMed]
36. Chen, L.-W.; Wang, S.-T.; Wang, L.-W.; Kao, Y.-C.; Chu, C.-L.; Wu, C.-C.; Hsieh, Y.-T.; Chiang, C.-H.; Huang, C.-C. Behavioral Characteristics of Autism Spectrum Disorder in Very Preterm Birth Children. *Mol. Autism* **2019**, *10*, 32. [CrossRef] [PubMed]
37. Talmi, Z.; Mankuta, D.; Raz, R. Birth Weight and Autism Spectrum Disorder: A Population-based Nested Case–Control Study. *Autism Res.* **2020**. [CrossRef]
38. Huberman Samuel, M.; Meiri, G.; Dinstein, I.; Flusser, H.; Michaelovski, A.; Bashiri, A.; Menashe, I. Exposure to General Anesthesia May Contribute to the Association between Cesarean Delivery and Autism Spectrum Disorder. *J. Autism Dev. Disord.* **2019**, *49*, 3127–3135. [CrossRef]
39. Zhang, T.; Sidorchuk, A.; Sevilla-Cermeño, L.; Vilaplana-Pérez, A.; Chang, Z.; Larsson, H.; Mataix-Cols, D.; Fernández de la Cruz, L. Association of Cesarean Delivery with Risk of Neurodevelopmental and Psychiatric Disorders in the Offspring: A Systematic Review and Meta-Analysis. *JAMA Netw. Open* **2019**, *2*, e1910236. [CrossRef] [PubMed]
40. OptumLabs. *OptumLabs and OptumLabs Data Warehouse (OLDW) Descriptions and Citation*; OptumLabs: Eden Prairie, MN, USA, 2020.
41. Palmsten, K.; Huybrechts, K.F.; Mogun, H.; Kowal, M.K.; Williams, P.L.; Michels, K.B.; Setoguchi, S.; Hernández-Díaz, S. Harnessing the Medicaid Analytic EXtract (Max) to Evaluate Medications in Pregnancy: Design Considerations. *PLoS ONE* **2013**, *8*, e67405. [CrossRef] [PubMed]
42. Veeravalli, N.; Thayer, S.; Bandoli, G. An unbreakable bond: Linking mothers and newborns in large, de-identified claims database. In Proceedings of the 2019 Annual Research Meeting, Washington, DC, USA, 3 June 2019.
43. Baio, J. Prevalence of Autism Spectrum Disorder among Children Aged 8 Years—Autism and Developmental Disabilities Monitoring Network, 11 Sites, United States, 2010. *MMWR Surveill. Summ. Morb. Mortal. Wkly. Rep. Surveill. Summ.* **2014**, *63*, 1–21.
44. Li, Q.; Andrade, S.E.; Cooper, W.O.; Davis, R.L.; Dublin, S.; Hammad, T.A.; Pawloski, P.A.; Pinheiro, S.P.; Raebel, M.A.; Scott, P.E.; et al. Validation of an Algorithm to Estimate Gestational Age in Electronic Health Plan Databases: Validity of Gestational Age Algorithm. *Pharmacoepidemiol. Drug Saf.* **2013**, *22*, 524–532. [CrossRef]
45. Ozonoff, S.; Young, G.S.; Carter, A.; Messinger, D.; Yirmiya, N.; Zwaigenbaum, L.; Bryson, S.; Carver, L.J.; Constantino, J.N.; Dobkins, K.; et al. Recurrence Risk for Autism Spectrum Disorders: A Baby Siblings Research Consortium Study. *Pediatrics* **2011**, *128*, e488–e495. [CrossRef]
46. Wright, R.E. Logistic regression. In *Reading and Understanding Multivariate Statistics*; Yarnold, P.R., Ed.; American Psychological Association: Washington, DC, USA, 1995; pp. 217–244.
47. Mukaka, M.M. Statistics Corner: A Guide to Appropriate Use of Correlation Coefficient in Medical Research. *Malawi Med. J. Med. Assoc. Malawi* **2012**, *24*, 69–71.
48. Pearson, K. Mathematical Contributions to the Theory of Evolution. III. Regression, Heredity, and Panmixia. *Philos. Trans. R. Soc. Math. Phys. Eng. Sci.* **1896**, *187*, 253–318. [CrossRef]
49. Hosmer, D.W.; Lemeshow, S.; Sturdivant, R.X. *Applied Logistic Regression*, 3rd ed.; Wiley Series in Probability and Statistics; Wiley: Hoboken, NJ, USA, 2013; ISBN 978-0-470-58247-3.
50. Risch, N.; Hoffmann, T.J.; Anderson, M.; Croen, L.A.; Grether, J.K.; Windham, G.C. Familial Recurrence of Autism Spectrum Disorder: Evaluating Genetic and Environmental Contributions. *Am. J. Psychiatry* **2014**, *171*, 1206–1213. [CrossRef] [PubMed]
51. Wood, C.L.; Warnell, F.; Johnson, M.; Hames, A.; Pearce, M.S.; McConachie, H.; Parr, J.R. Evidence for ASD Recurrence Rates and Reproductive Stoppage from Large UK ASD Research Family Databases: ASD Reproductive Stoppage. *Autism Res.* **2015**, *8*, 73–81. [CrossRef]
52. Grønborg, T.K.; Hansen, S.N.; Nielsen, S.V.; Skytthe, A.; Parner, E.T. Stoppage in Autism Spectrum Disorders. *J. Autism Dev. Disord.* **2015**, *45*, 3509–3519. [CrossRef] [PubMed]
53. Hoffmann, T.J.; Windham, G.C.; Anderson, M.; Croen, L.A.; Grether, J.K.; Risch, N. Evidence of Reproductive Stoppage in Families with Autism Spectrum Disorder: A Large, Population-Based Cohort Study. *JAMA Psychiatry* **2014**, *71*, 943. [CrossRef]
54. Bhasin, T.K.; Schendel, D. Sociodemographic Risk Factors for Autism in a US Metropolitan Area. *J. Autism Dev. Disord.* **2007**, *37*, 667–677. [CrossRef] [PubMed]
55. Durkin, M.S.; Maenner, M.J.; Meaney, F.J.; Levy, S.E.; DiGuiseppi, C.; Nicholas, J.S.; Kirby, R.S.; Pinto-Martin, J.A.; Schieve, L.A. Socioeconomic Inequality in the Prevalence of Autism Spectrum Disorder: Evidence from a U.S. Cross-Sectional Study. *PLoS ONE* **2010**, *5*, e11551. [CrossRef] [PubMed]
56. Wu, S.; Wu, F.; Ding, Y.; Hou, J.; Bi, J.; Zhang, Z. Advanced Parental Age and Autism Risk in Children: A Systematic Review and Meta-Analysis. *Acta Psychiatr. Scand.* **2017**, *135*, 29–41. [CrossRef] [PubMed]
57. Sandin, S.; Hultman, C.M.; Kolevzon, A.; Gross, R.; MacCabe, J.H.; Reichenberg, A. Advancing Maternal Age Is Associated with Increasing Risk for Autism: A Review and Meta-Analysis. *J. Am. Acad. Child Adolesc. Psychiatry* **2012**, *51*, 477–486.e1. [CrossRef]
58. Sandin, S.; Schendel, D.; Magnusson, P.; Hultman, C.; Surén, P.; Susser, E.; Grønborg, T.; Gissler, M.; Gunnes, N.; Gross, R.; et al. Autism Risk Associated with Parental Age and with Increasing Difference in Age between the Parents. *Mol. Psychiatry* **2016**, *21*, 693–700. [CrossRef] [PubMed]

59. Curran, E.A.; Cryan, J.F.; Kenny, L.C.; Dinan, T.G.; Kearney, P.M.; Khashan, A.S. Obstetrical Mode of Delivery and Childhood Behavior and Psychological Development in a British Cohort. *J. Autism Dev. Disord.* **2016**, *46*, 603–614. [CrossRef]
60. Langridge, A.T.; Glasson, E.J.; Nassar, N.; Jacoby, P.; Pennell, C.; Hagan, R.; Bourke, J.; Leonard, H.; Stanley, F.J. Maternal Conditions and Perinatal Characteristics Associated with Autism Spectrum Disorder and Intellectual Disability. *PLoS ONE* **2013**, *8*, e50963. [CrossRef] [PubMed]
61. Curran, E.A.; O'Neill, S.M.; Cryan, J.F.; Kenny, L.C.; Dinan, T.G.; Khashan, A.S.; Kearney, P.M. Research Review: Birth by Caesarean Section and Development of Autism Spectrum Disorder and Attention-Deficit/Hyperactivity Disorder: A Systematic Review and Meta-Analysis. *J. Child Psychol. Psychiatry* **2015**, *56*, 500–508. [CrossRef] [PubMed]
62. Curran, E.A.; Dalman, C.; Kearney, P.M.; Kenny, L.C.; Cryan, J.F.; Dinan, T.G.; Khashan, A.S. Association between Obstetric Mode of Delivery and Autism Spectrum Disorder: A Population-Based Sibling Design Study. *JAMA Psychiatry* **2015**, *72*, 935. [CrossRef] [PubMed]
63. Isaksson, J.; Pettersson, E.; Kostrzewa, E.; Diaz Heijtz, R.; Bölte, S. Brief Report: Association between Autism Spectrum Disorder, Gastrointestinal Problems and Perinatal Risk Factors within Sibling Pairs. *J. Autism Dev. Disord.* **2017**, *47*, 2621–2627. [CrossRef] [PubMed]
64. Chien, L.-N.; Lin, H.-C.; Shao, Y.-H.J.; Chiou, S.-T.; Chiou, H.-Y. Risk of Autism Associated with General Anesthesia during Cesarean Delivery: A Population-Based Birth-Cohort Analysis. *J. Autism Dev. Disord.* **2015**, *45*, 932–942. [CrossRef]
65. Timofeev, J.; Reddy, U.M.; Huang, C.-C.; Driggers, R.W.; Landy, H.J.; Laughon, S.K. Obstetric Complications, Neonatal Morbidity, and Indications for Cesarean Delivery by Maternal Age. *Obstet. Gynecol.* **2013**, *122*, 1184–1195. [CrossRef] [PubMed]
66. Mylonas, I.; Friese, K. Indications for and Risks of Elective Cesarean Section. *Dtsch. Aerzteblatt Online* **2015**. [CrossRef] [PubMed]
67. Moya-Pérez, A.; Luczynski, P.; Renes, I.B.; Wang, S.; Borre, Y.; Anthony Ryan, C.; Knol, J.; Stanton, C.; Dinan, T.G.; Cryan, J.F. Intervention Strategies for Cesarean Section–Induced Alterations in the Microbiota-Gut-Brain Axis. *Nutr. Rev.* **2017**, *75*, 225–240. [CrossRef]
68. Shin, H.; Pei, Z.; Martinez, K.A.; Rivera-Vinas, J.I.; Mendez, K.; Cavallin, H.; Dominguez-Bello, M.G. The First Microbial Environment of Infants Born by C-Section: The Operating Room Microbes. *Microbiome* **2015**, *3*, 59. [CrossRef]
69. O'Shea, T.M.; Klebanoff, M.A.; Signore, C. Delivery after Previous Cesarean: Long-Term Outcomes in the Child. *Semin. Perinatol.* **2010**, *34*, 281–292. [CrossRef]
70. Knight, H.; Gurol-Urganci, I.; van der Meulen, J.; Mahmood, T.; Richmond, D.; Dougall, A.; Cromwell, D. Vaginal Birth after Caesarean Section: A Cohort Study Investigating Factors Associated with Its Uptake and Success. *BJOG Int. J. Obstet. Gynaecol.* **2014**, *121*, 183–192. [CrossRef] [PubMed]
71. Lydon-Rochelle, M.T.; Cahill, A.G.; Spong, C.Y. Birth After Previous Cesarean Delivery: Short-Term Maternal Outcomes. *Semin. Perinatol.* **2010**, *34*, 249–257. [CrossRef]
72. Jackson, S.; Fleege, L.; Fridman, M.; Gregory, K.; Zelop, C.; Olsen, J. Morbidity Following Primary Cesarean Delivery in the Danish National Birth Cohort. *Am. J. Obstet. Gynecol.* **2012**, *206*, 139.e1–139.e5. [CrossRef]
73. Keag, O.E.; Norman, J.E.; Stock, S.J. Long-Term Risks and Benefits Associated with Cesarean Delivery for Mother, Baby, and Subsequent Pregnancies: Systematic Review and Meta-Analysis. *PLoS Med.* **2018**, *15*, e1002494. [CrossRef]
74. Miller, E.S.; Hahn, K.; Grobman, W.A. Consequences of a Primary Elective Cesarean Delivery across the Reproductive Life. *Obstet. Gynecol.* **2013**, *121*, 789–797. [CrossRef] [PubMed]
75. Silver, R.M. Delivery after Previous Cesarean: Long-Term Maternal Outcomes. *Semin. Perinatol.* **2010**, *34*, 258–266. [CrossRef]
76. Andalib, S.; Emamhadi, M.R.; Yousefzadeh-Chabok, S.; Shakouri, S.K.; Høilund-Carlsen, P.F.; Vafaee, M.S.; Michel, T.M. Maternal SSRI Exposure Increases the Risk of Autistic Offspring: A Meta-Analysis and Systematic Review. *Eur. Psychiatry* **2017**, *45*, 161–166. [CrossRef] [PubMed]
77. Boukhris, T.; Sheehy, O.; Mottron, L.; Bérard, A. Antidepressant Use during Pregnancy and the Risk of Autism Spectrum Disorder in Children. *JAMA Pediatr.* **2016**, *170*, 117. [CrossRef]
78. Bölte, S.; Girdler, S.; Marschik, P.B. The Contribution of Environmental Exposure to the Etiology of Autism Spectrum Disorder. *Cell. Mol. Life Sci.* **2019**, *76*, 1275–1297. [CrossRef] [PubMed]
79. Mezzacappa, A.; Lasica, P.-A.; Gianfagna, F.; Cazas, O.; Hardy, P.; Falissard, B.; Sutter-Dallay, A.-L.; Gressier, F. Risk for Autism Spectrum Disorders According to Period of Prenatal Antidepressant Exposure: A Systematic Review and Meta-Analysis. *JAMA Pediatr.* **2017**, *171*, 555. [CrossRef]
80. Zhou, X.-H.; Li, Y.-J.; Ou, J.-J.; Li, Y.-M. Association between Maternal Antidepressant Use during Pregnancy and Autism Spectrum Disorder: An Updated Meta-Analysis. *Mol. Autism* **2018**, *9*, 21. [CrossRef]
81. Andrade, C. Antidepressant Exposure during Pregnancy and Risk of Autism in the Offspring, 1: Meta-Review of Meta-Analyses: (Clinical and Practical Psychopharmacology). *J. Clin. Psychiatry* **2017**, *78*, e1047–e1051. [CrossRef]
82. Hagberg, K.W.; Robijn, A.L.; Jick, S.S. Maternal Depression and Antidepressant Use during Pregnancy and the Risk of Autism Spectrum Disorder in Offspring. *Clin. Epidemiol.* **2018**, *10*, 1599–1612. [CrossRef] [PubMed]
83. Kaplan, Y.C.; Keskin-Arslan, E.; Acar, S.; Sozmen, K. Maternal SSRI Discontinuation, Use, Psychiatric Disorder and the Risk of Autism in Children: A Meta-analysis of Cohort Studies. *Br. J. Clin. Pharmacol.* **2017**, *83*, 2798–2806. [CrossRef]
84. Kobayashi, T.; Matsuyama, T.; Takeuchi, M.; Ito, S. Autism Spectrum Disorder and Prenatal Exposure to Selective Serotonin Reuptake Inhibitors: A Systematic Review and Meta-Analysis. *Reprod. Toxicol.* **2016**, *65*, 170–178. [CrossRef]

85. Magdalena, H.; Beata, K.; Justyna, P.; Agnieszka, K.-G.; Szczepara-Fabian, M.; Buczek, A.; Ewa, E.-W. Preconception Risk Factors for Autism Spectrum Disorder—A Pilot Study. *Brain Sci.* **2020**, *10*, 293. [CrossRef]
86. Sorensen, M.J.; Christensen, J.; Parner, E.T.; Grønborg, T.K.; Vestergaard, M.; Schendel, D.; Pedersen, L.H. Antidepressant Exposure in Pregnancy and Risk of Autism Spectrum Disorders. *Clin. Epidemiol.* **2013**, 449. [CrossRef]
87. Xie, S.; Karlsson, H.; Dalman, C.; Widman, L.; Rai, D.; Gardner, R.M.; Magnusson, C.; Schendel, D.E.; Newschaffer, C.J.; Lee, B.K. Family History of Mental and Neurological Disorders and Risk of Autism. *JAMA Netw. Open* **2019**, *2*, e190154. [CrossRef] [PubMed]
88. Vega, M.L.; Newport, G.C.; Bozhdaraj, D.; Saltz, S.B.; Nemeroff, C.B.; Newport, D.J. Implementation of Advanced Methods for Reproductive Pharmacovigilance in Autism: A Meta-Analysis of the Effects of Prenatal Antidepressant Exposure. *Am. J. Psychiatry* **2020**, *177*, 506–517. [CrossRef]
89. Ornoy, A.; Weinstein-Fudim, L.; Ergaz, Z. Prenatal Factors Associated with Autism Spectrum Disorder (ASD). *Reprod. Toxicol.* **2015**, *56*, 155–169. [CrossRef]
90. Xu, G.; Jing, J.; Bowers, K.; Liu, B.; Bao, W. Maternal Diabetes and the Risk of Autism Spectrum Disorders in the Offspring: A Systematic Review and Meta-Analysis. *J. Autism Dev. Disord.* **2014**, *44*, 766–775. [CrossRef] [PubMed]
91. Kong, L.; Norstedt, G.; Schalling, M.; Gissler, M.; Lavebratt, C. The Risk of Offspring Psychiatric Disorders in the Setting of Maternal Obesity and Diabetes. *Pediatrics* **2018**, *142*, e20180776. [CrossRef]
92. Wan, H.; Zhang, C.; Li, H.; Luan, S.; Liu, C. Association of Maternal Diabetes with Autism Spectrum Disorders in Offspring: A Systemic Review and Meta-Analysis. *Medicine* **2018**, *97*, e9438. [CrossRef]
93. Xiang, A.H.; Wang, X.; Martinez, M.P.; Walthall, J.C.; Curry, E.S.; Page, K.; Buchanan, T.A.; Coleman, K.J.; Getahun, D. Association of Maternal Diabetes with Autism in Offspring. *JAMA* **2015**, *313*, 1425. [CrossRef] [PubMed]
94. Li, M.; Fallin, M.D.; Riley, A.; Landa, R.; Walker, S.O.; Silverstein, M.; Caruso, D.; Pearson, C.; Kiang, S.; Dahm, J.L.; et al. The Association of Maternal Obesity and Diabetes with Autism and Other Developmental Disabilities. *Pediatrics* **2016**, *137*, e20152206. [CrossRef]
95. Carpita, B.; Muti, D.; Dell'Osso, L. Oxidative Stress, Maternal Diabetes, and Autism Spectrum Disorders. *Oxid. Med. Cell. Longev.* **2018**, *2018*, 1–9. [CrossRef]
96. Levine, S.Z.; Kodesh, A.; Viktorin, A.; Smith, L.; Uher, R.; Reichenberg, A.; Sandin, S. Association of Maternal Use of Folic Acid and Multivitamin Supplements in the Periods before and during Pregnancy with the Risk of Autism Spectrum Disorder in Offspring. *JAMA Psychiatry* **2018**, *75*, 176. [CrossRef]
97. Surén, P.; Roth, C.; Bresnahan, M.; Haugen, M.; Hornig, M.; Hirtz, D.; Lie, K.K.; Lipkin, W.I.; Magnus, P.; Reichborn-Kjennerud, T.; et al. Association between Maternal Use of Folic Acid Supplements and Risk of Autism Spectrum Disorders in Children. *JAMA* **2013**, *309*, 570. [CrossRef] [PubMed]
98. Peretti, S.; Mariano, M.; Mazzocchetti, C.; Mazza, M.; Pino, M.C.; Verrotti Di Pianella, A.; Valenti, M. Diet: The Keystone of Autism Spectrum Disorder? *Nutr. Neurosci.* **2019**, *22*, 825–839. [CrossRef]
99. Raghavan, R.; Selhub, J.; Paul, L.; Ji, Y.; Wang, G.; Hong, X.; Zuckerman, B.; Fallin, M.D.; Wang, X. A Prospective Birth Cohort Study on Cord Blood Folate Subtypes and Risk of Autism Spectrum Disorder. *Am. J. Clin. Nutr.* **2020**, nqaa208. [CrossRef]
100. Raghavan, R.; Riley, A.W.; Volk, H.; Caruso, D.; Hironaka, L.; Sices, L.; Hong, X.; Wang, G.; Ji, Y.; Brucato, M.; et al. Maternal Multivitamin Intake, Plasma Folate and Vitamin B 12 Levels and Autism Spectrum Disorder Risk in Offspring. *Paediatr. Perinat. Epidemiol.* **2018**, *32*, 100–111. [CrossRef]
101. Frye, R.E.; Slattery, J.C.; Quadros, E.V. Folate Metabolism Abnormalities in Autism: Potential Biomarkers. *Biomark. Med.* **2017**, *11*, 687–699. [CrossRef]
102. Emberti Gialloreti, L.; Mazzone, L.; Benvenuto, A.; Fasano, A.; Alcon, A.G.; Kraneveld, A.; Moavero, R.; Raz, R.; Riccio, M.P.; Siracusano, M.; et al. Risk and Protective Environmental Factors Associated with Autism Spectrum Disorder: Evidence-Based Principles and Recommendations. *J. Clin. Med.* **2019**, *8*, 217. [CrossRef]
103. Burstyn, I.; Sithole, F.; Zwaigenbaum, L. Autism Spectrum Disorders, Maternal Characteristics and Obstetric Complications among Singletons Born in Alberta, Canada. *Chronic Dis. Can.* **2010**, *30*, 125–134. [CrossRef]
104. Dodds, L.; Fell, D.B.; Shea, S.; Armson, B.A.; Allen, A.C.; Bryson, S. The Role of Prenatal, Obstetric and Neonatal Factors in the Development of Autism. *J. Autism Dev. Disord.* **2011**, *41*, 891–902. [CrossRef]
105. Lyall, K.; Pauls, D.L.; Spiegelman, D.; Ascherio, A.; Santangelo, S.L. Pregnancy Complications and Obstetric Suboptimality in Association with Autism Spectrum Disorders in Children of the Nurses' Health Study II. *Autism Res.* **2012**, *5*, 21–30. [CrossRef]
106. Fang, S.-Y.; Wang, S.; Huang, N.; Yeh, H.-H.; Chen, C.-Y. Prenatal Infection and Autism Spectrum Disorders in Childhood: A Population-Based Case-Control Study in Taiwan: Prenatal Infection and Autism. *Paediatr. Perinat. Epidemiol.* **2015**, *29*, 307–316. [CrossRef]
107. Jenabi, E.; Karami, M.; Khazaei, S.; Bashirian, S. The Association between Preeclampsia and Autism Spectrum Disorders among Children: A Meta-Analysis. *Korean J. Pediatr.* **2019**, *62*, 126–130. [CrossRef]
108. Khazaei, S. The Association between Placenta Previa and the Risk of Preeclampsia: A Meta-Analysis. *Erciyes Med. J.* **2019**. [CrossRef]
109. Buchmayer, S.; Johansson, S.; Johansson, A.; Hultman, C.M.; Sparen, P.; Cnattingius, S. Can Association between Preterm Birth and Autism Be Explained by Maternal or Neonatal Morbidity? *Pediatrics* **2009**, *124*, e817–e825. [CrossRef]
110. Ng, M.; de Montigny, J.G.; Ofner, M.; Do, M.T. Environmental Factors Associated with Autism Spectrum Disorder: A Scoping Review for the Years 2003-2013. *Health Promot. Chronic Dis. Prev. Can. Res. Policy Pract.* **2017**, *37*, 1–23. [CrossRef]

111. Agrawal, S.; Rao, S.C.; Bulsara, M.K.; Patole, S.K. Prevalence of Autism Spectrum Disorder in Preterm Infants: A Meta-Analysis. *Pediatrics* **2018**, *142*, e20180134. [CrossRef]
112. Fezer, G.F.; de Matos, M.B.; Nau, A.L.; Zeigelboim, B.S.; Marques, J.M.; Liberalesso, P.B.N. Características Perinatais de Crianças Com Transtorno Do Espectro Autista. *Rev. Paul. Pediatr.* **2017**, *35*, 130–135. [CrossRef]
113. Goldin, R.L.; Matson, J.L. Premature Birth as a Risk Factor for Autism Spectrum Disorder: Brief Report. *Dev. Neurorehabilit.* **2015**, *19*, 1–4. [CrossRef]
114. Peralta-Carcelen, M.; Schwartz, J.; Carcelen, A.C. Behavioral and Socioemotional Development in Preterm Children. *Clin. Perinatol.* **2018**, *45*, 529–546. [CrossRef] [PubMed]
115. Pinto-Martin, J.A.; Levy, S.E.; Feldman, J.F.; Lorenz, J.M.; Paneth, N.; Whitaker, A.H. Prevalence of Autism Spectrum Disorder in Adolescents Born Weighing <2000 Grams. *Pediatrics* **2011**, *128*, 883–891. [CrossRef] [PubMed]
116. Verhaeghe, L.; Dereu, M.; Warreyn, P.; De Groote, I.; Vanhaesebrouck, P.; Roeyers, H. Erratum to: Extremely Preterm Born Children at Very High Risk for Developing Autism Spectrum Disorder. *Child Psychiatry Hum. Dev.* **2016**, *47*, 1009. [CrossRef]
117. Leavey, A.; Zwaigenbaum, L.; Heavner, K.; Burstyn, I. Gestational Age at Birth and Risk of Autism Spectrum Disorders in Alberta, Canada. *J. Pediatr.* **2013**, *162*, 361–368. [CrossRef] [PubMed]
118. Bilbo, S.D.; Block, C.L.; Bolton, J.L.; Hanamsagar, R.; Tran, P.K. Beyond Infection—Maternal Immune Activation by Environmental Factors, Microglial Development, and Relevance for Autism Spectrum Disorders. *Exp. Neurol.* **2018**, *299*, 241–251. [CrossRef] [PubMed]
119. Hallmayer, J.; Glasson, E.J.; Bower, C.; Petterson, B.; Croen, L.; Grether, J.; Risch, N. On the Twin Risk in Autism. *Am. J. Hum. Genet.* **2002**, *71*, 941–946. [CrossRef]
120. Van Naarden Braun, K.; Schieve, L.; Daniels, J.; Durkin, M.; Giarelli, E.; Kirby, R.S.; Lee, L.-C.; Newschaffer, C.; Nicholas, J.; Pinto-Martin, J. Relationships between Multiple Births and Autism Spectrum Disorders, Cerebral Palsy, and Intellectual Disabilities: Autism and Developmental Disabilities Monitoring (ADDM) Network-2002 Surveillance Year. *Autism Res.* **2008**, *1*, 266–274. [CrossRef]
121. Penner, M.; Rayar, M.; Bashir, N.; Roberts, S.W.; Hancock-Howard, R.L.; Coyte, P.C. Cost-Effectiveness Analysis Comparing Pre-Diagnosis Autism Spectrum Disorder (ASD)-Targeted Intervention with Ontario's Autism Intervention Program. *J. Autism Dev. Disord.* **2015**, *45*, 2833–2847. [CrossRef] [PubMed]
122. Peters-Scheffer, N.; Didden, R.; Korzilius, H.; Matson, J. Cost Comparison of Early Intensive Behavioral Intervention and Treatment as Usual for Children with Autism Spectrum Disorder in the Netherlands. *Res. Dev. Disabil.* **2012**, *33*, 1763–1772. [CrossRef] [PubMed]

Journal of *Personalized Medicine*

MDPI

Case Report

Genomics as a Clinical Decision Support Tool: Successful Proof of Concept for Improved ASD Outcomes

Heather Way [1], Grant Williams [2], Sharon Hausman-Cohen [2,*] and Jordan Reeder [2]

1 The Australian Centre for Genomic Analysis, Brisbane, QLD 4069, Australia; drheatherway@tacga.com.au
2 IntellxxDNA™, Austin, TX 78731, USA; gwilliams@intellxxdna.com (G.W.); jreeder@intellxxdna.com (J.R.)
* Correspondence: sharonmd@intellxxdna.com; Tel.: +1-512-717-3300

Abstract: Considerable evidence is emerging that Autism Spectrum Disorder (ASD) is most often triggered by a range of different genetic variants that interact with environmental factors such as exposures to toxicants and changes to the food supply. Up to 80% of genetic variations that contribute to ASD found to date are neither extremely rare nor classified as pathogenic. Rather, they are less common single nucleotide polymorphisms (SNPs), found in 1–15% or more of the population, that by themselves are not disease-causing. These genomic variants contribute to ASD by interacting with each other, along with nutritional and environmental factors. Examples of pathways affected or triggered include those related to brain inflammation, mitochondrial dysfunction, neuronal connectivity, synapse formation, impaired detoxification, methylation, and neurotransmitter-related effects. This article presents information on four case study patients that are part of a larger ongoing pilot study. A genomic clinical decision support (CDS) tool that specifically focuses on variants and pathways that have been associated with neurodevelopmental disorders was used in this pilot study to help develop a targeted, personalized prevention and intervention strategy for each child. In addition to an individual's genetic makeup, each patient's personal history, diet, and environmental factors were considered. The CDS tool also looked at genomic SNPs associated with secondary comorbid ASD conditions including attention deficit hyperactivity disorder (ADHD), obsessive-compulsive disorder (OCD), anxiety, and pediatric autoimmune neuropsychiatric disorder associated with streptococcal infections/pediatric acute-onset neuropsychiatric syndrome (PANDAS/PANS). The interpreted genomics tool helped the treating clinician identify and develop personalized, genomically targeted treatment plans. Utilization of this treatment approach was associated with significant improvements in socialization and verbal skills, academic milestones and intelligence quotient (IQ), and overall increased ability to function in these children, as measured by autism treatment evaluation checklist (ATEC) scores and parent interviews.

Keywords: autism spectrum disorder (ASD); genomics; personalized treatment strategy; single nucleotide polymorphisms; clinical decision support tool; ADHD; PANDAS; OCD; anxiety

Citation: Way, H.; Williams, G.; Hausman-Cohen, S.; Reeder, J. Genomics as a Clinical Decision Support Tool: Successful Proof of Concept for Improved ASD Outcomes. *J. Pers. Med.* **2021**, *11*, 596. https://doi.org/10.3390/jpm11070596

Academic Editor: Richard E. Frye

Received: 21 May 2021
Accepted: 22 June 2021
Published: 24 June 2021

Publisher's Note: MDPI stays neutral with regard to jurisdictional claims in published maps and institutional affiliations.

Copyright: © 2021 by the authors. Licensee MDPI, Basel, Switzerland. This article is an open access article distributed under the terms and conditions of the Creative Commons Attribution (CC BY) license (https://creativecommons.org/licenses/by/4.0/).

1. Introduction

Autism spectrum disorders (ASDs) are a group of neurodevelopmental syndromes characterized by deficits in social interaction and communication, as well as repetitive behaviors and restricted interests. ASD rates have increased tremendously over the last few decades from 3 per 1000 children in 1996 to 19 per 1000 children in 2016 [1,2]. While there are forms of ASD caused by pathogenic (disease-causing) genetic mutations, this represents only a small portion of individuals with ASD.

Considerable evidence is emerging that ASD is triggered by the interaction between a variety of single nucleotide polymorphisms (SNPs) and environmental factors such as toxicant exposures, changes to food supplies, and the gut microbiome [3]. In a 2020 study, only 19.7% of individuals with ASD were found to have rare pathogenic variants or copy number variants contributing to or causal of their ASD diagnosis [4]. This indicates that

ASD is much closer to what is seen with other chronic illnesses, where a multitude of less common SNPs (found in 1–15% of the population) are likely the main contributors. Additional contributing SNPs may have a much higher population frequency. While individually these SNPs are not disease-causing, they can contribute in an additive manner to the manifestations commonly associated with ASD.

The use of genomics for clinical decision support is a novel approach to medicine that has become feasible only within the last few years. This is in part due to improvements in genetic testing technology as well as advances in the literature regarding the mechanisms of how supplements, nutrients, and other interventions interact with the genome and molecular pathways. This article illustrates how a genomically targeted and personalized medicine approach was successfully used at the Australian Centre for Genomic Analysis (TACGA). While a number of ASD treatment centers across the world incorporate a functional medicine and integrative approach, this is the first time to our knowledge that a specialized neurodevelopmental genomic clinical decision support (CDS) tool has been used systematically to achieve marked improvements in ASD related symptoms. Additionally, as a CDS, the SNPs that were presented and prioritized were actionable. For example, there have been many reports demonstrating the association between elevated tumor necrosis factor alpha (TNFa) and ASD [5], but few studies were identified that connect supplements known to cross the blood–brain barrier and lower TNFa-based inflammation to their usage in response to genetic predisposition to higher TNFa levels.

2. Materials and Methods

The four patients presented in this study are a subset of an ongoing pilot study composed of approximately 100 patients and are meant to be illustrative of and give insight into the process used for improving outcomes. Each of the four individuals received treatment for ASD at The Australian Centre for Genomic Analysis (TACGA), which began using genomics in a simplistic manner beginning in 2012. Children who came to TACGA prior to 2018 were evaluated using a basic 54 SNP "health and well-being" panel that included information relating to inflammation, oxidative stress, vitamin D, detoxification and methylation. In 2018, the original version of a neurodevelopmental report (designed to help with non-syndromic ASD) from IntellxxDNA™ (IXXD)—a clinical decision support tool—became available.

IXXD is a more specific CDS tool that offers various versions of its report, including one that focuses on pediatric developmental issues such as ASD, obsessive–compulsive disorder (OCD), pediatric autoimmune neuropsychiatric disorder associated with streptococcal infections (PANDAS), attention deficit hyperactivity disorder (ADHD), and anxiety. This tool was used to analyze DNA specimens from subjects, which consisted of both new and existing TACGA patients. For existing patients, IXXD was implemented as add-on therapy in order to obtain additional improvements in neurodevelopmental outcomes. DNA was collected via buccal cells and analyzed at Rutgers University Cell and DNA Repository (RUCDR) using a customized version of the Affymetrix precision medicine microarray.

Genomic information was presented to the clinician as formatted by IXXD, which was a curated collection of the genomic research. Discussions on gene and SNP function, as well as genomically targeted potential intervention strategies (including nutrients, supplements, and lifestyle modifications) were presented to the ordering provider. In keeping with being a clinical decision support tool, all information was referenced. IXXD reported a particular supplement, food, or nutrient as a potential intervention if it (1) mechanistically addressed both the gene function and SNP impact on the given pathway, and (2) had evidence for improvement of ASD and/or various neurodevelopmental parameters. IXXD nutritional handouts were also incorporated into treatment plans, so that genomics could be addressed with nutrition when possible. A variety of potential intervention options were presented by the CDS, but all treatment decisions were made by the ordering clinician.

The degree of improvements in ASD outcomes were gauged using autism treatment evaluation checklist (ATEC) scores, intelligence quotient (IQ) scores, behavioral improvements, and other parental reporting. In addition to genetic profiling and behavioral observations, TACGA protocol also called for pre- and post-treatment measurement of vitamins, homocysteine, interleukins, and various additional blood markers.

Due to this being a pilot study, there was no specified control group. However, there were individuals evaluated who had previously been optimized with standard TACGA care, who were then given the opportunity to have their genomics evaluated to further improve outcomes. Supplements, nutrients, and dietary modifications were all items that had previously been discussed in the published medical literature and were available over the counter. Thus, consent in this pilot study was obtained via parental discussion.

A detailed discussion on how the CDS tool works is necessary due to this being the first presentation of the IntellxxDNA platform in the ASD literature. For illustration purposes, the Src homology 3 (SH3) and multiple ankyrin repeat domains 3 (SHANK3) variant discussed in the first case study below will be used as an example. Each sentence in quotations below and any accompanying information is linked to references in the live tool. To make the IXXD tool a useful resource for clinicians, genomic reports begin by discussing the gene function and how the variant of interest impacts protein functionality. For example, it would be relayed that SHANK3 "is part of the molecular scaffolding or platform where synapses, especially glutamate receptors of post synaptic nerves, are assembled." IXXD also provides clinicians with references supporting that the SNP conveys a decrease in SHANK3 expression, along with information linking the associated disorganization of synapses, pervasive developmental disorders, and ASD-like symptoms. Extensive discussions on how each of the SNPs can be modulated are also included. In this example, it is known that SHANK3 is destabilized and broken down by the extracellular signal-regulated kinase 2 (ERK2) protein. Therefore, inhibiting ERK2 with supplements such as curcumin, resveratrol, or a high butyrate diet are presented as potential interventions as they can help raise SHANK3 levels. Additionally, IXXD relays the cofactors that are needed in the molecular pathway, as they can also be modified to improve function. An excerpt from the referenced discussion of SHANK3 modulation in the CDS tool is as follows: "The protein encoded by SHANK3 is regulated by zinc, and zinc deficiency depletes synaptic pools of SHANK3. Melatonin increases SHANK3 protein concentrations. Blue light protection can be beneficial for maintaining proper melatonin levels. ERK2 inhibitors will increase SHANK3 protein indirectly by decreasing the degradation of SHANK3. Butyrate is an ERK2 inhibitor. A ketotic diet is one way to increase beta-hydroxybutyrate levels, but high butyrate foods (see patient dietary handout list), in addition to butyrate supplements, can also be beneficial. Resveratrol is also an ERK2 inhibitor and has data in children with ASD. Physical activity has also been shown to increase SHANK3 protein concentrations in the thalamus and cortex." This detailed information is given for every SNP in the report and differs in complexity, depending on the nature of the SNP itself. Discussions range from complicated SNPs such as SHANK3 and NAD(P)H quinone dehydrogenase 1 (NQO1), down to simple mechanisms such as the nutritional factor phosphatidylethanolamine N-methyltransferase (PEMT) for the choline pathway.

3. Results

3.1. CJM Case Study

3.1.1. Medical History and Background

The following is a case study of a male patient who initially made significant gains when following TACGA protocol, but later plateaued. His DNA was reevaluated using the IXXD CDS that targeted specific neurodevelopmental and neurobehavioral pathways.

This case study patient, referred to as CJM to protect his identity, was diagnosed ASD level 3 (highest level, requiring substantial support) at age three and intellectually impaired with an IQ of 54 at age seven. On a gluten free/dairy free diet since age five. First presented to the clinic at age 12 with an ATEC score of 117 (neurotypical ATEC score is about 10 or less). He was classified as non-verbal with some occasional rudimentary language in the form of two or three word strings when it suited him, and was unable to follow multiple instructions. Behavioral issues included self-harm, aggressiveness to peers and family, running away, and bed wetting. Also noted was no desire to socialize, lack of attention (2–3 min), lethargy and very low mental energy (less than 2 min), and significant sensory defensiveness around noise, clothing and stimming. Additionally, he displayed hyperactivity at times, a lack of eye contact, and chronic constipation (permanently on laxatives).

In 2015, he was screened using the initial TACGA protocol. He had SNPs relating to interleukin 1 (IL1a and IL1b), vitamin D receptors (VDR) and detoxification pathways. Alongside dietary changes and a gut healing protocol, the interventions were as follows: fish oil (2 g eicosapentaenoic acid + docosahexaenoic acid), broccoli sprouts (releasing 16 mg sulforaphane), vitamin D (3000 IU), anti-inflammatory probiotics, fermented foods in diet, zinc, and D-ribose-L-cysteine (glutathione precursor).

Over the next 12 months, his family reported considerable improvements in both receptive and expressive language. Behavior significantly improved, stimming reduced, and constipation had resolved. His ATEC had reduced to 71, but he subsequently plateaued. Residual symptoms included lack of attention and focus (15 min), lethargy/became mentally tired very quickly (10–15 min), impaired cognitive abilities, bed wetting (still nightly), and some sensory issues (mostly when tired). Language skills were improved, and he was able to talk in phrases and understand most general words, but he struggled to have meaningful conversations. IXXD's neurodevelopmental report became available for alpha testing in November 2018, and his family decided to pursue this option shortly after in an attempt to break through the plateau.

3.1.2. Genomic CDS Results and Interpretation

Various genomic pathways, including SNPs reported in the literature to contribute to neurodevelopment and cognitive dysfunction, were discovered and appropriately addressed. CJM was found to be homozygous for a relatively rare variant (c.1304 + 48C > T) in the SHANK3 gene, which is found in less than 4% of the population and is highly associated with increased ASD risk. Deletions and variations within the SHANK3 pathway have been associated with ASD [6], and this particular SNP has been associated with an odds ratio (OR) of 5.5 for ASD and an OR of 12.6 for pervasive developmental disorder [7]. This SNP appears to lead to decreased protein activity. SHANK3 variants (or deletions) causing decreased activity are associated with less ability to form glutamatergic nerve connections during brain development and throughout childhood [7]. Furthermore, SHANK3 contributes to delayed or absent speech, lower muscle tone, and altered social interactions [8]. Interventions targeted towards decreasing the breakdown of this scaffolding protein, as discussed in the genomic CDS, were introduced. Some of these interventions included increasing cofactors, such as zinc, that stabilized the SHANK3 protein [9]. Other interventions related to inhibiting ERK2, which is responsible for breaking down SHANK3, included melatonin [10], resveratrol [11], and using blue light filtering glasses (to block decreases in melatonin levels) [12].

This patient also had multiple SNPs that relate to memory and cognition, including mitochondrial membrane issues that predispose him to more oxidative stress and mitochondrial dysfunction. Additionally, CJM had SNPs that disrupt his natural ability to synthesize phosphatidylcholine, which is an essential nutrient for the synthesis of acetylcholine that is also involved in pathways relating to phospholipid membrane production [13]. He was started on citicoline for this PEMT variant, alongside and a variety of supplements for mitochondrial support that included a combined formulation of ubiquinol (UBQH) + pyrroloquinoline quinone (PQQ) and acetyl-L-carnitine. Additionally, targeted anti-inflammatory interventions were addressed with supplements, and dietary changes to support mitochondrial function were instituted (more coconut oil and mildly ketogenic).

ADHD is a frequent comorbidity to ASD [14]. CJM was homozygous for an ADHD-associated SNP found in approximately 7% of the population. This particular SNP can lead to higher glutamate and dopamine, and lower gamma aminobutyric acid (GABA) via serotonin dysregulation [15]. Variants are known to contribute to inattentive ADHD traits [16], reduced impulse control and increased impulsivity [17], and antisocial personality traits [18]. Additional variants were present in pathways that contribute to attention and focus, language delays, and difficulties with auditory processing. Targeted interventions including L-theanine, magnesium threonate, and magnesium citrate were introduced to address some of these additional variants. Over 600 clinically relevant SNPs were evaluated with the neurodevelopmentally focused genomic CDS. Due to the intended brief nature of this case study report, however, we will not go into each of these pathways in great detail.

3.1.3. Effects of Implemented Interventions on CJM

Patient's bedwetting stopped completely, stimming ceased, cognition dramatically improved, and he is now fully conversational. These new interventions for the multiple mitochondrial related pathways markedly improved his mitochondrial function and energy to the point that he is now able to play tennis and attend the gym regularly.

The changes in this young man's life have been astonishing. His ATEC score decreased to 21 and IQ increased to 70. CJM was no longer officially classified as intellectually impaired and was legally, according to Australian guidelines, eligible to attend a mainstream school. The patient became class "captain", attended the end of year prom, passed his driver's license exam, and was even able to attain part-time employment, working in a gluten free café. Independence became a reality. CJM is now holding meaningful conversations with family, peers, teachers and employer, who are all thrilled with his progress.

3.2. *JD1 and JD2 Case Study*

3.2.1. Medical History and Background

The next two case study patients, referred to as JD1 and JD2, are interesting in that they involve identical twins who presented to the clinic in 2019 at age six. Both patients were reported by the parents to have severely regressed following an early childhood vaccination. Clinically, the children appeared to have symptoms relating to mitochondrial dysfunction and had difficulties with verbal communication.

Although they were identical twins presenting clinically with ASD, one child had additional symptoms more characteristic of ADHD, while the other clinically suffered from severe anxiety and OCD. Both were prone to recurrent PANDAS/PANS flares and OCD symptoms were present and increased during these infections. Prior to genomic interventions, both patients were taking melatonin and low dose naltrexone. IXXD's neurodevelopmental report was used to elucidate and address some of the root causes not only of ASD, but also of PANDAS/PANS, attention and focus, and anxiety-related symptoms. A table of symptoms prior to and after treatment is presented below (Table 1).

Table 1. JD1 and JD2 symptoms before and after personalized treatment.

	JD1 Pre-Treatment Symptoms	JD1 Post-Treatment Symptoms	JD2 Pre-Treatment Symptoms	JD2 Post-Treatment Symptoms
Behavior	• Severe anxiety • OCD • Obsessed with details • Lining things up • Severe constipation • Not toilet trained • Poor sleep • Low energy	• Anxiety resolved • Not afraid anymore • Fully toilet trained, dry at night • Sleeping well through the night • High energy, jumping on trampoline	• Hyperactivity • Difficulty concentrating • Self-harming • Meltdowns and rage • Poor sleep, night waking • Night wetting • Low energy	↑ No longer hyperactive Δ Still some difficulty concentrating ↑ Better moods ↑ Sleeping much improved through the night, rarely night wetting ↑ High energy
Speech	• Non-verbal • Very low receptive language	↑ Speaking in 3–4-word phrases ↑ Initiating conversation with parents ↑ Receptive language good	• Considered non-verbal • Some echolalia and echolalic "singing"	– Still considered non-verbal – Some echolalia and echolalic "singing" ↑ Listening to commands
Sensory and Cognitive	• Very fussy eater, malnourished • Severe anorexia • Fear of food • Rigid rituals around eating food • Stimming • Low fine motor skills • Low gross motor skills	↑ Eating really well, eats anything in sight ↑ Improved fine motor skills ↑ Vastly improved gross motor skills, dressing himself, riding a scooter	• Eats well • Low fine motor skills • Low gross motor skills	↑ Improved fine motor skills ↑ Vastly improved gross motor skills, riding a scooter
Social	• Very shy, "in his shell" • No eye contact • Not engaging with peers or family	↑ Very friendly ↑ Good eye contact ↑ Engaging with family and peers ↑ Playing with brother	• Won't participate in group activities	↑ Much more social ↑ Participates in group activities ↑ Playing with brother
PANDAS—Regular Flares	• OCD • Facial tics • Choreiform hand movements • Very high Streptococcus in bloodwork & stool	Δ Still some flares ↑ Markedly less OCD ↑ Facial tics gone Δ Some choreiform hand movements	• OCD • Verbal tics and humming • Very high Streptococcus in bloodwork & stool	Δ Still some flares ↑ Markedly less OCD Δ Occasional Verbal tics and humming

JD1-case study patient; JD2-case study patient; OCD-obsessive compulsive disorder; PANDAS-pediatric autoimmune neuropsychiatric disorders associated with streptococcal infections. Note: ↑ = Significant symptom improvement after treatment; Δ = slight changes/some improvement noted after treatment; – = no change noted after treatment.

3.2.2. CDS Results and Interpretation

Genetic analysis identified the presence of many different SNPs that correlated with symptoms shared between the twins. The children had a SNP in the mannose-binding lectin 2 gene (MBL2), which plays a role in the complement pathway, a component of the immune system. The T allele of this MBL2 SNP has been associated with significantly reduced MBL2 levels [19]. This correlates with a lower capacity to recognize foreign invaders (such as Streptococcus infections) and a higher risk for PANDAS (OR = 4.15) [19]. The abnormal immune response from these same SNPs has also been associated with brain autoimmune activity [20], reduced blood–brain barrier function [20], tics, and an increased risk of OCD symptoms [19]. To help address this, a combination of lignite to help tighten the tight junctions of the gut [21], vitamin D [22], probiotics [23], and prebiotics [24] were added to the treatment protocol of JD1 and JD2.

The OCD risk was believed to be exacerbated by the presence of two variants in the solute carrier family 1 member 1 gene (SLC1A1). This solute carrier SNP, particularly in homozygotes, appears to contribute to higher glutamate levels [25] and has been shown to be associated with increased risk of OCD behaviors such as hoarding, ordering and lining things up (OR = 2.01) [26]. Targeted interventions including N-acetylcysteine (NAC) [27], L-theanine [28], vitamin D [29] and vitamin B12 [29] were used to address this pathway. Additional SNPs associated with OCD comorbid with tic disorder and severe bed wetting issues (OR = 2.68) [30] were also discovered in JD1 and JD2. As presented in the genomic CDS, there was overlap in potential interventions between SLC1A1 and the additional SNPs (i.e., some of the same supplements could be used to address both pathways).

The twins were revealed to have some SNPs that are fairly uncommon, as is the case with most TACGA patients presenting with ASD. They were shown to be homozygous for a rare protein kinase SNP found in just 5% of the population. Variants have been associated with increased ASD risk (OR = 1.86) [31], and are involved in pathways relating to cell differentiation, autophagy and survival, and brain development and remodeling [32]. Resveratrol and NAD+ were incorporated into the treatment protocol since both have been shown in studies to help autophagy pathways [33,34].

SNPs contributing to mitochondrial dysfunction were present in JD1 and JD2 and were believed to impact severe fatigue, and may have also contributed to some of their muscle weakness, as evidenced by trouble holding own posture and pencil grip. Genetic analysis revealed that both children had a variant in NQO1 that is associated with an approximate 67% reduction in enzymatic activity [35]. This contributed to mitochondrial dysfunction, oxidative stress, and impaired ability to clear environmental toxins [35]. To combat this SNP's low NQO1-conveying effects, both patients were started on sulforaphane, which is known to upregulate NQO1 activity [36]. Additionally, NQO1 is needed to convert coenzyme Q10 (CoQ10) to its active form ubiquinol [37]. Therefore, ubiquinol was also used to address this pathway.

Variants relating to vitamins, ADHD, neurotransmitter balance and various other molecular pathways were also present in these patients. For the purposes of brevity, a comprehensive discussion of these additional pathways is not included in this case study report. To address some of these other pathways, the twins' personalized treatment plan included pycnogenol, ashwagandha, pyridoxal-5-phosphate (P5P) and specific soil-borne probiotics.

3.2.3. Post-Treatment Symptoms and Improvements

Highly significant improvements were seen in both JD1 and JD2. Gains in speech and socialization with family and peers were evident. Improvements in sleep were noted, bed wetting ceased, and increased energy levels were obvious. Fine and gross motor skills were improved; the children gained the ability to dress themselves and developed enough coordination to be able to ride scooters. The PANDAS flares decreased in frequency, and marked reductions were noticed regarding OCD and tics. JD1's anxiety resolved, and he was no longer a picky eater. Parents relayed that he was "eating everything in front of him". These improvements led to an increase in his weight, and he was no longer considered malnourished. JD2, on the other hand, showed marked improvements relating to ADHD symptoms. ATEC scores in both children have noticeably improved; JD1 showed a 41% reduction in ATEC scores (from 85 to 50), and JD2 showed a 44% reduction (from 97 to 54). ATEC scores continue to improve with each passing month the twins remain on the protocol. Table 1 shows post-treatment symptoms and improvements.

3.3. AD Case Study

3.3.1. Medical History and Background

This final case study patient, referred to as AD, will be briefly touched upon. In this case, the patient's mother chose to go very slowly with supplements—targeted potential interventions were added one at a time. Thus, even though treatment was initiated late in 2019 when his genomic results were initially received, his regimen is continuing to be optimized at time of publication. However, this case is also important in that the CDS allowed better prioritization of interventions, rather than the usual trial and error approach.

Prior to genomics, patient had an ATEC score of 54. Clinically, this male four-year-old exhibited significant language delays with only five words at the age of three, developed a stutter, very frequent hand flapping, tics, eye rolling, stimming triggered by excitement, seizures, inappropriate socializing, and found it hard to focus or concentrate. Child had many chest infections, adenoid surgery, and over 20 rounds of antibiotics and steroids in the previous 12 months. Patient was not on any supplements when he presented to the clinic.

3.3.2. IXXD Genomic Results and Interpretation

AD had many variants known to be of clinical significance in the pathways discussed in both case study patients above, including those associated with the language center and mitochondrial pathways. In addition to the aforementioned pathways and SNPs, it was discovered that the patient had glutamate receptor SNPs as well as two copies of an alcohol dehydrogenase 5 (ADH5) SNP that has been associated with ASD (OR = 1.54) [38]. ADH5 is a glutathione dependent enzyme that is primarily responsible for removing formaldehyde and is also important for protecting natural lipids from peroxidation [38,39]. Formaldehyde is a natural by-product of white blood cells and myeloperoxidase, and when formaldehyde is not properly removed (as would be the case in individuals homozygous for this SNP) it can build up in the brain and become neurotoxic [10,41]. This child's high rate of infections likely contributed to high neutrophil/myeloperoxidase (MPO) activation and higher levels of formaldehyde. In addition to supporting glutathione levels, since this enzyme is glutathione dependent [42], a list of foods shown to upregulate ADH5 was given the patient's mother. This list included foods such as pomegranate, watermelon, and tomatoes [43]. AD's mother was also informed regarding foods that could exacerbate the negative effects of this genomic pathway. For example, it was recommended to avoid foods artificially sweetened with aspartame, since aspartame is converted to formaldehyde [44]. These types of food and supplement interventions were taken from information listed in the referenced IXXD CDS.

Genomic CDS testing revealed that this child was homozygous for the same NQO1 SNP discussed in the case above (but case above only had one copy). Two copies of this SNP are found in approximately 4% of the population and lead to a significant reduction in enzymatic activity (approximately 97%) [35]. This drastic impairment in NQO1 activity contributes to significant mitochondrial dysfunction, increased oxidative stress, and markedly reduced detoxification [37]. As discussed above, NQO1 variants can contribute to decreased levels of the activated form of CoQ10 [37,45]. Being homozygous for this SNP dramatically impaired his ability to detoxify benzene, solvents, and many other pollutants [46]. High levels of these toxicants have been shown to contribute to increased DNA damage when exposed to various pollutants [47]. Unsurprisingly, the patient had extremely high levels of gasoline additives detected in his GPL Tox screen results, which was addressed as well.

Patient was also found to be homozygous for a well-known haplotype in the brain derived neurotrophic factor (BDNF) gene, which is found in approximately 4% of the population. This growth factor has been shown to be very important for memory and mood [48]. These BDNF SNPs contribute to decreased ability to cleave pro-BDNF to the truncated, mature form of BDNF [49]. While the mature form of BDNF is synaptogenic, the pro-BDNF form induces neuronal apoptosis and is synaptoclastic [49]. Furthermore, higher levels of pro-BNDF levels have been observed in patients with ASD [50]. Regular aerobic exercise was encouraged to help increase the conversion of pro- to mature BDNF [51]. A high butyrate diet and butyrate supplement was also implemented to address this pathway [52].

A personalized, genomically targeted treatment plan was developed. Regimen included moderately high dose UBQH-PQQ, sulforaphane, fish oil, L-theanine, butyrate, magnesium threonate, and a few other supplements. Regular aerobic exercise was also encouraged.

3.3.3. Post-Genomic Testing Improvements

ATEC scores with above interventions improved by 54% (scores decreased from 54 to 25) and continue to improve (as per communication with mother). Regarding symptom improvements, speech and socializing improved very quickly upon reducing inflammation and oxidative stress, working on detox pathways, and addressing gut health. Additionally, and remarkably, after adherence to the personalized list of supplements discussed above for only a few weeks, his seizures stopped. Hyperactive behavior continues to decrease, and tics and stims are improving. Parents continue to notice improvements on a weekly basis and are very happy with the progress to date.

4. Discussion

Non-syndromic ASD is clearly due to a multitude of contributing genomic factors that interact with environmental factors. The CDS tool used in this study also looked at genomic SNPs associated with secondary comorbid ASD conditions, given that they are pervasive amongst individuals with ASD. Comorbid conditions investigated by IXXD include ADHD, OCD, anxiety, PANDAS/PANS, gastrointestinal issues, food intolerances and nutrient deficiencies. The genomic and environmental factors, however, significantly vary from person to person. Outcomes trials have shown benefit for methyl-B12 [53], sulforaphane [54], luteolin [55], quercetin [56], melatonin [57], vitamin D [58], omega-3s [59], L-theanine [60] and dozens of other supplements in the treatment of ASD and comorbid conditions. Determining which potential interventions would be the most likely to result in improved ASD outcomes in a particular individual, however, has been a difficult hurdle to clear. Evidence-based genomic clinical decision support tools that focus on variants associated with neurodevelopmental, nutritional, toxicant clearing, and inflammatory pathways can help in prioritization and choice of interventions.

These case studies demonstrate that a well-referenced genomic CDS can be used as a tool to aid in the understanding of some of the gene variants contributing to the patient's neurodevelopmental disorder. This enables clinicians to address root causes and truly personalize treatment strategies, allowing for the achievement of more robust improvements as well as potentially faster improved outcomes in children with ASD. Initial results from the Australian Centre for Genomic Analysis practice using the IXXD tool, as illustrated by these cases, have been extremely promising. This short case series provides optimism for the role of genomics in improving function and quality of life in children with ASD and neurodevelopmental disorders and suggests that genomics in the form of a CDS can decrease the burden of the trial-and-error method.

The first limitation of this case study report is that only four cases were discussed. It will be important to analyze the collective data (ATEC scores, IQ scores, behavioral observations, etc.) from the complete cohort of approximately 100 patients. In this future analysis it will be important to separate out the results from individuals with access to the IXXD neurodevelopmental genomics CDS tool from the beginning, versus individuals who were previously optimized using the center's previous treatment methods and then plateaued.

A second limitation of this method of addressing neurodevelopmental disorders is that some patients will respond better than others to genomic CDS tools. Additional research must therefore be conducted. Next steps, which are currently in progress, include being able to reproduce the ability to obtain significant improvements in ATEC or other ASD rating scales in private physicians' offices in ASD centers across the country. In further research, controlled trials comparing the use of genomics to traditional care in ASD would be beneficial. Another limitation of this method is that it is a relatively new field not taught in residency or fellowships, and thus in order for genomics to be used systematically on a larger scale, clinicians will require dedicated time for study and continuing education. Nonetheless, genomics as a CDS tool can shift the paradigm of care for individuals with non-syndromic ASD and allow for higher functioning and better, quicker outcomes.

An additional limitation to this type of personalized medicine is the treatment cost. Utilization of a tailored, genomically-targeted approach is an investment for the family or whomever else is covering the ASD-related expenses. The cost of the IXXD tool used in this study was $900 per patient. The cost of working intensely with a clinical team that is experienced in functional or integrative medicine, genomic interpretation, and nutrition generally ranges from $2000 to $5000 per year. Currently, insurance coverage for genomic testing is most often limited to specific instances (cancer treatment, pharmacogenomics in some situations, whole genomic sequencing for diagnostic purposes). Therefore, the financial responsibility of this IXXD approach is borne by the families. This cost, however, pales in comparison to the multitude of fees that families of children with ASD incur (financing a caregiver, providing special education, loss of wages of family members, etc.). As illustrated in the cases above, there is potential for a significant financial, long-term benefit when a child can improve overall function, attend schools, and join the workforce rather than being fully reliant on caregivers. Ultimately, as additional studies are published showing the benefit of this precision medicine approach, the potential for this type of CDS targeted treatment to become mainstream and covered by insurance is likely to increase.

Author Contributions: Conceptualization, S.H.-C. and H.W.; methodology, H.W.; software, S.H.-C. and G.W.; writing—original draft preparation, H.W. and G.W.; writing—reviewing and editing, G.W., J.R. and S.H.-C. All authors have read and agreed to the published version of the manuscript.

Funding: This research received no external funding.

Institutional Review Board Statement: Ethical review and approval were waived for this study, due the study being a case report only with no double-blind or placebo control and with explicit parental consent obtained as below. All interventions in the study consisted of foods and supplements available over the counter.

Informed Consent Statement: Written parental consent was obtained for all subjects involved in the study. Consent discussed the risk, benefits, and limitations of genomics when genomics were ordered. Written informed parental consent was also obtained for each participant to participate in the study and publish this paper.

Data Availability Statement: Relevant genomics and data presented in paper. Full access to genomics is part of an online resource available to ordering clinicians and is not available in downloadable or printable form.

Acknowledgments: Amanda Mullard at TACGA for both administrative support and other support in collecting genomic information and assisting with implementation of plan.

Conflicts of Interest: Heather Way declares no conflict of interest. She was the sole investigator and clinician responsible for collection and interpretation of data as well as determination and implementation of the personalized plan for each child. Grant Williams and Jordan Reeder are employees at IntellxxDNA™, which was the genomics clinical decision support tool used in this study, but have no financial interests. Sharon Hausman-Cohen is the medical director of IntellxxDNA™ and does have ownership interest.

References

1. Yeargin-Allsopp, M.; Rice, C.; Karapurkar, T.; Doernberg, N.; Boyle, C.; Murphy, C. Prevalence of Autism in a US Metropolitan Area. *JAMA* **2003**, *289*, 49–55. [CrossRef]
2. CDC. Data and Statistics on Autism Spectrum Disorder | CDC. Centers for Disease Control and Prevention. 2020. Available online: https://www.cdc.gov/ncbddd/autism/data.html (accessed on 17 August 2020).

3. Santocchi, E.; Guiducci, L.; Fulceri, F.; Billeci, L.; Buzzigoli, E.; Apicella, F.; Calderoni, S.; Grossi, E.; Morales, M.A.; Muratori, F. Gut to brain interaction in Autism Spectrum Disorders: A randomized controlled trial on the role of probiotics on clinical, biochemical and neurophysiological parameters. *BMC Psychiatry* **2016**, *16*, 183. [CrossRef] [PubMed]
4. Husson, T.; Lecoquierre, F.; Cassinari, K.; Charbonnier, C.; Quenez, O.; Goldenberg, A.; Guerrot, A.-M.; Richard, A.-C.; Drouin-Garraud, V.; Brehin, A.-C.; et al. Rare genetic susceptibility variants assessment in autism spectrum disorder: Detection rate and practical use. *Transl. Psychiatry* **2020**, *10*, 77. [CrossRef]
5. Xie, J.; Huang, L.; Li, X.; Li, H.; Zhou, Y.; Zhu, H.; Pan, T.; Kendrick, K.M.; Xu, W. Immunological cytokine profiling identifies TNF-α as a key molecule dysregulated in autistic children. *Oncotarget* **2017**, *8*, 82390–82398. [CrossRef] [PubMed]
6. Lutz, A.-K.; Pfaender, S.; Incearap, B.; Ioannidis, V.; Ottonelli, I.; Föhr, K.J.; Cammerer, J.; Zoller, M.; Higelin, J.; Giona, F.; et al. Autism-associated SHANK3 mutations impair maturation of neuromuscular junctions and striated muscles. *Sci. Transl. Med.* **2020**, *12*, eaaz3267. [CrossRef] [PubMed]
7. Boccuto, L.; Lauri, M.; Sarasua, S.M.; Skinner, C.D.; Buccella, D.; Dwivedi, A.; Orteschi, D.; Collins, J.S.; Zollino, M.; Visconti, P.; et al. Prevalence of SHANK3 variants in patients with different subtypes of autism spectrum disorders. *Eur. J. Hum. Genet.* **2013**, *21*, 310–316. [CrossRef] [PubMed]
8. Wang, L.; Adamski, C.J.; Bondar, V.V.; Craigen, E.; Collette, J.R.; Pang, K.; Han, K.; Jain, A.; Jung, S.Y.; Liu, Z.; et al. A kinome-wide RNAi screen identifies ERK2 as a druggable regulator of Shank3 stability. *Mol. Psychiatry* **2020**, *25*, 2504–2516. [CrossRef] [PubMed]
9. Hagmeyer, S.; Sauer, A.K.; Grabrucker, A.M. Prospects of Zinc Supplementation in Autism Spectrum Disorders and Shankopathies Such as Phelan McDermid Syndrome. *Front. Synaptic Neurosci.* **2018**, *10*, 11. [CrossRef]
10. Ren, D.-L.; Sun, A.-A.; Li, Y.-J.; Chen, M.; Ge, S.-C.; Hu, B. Exogenous melatonin inhibits neutrophil migration through suppression of ERK activation. *J. Endocrinol.* **2015**, *227*, 49–60. [CrossRef] [PubMed]
11. Hendouei, F.; Moghaddam, H.S.; Mohammadi, M.R.; Taslimi, N.; Rezaei, F.; Akhondzadeh, S. Resveratrol as adjunctive therapy in treatment of irritability in children with autism: A double-blind and placebo-controlled randomized trial. *J. Clin. Pharm. Ther.* **2019**, *45*, 324–334. [CrossRef]
12. Sasseville, A.; Paquet, N.; Sevigny, J.; Hebert, M. Blue blocker glasses impede the capacity of bright light to suppress melatonin production. *J. Pineal Res.* **2006**, *41*, 73–78. [CrossRef]
13. Resseguie, M.E.; da Costa, K.-A.; Galanko, J.A.; Patel, M.; Davis, I.J.; Zeisel, S.H. Aberrant Estrogen Regulation of PEMT Results in Choline Deficiency-associated Liver Dysfunction. *J. Biol. Chem.* **2011**, *286*, 1649–1658. [CrossRef] [PubMed]
14. Eleitner, Y. The Co-Occurrence of Autism and Attention Deficit Hyperactivity Disorder in Children—What Do We Know? *Front. Hum. Neurosci.* **2014**, *8*, 268. [CrossRef]
15. Tiger, M.; Varnäs, K.; Okubo, Y.; Lundberg, J. The 5-HT1B receptor—A potential target for antidepressant treatment. *Psychopharmacology* **2018**, *235*, 1317–1334. [CrossRef]
16. Bidwell, L.C.; Gray, J.C.; Weafer, J.; Palmer, A.A.; De Wit, H.; MacKillop, J. Genetic influences on ADHD symptom dimensions: Examination of a priori candidates, gene-based tests, genome-wide variation, and SNP heritability. *Am. J. Med. Genet. Part B Neuropsychiatr. Genet.* **2017**, *174*, 458–466. [CrossRef] [PubMed]
17. Van Rooij, D.; Hartman, C.A.; Van Donkelaar, M.M.; Bralten, J.; Von Rhein, D.; Hakobjan, M.; Franke, B.; Heslenfeld, D.J.; Oosterlaan, J.; Rommelse, N.; et al. Variation in serotonin neurotransmission genes affects neural activation during response inhibition in adolescents and young adults with ADHD and healthy controls. *World J. Biol. Psychiatry* **2015**, *16*, 625–634. [CrossRef]
18. Herman, A.; Balogh, K.N. Polymorphisms of the serotonin transporter and receptor genes: Susceptibility to substance abuse. *Subst. Abus. Rehabilit.* **2012**, *3*, 49–57. [CrossRef]
19. Celik, G.G.; Tas, D.A.; Tahiroglu, A.Y.; Erken, E.; Seydaoglu, G.; Ray, P.C.; Avci, A. Mannose-Binding Lectin2 gene polymorphism in PANDAS patients. *Arch. Neuropsychiatry* **2018**, *56*, 99–105. [CrossRef]
20. Platt, M.P.; Agalliu, D.; Cutforth, T. Hello from the Other Side: How Autoantibodies Circumvent the Blood–Brain Barrier in Autoimmune Encephalitis. *Front. Immunol.* **2017**, *8*, 442. [CrossRef] [PubMed]
21. Roberts, D.A.; Bush, Z. Protective Effects of Lignite Extract Supplement on Intestinal Barrier Function in Glyphosate-Mediated Tight Junction Injury. *J. Clin. Nutr. Diet.* **2017**, 3. [CrossRef]
22. Aranow, C. Vitamin D and the Immune System. *J. Investig. Med.* **2011**, *59*, 881–886. [CrossRef] [PubMed]
23. Yan, F.; Polk, D. Probiotics and immune health. *Curr. Opin. Gastroenterol.* **2011**, *27*, 496–501. [CrossRef] [PubMed]
24. Galdeano, C.M.; Cazorla, S.I.; Dumit, J.M.L.; Vélez, E.; Perdigón, G. Beneficial Effects of Probiotic Consumption on the Immune System. *Ann. Nutr. Metab.* **2019**, *74*, 115–124. [CrossRef]
25. Arnold, P.D.; Sicard, T.; Burroughs, E.; Richter, M.A.; Kennedy, J.L. Glutamate Transporter Gene SLC1A1 Associated With Obsessive-compulsive Disorder. *Arch. Gen. Psychiatry* **2006**, *63*, 769–776. [CrossRef]
26. Andrade, J.B.D.S.; Giori, I.G.; Melo-Felippe, F.B.; Vieira-Fonseca, T.; Fontenelle, L.F.; Kohlrausch, F.B. Glutamate transporter gene polymorphisms and obsessive-compulsive disorder: A case-control association study. *J. Clin. Neurosci.* **2019**, *62*, 53–59. [CrossRef]
27. Oliver, G.; Dean, O.; Camfield, D.; Blair-West, S.; Ng, C.; Berk, M.; Sarris, A.J. N-Acetyl Cysteine in the Treatment of Obsessive Compulsive and Related Disorders: A Systematic Review. *Clin. Psychopharmacol. Neurosci.* **2015**, *13*, 12–24. [CrossRef]
28. Nathan, P.J.; Lu, K.; Gray, M.; Oliver, C. The neuropharmacology of L-theanine(N-ethyl-L-glutamine): A possible neuroprotective and cognitive enhancing agent. *J. Herb. Pharmacother.* **2006**, *6*, 21–30. [CrossRef] [PubMed]

29. Karcı, C.K.; Celik, G.G. Nutritional and herbal supplements in the treatment of obsessive compulsive disorder. *Gen. Psychiatry* **2020**, *33*, e100159. [CrossRef] [PubMed]
30. Wei, C.-C.; Wan, L.; Lin, W.-Y.; Tsai, F.-J. Rs 6313 polymorphism in 5-hydroxytryptamine receptor 2A gene association with polysymptomatic primary nocturnal enuresis. *J. Clin. Lab. Anal.* **2010**, *24*, 371–375. [CrossRef]
31. Kuo, P.-H.; Chuang, L.-C.; Su, M.-H.; Chen, C.-H.; Chen, C.-H.; Wu, J.-Y.; Yen, C.-J.; Wu, Y.-Y.; Liu, S.-K.; Chou, M.-C.; et al. Genome-Wide Association Study for Autism Spectrum Disorder in Taiwanese Han Population. *PLoS ONE* **2015**, *10*, e0138695. [CrossRef] [PubMed]
32. Zhou, C.; Qian, X.; Hu, M.; Zhang, R.; Liu, N.; Huang, Y.; Yang, J.; Zhang, J.; Bai, H.; Yang, Y.; et al. STYK1 promotes autophagy through enhancing the assembly of autophagy-specific class III phosphatidylinositol 3-kinase complex I. *Autophagy* **2020**, *16*, 1786–1806. [CrossRef] [PubMed]
33. Aman, Y.; Qiu, Y.; Tao, J.; Fang, E.F. Therapeutic potential of boosting NAD+ in aging and age-related diseases. *Transl. Med. Aging* **2018**, *2*, 30–37. [CrossRef]
34. Tian, Y.; Song, W.; Li, D.; Cai, L.; Zhao, Y. Resveratrol as A Natural Regulator Of Autophagy For Prevention And Treatment of Cancer. *Onco Targets Ther.* **2019**, *12*, 8601–8609. [CrossRef]
35. Lajin, B.; Alachkar, A. The NQO1 polymorphism C609T (Pro187Ser) and cancer susceptibility: A comprehensive meta-analysis. *Br. J. Cancer* **2013**, *109*, 1325–1337. [CrossRef] [PubMed]
36. Houghton, C.A.; Fassett, R.G.; Coombes, J.S. Sulforaphane and Other Nutrigenomic Nrf2 Activators: Can the Clinician's Expectation Be Matched by the Reality? *Oxidative Med. Cell. Longev.* **2016**, *2016*, 7857186. [CrossRef]
37. Ross, D.; Siegel, D. Functions of NQO1 in Cellular Protection and CoQ10 Metabolism and its Potential Role as a Redox Sensitive Molecular Switch. *Front. Physiol.* **2017**, *8*, 595. [CrossRef] [PubMed]
38. Bowers, K.; Li, Q.; Bressler, J.; Avramopoulos, D.; Newschaffer, C.; Fallin, M.D. Glutathione pathway gene variation and risk of autism spectrum disorders. *J. Neurodev. Disord.* **2011**, *3*, 132–143. [CrossRef]
39. Orywal, K.; Szmitkowski, M. Alcohol dehydrogenase and aldehyde dehydrogenase in malignant neoplasms. *Clin. Exp. Med.* **2017**, *17*, 131–139. [CrossRef]
40. Nakamura, J.; Shimomoto, T.; Collins, L.B.; Holley, D.W.; Zhang, Z.; Barbee, J.M.; Sharma, V.; Tian, X.; Kondo, T.; Uchida, K.; et al. Evidence that endogenous formaldehyde produces immunogenic and atherogenic adduct epitopes. *Sci. Rep.* **2017**, *7*, 10787. [CrossRef]
41. Nakamura, J.; Holley, D.W.; Kawamoto, T.; Bultman, S.J. The failure of two major formaldehyde catabolism enzymes (ADH5 and ALDH2) leads to partial synthetic lethality in C57BL/6 mice. *Genes Environ.* **2020**, *42*, 21. [CrossRef]
42. Barnett, S.D.; Buxton, I.L.O. The role of S-nitrosoglutathione reductase (GSNOR) in human disease and therapy. *Crit. Rev. Biochem. Mol. Biol.* **2017**, *52*, 340–354. [CrossRef] [PubMed]
43. Srinivasan, S.; Dubey, K.K.; Singhal, R.S. Influence of food commodities on hangover based on alcohol dehydrogenase and aldehyde dehydrogenase activities. *Curr. Res. Food Sci.* **2019**, *1*, 8–16. [CrossRef]
44. Jacob, S.E.; Stechschulte, S. Formaldehyde, aspartame, and migraines: A possible connection. *Dermatitis* **2008**, *19*, E10–E11. [PubMed]
45. Hausman-Cohen, S.R.; Hausman-Cohen, L.J.; Williams, G.E.; Bilich, C.E. Genomics of detoxification: How genomics can be used for targeting potential intervention and prevention strategies including nutrition for environmentally acquired illness. *J. Am. Coll. Nutr.* **2020**, *39*, 94–102. [CrossRef] [PubMed]
46. Kim, S.; Lan, Q.; Waidyanatha, S.; Chanock, S.; Johnson, B.A.; Vermeulen, R.; Smith, M.T.; Zhang, L.; Li, G.; Shen, M.; et al. Genetic polymorphisms and benzene metabolism in humans exposed to a wide Range of air concentrations. *Pharmacogenet. Genom.* **2007**, *17*, 789–801. [CrossRef] [PubMed]
47. Lan, Q.; Zhang, L.; Li, G.; Vermeulen, R.; Weinberg, R.S.; Dosemeci, M.; Rappaport, S.M.; Shen, M.; Alter, B.P.; Wu, Y.; et al. Hematotoxicity in Workers Exposed to Low Levels of Benzene. *Science* **2004**, *306*, 1774–1776. [CrossRef]
48. Binder, D.K.; Scharfman, H.E. Mini Review. *Growth Factors* **2004**, *22*, 123–131. [CrossRef] [PubMed]
49. Sheikh, H.I.; Hayden, E.P.; Kryski, K.R.; Smith, H.J.; Singh, S.M. Genotyping the BDNF rs6265 (val66met) polymorphism by one-step amplified refractory mutation system PCR. *Psychiatr. Genet.* **2010**, *20*, 109–112. [CrossRef]
50. Garcia, K.L.; Yu, G.; Nicolini, C.; Michalski, B.; Garzon, D.J.; Chiu, V.S.; Tongiorgi, E.; Szatmari, P.; Fahnestock, M. Altered Balance of Proteolytic Isoforms of Pro-Brain-Derived Neurotrophic Factor in Autism. *J. Neuropathol. Exp. Neurol.* **2012**, *71*, 289–297. [CrossRef]
51. Sleiman, S.F.; Henry, J.; Al-Haddad, R.; El Hayek, L.; Haidar, E.A.; Stringer, T.; Ulja, D.; Karuppagounder, S.S.; Holson, E.B.; Ratan, R.R.; et al. Exercise promotes the expression of brain derived neurotrophic factor (BDNF) through the action of the ketone body β-hydroxybutyrate. *eLife* **2016**, *5*, e15092. [CrossRef]
52. Varela, R.B.; Valvassori, S.S.; Lopes-Borges, J.; Mariot, E.; Dal-Pont, G.C.; Amboni, R.T.; Bianchini, G.; Quevedo, J. Sodium butyrate and mood stabilizers block ouabain-induced hyperlocomotion and increase BDNF, NGF and GDNF levels in brain of Wistar rats. *J. Psychiatr. Res.* **2015**, *61*, 114–121. [CrossRef]
53. Zhang, Y.; Hodgson, N.W.; Trivedi, M.S.; Abdolmaleky, H.M.; Fournier, M.; Cuenod, M.; Do, K.Q.; Deth, R.C. Decreased Brain Levels of Vitamin B12 in Aging, Autism and Schizophrenia. *PLoS ONE* **2016**, *11*, e0146797. [CrossRef] [PubMed]

54. Lynch, R.; Diggins, E.L.; Connors, S.L.; Zimmerman, A.W.; Singh, K.; Liu, H.; Talalay, P.; Fahey, J.W. Sulforaphane from Broccoli Reduces Symptoms of Autism: A Follow-up Case Series from a Randomized Double-blind Study. *Glob. Adv. Health Med.* **2017**, *6*. [CrossRef]
55. Theoharides, T.C.; Kavalioti, M. Effect of stress on learning and motivation-relevance to autism spectrum disorder. *Int. J. Immunopathol. Pharmacol.* **2019**, *33*. [CrossRef]
56. Costa, L.G.; Giordano, G.; Cole, T.B.; Marsillach, J.; Furlong, C.E. Paraoxonase 1 (PON1) as a genetic determinant of susceptibility to organophosphate toxicity. *Toxicology* **2013**, *307*, 115–122. [CrossRef] [PubMed]
57. Gagnon, K.; Godbout, R. Melatonin and Comorbidities in Children with Autism Spectrum Disorder. *Curr. Dev. Disord. Rep.* **2018**, *5*, 197–206. [CrossRef] [PubMed]
58. Jia, F.; Wang, B.; Shan, L.; Xu, Z.; Staal, W.G.; Du, L. Core Symptoms of Autism Improved After Vitamin D Supplementation. *Pediatrics* **2014**, *135*, e196–e198. [CrossRef]
59. Caughey, G.; Mantzioris, E.; Gibson, R.; Cleland, L.G.; James, M.J. The effect on human tumor necrosis factor alpha and interleukin 1 beta production of diets enriched in n-3 fatty acids from vegetable oil or fish oil. *Am. J. Clin. Nutr.* **1996**, *63*, 116–122. [CrossRef]
60. Ahn, J.; Ahn, H.S.; Cheong, J.H.; Pena, I.D. Natural Product-Derived Treatments for Attention-Deficit/Hyperactivity Disorder: Safety, Efficacy, and Therapeutic Potential of Combination Therapy. *Neural Plast.* **2016**, *2016*, 1320423. [CrossRef]

Journal of
Personalized
Medicine

Case Report

The Temple Grandin Genome: Comprehensive Analysis in a Scientist with High-Functioning Autism

Rena J. Vanzo [1,*,†], Aparna Prasad [1,†], Lauren Staunch [1], Charles H. Hensel [1], Moises A. Serrano [1], E. Robert Wassman [1], Alexander Kaplun [2], Temple Grandin [3] and Richard G. Boles [4]

1 Lineagen, Inc., Salt Lake City, UT 84109, USA; aparna.ambastha@gmail.com (A.P.); laurenstaunch@gmail.com (L.S.); ghensel3@comcast.net (C.H.H.); mserrano@lineagen.com (M.A.S.); drwassman@icloud.com (E.R.W.)
2 Variantyx, Inc., Framingham, MA 01701, USA; alex.kaplun@variantyx.com
3 Department of Animal Science, Colorado State University, Fort Collins, CO 80523, USA; Cheryl.Miller@ColoState.EDU
4 The Center for Neurological and Neurodevelopmental Health, Voorhees, NJ 08043, USA; drboles@molecularmito.com
* Correspondence: rvanzo@lineagen.com
† These authors contributed equally to this work.

Abstract: Autism spectrum disorder (ASD) is a heterogeneous condition with a complex genetic etiology. The objective of this study is to identify the complex genetic factors that underlie the ASD phenotype and other clinical features of Professor Temple Grandin, an animal scientist and woman with high-functioning ASD. Identifying the underlying genetic cause for ASD can impact medical management, personalize services and treatment, and uncover other medical risks that are associated with the genetic diagnosis. Prof. Grandin underwent chromosomal microarray analysis, whole exome sequencing, and whole genome sequencing, as well as a comprehensive clinical and family history intake. The raw data were analyzed in order to identify possible genotype-phenotype correlations. Genetic testing identified variants in three genes (*SHANK2*, *ALX1*, and *RELN*) that are candidate risk factors for ASD. We identified variants in *MEFV* and *WNT10A*, reported to be disease-associated in previous studies, which are likely to contribute to some of her additional clinical features. Moreover, candidate variants in genes encoding metabolic enzymes and transporters were identified, some of which suggest potential therapies. This case report describes the genomic findings in Prof. Grandin and it serves as an example to discuss state-of-the-art clinical diagnostics for individuals with ASD, as well as the medical, logistical, and economic hurdles that are involved in clinical genetic testing for an individual on the autism spectrum.

Keywords: autism spectrum disorder; genetic testing; chromosomal microarray analysis; whole exome sequencing; whole genome sequencing; clinical utility; polygenic risk scores; Temple Grandin

Citation: Vanzo, R.J.; Prasad, A.; Staunch, L.; Hensel, C.H.; Serrano, M.A.; Wassman, E.R.; Kaplun, A.; Grandin, T.; Boles, R.G. The Temple Grandin Genome: Comprehensive Analysis in a Scientist with High-Functioning Autism. *J. Pers. Med.* **2021**, *11*, 21. https://doi.org/10.3390/jpm11010021

Received: 13 November 2020
Accepted: 24 December 2020
Published: 29 December 2020

Publisher's Note: MDPI stays neutral with regard to jurisdictional claims in published maps and institutional affiliations.

Copyright: © 2020 by the authors. Licensee MDPI, Basel, Switzerland. This article is an open access article distributed under the terms and conditions of the Creative Commons Attribution (CC BY) license (https://creativecommons.org/licenses/by/4.0/).

1. Introduction

Autism spectrum disorder (ASD) is one of the most common neurodevelopmental disorders characterized by impairments in communication and social interaction and the presence of restrictive and repetitive behaviors [1]. The American College of Medical Genetics and Genomics (ACMG) recommends genetic evaluation for individuals with ASD [2]. Discovering the underlying genetic cause for ASD can improve the care and management by personalizing services and treatment, including addressing the medical risks that are associated with the genetic diagnosis [3]. We performed chromosomal microarray (CMA), as well as whole exome and genome sequencing (WES, WGS), on our co-author, Prof. Temple Grandin (T.G.), a widely recognized animal scientist and woman with high-functioning ASD, who is renowned for her insights on the condition. While using this report of the genomic findings in T.G., we create a discourse on state-of-the-art diagnostics for individuals with ASD. Predictably, we found many variants of uncertain significance (VUSs).

However, we also identified the variants that were previously reported in the literature as pathogenic/disease-causing and overlap with her clinical features. Furthermore, many of these variants lie in genes that will personalize medical management and guide potential therapeutic options, which underscores the importance of clinical genetic testing in those with ASD.

2. Materials and Methods

2.1. Case Report

T.G. was a full-term female infant born in 1947 after an uncomplicated pregnancy, labor, and delivery. She had normal muscle tone and early motor milestones. However, she did not make eye contact and had touch sensitivity and aversion, including stiffening up when held by others. Even based on these specific features, ASD was not suggested as the diagnostic entity had only been described four years previously [4]. A neurologist performed an electroencephalogram and ruled out petite mal epilepsy, and a hearing test was normal. T.G. was diagnosed with "minimal brain damage" at two years old. At two and a half years old, expressive and receptive language delays were noted (she was non-verbal), and she was enrolled in speech therapy. With intensive treatment and emphasis on turn-taking games, she began speaking at age three and a half and was fully verbal by age four. She maintained typical autistic behaviors, such as repetitively dribbling sand through her hands at the beach and tantrums after sudden loud noises. The associated issues included stuttering and challenges with auditory and sensory integration. In particular, touch aversion improved with the use of a squeezing machine during childhood, which T.G. designed and has adapted in order to improve ethical animal husbandry management [5]. She also reported difficulties with social interactions in childhood and adolescence. The diagnosis of autism came later in elementary school by a psychiatrist. At age nine years and at age twelve years, her IQ was tested with the Wechsler. Her full-scale IQ was 120 on the first test and 137 on the second test. The measurement of cognitive abilities ranged from disability to gifted; for example, cognitive skills that require visualization, including block design and puzzle completion, were superior, whereas auditory integration was reduced [5,6]. T.G. received a Ph.D. and has been highly successful in her career regarding animal behavior-informed agriculture design prior to her career lecturing on ASD. Despite the absence of formal testing for ASD (based on age), T.G. meets current diagnostic criteria for ASD, given her childhood clinical history. The family history is unremarkable for specific diagnoses of ASD or intellectual disability in other family members. However, T.G.'s maternal grandmother was medicated for anxiety, and T.G. suspects that her father had high-functioning ASD. Both of T.G.'s parents held college degrees, and her maternal grandfather had particular academic success as an MIT-trained engineer and co-inventor of the autopilot for airplanes. The remainder of the family history is non-contributory without a suggested inheritance pattern; further details on family history is withheld in order to maintain privacy.

T.G. reports a substantial, decades-long history of chronic myalgia, muscle rigidity, paresthesia, and hyperesthesia of the feet, as well as sudden episodes of feeling "boiling hot". She reports coordination difficulties and tires easily with exercise, reportedly since childhood. She experiences insomnia and requires physical exercise at bedtime ("100 sit-ups") to sleep. Severe anxiety and panic attacks have been major life-long issues that have moderately improved on desipramine (50 mg/day since 1980). Desipramine also alleviated colitis-like symptoms. Her diet is high in animal protein, and its reduction or elimination results in perceived irritability. A peculiar rash with eczema- and psoriasis-like features, which had been present since early childhood and diagnosed in adolescence as eczema, responds to topical steroids. She has a widow's peak (a V-shaped growth of hair in the center of the forehead). Cranial MRI identified the asymmetry of the ventricles and a reduction in cerebellum size [7].

T.G. has microdontia and hypodontia, including six missing adult teeth (two on bottom, four on top, bilaterally symmetrical) which are absent on x-ray; she did not lose the corresponding deciduous teeth until the third to sixth decades. Two dentists have commented that she has a high arched palate. Additional ectodermal dysplasia (ED)-related manifestations include soft and very brittle nails, hyperhidrosis, and body hair loss since the fifth decade of life.

2.2. Sample and Genetic Analysis

We obtained written consent from T.G. to disclose her name and health information for this study and publication. We did not have access to parental samples. Genomic DNA was extracted from an oral swab (OC-100Dx, DNA Genotek, Kantana, ON, Canada) using the PureGene extraction kit (Qiagen, Inc., Valencia, CA, USA). DNA extraction and all the analyses were performed in CAP and CLIA certified laboratories. Table 1 presents details regarding the various genetic testing technologies utilized in this study.

Table 1. Genetic testing methodologies utilized for Prof. Grandin in this study.

Genetic Test	Technology	Interpretation
Chromosomal microarray (CMA)	Custom-designed [1] Affymetrix microarray [8].	Chromosome Analysis Suite v2.0.1 software (Thermo Fisher Scientific, Santa Clara, CA)
Whole exome sequencing (WES)	Enrichment: Ion AmpliSeq™ Exome Kit (Thermo Fisher Scientific) Sequencing: Ion Proton sequencing system (Thermo Fisher Scientific) with 200 bp amplicon read technology. Genome Reference Consortium Human Build 37 (GRCh37, hg19) using the Ion Torrent Suite software v4.2 (Thermo Fisher Scientific)	Clinical Sequence Analyzer tool from WuXi NextCode [2] (https://www.wuxinextcode.com) Non-sense, missense and splice site variants were analyzed and were assessed for predicted deleterious effects using the Variant Effect Predictor (VEP) score [9].
Whole genome sequencing (WGS)	2 × 150 bp reads on Illumina next-generation sequencing systems (mean coverage of 30x in the target region, including coding exons and 10 bp of flanking intronic sequence of the known protein-coding Ref-Seq genes) [3] Alignment to human reference genome hg19 and GRCh38	Primary data analysis: Illumina DRAGEN Bio-IT Platform v2.03, interpreted on internal proprietary software from Variantyx, Framingham, MA, USA. Secondary and tertiary data analysis: Internal laboratory systems and Biodiscovery's NxClinical v4.3 or Illumina DRAGEN Bio-IT Platform v2.03 for CNV and absence of heterozygosity Detection and annotation of structural variants: The variants were called and annotated using Variantyx Genomic Intelligence structural variant pipeline [10].

Caption. [1] Affymetrix CytoScan-HD microarray plus 88,435 custom probes added to improve detection of copy number variants (CNVs) associated with neurodevelopmental disorders [8]. [2] Default settings used [3] >97% coverage of 22,000 genes in the genome at >30x.

3. Results

In our testing population on the aforementioned custom array, we have historically observed that 28% of patients with neurodevelopmental disorders have one or more abnormal or potentially abnormal copy number variants (CNVs) [11]. In the case of T.G., we did not identify any pathogenic or likely pathogenic CNVs on either custom CMA or WGS, as reported through our clinical pipeline and ACMG reporting criteria [12], and the results were consistent with a normal female chromosome complement. However, out of over 4000 structural variants of different types (including deletions, duplications, inversions, LOH, break points, and insertions of transposable elements; see Table S2 for complete list) some of the variants of unknown significance could be relevant to patient's phenotype given their relevance to brain pathology. Two of these variants are discussed in more detail below, both being located on the q arm of chromosome 9.

One of them, a heterozygous duplication of chr9q34.3q34.3x3(138,014,000–138,228,000) is about 200 kbp long and it includes several noncoding genes and exons 19 to 47 of a calcium channel gene CACNA1B. *CACNA1B* is associated with Neurodevelopmental disorder with seizures and nonepileptic hyperkinetic movements, according to OMIM. The disease is autosomal recessive, and while the deletion has a 0.00035 allele frequency in general population (four cases out of 11,295 in DGV database), one cannot completely exclude mild phonotype in heterozygotes.

Another candidate structural variant is a 1656 bp heterozygous deletion of chr9q34.13q34.13 x1(131,153,102–131,154,758), which is not found in the general population. The deletion affects exon 3 of non-coding gene RP11-544A12.4. Interestingly, this gene overlaps *NUP214*, which is located on the opposite DNA strand and, according to OMIM, is associated with susceptibility to acute infection-induced encephalopathy-9. However, the facts that disease is recessive and for *NUP214* the deletion is entirely intronic suggest that this variant is a less feasible candidate to be causative, at least not by itself.

WGS interpretation also revealed that CGG repeats that correspond to fragile X syndrome are 30,30 (a frequent normal genotype).

Three sequence variants of interest were identified in suspected or known ASD risk genes SHANK2, ALX1, and RELN (Table 2). Nevertheless, as of November 2020, none of these variants met the ACMG guidelines for "pathogenic" or "likely pathogenic" designation and, thus, are clinically classified as variants of uncertain significance (VUS) [12]. A heterozygous missense variant in *SHANK2* (p.H64R) was identified. This missense variant is a change from histidine to arginine. The histidine at this location does not lie in any well-defined protein domains. However, histidine is present at this location in primates. Further, the substitution of histidine to arginine is predicted by SIFT to be deleterious. This suggests that the his to arg amino acid substitution may alter protein function. Additionally, the variant is only observed in seven of 184,874 reference alleles (allele frequency: 3.79×10^{-5}) in the Genome Aggregation Database, a database of approximately 141,000 individuals without severe genetic conditions (gnomAD) [13,14]. Several studies suggest a role for *SHANK2* in ASD and/or intellectual disability (ID). In one publication, a patient with ASD harbored a *de novo* nonsense variant in *SHANK2*, while two additional, unrelated patients with ASD and mild-to-moderate intellectual disability had *de novo* deletions in *SHANK2* [15]. This study suggests that the haploinsufficiency of the SHANK2 gene may affect synaptic function and predispose to ASD and/or ID. In a subsequent study, a novel *de novo SHANK2* deletion was identified in another patient with ASD. Further, sequencing identified a significant enrichment of variants affecting conserved amino acids in *SHANK2* (3.4% of autism cases and 1.5% of controls, $P = 0.004$, OR = 2.37) [16]. In neuronal cell cultures, the variants that were identified in patients were associated with reduced synaptic density at dendrites when compared to variants that were only detected in controls. Interestingly, the three patients with *de novo* deletions identified in the two aforementioned studies also carry inherited CNVs at 15q11-q13 previously associated with neuropsychiatric disorders [17–19]. These data strengthen the role of synaptic gene dysfunction in ASD and support the "multiple hit model", suggesting that a better knowledge of these genetic interactions will be important in understanding the complex inheritance pattern of ASD [18,20].

A heterozygous missense variant (p.R64L) was identified in the ALX1 gene. *ALX1* encodes a transcription factor that plays a role in development, including proper neural crest migration in animal models [21]. Bi-allelic loss-of-function variants in *ALX1* cause frontonasal dysplasia, while gain-of-function variants are hypothesized to impact neurodevelopment [22,23]. T.G.'s craniofacial finding of a "widow's peak" could be related to this variant, as neural crest cells can be found in hair follicles [24]. This variant was found in 1203 of the 280,730 reference alleles (allele frequency: 0.004285) in the gnomAD database [14]. Additionally, the variant identified in T.G. was one of several potential ASD risk variants that were identified in two unrelated multiplex families [25]. In one family, this variant was shared by two siblings with ASD and it was inherited from their unaffected father. In the second family, the variant was found in an individual with ASD and it was not found in his two brothers with ASD, but was inherited from his unaffected father. Importantly, reportedly unaffected parents were not phenotyped in detail in that publication.

The authors showed the *ALX1* variant was observed multiple times in their population study (27/1541 cases and 58/5785 controls), yielding an odds ratio of 1.75 (95% confidence interval 1.11 to 2.77; $p = 0.022$; on page 7 of Matsunami et al., 2014 [25]). Although this specific variant has been observed in a supposedly unaffected control population, its higher prevalence in individuals with ASD when compared to those without ASD supports it as a potential risk factor. Further research is needed in order to confirm the impact of this variant on gene function and the role of *ALX1* in ASD susceptibility.

A heterozygous missense variant in the RELN gene (p.T1002S) was also identified in T.G. *RELN* encodes the reelin protein, which is thought to control interactions between cells for cell positioning and neuronal migration. Although the serine for threonine substitution is conservative and does not lie within any known protein domain, this variant was not present in the gnomAD database and it is conserved across different vertebrate species, except lamprey (PhyloP 1.048) [14]. Variants in *RELN* are associated with autosomal recessive lissencephaly with cerebellar hypoplasia (OMIM). In addition, *de novo* variants in *RELN* have been observed in individuals with ASD in several studies [26–28].

MEFV is a fourth gene that harbored variants with clinical overlap for T.G. Two heterozygous variants, p.R408Q and p.P369S, were identified in T.G. and they have been reported to be disease-associated. Allele frequencies in the gnomAD database are 0.00001595 (four out of 250,794 reference alleles) and 0.01470 (4150 out of 282,228 reference alleles, respectively [14]. The MEFV gene encodes a protein, called pyrin, whose function is not fully understood, but appears to direct the migration of white blood cells to sites of inflammation and downregulate the inflammatory response following the improvement of infection or injury. Over 80 variants in *MEFV* have been associated with familial Mediterranean fever (FMF), a highly complex and variable condition that can exhibit either autosomal dominant or autosomal recessive inheritance [29]. Studies suggest these variants are in linkage disequilibrium and are, thus, in cis [30]; indeed, a review of the WGS read data that were utilized in this study (2×150 bp) was long enough to confirm cis phasing.]. Despite having ClinVar associations that range from "benign" to "pathogenic", these variants, when found together, have been published as associated with disease and they are often included in clinical gene panels that are designed to test for FMF [31,32]. Most of the patients with both variants are reported to have an atypical clinical presentation. Although T.G. does not strictly meet the Tel-Hashomer clinical criteria for FMF, she has symptoms that are consistent with the atypical presentation of the condition seen in those with the same genotype, including frequent intermittent hot spells, muscles that are stiff and sore, episodes of calor, and paresthesia in both feet, and lifelong skin rashes that are diagnosed as eczema [32]. FMF has not been reported to be associated with ASD; however, inflammation is one of many pathways implemented in ASD pathogenesis and, thus, we cannot exclude these variants as being risk factors for ASD in T.G.

Further, *WNT10A* is another gene harboring a variant with overlap to T.G.'s phenotype. A homozygous variant (p.F228I) has been previously reported as pathogenic. *WNT10A* is a member of the WNT gene family, which encodes proteins that are implicated in several developmental processes, including the regulation of cell fate and patterning during embryogenesis [33]. Although p.F228I is a conservative amino acid substitution, the amino acid at this position is conserved across different species (PhyloP 0.964) and the variant has been predicted to be deleterious to the protein structure or function by in silico prediction tools. The variant identified here has been reported previously, either in the homozygous state or in trans with a second pathogenic variant, in individuals with either isolated oligodontia, tooth agenesis, or with other features of ED [34–38]. The p.F228I variant that is identified in T.G. is observed at a relatively high frequency in the general population (heterozygous carrier frequency: 0.0137, homozygote frequency: 0.000153 in the gnomAD database) [14]. Oligodontia is observed in approximately 0.14% of the population and, in one study, it was shown that variants in *WNT10A* were present in more than half of the cases of isolated oligodontia [38,39]. The variant in WNT10A possibly explains the multiple ED-like manifestations in T.G. involving her teeth, nails, hair, and sweat glands.

Table 2. Rare missense variants that are potentially relevant to T.G.'s phenotype, identified on both whole exome and whole genome sequencing.

	Gene	Chromosome [GRCh37]	ISCN	HGVS Protein Reference	SIFT Predicted Effect	Clinical Classification	dbSNP/dbVar ID	gnomAD Allele Frequency (v2.1.1; GRCh37)	Genotype in T.G.	Symptoms with Overlap
1	*ALX1*	12: 85674230	NM_006982.3:c.191G>T	p.Arg64Leu	Deleterious	VUS	rs115596276	0.004285	Het	ASD
2	*RELN*	7: 103251145	NM_005045.4:c.3005C>G	p.Thr1002Ser	Tolerable	VUS	rs1376812440	NA	Het	ASD
3	*SHANK2*	11:70858182	NM_012309.4:c.191T>C	p.His64Arg	Deleterious	VUS	rs200995537	0.0000379	Het	ASD
4	*MEFV*	16: 3299468	NM_000243.3:c.1223G>A	p.Arg408Gln	Tolerable	Pathogenic	rs11466024	0.00001595	Het	FMF
5	*MEFV*	16: 3299586	NM_000243.3:c.1105C>T	p.Pro369Ser	Deleterious	Pathogenic	rs11466023	0.01470	Het	FMF
6	*WNT10A*	2:219755011	NM_025216.3:c.682T>A	p.Phe228Ile	Deleterious	Pathogenic	rs121908120	0.0137	Homo	ED

Caption. VUS-variant of uncertain clinical significance; NA-not available; Het-Heterozygous; Homo- Homozygous; ASD-autism spectrum disorder; FMF-familial Mediterranean fever; ED-ectodermal dysplasia; rows 1–3 strong evidence to support autism susceptibility; rows 4–6 lists published pathogenic variants with excellent clinical correlation. Based on review of WGS raw data, *MEFV* variants are in *cis*. Note: *VKORC1* and *CYP2C9* variants described in the text are polymorphisms and thus not represented in the rare variant table above.

Please see Supplementary Table S1 for additional variants, which were identified in both the whole exome and whole genome sequencing assays that were run independently, with additional clinical overlap that potentially contributes to T.G.'s ASD, sleep pathogenesis, anxiety, mitochondrial function, and more, including some with potential therapeutic targets.

From a proactive standpoint, sequencing also identified a *CYP2C9* genotype that was associated with slowed metabolism of many drugs, including the anticoagulant warfarin [40]. This information, coupled with T.G.'s heterozygous status of the *VKORC1* 1639G>A variant also revealed by this testing, provides specific dosing information if warfarin is prescribed to reduce the risk adverse events. Furthermore, this *CYP2C9* genotype is also correlated with slowed metabolism of the anti-epileptic drug phenytoin, which would impact the dosing recommendations; this is critical information, given that there is a high rate of comorbidity between epilepsy/seizures and ASD [41,42].

Given the presence of multiple genetic variants potentially contributing to the manifestation of ASD in T.G., we sought to explore her data through a currently available polygenic risk score (PRS) algorithm (impute.me). This algorithm showed that T.G.'s PRS for ASD is lower than 99% and greater than 1% of the general population by assessing 17 single nucleotide polymorphisms (SNPs) that were previously reported to be associated with ASD [43].

4. Discussion

We present this case of a female scientist, Prof. Temple Grandin, with high-functioning ASD and other clinical sequelae, who was referred for clinical diagnostic testing. Through various test methodologies, we identified variants of unknown significance in three ASD risk genes (*SHANK2*, *ALX1*, and *RELN*) and other variants that impact genes that are possibly relevant to ASD pathology. This supports the concept of a polygenic model in ASD. Surprisingly, the PRS model used for T.G. showed her risk for ASD in the 1st centile of the general population. The tool did provide a pie chart indicating that the genetic liability captured by this assessment is very small (~1%), which echoes the disclaimer supplied in other publications regarding the limitations of PRS for clinical application [44]. There are several potential reasons for the contradictory ASD PRS score in T.G., given her clinical diagnosis. The SNPs that were used to generate the score in the impute.me tool were derived from case cohort individuals diagnosed with ASD prior to 2014 [43]. Importantly, Asperger disorder was a diagnostic entity until 2013, according to the American Psychiatric Association's Diagnostic and Statistical Manual of Mental Disorders (DSM). Therefore, the case cohort whose data are represented in the tool is likely more representative of those individuals who are lower functioning, which is in stark contrast to the phenotype of T.G. Additionally, we, as a community, do not yet know all of the genes and variants contributing to ASD. Additionally, finally, some co-occurring traits in those with ASD are also clearly polygenic (IQ and anxiety for instance) and may skew the algorithmic outcomes. In summary, a low PRS score, at least for ASD, cannot be used to rule out the potential for a future clinical diagnosis.

While T.G. herself does not harbor any known, identifiable ASD-related variants that garner specific medical management changes, this is a possibility for others with ASD and genetic testing should be pursued as a standard of care in line with ACMG and other medical guidelines [45]. Importantly, genetic testing did identify actionable variants that contribute to T.G.'s clinical symptomatology and can be specifically addressed in order to improve her functional symptoms and prevent further medical issues. Of note, prior to testing, additional neurological and non-neurological symptoms were attributed to a broader diagnosis of ASD and not specifically addressed based on underlying genetic etiology. This is critical for medical action, as well as family understanding, coping, and improved quality of life.

For example, clinical features that disturb T.G.'s activities of daily living are longstanding calor and paresthesia in both feet. These correlate with the two identified *MEFV* variants that were reported in cases with atypical familial Mediterranean fever. FMF is a treatable condition, and T.G. has since been referred to see a specialist. In addition, the homozygous pathogenic variant in *WNT10A* is likely to explain T.G.'s multiple ED-related symptoms. Dentists and orthodontists incorporate specific management decisions for individuals with ED-related disorders. Fortunately, T.G. herself chose not to have dental implants; the avoidance of dental implants would have been advised previously had a diagnosis of ED been known at the time. Moreover, genetic testing has provided actionable guidelines for the future prescription of certain pharmacologic treatments that were impacted by *CYP2C9* metabolism. There are a variety of other findings for T.G. with currently less well-supported medical literature that will advance with time. For example, will some combination of CNVs and SNVs that are currently classified as benign emerge as a risk susceptibility for ASD? In the future, will the reclassification of VUS to pathogenic or likely pathogenic variants trigger medical action that prevents medical morbidity or mortality? A reinterpretation of the raw data and integration with medical care can be pursued based on T.G.'s medical course and preferences in the future.

The power of clinically available genetic testing for those with ASD with or without co-occurring morbidities can be substantial for neurologic and non-neurologic precision medicine, as shown in this study. However, there are associated challenges that we must address as a medical community to make this process more impactful. One is a lack of trained clinical experts that are comfortable in reading vast amounts of genetic data and translating it in order to inform disease-associated factors and treatment options. Efforts should be made to train physicians and other healthcare providers in the practical use of genomics, as the future of health care depends on its understanding and application, including the limitations of using PRS models to predict future presence and severity for ASD. A second challenge is that the feasibility of a "genomics board" (akin to that of a multidisciplinary "tumor board", which is standard in oncologic care) is hindered by state medical licensing and telemedicine laws. Genetic counselors (GCs) are essential in this process and growing in number, but they typically have long wait lists or their own state licensure barriers that encumber integrated care. Peer-to-peer consultation between physicians and GCs is not precluded by such laws; however, including the family in the discussion constitutes the practice of medicine in most jurisdictions. Third, market forces have resulted in low-cost exome and genome testing. However, careful report generation and detailed discussion with the patient's attending providers takes substantial professional time and it is not practical under the current cost structures. Paradoxically, this results in healthcare providers being unaware of or unable to utilize the resulting complex genetic reports in order to improve clinical care and leads insurance companies to deny coverage for lack of clinical application. We propose that payer policies should be devised to commensurately compensate parties that are involved in sequencing and variant interpretation, as well as physicians and GCs for effective use of the data and the treatment of the patients.

To summarize, these data support the concept that the genetic etiology of high-functioning ASD in T.G. could result from a combination of multiple genetic factors interacting in order to yield the observed clinical features. We demonstrated that comprehensive clinical phenotype information and genomics-trained providers/laboratorians are critical in the interpretation of genomic variants that were identified through these high-throughput genomic technologies. The genomic analysis that was carried out in this study provides a basis for at least part of T.G.'s clinical features and delivers suggestions for effective management of some of the symptoms. While improvements can be made to the process and application of genetic testing for individuals with ASD, it is effective and critical, as it currently exists for optimal medical and improved personal and family quality of life.

Supplementary Materials: The following are available online at https://www.mdpi.com/2075-4426/11/1/21/s1, Table S1: Detailed Sequence Variant Spreadsheet, Table S2: Detailed Structural Variant Spreadsheet.

Author Contributions: Conceptualization, R.J.V., C.H.H., E.R.W., T.G., R.G.B.; resources, R.J.V., L.S., E.R.W., T.G., R.G.B.; data curation, A.P., M.A.S., A.K.; writing—original draft preparation, R.J.V., A.P.; writing—review and editing, R.J.V., A.P., L.S., M.A.S., R.G.B.; visualization, R.J.V., E.R.W., T.G., A.K., R.G.B.; supervision, R.J.V., C.H.H., E.R.W., R.G.B.; project administration, R.J.V.; funding acquisition, R.J.V., C.H.H., E.R.W., T.G., R.G.B. All authors have read and agreed to the published version of the manuscript.

Funding: This study was funded by Lineagen, Inc.

Institutional Review Board Statement: The study was conducted according to the guidelines of the Declaration of Helsinki and approved by Western Institutional Review Board (protocol code 20162032 and date of approval 11/1/2018).

Informed Consent Statement: Informed consent was obtained from all subjects involved in the study.

Data Availability Statement: The data presented in this study are available in the supplemental materials of this manuscript submission.

Acknowledgments: We thank members of our CAP/CLIA laboratory partners (including Predictive Laboratories, formerly known as Taueret Laboratories, LLC and PerkinElmer Genomics) for their assistance in processing and analyzing this sample and the team at Variantyx, Inc. for providing access to its Genomic Intelligence®software for WGS analysis. We also thank Jehannine Austin for providing expert guidance regarding the impute.me website and utility of polygenic risk scores as well as the entire Lineagen team for upholding our vision and mission to improve the lives of all individuals with autism spectrum disorder.

Conflicts of Interest: A.P., C.H.H., E.R.W., and L.S. were employees of Lineagen. M.A.S. and R.J.V. are employees and shareholders of Bionano Genomics, Lineagen's owner. A.K. is an employee and shareholder of Variantyx, Inc. T.G. and R.G.B. have no conflicts to declare.

References

1. Veenstra-Vanderweele, J.; Christian, S.L.; Cook, E.H. Autism as a paradigmatic complex genetic disorder. *Annu. Rev. Genom. Hum. Genet.* **2004**, *5*, 379–405. [CrossRef] [PubMed]
2. Schaefer, G.B.; Mendelsohn, N.J.; Professional Practice and Guidelines Committee. Clinical genetics evaluation in identifying the etiology of autism spectrum disorders: 2013 guideline revisions. *Genet. Med. Off. J. Am. Coll. Med. Genet.* **2013**, *15*, 399–407. [CrossRef]
3. Çöp, E.; Yurtbaşi, P.; Öner, Ö.; Münir, K.M. Genetic testing in children with autism spectrum disorders. *Anadolu Psikiyatr. Derg.* **2015**, *16*, 426–432. [CrossRef] [PubMed]
4. Kanner, L. Autistic disturbances of affective contact. *Nerv. Child* **1943**, *2*, 217–250.
5. Grandin, T. *Thinking in Pictures: And Other Reports from My Life with Autismi*, 1st ed.; Doubleday: New York, NY, USA, 1995.
6. Grandin, T. How does visual thinking work in the mind of a person with autism? A personal account. *Philos. Trans. R. Soc. Lond. Ser. B Biol. Sci.* **2009**, *364*, 1437–1442. [CrossRef]
7. Grandin, T.; Panek, R. *The Autistic Brain*; Houghton Mifflin Harcourt: New York, NY, USA, 2013.
8. Hensel, C.; Vanzo, R.; Martin, M.; Dixon, S.; Lambert, C.; Levy, B.; Nelson, L.; Peiffer, A.; Ho, K.S.; Rushton, P.; et al. Analytical and Clinical Validity Study of FirstStepDx PLUS: A Chromosomal Microarray Optimized for Patients with Neurodevelopmental Conditions. *PLoS Curr.* **2017**, *9*. [CrossRef]
9. McLaren, W.; Pritchard, B.; Rios, D.; Chen, Y.; Flicek, P.; Cunningham, F. Deriving the consequences of genomic variants with the Ensembl API and SNP Effect Predictor. *Bioinformatics* **2010**, *26*, 2069–2070. [CrossRef]
10. Neerman, N.; Faust, G.; Meeks, N.; Modai, S.; Kalfon, L.; Falik-Zaccai, T.; Kaplun, A. A clinically validated whole genome pipeline for structural variant detection and analysis. *BMC Genom.* **2019**, *16*, 545. [CrossRef]
11. Ho, K.S.; Wassman, E.R.; Baxter, A.L.; Hensel, C.; Martin, M.M.; Prasad, A.; Twede, H.; Vanzo, R.J.; Butler, M.G. Chromosomal Microarray Analysis of Consecutive Individuals with Autism Spectrum Disorders Using an Ultra-High Resolution Chromosomal Microarray Optimized for Neurodevelopmental Disorders. *Int. J. Mol. Sci.* **2016**, *17*, 2070. [CrossRef]
12. Richards, S.; Aziz, N.; Bale, S.; Bick, D.; Das, S.; Gastier-Foster, J.; Grody, W.W.; Hegde, M.; Lyon, E.; Spector, E.; et al. Standards and guidelines for the interpretation of sequence variants: A joint consensus recommendation of the American College of Medical Genetics and Genomics and the Association for Molecular Pathology. *Genet. Med. Off. J. Am. Coll. Med. Genet.* **2015**, *17*, 405–424. [CrossRef]
13. Ng, P.C.; Henikoff, S. Predicting deleterious amino acid substitutions. *Genome Res.* **2001**, *11*, 863–874. [CrossRef] [PubMed]
14. Lek, M.; Karczewski, K.J.; Minikel, E.V.; Samocha, K.E.; Banks, E.; Fennell, T.; O'Donnell-Luria, A.H.; Ware, J.S.; Hill, A.J.; Cummings, B.B.; et al. Analysis of protein-coding genetic variation in 60,706 humans. *Nature* **2016**, *536*, 285–291. [CrossRef] [PubMed]

15. Berkel, S.; Marshall, C.; Weiss, B.; Howe, J.L.; Roeth, R.; Moog, U.; Endris, V.; Roberts, W.; Szatmari, P.; Pinto, D.; et al. Mutations in the SHANK2 synaptic scaffolding gene in autism spectrum disorder and mental retardation. *Nat. Genet.* **2010**, *42*, 489–491. [CrossRef] [PubMed]
16. Leblond, C.S.; Heinrich, J.; Delorme, R.; Proepper, C.; Betancur, C.; Huguet, G.; Konyukh, M.; Chaste, P.; Ey, E.; Rastam, M.; et al. Genetic and functional analyses of SHANK2 mutations suggest a multiple hit model of autism spectrum disorders. *PLoS Genet.* **2012**, *8*, e1002521. [CrossRef] [PubMed]
17. Bucan, M.; Abrahams, B.S.; Wang, K.; Glessner, J.T.; Herman, E.I.; Sonnenblick, L.I.; Retuerto, A.I.A.; Imielinski, M.; Hadley, D.; Bradfield, J.P.; et al. Genome-wide analyses of exonic copy number variants in a family-based study point to novel autism susceptibility genes. *PLoS Genet.* **2009**, *5*, e1000536. [CrossRef] [PubMed]
18. Ingason, A.; Kirov, G.; Giegling, I.; Hansen, T.; Isles, A.R.; Jakobsen, K.D.; Kristinsson, K.T.; Le Roux, L.; Gustafsson, O.; Craddock, N.; et al. Maternally derived microduplications at 15q11-q13: Implication of imprinted genes in psychotic illness. *Am. J. Psychiatry* **2011**, *168*, 408–417. [CrossRef]
19. Stewart, L.R.; Hall, A.L.; Kang, S.-H.L.; Shaw, C.A.; Beaudet, A.L. High frequency of known copy number abnormalities and maternal duplication 15q11-q13 in patients with combined schizophrenia and epilepsy. *BMC Med Genet.* **2011**, *12*, 154. [CrossRef]
20. Guo, H.; Wang, T.; Wu, H.; Long, M.; Coe, B.P.; Li, H.; Xun, G.; Ou, J.; Chen, B.; Duan, G.; et al. Inherited and multiple de novo mutations in autism/developmental delay risk genes suggest a multifactorial model. *Mol. Autism* **2018**, *9*, 64. [CrossRef]
21. Dee, C.T.; Szymoniuk, C.R.; Mills, P.E.D.; Takahashi, T. Defective neural crest migration revealed by a Zebrafish model of Alx1-related frontonasal dysplasia. *Hum. Mol. Genet.* **2013**, *22*, 239–251. [CrossRef]
22. Uz, E.; Alanay, Y.; Aktaş, D.; Vargel, I.; Gucer, S.; Tuncbilek, G.; Von Eggeling, F.; Yilmaz, E.; Deren, O.; Posorski, N.; et al. Disruption of ALX1 causes extreme microphthalmia and severe facial clefting: Expanding the spectrum of autosomal-recessive ALX-related frontonasal dysplasia. *Am. J. Hum. Genet.* **2010**, *86*, 789–796. [CrossRef]
23. Liao, H.-M.; Fang, J.-S.; Chen, Y.-J.; Wu, K.-L.; Lee, K.-F.; Chen, C.-H. Clinical and molecular characterization of a transmitted reciprocal translocation t(1;12)(p32.1;q21.3) in a family co-segregating with mental retardation, language delay, and microcephaly. *BMC Med Genet.* **2011**, *12*, 70. [CrossRef] [PubMed]
24. Sieber-Blum, M.; Grim, M.; Hu, Y.F.; Szeder, V. Pluripotent neural crest stem cells in the adult hair follicle. *Dev. Dyn. Off. Publ. Am. Assoc. Anat.* **2004**, *231*, 258–269. [CrossRef]
25. Matsunami, N.; Hensel, C.; Baird, L.; Stevens, J.; Otterud, B.; Leppert, T.; Varvil, T.; Hadley, D.; Glessner, J.; Pellegrino, R.; et al. Identification of rare DNA sequence variants in high-risk autism families and their prevalence in a large case/control population. *Mol. Autism* **2014**, *5*, 5. [CrossRef] [PubMed]
26. De Rubeis, S.; Menachem, F.; Goldberg, A.P.; Poultney, C.S.; Samocha, K.; Cicek, A.E.; Kou, Y.; Liu, L.; Fromer, M.; Walker, S.; et al. Synaptic, transcriptional and chromatin genes disrupted in autism. *Nature* **2014**, *515*, 209–215. [CrossRef] [PubMed]
27. Iossifov, I.; Ronemus, M.; Levy, D.; Wang, Z.; Hakker, I.; Rosenbaum, J.; Yamrom, B.; Lee, Y.-H.; Narzisi, G.; Leotta, A.; et al. De novo gene disruptions in children on the autistic spectrum. *Neuron* **2012**, *74*, 285–299. [CrossRef] [PubMed]
28. Stessman, H.A.F.; Xiong, B.; Coe, B.P.; Wang, T.; Hoekzema, K.; Fenckova, M.; Kvarnung, M.; Gerdts, J.; Trinh, S.; Cosemans, N.; et al. Targeted sequencing identifies 91 neurodevelopmental-disorder risk genes with autism and developmental-disability biases. *Nat. Genet.* **2017**, *49*, 515–526. [CrossRef] [PubMed]
29. Shohat, M. Familial Mediterranean Fever. In *GeneReviews® [Internet]*; Adam, M.P., Ardinger, H.H., Pagon, R.A., Wallace, S.E., Bean, L.J.H., Stephens, K., Amemiya, A., Eds.; University of Washington: Seattle, WA, USA, 2000. Available online: http://www.ncbi.nlm.nih.gov/books/NBK1227/ (accessed on 16 December 2019).
30. Ryan, J.G.; Masters, S.L.; Booty, M.G.; Habal, N.; Alexander, J.D.; Barham, B.K.; Remmers, E.F.; Barron, K.S.; Kastner, D.L.; Aksentijevich, I. Clinical features and functional significance of the P369S/R408Q variant in pyrin, the familial Mediterranean fever protein. *Ann. Rheum. Dis.* **2010**, *69*, 1383–1388. [CrossRef]
31. Landrum, M.J.; Lee, J.M.; Benson, M.; Brown, G.R.; Chao, C.; Chitipiralla, S.; Gu, B.; Hart, J.; Hoffman, D.; Jang, W.; et al. ClinVar: Improving access to variant interpretations and supporting evidence. *Nucleic Acids Res.* **2018**, *46*, D1062–D1067. [CrossRef]
32. Livneh, A.; Langevitz, P.; Zemer, D.; Zaks, N.; Kees, S.; Lidar, T.; Migdal, A.; Padeh, S.; Pras, M. Criteria for the diagnosis of familial Mediterranean fever. *Arthritis Rheum.* **1997**, *40*, 1879–1885. [CrossRef]
33. Lee, H.-Y.; Kléber, M.; Hari, L.; Brault, V.; Suter, U.; Taketo, M.M.; Kemler, R.; Sommer, L. Instructive role of Wnt/beta-catenin in sensory fate specification in neural crest stem cells. *Science* **2004**, *303*, 1020–1023. [CrossRef]
34. Bohring, A.; Stamm, T.; Spaich, C.; Haase, C.; Spree, K.; Hehr, U.; Hoffmann, M.; Ledig, S.; Sel, S.; Wieacker, P.; et al. WNT10A mutations are a frequent cause of a broad spectrum of ectodermal dysplasias with sex-biased manifestation pattern in heterozygotes. *Am. J. Hum. Genet.* **2009**, *85*, 97–105. [CrossRef] [PubMed]
35. Dinckan, N.; Du, R.; Petty, L.; Coban-Akdemir, Z.; Jhangiani, S.; Paine, I.; Baugh, E.; Erdem, A.; Kayserili, H.; Doddapaneni, H.; et al. Whole-Exome Sequencing Identifies Novel Variants for Tooth Agenesis. *J. Dent. Res.* **2018**, *97*, 49–59. [CrossRef] [PubMed]
36. Kantaputra, P.; Sripathomsawat, W. WNT10A and isolated hypodontia. *Am. J. Med Genet. Part A* **2011**, *155A*, 1119–1122. [CrossRef] [PubMed]
37. Plaisancié, J.; Bailleul-Forestier, I.; Gaston, V.; Vaysse, F.; Lacombe, D.; Holder-Espinasse, M.; Abramowicz, M.; Coubes, C.; Plessis, G.; Faivre, L.; et al. Mutations in WNT10A are frequently involved in oligodontia associated with minor signs of ectodermal dysplasia. *Am. J. Med Genet. Part A* **2013**, *161A*, 671–678. [CrossRef] [PubMed]

38. van den Boogaard, M.-J.; Créton, M.; Bronkhorst, Y.; van der Hout, A.; Hennekam, E.; Lindhout, D.; Cune, M.; Ploos van Amstel, H.K. Mutations in WNT10A are present in more than half of isolated hypodontia cases. *J. Med Genet.* **2012**, *49*, 327–331. [CrossRef] [PubMed]
39. Nieminen, P. Genetic basis of tooth agenesis. *J. Exp. Zool. Part B Mol. Dev. Evol.* **2009**, *312B*, 320–342. [CrossRef] [PubMed]
40. JoJohnson, J.A.; Caudle, K.E.; Gong, L.; Whirl-Carrillo, M.; Stein, C.M.; Scott, S.A.; Lee, M.T.M.; Gage, B.F.; Kimmel, S.E.; Perera, M.A.; et al. Clinical Pharmacogenetics Implementation Consortium (CPIC) Guideline for Pharmacogenetics-Guided Warfarin Dosing: 2017 Update. *Clin. Pharmacol. Ther.* **2017**, *102*, 397–404. [CrossRef]
41. Caudle, K.E.; Rettie, A.E.; Whirl-Carrillo, M.; Smith, L.H.; Mintzer, S.; Lee, M.T.M.; Klein, T.E.; Callaghan, J.T. Clinical pharmacogenetics implementation consortium guidelines for CYP2C9 and HLA-B genotypes and phenytoin dosing. *Clin. Pharmacol. Ther.* **2014**, *96*, 542–548. [CrossRef]
42. Sundelin, H.E.K.; Larsson, H.; Lichtenstein, P.; Almqvist, C.; Hultman, C.M.; Tomson, T.; Ludvigsson, J.F. Autism and epilepsy: A population-based nationwide cohort study. *Neurology* **2016**, *87*, 192–197. [CrossRef]
43. Grove, J.; Ripke, S.; Als, T.D.; Mattheisen, M.; Walters, R.K.; Won, H.; Pallesen, J.; Agerbo, E.; A Andreassen, O.; Anney, R.; et al. Identification of common genetic risk variants for autism spectrum disorder. *Nat Genet.* **2019**, *51*, 431–444. [CrossRef]
44. Wray, N.R.; Lin, T.; Austin, J.; McGrath, J.J.; Hickie, I.B.; Murray, G.K.; Visscher, P.M. From Basic Science to Clinical Application of Polygenic Risk Scores: A Primer. *JAMA Psychiatry* **2020**. [CrossRef] [PubMed]
45. Henderson, L.B.; Applegate, C.D.; Wohler, E.; Sheridan, M.B.; Hoover-Fong, J.; Batista, D.A.S. The impact of chromosomal microarray on clinical management: A retrospective analysis. *Genet. Med. Off. J. Am. Coll. Med Genet.* **2014**, *16*, 657–664. [CrossRef] [PubMed]

Journal of *Personalized Medicine*

MDPI

Review

The Relationship between Autism and Ehlers-Danlos Syndromes/Hypermobility Spectrum Disorders

Emily L. Casanova [1,*], Carolina Baeza-Velasco [2,3], Caroline B. Buchanan [4] and Manuel F. Casanova [1,5]

1. School of Medicine Greenville, University of South Carolina, Greenville, SC 29615, USA; m0casa02@louisville.edu
2. Laboratory of Psychopathology and Health Processes, University of Paris, 92100 Boulogne Billancourt, France; carolina.baeza-velasco@u-paris.fr
3. Department of Emergency Psychiatry and Acute Care, CHU Montpellier, 34000 Montpellier, France
4. Greenwood Genetic Center, Greenville, SC 29605, USA; cbuchanan@ggc.org
5. Department of Psychiatry and Behavioral Sciences, University of Louisville, Louisville, KY 40292, USA

* Correspondence: scienceoveracuppa@gmail.com

Received: 12 November 2020; Accepted: 29 November 2020; Published: 1 December 2020

Abstract: Considerable interest has arisen concerning the relationship between hereditary connective tissue disorders such as the Ehlers-Danlos syndromes (EDS)/hypermobility spectrum disorders (HSD) and autism, both in terms of their comorbidity as well as co-occurrence within the same families. This paper reviews our current state of knowledge, as well as highlighting unanswered questions concerning this remarkable patient group, which we hope will attract further scientific interest in coming years. In particular, patients themselves are demanding more research into this growing area of interest, although science has been slow to answer that call. Here, we address the overlap between these two spectrum conditions, including neurobehavioral, psychiatric, and neurological commonalities, shared peripheral neuropathies and neuropathologies, and similar autonomic and immune dysregulation. Together, these data highlight the potential relatedness of these two conditions and suggest that EDS/HSD may represent a subtype of autism.

Keywords: autism spectrum disorder; Ehlers-Danlos syndrome; hypermobility spectrum disorders; autonomic disorder; mast cell activation syndrome

1. Introduction

Autism is a complex spectrum condition. Most of the autistic population is considered "idiopathic" with causes unknown, likely the result of complex polygenic and environmental interactions [1–4]. Meanwhile, a substantial minority on the autism spectrum display rare genetic variants that appear to be the primary cause of their conditions [5]. Often the autistic phenotype associated with these rare variants is secondary to a genetic syndrome (aka, syndromic autism) and is accompanied by intellectual disability and other physical impairments such as multiple congenital anomalies [6]. Popular examples of syndromic autism include fragile X syndrome (FXS) (1–5:10,000) and tuberous sclerosis (TSC) (1–5:10,000), but also include even less well known and even rarer syndromes such as Lowe syndrome (OCRL) (1:500,000) and mucopolysaccharidosis type 3 (MPS3) (1–9:1,000,000) [7,8]. To date, there are more than 60 monogenic syndromes with high penetrance for autism, as well as other forms of syndromic autism that are the result of larger chromosomal abnormalities [6,9,10]. The severity of the autism phenotype varies across the entire spectrum, although individuals with rare (often de novo) deleterious gene variants tend to be more severely affected; meanwhile, individuals of average or above-average cognitive ability tend to harbor a higher polygenic load of small effect variants, which are often inherited and may also be linked with the broader autism phenotype (BAP) in parents and siblings (reviewed in [11,12]).

Like autism, Ehlers-Danlos syndromes (EDS)/hypermobility spectrum disorders (HSD) appear to be complex spectrum conditions and are classed as hereditary connective tissue disorders (HCTD). According to the International EDS Consortium [13], there are currently 14 recognized subtypes of EDS, 13 of which are considered "rare," each occurring in no more than 1:2000 individuals and usually far rarer. All are associated with rare gene variants, often targeting collagen pathway genes [13,14]. Meanwhile, although there are currently no accurate prevalence rates or known genetic associations for the remaining subtype, hypermobile EDS (hEDS), clinical opinion and the fact that it makes up 80–90% of EDS cases strongly suggests it is a common condition. It is therefore probable the majority of hEDS cases are associated with small effect polygenic risk factors and environmental exigencies [15,16]. A whole genome/exome sequencing investigation, the Hypermobile Ehlers-Danlos Genetic Evaluation (HEDGE) study, is currently underway that will hopefully help to address some of these questions [17].

Previous research indicates that the new diagnostic entity known as generalized hypermobility spectrum disorder (G-HSD) (which partly takes the place of joint hypermobility syndrome or JHS) occurs in roughly 0.75–2% of the population and is defined by generalized joint hypermobility and chronic musculoskeletal pain and/or instability [15]. Many individuals with a current diagnosis of G-HSD could have previously received an EDS diagnosis, but since stricter changes to the nosology in 2017 patients must now meet additional criteria involving features such as the skin, hernias/prolapses, Marfanoid habitus, and heart malformations [15]. There is considerable ongoing debate amongst the patient and medical communities as to whether these additional clinical signs truly delineate two unique entities (hEDS vs. G-HSD) or are an arbitrary line drawn in the diagnostic sand. Research seems to indicate that the two conditions blend into one another and the diagnoses are poor predictors of overall physical impairment and prognosis, suggesting criteria may well change again in future [18–20].

2. Autism and Ehlers-Danlos Syndrome Comorbidity and Familial Co-Occurrence

There is a small but growing body of literature highlighting the overlap between autism and EDS/HSD. Early research includes mainly case studies [21–23], but later research has provided population-level evidence of a relationship [24]. There has also been a number of studies investigating joint hypermobility (irrespective of HCTD) and its relationship to neurodevelopmental conditions such as autism and ADHD [25–28].

Unfortunately, because these two spectrum conditions tend to be diagnosed and treated by different clinical professionals, it is not often that their comorbidity is recognized, likely leading to significant underdiagnosis [28]. For instance, although developmental-behavioral pediatricians may test for hypotonia and joint laxity in autistic children during initial assessment, unless signs are severe and suggestive of an underlying genetic disorder they are usually ascribed to the autism itself, a result of diagnostic overshadowing.

In addition, it is well-recognized that females with autism are an underdiagnosed population, particularly those who fall within the intellectually-abled end of the spectrum as they may have a different symptom presentation, are usually more skilled at social masking or rehearsed mimickry, and may experience different psychiatric comorbidities than their male counterparts [29–31]. Because hEDS is overwhelmingly diagnosed in women, it is therefore likely that autism spectrum conditions are underrecognized in this clinical subpopulation [32].

Preliminary work from Casanova et al. [16] also suggests that autism and EDS/HSD co-occur within the same families. The researchers found that more than 20% of mothers with EDS/HSD reported having autistic children—a rate not significantly different from those reported by mothers who themselves are on the autism spectrum. In addition, the rates of autism in the children shared a significant positive relationship with the severity of maternal immune disorders in EDS/HSD, suggesting that the mother's immune system may play an additional role in autism susceptibility in these connective tissue disorders. Interestingly, maternal immune activation (MIA) appears to play a significant role in many cases of idiopathic autism, suggesting a shared mechanism of risk [33]. We will discuss these relationships in greater detail later in the manuscript.

3. The Genetics of Hypermobility

The majority of gene mutations associated with the rarer forms of EDS involves fibrillar collagens, proteins that modify collagen, or enzymes involved in collagen processing [13]. Interestingly, one type of EDS, known as the periodontal type, is associated with variants in two different complement genes involved in the innate immune system, leading to chronic activation of the complement system independent of microbial triggers [34]. Although *C1R* and *C1S* are not collagen-related genes per se, synthesis of types I and III procollagen is nevertheless impaired in this form of EDS, suggesting upstream effects [35].

Recently, Tassanakijpanich et al. [36] (unpublished data) have collected a series of case studies identifying a fully presenting hEDS phenotype in adult female fragile X premutation carriers, including a case with Marfanoid habitus, arachnodactyly, and right ventricular dilation. Previous reports have linked hypermobility with fragile X syndrome (FXS) and fragile X-associated disorders, although most studies have focused on hypermobility within the distal small joints and have not addressed generalized hypermobility as often [37]. (As a note, most genetics centers do not include the Beighton assessment for generalized joint hypermobility within their fragile X protocols, which may help explain why some aspects of joint hypermobility are overlooked.)

Although data are still preliminary, the presence of an EDS-like phenotype associated with the *FMR1* gene, a negative regulator of protein translation, suggests upregulated protein translation may lead to collagen dysregulation. For instance, matrix metallopeptidase 9 (MMP9) levels are disturbed in FXS as a direct consequence of low or absent Fragile X Mental Retardation Protein (FMRP) [38]. MMP9 is a known regulator of various types of fibrillar collagen, suggesting that collagen synthesis and/or secretion may be altered in FXS and fragile X-associated disorders [39]. Because FMRP negatively regulates a wide variety of proteins, it is likely that it has other indirect effects on collagen synthesis and modification in addition to MMP9. Interestingly, Rett syndrome, which is associated with *MECP2* deletions, is also associated with joint hypermobility [40]. The MECP2 protein, like FMRP, is a major (positive) regulator of collagen deposition and Rett syndrome fibroblasts exhibit a notable reduction in collagen I synthesis, once again linking upstream dysregulation of collagen to the hypermobile phenotype [41,42].

It is intriguing, and perhaps unsurprising in the context of this paper, that both of the above-mentioned syndromes share strong ties with autism. In fact, there is a substantial list of syndromic forms of autism that share a hypermobile phenotype. We have collected 35 such monogenic syndromes from the Online Mendelian Inheritance in Man (OMIM) [43] database with strong associations to autism and hypermobility (OMIM search terms: "joint (hypermobility OR hyperlaxity OR laxity OR hyperextensibility) AND autism") (Table 1). Syndromes that had tenuous associations with either autism or hypermobility, were extremely low in patient numbers, or involved multigene deletions/duplications were removed (see Supplementary File S1, Table S5). We likewise collected the 12 different rare subtypes of EDS with their 19, respectively, associated genes into a similar list (hEDS is absent due to lack of gene associations) (Table 1).

Table 1. Genetic syndromes and their associated genes derived from the Online Mendelian Inheritance in Man (OMIM) database. These syndromes are either associated with autism and hypermobility or the Ehlers-Danlos syndromes. Autosomal dominant = AD; autosomal recessive = AR; X-linked dominant = XLD; X-linked recessive = XLR; unknown inheritance pattern = ?.

OMIM #	Syndrome	Gene/Locus	Inheritance	Group
606053	Intellectual Developmental Disorder with Autism and Speech Delay	*TBR1*	AD	Autism/hypermobility
616603	Cutis Laxa, Autosomal Dominant 3	*ALDH18A1*	AD	Autism/hypermobility
618906	Intellectual Developmental Disorder with Autistic Features and Language Delay, with or without Seizures	*TANC2*	AD	Autism/hypermobility
300624	Fragile X Syndrome	*FMR1*	XLD	Autism/hypermobility
618718	Neurodevelopmental Disorder with Behavioral Abnormalities, Absent Speech, and Hypotonia	*NTNG2*	AR	Autism/hypermobility
610443	Koolen-De Vries Syndrome	*KANSL1*	AD	Autism/hypermobility
615873	Helsmoortel-Van der AA Syndrome	*ADNP*	AD	Autism/hypermobility
615828	Vulto-Van Silfhout-De Vries Syndrome	*DEAF1*	AD	Autism/hypermobility
300958	Intellectual Developmental Disorder, X-linked, Syndromic, Snijders Blok Type	*DDX3X*	XLD, XLR	Autism/hypermobility
618505	Neurodevelopmental Disorder with Coarse Facies and Mild Distal Skeletal Abnormalities	*KDM6B*	AD	Autism/hypermobility
617804	Neurodevelopmental Disorder with Severe Motor Impairment and Absent Language	*DHX30*	AD	Autism/hypermobility
180849	Rubinstein-Taybi Syndrome 1	*CREBBP*	AD	Autism/hypermobility
617140	ZTTK Syndrome	*SON*	AD	Autism/hypermobility
617101	Intellectual Developmental Disorder with Persistence of Fetal Hemoglobin	*BLC11A*	AD	Autism/hypermobility
618354	Neurodevelopmental Disorder and Language Delay with or without Structural Brain Abnormalities	*PPP2CA*	AD	Autism/hypermobility
618205	Snijders Blok-Campeau Syndrome	*CHD3*	AD	Autism/hypermobility
616364	White-Sitton Syndrome	*POGZ*	AD	Autism/hypermobility
613406	Witteveen-Kolk Syndrome	*SIN3A*	AD	Autism/hypermobility
617062	Oku-Chung Neurodevelopmental Syndrome	*CSNK2A1*	AD	Autism/hypermobility
618659	Neurodevelopmental Disorder with Dysmorphic Facies and Dystal Skeletal Anomalies	*ZMIZ1*	AD	Autism/hypermobility
617635	Mental Retardation, Autosomal Dominant 47	*STAG1*	AD	Autism/hypermobility
617991	Chung-Jansen Syndrome	*PHIP*	AD	Autism/hypermobility
618050	Mental Retardation, Autosomal Dominant 57	*TLK2*	AD	Autism/hypermobility

Table 1. *Cont.*

OMIM #	Syndrome	Gene/Locus	Inheritance	Group
618707	Neurodevelopmental Disorder with Absent Language and Variable Seizures	*WASF1*	AD	Autism/hypermobility
300986	Mental Retardation, X-linked, Syndromic, Bain Type	*HNRNPH2*	XLD	Autism/hypermobility
617164	Short Stature, Rhizomelic, with Microcephaly, Micrognathia, and Developmental Delay	*ARCN1*	AD	Autism/hypermobility
618089	Intellectual Developmental Disorder with Dysmorphic Facies and Behavioral Abnormalities	*FBXO11*	AD	Autism/hypermobility
618709	Neurodevelopmental Disorder with Nonspecific Brain Abnormalities, with or without Seizures	*DLL1*	AD	Autism/hypermobility
619000	Intellectual Developmental Disorder with Seizures and Language Delay	*SETB1B*	?	Autism/hypermobility
617360	Congenital Heart Defects, Dysmorphic Facial Features, and Intellectual Developmental Disorder	*CDK13*	AD	Autism/hypermobility
300966	Mental Retardation, X-linked, Syndromic 33	*TAF1*	XLR	Autism/hypermobility
618748	Intellectual Developmental Disorder with Hypotonia and Behavioral Abnormalities	*CDK8*	AD	Autism/hypermobility
606232	Phelan-McDermid Syndrome	*SHANK3*	AD	Autism/hypermobility
619033	Vissers-Bodmer Syndrome	*CNOT1*	?	Autism/hypermobility
613684	Rubinstein-Taybi Syndrome 2	*EP300*	AD	Autism/hypermobility
130000	Ehlers-Danlos Syndrome, Classic Type 1	*COL5A1*	AD	Ehlers-Danlos syndrome
130010	Ehlers-Danlos Syndrome, Classic Type, 2	*COL5A2*	AD	Ehlers-Danlos syndrome
606408	Ehlers-Danlos Syndrome, Classic-like	*TNXB*	AR	Ehlers-Danlos syndrome
225320	Ehlers-Danlos Syndrome, Cardiac Valvular Type	*COL1A2*	AR	Ehlers-Danlos syndrome
130050	Ehlers-Danlos, Vascular Type	*COL3A1*	AD	Ehlers-Danlos syndrome
130060	Ehlers-Danlos Syndrome, Arthrochalasia Type, 1	*COL1A1*	AD	Ehlers-Danlos syndrome
617821	Ehlers-Danlos Syndrome, Arthrochalasia Type, 2	*COL1A2*	AD	Ehlers-Danlos syndrome
225410	Ehlers-Danlos Syndrome, Dermatosparaxis Type	*ADAMTS2*	AR	Ehlers-Danlos syndrome
225400	Ehlers-Danlos Syndrome, Kyphoscoliotic Type, 1	*PLOD1*	AR	Ehlers-Danlos syndrome
614557	Ehlers-Danlos Syndrome, Kyphoscoliotic Type, 2	*FKBP14*	AR	Ehlers-Danlos syndrome
130070	Ehlers-Danlos Syndrome, Spondylodysplastic Type, 1	*B4GALT7*	AR	Ehlers-Danlos syndrome
615349	Ehlers-Danlos Syndrome Spondylodysplastic Type, 2	*B4GALT6*	AR	Ehlers-Danlos syndrome
613350	Ehlers-Danlos Syndrome, Spondylodysplastic Type, 3	*SLC39A13*	AR	Ehlers-Danlos syndrome

Table 1. *Cont.*

OMIM #	Syndrome	Gene/Locus	Inheritance	Group
130080	Ehlers-Danlos Syndrome, Periodontal Type, 1	*C1R*	AD	Ehlers-Danlos syndrome
617174	Ehlers-Danlos Syndrome, Periodontal Type, 2	*C1S*	AD	Ehlers-Danlos syndrome
616471	Bethlem Myopathy 2	*COL12A1*	AR	Ehlers-Danlos syndrome
229200	Brittle Cornea Syndrome 1	*ZNF469*	AR	Ehlers-Danlos syndrome
614170	Brittle Cornea Syndrome 2	*PRDM5*	AR	Ehlers-Danlos syndrome
610776	Ehlers-Danlos Syndrome, Musculocontractural Type, 1	*CHST14*	AR	Ehlers-Danlos syndrome
615539	Ehlers-Danlos Syndrome, Musculocontractural Type, 2	*DSE*	AR	Ehlers-Danlos syndrome

We took the 35 autism/hypermobility (A–H) genes, together with the 19 EDS genes, and ran them through GeneMANIA to produce an extended gene interaction network based on direct physical interactions between proteins, shared pathway involvement, and genetic interactions [44] (see Supplementary File S1, Table S4). As can be seen in Figure 1, the EDS and A–H genes cluster extensively, suggesting substantial interactions between these gene networks and a potential mechanism for phenotypic overlap between autism and hypermobility-related disorders.

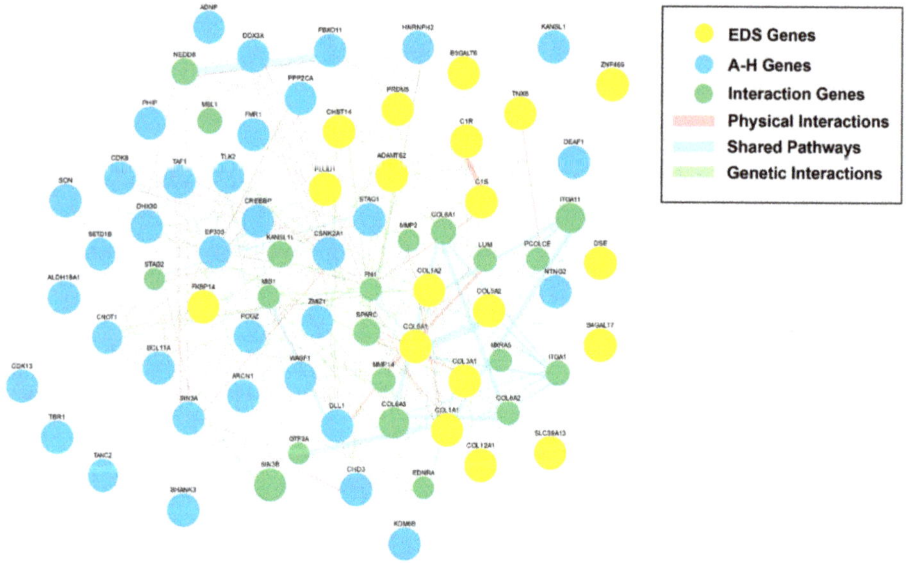

Figure 1. An extended interaction network of genes that are associated with OMIM syndromes comorbid with autism and hypermobility (A–H) (blue) and the Ehlers-Danlos syndromes (EDS) (yellow). An extended interaction network of nodes is shown in green. Direct physical interactions between gene nodes are shown in pink, shared pathways are shown in light blue, and genetic interactions are shown in light green. Note the substantial overlap between A–H and EDS genes, suggesting an extended interactive network and a possible explanation for phenotypic overlap.

These data indicate that, in future, our genetic concept of collagen-related disorders may expand significantly beyond the Ehlers-Danlos syndromes as we currently know them. Undoubtedly, their heterogeneity may become more apparent as whole genome sequencing studies continue to be performed.

4. Symptom Overlap between Autism and Ehlers-Danlos Syndromes/Hypermobility Spectrum Disorders

Although the criteria of these two complex spectrum conditions appear different on paper (one is defined by neurobehavioral symptomology, while the other is defined by structural manifestations of connective tissue impairment), they share not only comorbidity and familial co-occurrence but symptom overlap. In this section, we will review these similarities.

4.1. The Nervous System

4.1.1. Neurobehavioral, Psychiatric, and Neurological Features

It is well known that high rates of comorbidity exist between various neurodevelopmental conditions (e.g., autism, attention-deficit/hyperactivity disorder (ADHD), learning disorders, and motor disorders), which is more the norm than the exception. Indeed, up to 78% of children with autism present with comorbid ADHD [45]. In addition, autism is more frequent among people with learning disabilities and these share an inverse relationship with IQ [46]. As we see in autism, neurodevelopmental comorbidities also frequently co-occur in EDS/HSD [47,48]. In a study involving a large cohort of patients with EDS (N = 1771) and JHS (N = 10,019), the researchers observed an increased risk for ADHD in both samples, as well as in unaffected siblings [24]. Later, Piedimonte et al. [49], who explored developmental attributes in a group of 23 children with different HCTD (22 with EDS/HSD and one with Loeys-Dietz syndrome), observed that 61% presented with some kind of comorbid neurodevelopmental disorder (26% developmental coordination disorder (DCD); 22% learning disorder, 9% ADHD, and 4% ADHD plus DCD). Tourette syndrome, which also co-occurs with autism [50], has recently been associated with generalized joint laxity, orthostatic intolerance, and pain [26], as well as other neurodevelopmental conditions such as ADHD and autism. In addition, Adib et al. [51], Ghibellini et al. [52] and Piedimonte et al. [49] highlighted the presence of learning disorders in children with EDS/HSD.

Neurodevelopmental issues in EDS/HSD may also be related to proprioceptive impairment, which alters coordination and posture, and likewise may be involved in the acquisition of verbal communication and motor competence [52]. Baeza-Velasco et al. [28,48] have proposed that in order to maintain motor competence despite proprioceptive impairment, executive function may be overwhelmed in those affected, leading to some symptoms reminiscent of ADHD. In addition, pain and dysautonomia, which are frequently experienced by people with EDS/HSD, have also been associated with cognitive deficits in attention and concentration [53,54]. Thus, certain features present in EDSH/HSD, such as hypermobility, dysautonomia, chronic pain, and proprioceptive impairment, may have consequences in terms of motor, cognitive, and behavioral skills, and may ultimately affect aspects of neurodevelopment [28,48,55]. These hypotheses require further scientific exploration.

Other psychiatric features that are common in both autism and EDS/HSD include: anxiety, depression, bipolar disorder, eating disorders, and suicidal behaviors [24,56–62]. In particular, anxiety and mood disorders share strong links with autonomic dysregulation (which we will discuss in further sections) and may be related to sympathetic hyperarousal/parasympathetic hypoarousal and the chronic fatigue that often results [63,64].

Certain neurological conditions are also more common in both EDS/HSD and autism. In autism, for instance, the lifetime risk for developing epilepsy ranges between 2.7% to 44.4%, which is a seven-fold increased risk compared to the general population [65]. Individuals with intellectual disability experience the highest rates of epilepsy at approximately 22%; however, autistic people without intellectual disability still develop epilepsy at a rate of about 8% as compared to 0.75–1.1% within the general population [65–67]. In addition, abnormal electroencephalograms (EEG), even in the absence of epilepsy, have been reported in up to 60% of those with autism [66].

Seizure disorders have also been reported in EDS/HSD, particularly in association with certain subtypes such as an EDS-like disorder associated with mutations in the *FLNA* gene [68]. This form of

EDS often presents with periventricular heterotopias, a structural anomaly that has also been noted in autism [69,70]. Raw data from our own previous study [16] likewise indicate that, compared to sex-matched controls, women with EDS/HSD report higher rates of epilepsy (5% vs. 1%), a figure that is similar to those with autism without intellectually disability (Mann–Whitney U, one-tailed, $W = 17284.5$, $p = 0.042$, EDS/HSD N = 367, control N = 98). (See Supplementary File S1, Table S6 for abbreviated raw data). It should be noted, however, that some individuals within our study—though not all—reported seizure disorders following some form of head trauma [16]. Higher rates of head trauma in this clinical population have been reported in our study and others [71], possibly related to events of syncope or even coordination issues and increased numbers of accidents. Interestingly, a longitudinal study utilizing data from the Taiwanese National Health Insurance Research Database reported links between traumatic brain injury (TBI) and various neurodevelopmental conditions, including autism [72], suggesting TBI-related epilepsy may be underappreciated in these neurodevelopmental conditions.

Like epilepsy, sleep disorders are also overrepresented in both of these clinical populations. Within autism, although sleep problems persist across age groups, the types of sleep problems may vary. In younger children, bedtime resistance, sleep-related anxiety, night wakings, and parasomnias appear to be the most common issues. Meanwhile, older children and adolescents are more likely to experience delays in sleep onset, decreased sleep duration, and sleepiness during the daytime hours [73,74].

In EDS/HSD, insomnia, hypersomnia, and periodic limb movement disorder are often present; however, this population also tends to have problems sleep-disordered breathing (SDB), including obstructive sleep apnea (OSA) [75,76]. In particular, individuals with OSA report excessive fatigue and daytime sleepiness, which can be helped by nasal continuous positive airway pressure (CPAP) [76,77]. By comparison, although SDB has been little studied in autism, one report by Elrod et al. [78] indicated that individuals with autism had higher rates of SDB as compared to controls. These findings suggest that—like TBI—apneas, hypopneas, and other insufficiencies in ventilation may warrant further investigation in the autism population.

4.1.2. Coordination Problems and Sensory Issues

As briefly discussed in the previous section, motor coordination is significantly impaired in autism and may be apparent from an early age [79]. Delays in motor milestones have been consistently reported by parents, as well as noted in experimental studies (reviewed in [80]). In addition, these deficits may become more apparent with age and lead to notable developmental coordination concerns in the majority of children on the spectrum, including females [81–83].

Children with developmental coordination disorder (DCD) (without a diagnosis of autism) experience significant proprioceptive impairment, which appears to be at the root of the condition [84–86]. Some studies have reported a similar proprioceptive impairment in autism, suggesting links with the coordination issues observed [87,88]. Like autism, EDS/HSD also frequently presents with coordination and proprioceptive deficits and may lead to further complications and injury in these HCTD [52,89,90]. Given the neurodevelopmental profile gradually being recognized in EDS/HSD, it is possible that issues with motor coordination and proprioception arise not only from connective tissue dysfunction but via a neurodevelopmental component as well [52].

In the context of specialized clinics for connective tissue disorders, a clear relationship between generalized joint hypermobility and a characteristic neurodevelopmental profile affecting coordination is emerging. The clinical features of these patients tend to overlap with those of developmental coordination disorder and can be associated with learning and other disabilities. Physical and psychological consequences of these additional difficulties add to the chief manifestations of the pre-existing connective tissue disorder, affecting the well-being and development of children and their families [52].

People with autism also typically experience sensory issues in the form of both hyper- and hypo-sensitivities, which depend on the individual, the organ involved, and even the surrounding environment. For instance, the sense of touch is often affected, although the presentation is variable. The majority of intellectually-abled (IQ > 70) autistic individuals tend to experience increased pain and touch sensitivity, particularly in areas innervated by small unmyelinated C-fibers [88]. Chien et al. [91] reported the presence of small C-fiber pathology (denervation) in more than half of their adult male cases, a finding that shared a U-shaped relationship with autism severity. Another small study by Silva and Schalock [92] investigated C-fiber innervation in the skin of four autistic children with hypoesthesia and allodynia, again finding reduced density of nerve fibers within the regions studied. Notably, small fiber neuropathy often leads to hyperalgesia and allodynia, due in part to hyperreactivity of the affected nerves to typical pain-modulating effectors like substance P [93]. Hypoesthesia is also common in conjunction with hyperresponsivity to non-painful or mildly painful stimuli.

Remarkably similar to the findings in autism, the vast majority of EDS/HSD individuals—including those with some of the rarer forms of EDS—experience neuropathic pain including generalized hyperalgesia and exhibit denervation of C-fibers upon skin biopsy [94–97]. The exact same features are found in a mouse model of classic EDS (cEDS) (*Col5a1*$^{+/-}$), including allodynia and hyperalgesia, as well as the denervation of small C-fibers seen in the human condition [98]. Although the mechanism is not well understood, it is clear that connective tissue dysfunction lies upstream of such peripheral neuropathies. In contrast, most sensory disturbances in autism have been presumed to derive from pathology of the central nervous system; however, the data reviewed here suggest that peripheral nerves may also be involved.

Autistic people also experience sensory sensitivities in other modalities, such as light and sound hypersensitivity [99]. Although these modalities have been little studied within EDS/HSD specifically, they do share overlap with a common comorbid condition known as postural orthostatic tachycardia syndrome (POTS), which often involves light and sound sensitivity as part of its neurological sequelae [100]. Interestingly, cardiac function (especially baroreflex activity), which is abnormal in POTS, has been shown to have a significant effect on the processing of sensory information in the brain, suggesting links between this form of dysautonomia and sensory abnormalities [101,102]. In the next section, we will also discuss a variety of neurological and spinal stability issues that are common to EDS/HSD that predispose towards sensory processing abnormalities and that, in some instances such as Chiari I malformation, share overlap with autism [103,104].

4.1.3. Autonomic Dysregulation

There is a large body of literature describing autonomic dysregulation in autism. The profile in autism is typified by high basal sympathetic (fight or flight) tone, lower parasympathetic (rest and digest) activation, and low sympathetic reactivity to certain stimuli including tests of orthostatic tolerance [105–108]. However, a small percentage of more severely affected cases tend to have sympathetic under activation except when engaging in self-injurious behaviors, which suggests these behaviors are a form of autonomic self-regulation. Similarly, in others on the spectrum with sympathetic hyperarousal, stimulatory behaviors are a means of self-calming [107].

Sympathetic hyperarousal can be inferred in this population from higher basal heart rate, increased pupillary size, and higher respiration rate, all of which have been regularly reported in autism [105,109,110]. Autistic people also have higher sympathetic tone during certain stages of sleep (N2, N3, REM) suggesting potential sleep disturbance, and during social interactions with peers [111,112]. Interestingly, when pets are included in these peer interactions, children with autism exhibit comparatively lower sympathetic arousal, suggesting animal therapy may be a useful technique in mediating autonomic dysregulation [112].

As mentioned, autistic people tend to have lower parasympathetic tone, which is most exaggerated during the morning hours [113]. In addition, usually the lower the parasympathetic tone the greater the symptoms of anxiety and the poorer the social skills [63,114]. Children with autism who have lower tone also tend to have more lower gastrointestinal problems such as constipation, which are particularly common in children who experience regression or skills loss [115].

Despite the breadth of literature on autonomic dysregulation in autism, the available treatments are comparatively few. The beta blocker, propranolol, has been used with some modest success in order to treat various symptoms in autism, with positive effects on autonomic symptoms, although randomized controlled trials are still needed [116]. Unfortunately, its use is contraindicated in individuals with asthma, which is a condition that may share greater comorbidity with dysautonomias in pediatric populations [117]. Our group has also had significant success treating dysautonomia in autism using low-frequency repetitive transcranial magnetic stimulation (rTMS), with the hopes of expanding its use to other autonomic disorders in future [118,119].

As with autism, dysautonomias are common extraarticular manifestations in EDS, particularly in the hypermobile type, and they significantly influence quality of life for these individuals. According to one study, the extent of autonomic burden in hEDS is similar to that seen in fibromyalgia, both of which are comparatively more severe than that found in classic and vascular types of EDS [120]. Similar to the profile in autism, hEDS patients typically exhibit high resting sympathetic tone but blunted sympathetic reactivity to certain stimuli (e.g., valsalva maneuver, tilt test) [120,121]. Some individuals with these conditions, particularly those with POTS (mentioned in the previous section), also seem to exhibit a weakened baroreflex response due to dysregulated vagal (parasympathetic) efferent activity [102].

Clinical manifestations of these autonomic disorders include tachycardia, hypotension, gastrointestinal disorders (particularly those relating to motility), bladder dysfunction (e.g., urinary frequency), and poor temperature regulation. Although the dysautonomia present in autism does not typically receive a diagnostic label and is usually only symptomatically described, people with EDS frequently receive comorbid diagnoses of POTS, orthostatic hypotension (OH), mixed POTS/OH, orthostatic intolerance (OI), and neurally mediated hypotension (NMH) [122].

The first line of interventions for these types of autonomic disorders, particularly in those patients who are not experiencing significant disability, are primarily behavioral and focus on avoiding triggering factors (e.g., avoid standing for long periods of time in order to reduce blood pooling within the legs), increasing fluid intake (particularly with sodium to increase blood volume), taking salt tablets or adding more salt to the diet, wearing compression garments on the lower limbs, and performing regular cardiovascular exercise [122]. Unfortunately, cardiovascular exercise may be a challenge for some individuals with EDS/HSD due to connective tissue instability/inflammation, leading to further injury, thus placing some patients with comorbid autonomic disorders in a "catch 22".

Pharmacological treatments, which are often used in moderate-to-severely affected individuals, include medications such as the corticosteroid, fludrocortisone; the alpha-adrenergic agonist, midodrine and various beta blockers. Interestingly, for those individuals who also have endocrine disorders such as dysmenorrhea, menorrhagia, or menstrual irregularity, hormonal contraceptives can also be a first line of treatment for dysautonomias. In addition, intravenous normal saline is often helpful for individuals experiencing acute episodes or as weekly infusions for those intolerant of other treatment approaches [122].

There are a variety of neurological and spinal manifestations common to EDS/HSD that seem to predispose towards or worsen autonomic symptoms, particularly those that are related to instability and deformation of the brain stem/spinal cord. These include conditions such as Chiari I malformation, idiopathic intracranial hypertension, tethered cord, cerebrospinal fluid leaks, cranio-cervical instability, and atlantoaxial instability. In general, for those conditions in which surgical intervention is an option, surgery tends to significantly improve autonomic disorder severity [103].

Interestingly, research by Jayarao et al. [104] suggests that approximately 7% of autistic children who had an MRI for any reason exhibited evidence of Chiari I malformations, with about half of those children asymptomatic. Given, however, that most MRIs are performed in the supine rather than upright position, Chiari malformations may have been missed in some cases. Therefore, this series may be an underestimate—although the sample was likely biased considering the collection method (individuals prescribed MRI) [123]. The presence of Chiari in a significant minority of autistic patients, however, suggests the possibility of heritable disorders of connective tissue.

As discussed in the previous section, many autistic people display signs of small fiber neuropathy within the skin [91,92]. These same types of small unmyelinated C-fibers are intimately involved in the autonomic nervous system, suggesting that structural and functional damage may also be present within this system as well. Similarly, the vast majority of EDS patients exhibit small fiber neuropathy on skin biopsy, once again drawing potential links between the neuropathy within the somatosensory systems in EDS/HSD and autism and the autonomic disorders they experience [95].

4.2. Immune Dysregulation

The literature exploring immune dysregulation in autism is broad, ranging from upregulated pro-inflammatory cytokine levels in cerebrospinal fluid and blood, brain-specific autoantibodies (both in patients and mothers), and changes to immune cell function (e.g., downregulated T regulatory cells) [124,125]. The influence of the maternal immune system has also been explored in the form of human studies, cell lines, and maternal immune activation (MIA) animal models, illustrating the direct influences of maternal immunomodulators and autoantibodies on embryonic and fetal brain development (reviewed in [33]). Jones et al. [126], for example, found that mothers of children with both autism and intellectual disability (ID) produced significantly more cytokines and chemokines during pregnancy than mothers of autistic children without ID, indicating these immunomodulators may be playing an additional role in the severity of the children's conditions.

Cytokines and chemokines are known to derail preprogrammed brain development by altering cell proliferation, differentiation, and dendrite and synapse formation. For example, Smith et al. [127] found that maternal exposure during pregnancy to the immunostimulant, polyI:C (a toll-like receptor 3 agonist), resulted in thickening of the developing neocortex in the offspring—with the thickness of different layers varying according to the timing of exposure (i.e., earlier exposures tended to affect the lower layers, which develop earlier, while later exposures influenced the upper neocortical layers). Similarly, Gallagher et al. [128] found that maternal exposure to the inflammatory cytokine, interleukin 6 (IL-6), resulted in significant expansion of the forebrain neural progenitor pool of the offspring well into adulthood, suggesting permanent changes occurred affecting both the forebrain cell population and its epigenome. Cortical thickening has often been noted in autism on MRI [129,130].

Although EDS/HSD are typically thought of as collagen-based disorders, like autism there is evidence for significant immune involvement in these conditions. As discussed earlier, one type of EDS, known as the periodontal type, is the result of mutations in immune-mediating genes (*C1R*, *C1S*) that help regulate activation of the complement system. Mutations in these genes lead to chronic overactivation of this system, but further downstream also lead to reduced synthesis of procollagens I and III and ultimately the classic symptoms of EDS. Periodontal EDS strongly suggests that the immune system is an important mediator of connective tissue synthesis and therefore certain immune disorders may predispose towards the Ehlers-Danlos syndrome.

On the other hand, it is also possible that chronic collagen dysregulation and subsequent tissue injury may lead to chronic immune dysregulation, as evidenced by the mast cell-related disorders that are such a common comorbid feature in EDS/HSD [131]. For instance, one preliminary study by Chang and Vadas [132] found that all of the patients they studied with hEDS and/or POTS displayed symptoms indicative of mast cell activation, including cutaneous, gastrointestinal, naso-ocular, cardiovascular, respiratory, and central nervous system symptoms. In addition, the vast majority of these patients responded well to treatment with histamine receptor 1/2 blockers and mast cell stabilizers.

In support of this relationship, particularly within the hEDS phenotype, Chiarelli et al. [133] reported that while fibroblasts from classic and vascular EDS patients displayed perturbed collagen biosynthesis and processing, hEDS fibroblasts were typified by a pro-inflammatory myofibroblast-like state, suggesting a process of chronic abnormal wound repair. Therefore, the originating cause in many cases of hEDS may be upstream of collagen synthesis and mediated by the immune system. Both the immune system and connective tissue engage in significant crosstalk and it is therefore possible that impairment may arise anywhere along this reversible feedback loop, leading to a common phenotype [16,134,135]. For instance, in utilizing raw data reported originally in Casanova et al. [16], we show statistically similar profiles of immune-mediated symptoms as reported by female patients across hEDS, cEDS, and vascular EDS (vEDS) subgroups, suggesting that—at least in the case of cEDS and vED—primary collagen impairment also leads to immune dysregulation (Mann–Whitney U, 2-tailed, $W = 239–4960.5$, $p = 0.080–0.232$) (Figure 2). (See Supplementary_File_S1 "Tab7_EDS_Immune" for abbreviated dataset; see [16], Supplementary Materials for full raw datasets). Of relevance to the relationship between hEDS and fragile X premutation discussed earlier, immune-mediated disorders have also been reported in carriers, a finding linked with *FMR1* CGG repeat number [136–138].

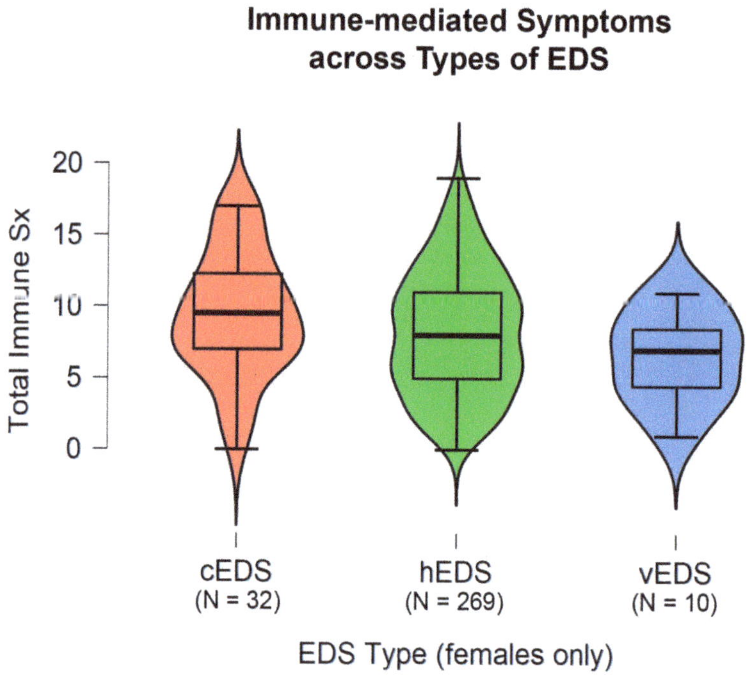

Figure 2. Violin plot indicating the number of reported immune-mediated symptoms across hypermobile EDS (hEDS), classic EDS (cEDS), and vascular EDS (vEDS). Data originally reported in Casanova et al., (2020). Only data for female participants were utilized for the analysis due to low numbers of males in the hEDS group, a condition that is extremely heavily sex skewed towards women.

As mentioned previously, Casanova et al. [16] also found that EDS/HSD mothers reported having unusually high rates of autistic children and that these EDS/HSD mothers tended to report more immune-mediated symptoms. This suggests that the maternal immune system may have played a role in autism susceptibility in these families. This work, however, is still preliminary and requires clinical studies to confirm these associations.

5. Conclusions

Although autism is defined neurobehaviorally and EDS/HSD by various articular and extra-articular connective tissue manifestations, these two conditions share considerable phenotypic overlap at various levels. Genetic data indicate similarities at the molecular, cellular, and tissue levels, as illustrated by numerous genetic syndromes with comorbid autism and hypermobility, which we have reviewed within this manuscript. EDS/HSD and autism comorbidity and familial co-occurrence lend further credence to this relationship, suggesting potential links via the maternal immune system

Meanwhile, these two spectrum conditions share a variety of secondary comorbidities, including similar neurobehavioral, psychiatric, and neurological phenotypes, such as ADHD, anxiety and mood disorders, proprioceptive impairment, sensory hyper-/hyposensitivities, eating disorders, suicidality, epilepsy, structural abnormalities such as Chiari I malformation and periventricular heterotopias, and sleep disorders—particularly those involving SDB. Relevant to these neurophenotypes are also common autonomic disorders (sympathetic hyperarousal, low parasympathetic tone) and immune disorders, which may influence cognition (e.g., anxiety, depression, fatigue, sleep disorders).

In consideration of the materials presented in this review, we (along with previous authors) have proposed that hereditary connective tissue disorders represent a subtype of autism whose prevalence is currently unknown, although the common nature of HSDs (and likely hEDS) suggests it may comprise a significant minority of autism cases. This relationship indicates that connective tissue impairment may influence brain development, either through direct and/or indirect means. Future studies will ideally involve in vitro and in vivo research to address these possibilities and further define the causative factors in autism susceptibility.

Precision Medicine and HCTD in Autism

Given the push towards personalized and precision medicine in clinical practice, we strongly recommend that the Beighton scoring system be integrated into the standard physical assessment for those individuals on or suspected to be on the autism spectrum [15,139]. Training is required in the use of this simple assessment which may be taught by physical therapists, geneticists, or rheumatologists, and we strongly recommend the use of a goniometer for accuracy and the use of important landmarks for measurement. Gauging hypermobility by eye, particularly for the larger joints like the knees and elbows, can easily be underestimated for those individuals falling within the 11–13° range, leading to false negatives and missed diagnoses. Therefore, the use of the goniometer and repeated measurements are highly recommended. For those individuals who meet criteria for generalized joint hypermobility, they should be referred to a genetics clinic for genetic testing and further assessment for HCTD in order to rule out more serious health conditions. In addition, those individuals with joint hypermobility may also benefit from referral to physical and occupational therapists who are familiar with working with hypermobility-related issues, as they may experience greater proprioceptive impairment and poorer overall body awareness [140,141].

Supplementary Materials: The following are available online at http://www.mdpi.com/2075-4426/10/4/260/s1, Supplementary File, Tables S1–S7. Tables S1–S5 concern Ehlers-Danlos syndromes (EDS) and autism/hypermobility genes and their extended gene interaction networks. Tables S6 and S7 concern raw data on epilepsy in EDS and number of immune-mediated symptoms, respectively.

Author Contributions: E.L.C. and C.B.-V. wrote original draft; C.B.B. provided expertise in Fragile X premutation and other hereditary connective tissue disorders; M.F.C. provided expertise in autism. All authors have read and agreed to the published version of the manuscript.

Funding: This research received no external funding.

Conflicts of Interest: The authors declare no conflict of interest.

References

1. Weiner, D.J.; Wigdor, E.M.; Ripke, S.; Walters, R.K.; Kosmicki, J.A.; Grove, J.; Samocha, K.E.; Goldstein, J.I.; Okbay, A.; Bybjerg-Grauholm, J.; et al. Polygenic transmission disequilibrium confirms that common and rare variation act additively to create risk for autism spectrum disorders. *Nat. Genet.* **2017**, *49*, 978–985. [CrossRef] [PubMed]
2. Klei, L.; Sanders, S.J.; Murtha, M.T.; Hus, V.; Lowe, J.K.; Willsey, A.J.; Moreno-De-Luca, D.; Timothy, W.Y.; Fombonne, E.; Geschwind, D.; et al. Common genetic variants, acting additively, are a major source of risk for autism. *Mol. Autism* **2012**, *3*, 1–13. [CrossRef] [PubMed]
3. Herbert, M.R. Contributions of the environment and environmentally vulnerable physiology to autism spectrum disorders. *Curr. Opin. Neurol.* **2010**, *23*, 103–110. [CrossRef] [PubMed]
4. Tordjman, S.; Somogyi, E.; Coulon, N.; Kermarrec, S.; Cohen, D.; Bronsard, G.; Bonnot, O.; Weismann-Arcache, C.; Botbol, M.; Lauth, B.; et al. Gene x environment interactions in autism spectrum disorders: Role of epigenetic mechanisms. *Front. Psychiatry* **2014**, *5*, 53. [CrossRef] [PubMed]
5. Stein, J.L.; Parikshak, N.N.; Geschwind, D.H. Rare inherited variation in autism: Beginning to see the forest and a few trees. *Neuron* **2013**, *77*, 209–211. [CrossRef]
6. Casanova, E.L.; Gerstner, Z.; Sharp, J.L.; Casanova, M.F.; Feltus, F.A. Widespread genotype-phenotype correlations in intellectual disability. *Front. Psychiatry* **2018**, *9*, 535. [CrossRef]
7. Oliver, C.; Berg, K.; Moss, J.; Arron, K.; Burbidge, C. Delineation of behavioral phenotypes in genetic syndromes: Characteristics of autism spectrum disorder, affect and hyperactivity. *J. Autism Dev. Disord.* **2011**, *41*, 1019–1032. [CrossRef]
8. Héron, B.; Mikaeloff, Y.; Froissart, R.; Caridade, G.; Maire, I.; Caillaud, C.; Levade, T.; Chabrol, B.; Feillet, F.; Ogier, H.; et al. Incidence and natural history of mucopolysaccharidosis type III in France and comparison with United Kingdom and Greece. *Am. J. Med. Genet. Part A* **2011**, *155*, 58–68. [CrossRef]
9. Wassink, T.H.; Piven, J.; Patil, S.R. Chromosomal abnormalities in a clinic sample of individuals with autistic disorder. *Psychiatr. Genet.* **2001**, *11*, 57–63. [CrossRef]
10. Jacquemont, M.L.; Sanlaville, D.; Redon, R.; Raoul, O.; Comier-Daire, V.; Lyonnet, S.; Amiel, J.; Le Merrer, M.; Heron, D.; De Blois, M.C.; et al. Array-based comparative genomic hybridization identifies high frequency of cryptic chromosomal rearrangements in patients with syndromic autism spectrum disorders. *J. Med. Genet.* **2006**, *43*, 843–849. [CrossRef]
11. Toma, C. Genetic variation across phenotypic severity of autism. *Trends Genet.* **2020**, *36*, 228–231. [CrossRef]
12. Nayar, K.; Sealock, J.M.; Maltman, N.; Bush, L.; Cook, E.H.; Davis, L.K.; Losh, M. Elevated polygenic burden for ASD is associated with the broad autism phenotype in mothers of individuals with ASD. *Biol. Psychiatry* **2020**, in press. [CrossRef]
13. Malfait, F.; Francomano, C.; Byers, P.; Belmont, J.; Berglund, B.; Black, J.; Bloom, L.; Bowen, J.M.; Brady, A.F.; Burrows, N.P.; et al. The 2017 international classification of the Ehlers-Danlos syndromes. *Am. J. Med. Genet. Part C Semin. Med. Genet.* **2017**, *175*, 8–26. [CrossRef] [PubMed]
14. Malfait, F.; Castori, M.; Francomano, C.A.; Giunta, C.; Kosho, T.; Byers, P.H. The Ehlers-Danlos syndromes. *Nat. Rev. Dis. Primers* **2020**, *6*, 63. [CrossRef] [PubMed]
15. Tinkle, B.; Castori, M.; Berglund, B.; Cohen, H.; Grahame, R.; Kazkaz, H.; Levy, H. Hypermobile Ehlers-Danlos syndrome (aka Ehlers-Danlos syndrome type III and Ehlers-Danlos syndrome hypermobility type): Clinical description and natural history. *Am. J. Med. Genet. Part C Semin. Med. Genet.* **2017**, *175*, 48–69. [CrossRef] [PubMed]
16. Casanova, E.L.; Sharp, J.L.; Edelson, S.M.; Kelly, D.P.; Sokhadze, E.M.; Casanova, M.F. Immune, autonomic, and endocrine dysregulation in autism and Ehlers-Danlos syndrome/hypermobility spectrum disorders versus unaffected controls. *J. Reatt. Ther. Dev. Divers.* **2020**, *2*, 82–95.
17. The Ehlers-Danlos Society. Hypermobile Ehlers-Danlos Genetic Evaluation (HEDGE) Study. Available online: https://www.ehlers-danlos.com/hedge/ (accessed on 25 September 2020).
18. Copetti, M.; Morlino, S.; Colombi, M.; Grammatico, P.; Fontana, A.; Castori, M. Severity classes in adults with hypermobile Ehlers-Danlos syndrome/hypermobility spectrum disorders: A pilot study of 105 Italian patients. *Rheumatology* **2019**, *58*, 1722–1730. [CrossRef] [PubMed]

19. Tinkle, B.T.; Bird, H.A.; Grahame, R.; Lavallee, M.; Levy, H.P.; Sillence, D. The lack of clinical distinction between the hypermobility type of Ehlers-Danlos syndrome and the joint hypermobility syndrome (a.k.a. hypermobility syndrome). *Am. J. Med. Genet. Part A* **2009**, *149*, 2368–2370. [CrossRef]
20. Castori, M.; Dordoni, C.; Valiante, M.; Sperduti, I.; Ritelli, M.; Morlino, S.; Chiarelli, N.; Celletti, C.; Venturini, M.; Camerota, F.; et al. Nosology and inheritance pattern(s) of joint hypermobility syndrome and Ehlers-Danlos syndrome, hypermobility type: A study of intrafamilial and interfamilial variability in 23 Italian pedigrees. *Am. J. Med. Genet. Part A* **2014**, *164*, 3010–3020. [CrossRef]
21. Fehlow, P.; Bernstein, K.; Tennstedt, A.; Walther, F. Early infantile autism and excessive aerophagy with symptomatic megacolon and ileus in a case of Ehlers-Danlos syndrome. *Padiatr. Grenzegebiete* **1993**, *31*, 259–267.
22. Sieg, K.G. Autism and Ehlers-Danlos syndrome. *J. Am. Med. Acad. Child Adolesc. Psychiatry* **1992**, *31*, 173. [CrossRef] [PubMed]
23. Takei, A.; Mera, K.; Sato, Y.; Haraoka, Y. High-functioning autistic disorder with Ehlers-Danlos syndrome. *Psychiatry Clin. Neurosci.* **2011**, *65*, 605–606. [CrossRef] [PubMed]
24. Cederlöf, M.; Larsson, H.; Lichtenstein, P.; Almqvist, C.; Serlachius, E.; Ludvigsson, J.F. Nationwide population-based cohort study of psychiatric disorders in individuals with Ehlers-Danlos syndrome or hypermobility syndrome and their siblings. *BMC Psychiatry* **2016**, *16*, 207. [CrossRef]
25. Eccles, J.A.; Iodice, V.; Dowell, N.G.; Owens, A.; Hughes, L.; Skipper, S.; Lycette, Y.; Humphries, K.; Harrison, N.A.; Mathias, C.J.; et al. Joint hypermobility and autonomic hyperactivity: Relevance to neurodevelopmental disorders. *J. Neurol. Neurosurg. Psychiatry* **2014**, *85*, e3. [CrossRef]
26. Csecs, J.L.; Iodice, V.; Rae, C.L.; Brooke, A.; Simmons, R.; Dowell, N.G.; Prowse, F.; Themelis, K.; Critchley, H.D.; Eccles, J.A. Increased rate of joint hypermobility in autism and related neurodevelopmental conditions is linked to dysautonomia and pain. *medRxiv* **2020**. [CrossRef]
27. Doğan, Ş.K.; Taner, Y.; Evcik, D. Benign joint hypermobility syndrome in patients with attention deficit/hyperactivity disorders. *Arch. Rheumatol.* **2011**, *26*, 187–192. [CrossRef]
28. Baeza-Velasco, C.; Cohen, D.; Hamonet, C.; Vlamynck, E.; Diaz, L.; Cravero, C.; Cappe, E.; Guinchat, V. Autism, joint hypermobility-related disorders and pain. *Front. Psychiatry* **2018**, *9*, 656. [CrossRef]
29. Gould, J.; Ashton-Smith, J. Missed diagnosis or misdiagnosis? Girls and women on the autism spectrum. *Good Autism Pract. (Gap)* **2011**, *12*, 34–41.
30. Green, R.M.; Travers, A.M.; Howe, Y.; McDougle, C.J. Women and autism spectrum disorder: Diagnosis and implications for treatment of adolescents and adults. *Curr. Psychiatry Rep.* **2019**, *21*, 22. [CrossRef]
31. Lai, M.C.; Lombardo, M.V.; Ruigrok, A.N.; Chakrabarti, B.; Auyeung, B.; Szatmari, P.; Happé, F.; Baron-Cohen, S.; MRC AIMS Consortium. Quantifying and exploring camouflaging in men and women with autism. *Autism* **2017**, *21*, 690–702. [CrossRef]
32. Castori, M.; Camerota, F.; Celletti, C.; Grammatico, P.; Padua, L. Ehlers-Danlos syndrome hypermobility type and the excess of affected females: Possible mechanisms and perspectives. *Am. J. Med. Genet. Part A* **2010**, *152*, 2406–2408. [CrossRef] [PubMed]
33. Careaga, M.; Murai, T.; Bauman, M.D. Maternal immune activation and autism spectrum disorder: From rodents to nonhuman and human primates. *Biol. Psychiatry* **2017**, *81*, 391–401. [CrossRef] [PubMed]
34. Gröbner, R.; Kapferer-Seebacher, I.; Amberger, A.; Redolfi, R.; Dalonneau, F.; Björck, E.; Milnes, D.; Bally, I.; Rossi, V.; Thielens, N.; et al. C1R mutations trigger constitutive complement 1 activation in periodontal Ehlers-Danlos syndrome. *Front. Immunol.* **2019**, *10*, 2537. [CrossRef]
35. Mataix, J.; Bañuls, J.; Muñoz, C.; Bermejo, A.; Climent, J.M. Periodontal Ehlers-Danlos syndrome associated with type III and I collagen deficiencies. *Br. J. Dermatol.* **2008**, *158*, 825–830. [CrossRef] [PubMed]
36. Tassanakijpanich, N.; McKenzie, F.J.; McLennan, Y.A.; Makhoul, E.; Tassone, F.; Jasoliya, M.J.; Romney, C.; Cortina Petrasic, I.; Napalinga, K.; Buchanan, C.; et al. Hypermobile Ehlers-Danlos syndrome (hEDS) phenotype in fragile X premutation carriers: Case series. **2020**. under submission.
37. Hagerman, R.J.; Van Housen, K.; Smith, A.C.; McGavran, L.; Opitz, J.M. Consideration of connective tissue dysfunction in the fragile X syndrome. *Am. J. Med. Genet.* **1984**, *17*, 111–121. [CrossRef] [PubMed]
38. Dziembowska, M.; Pretto, D.I.; Janusz, A.; Kaczmarek, L.; Leigh, M.J.; Gabriel, N.; Durbin-Johnson, B.; Hagerman, R.J.; Tassone, F. High MMP-9 activity levels in fragile X syndrome are lowered by minocycline. *Am. J. Med. Genet. Part A* **2013**, *161*, 1897–1903. [CrossRef]

39. Rao, V.H.; Kansal, V.; Stoupa, S.; Agrawal, D.K. MMP-1 and MMP-9 regulate epidermal growth factor-dependent collagen loss in human carotid plaque smooth muscle cells. *Physiol. Rep.* **2014**, *2*, e00224. [CrossRef]
40. Bisgaard, A.-M.; Schönewolf-Greulich, B.; Ravn, K.; Rønde, G. Is it possible to diagnose Rett syndrome before classical symptoms become obvious? Review of 24 Danish cases born between 2003 and 2012. *Eur. J. Paediatr. Neurol.* **2015**, *19*, 679–687. [CrossRef]
41. Hu, B.; Gharaee-Kermani, M.; Wu, Z.; Phan, S.H. Essential role of MeCP2 in the regulation of myofibroblast differentiation during pulmonary fibrosis. *Am. J. Pathol.* **2011**, *178*, 1500–1508. [CrossRef]
42. Signorini, C.; Leoncini, S.; De Felice, C.; Pecorelli, A.; Meloni, I.; Ariani, F.; Mari, F.; Amabile, S.; Paccagnini, E.; Gentile, M.; et al. Redox imbalance and morphological changes in skin fibroblasts in typical Rett syndrome. *Oxidative Med. Cell. Longev.* **2014**, *2014*, 195935. [CrossRef] [PubMed]
43. Online Mendelian Inheritance in Man, OMIM. McKusick-Nathans Institute of Genetic Medicine, Johns Hopkins University (Baltimore, MD). 2020. Available online: https://omim.org/ (accessed on 11 May 2020).
44. Warde-Farley, D.; Donaldson, S.L.; Comes, O.; Zuberi, K.; Badrawi, R.; Chao, P.; Franz, M.; Grouios, C.; Kazi, F.; Lopes, T.; et al. The GeneMANIA prediction server: Biological network integration for gene prioritization and predicting gene function. *Nucleic Acids Res.* **2010**, *38*, W214–W220. [CrossRef]
45. Brookman-Frazee, L.; Stadnick, N.; Chlebowski, C.; Baker-Ericzén, M.; Ganger, W. Characterizing psychiatric comorbidity in children with autism spectrum disorder receiving publicly funded mental health services. *Autism* **2017**, *22*, 938–952. [CrossRef] [PubMed]
46. O'Brien, G.; Pearson, J. Autism and learning disability. *Autism* **2004**, *8*, 125–140. [CrossRef] [PubMed]
47. Baeza-Velasco, C.; Grahame, R.; Bravo, J.F. A connective tissue disorder may underlie ESSENCE problems in childhood. *Res. Dev. Disabil.* **2017**, *60*, 232–242. [CrossRef] [PubMed]
48. Baeza-Velasco, C.; Sinibaldi, L.; Castori, M. Attention deficit/hyperactivity disorder, joint hypermobility related disorders and pain: Expanding body-mind connections to the developmental age. *Atten. Deficit Hyperact. Disord.* **2018**, *10*, 163–175. [CrossRef]
49. Piedimonte, C.; Penge, R.; Morlino, S.; Sperduti, I.; Terzani, A.; Giannini, M.T.; Colombi, M.; Grammatico, P.; Cardona, F.; Castori, M. Exploring relationships between joint hypermobility and neurodevelopment in children (4–13 years) with hereditary connective tissue disorders and developmental coordination disorder. *Am. J. Med. Genet. B* **2018**, *177*, 546–556. [CrossRef]
50. Darrow, S.M.; Grados, M.; Sandor, P.; Hirschtritt, M.E.; Illmann, C.; Osiecki, L.; Dion, Y.; King, R.; Pauls, D.; Budman, C.L.; et al. Autism Spectrum Symptoms in a Tourette's Disorder Sample. *J. Am. Acad. Child Adolesc. Psychiatry* **2017**, *56*, 610–617.e1. [CrossRef]
51. Adib, N.; Davies, R.; Grahame, R.; Woo, P.; Murray, K.J. Joint hypermobility syndrome in childhood. A not so benign multisystem disorder? *Rheumatology* **2005**, *44*, 744–750. [CrossRef]
52. Ghibellini, G.; Brancati, F.; Castori, M. Neurodevelopmental attributes of joint hypermobility syndrome/Ehlers-Danlos syndrome, hypermobility type: Update and perspectives. *Am. J. Med. Genet. Part C Semin. Med. Genet.* **2015**, *169*, 107–116. [CrossRef]
53. Karas, B.; Grubb, B.P.; Boehm, K.; Kip, K. The Postural Orthostatic Tachycardia Syndrome: A potentially treatable cause of chronic fatigue, exercise intolerance, and cognitive impairment in adolescents. *Pacing Clin. Electrophysiol.* **2000**, *23*, 344–351. [CrossRef] [PubMed]
54. Moriarty, O.; McGuire, B.E.; Finn, D.P. The effect of pain on cognitive function: A review of clinical and preclinical research. *Prog. Neurobiol.* **2011**, *93*, 385–404. [CrossRef] [PubMed]
55. Baeza-Velasco, C. Neurodiversity: Associations and implications in hypermobility spectrum disorders and Ehlers-Danlos syndrome. In Proceedings of the EDS ECHO Summit. Scientific Meeting on EDS, HSD and Co-Morbidities (Virtual Event), 2–3 October 2020.
56. Postorino, V.; Kerns, C.M.; Vivanti, G.; Bradshaw, J.; Siracusano, M.; Mazzone, L. Anxiety Disorders and Obsessive-Compulsive Disorder in Individuals with Autism Spectrum Disorder. *Curr. Psychiatry Rep.* **2017**, *19*, 92. [CrossRef] [PubMed]
57. Bulbena, A.; Baeza-Velasco, C.; Bulbena-Cabré, A.; Pailhez, G.; Critchley, H.; Chopra, P.; Mallorqui-Bagué, N.; Frank, C.; Porges, S. Psychiatric and psychological aspects in the Ehlers-Danlos syndrome. *Am. J. Med. Genet. Part C* **2017**, *175*, 237–245. [CrossRef]

58. Van Heijst, B.F.C.; Deserno, M.K.; Rhebergen, D.; Geurts, H.M. Autism and depression are connected: A report of two complementary network studies. *Autism* **2020**, *24*, 680–692. [CrossRef]
59. Munesue, T.; Ono, Y.; Mutoh, K.; Shimoda, K.; Nakatani, H.; Kikuchi, M. High prevalence of bipolar disorder comorbidity in adolescents and young adults with high-functioning autism spectrum disorder: A preliminary study of 44 outpatients. *J. Affect. Disord.* **2008**, *111*, 170–175. [CrossRef]
60. Vuiller, L.; Carter, Z.; Teixeira, A.R.; Moseley, R.L. Alexithymia may explain the relationship between autistic traits and eating disorder psychopathology. *Mol. Autism* **2020**, *11*, 63. [CrossRef]
61. Baeza-Velasco, C.; Lorente, S.; Tasa Vindral, B.; Guillaume, S.; Mora, M.; Espinoza, P. Gastrointestinal and eating problems in women with Ehlers-Danlos syndromes. **2020**. under submission.
62. Storch, E.A.; Sulkowski, M.L.; Nadeau, J.; Lewin, A.B.; Arnold, E.B.; Mutch, P.J.; Murphy, T.K. The phenomenology and clinical correlates of suicidal thoughts and behaviors in youth with autism spectrum disorders. *J. Autism Dev. Disord.* **2013**, *43*, 2450–2459. [CrossRef]
63. Bal, E.; Harden, E.; Lamb, D.; Van Hecke, A.V.; Denver, J.W.; Porges, S.W. Emotion recognition in children with autism spectrum disorders: Relations to eye gaze and autonomic state. *J. Autism Dev. Disord.* **2010**, *40*, 358–370. [CrossRef]
64. Anderson, J.W.; Lambert, E.A.; Sari, C.I.; Dawood, T.; Esler, M.D.; Vaddadi, G.; Lambert, G.W. Cognitive function, health-related quality of life, and symptoms of depression and anxiety sensitivity are impaired in patients with postural orthostatic tachycardia syndrome (POTS). *Front. Physiol.* **2014**, *5*, 230. [CrossRef] [PubMed]
65. Strasser, L.; Downes, M.; Kung, J.; Cross, J.H.; De Haan, M. Prevalence and risk factors for autism spectrum disorder in epilepsy: A systematic review and meta-analysis. *Dev. Med. Child Neurol.* **2018**, *60*, 19–29. [CrossRef] [PubMed]
66. Spence, S.J.; Schneider, M.T. The role of epilepsy and epileptiform EEGs in autism spectrum disorders. *Pediatrics Res.* **2009**, *65*, 599–606. [CrossRef]
67. Amiet, C.; Gourfinkel-An, I.; Bouzamondo, A.; Tordjman, S.; Baulac, M.; Lechat, P.; Mottron, L.; Cohen, D. Epilepsy in autism is associated with intellectual disability and gender: Evidence from a meta-analysis. *Biol. Psychiatry* **2008**, *64*, 577–582. [CrossRef] [PubMed]
68. Cortini, F.; Villa, C. Ehlers-Danlos syndromes and epilepsy: An updated review. *Seizure* **2018**, *57*, 1–4. [CrossRef] [PubMed]
69. Castori, M.; Voermans, N.C. Neurological manifestations of Ehlers-Danlos syndrome(s): A review. *Iran. J. Neurol.* **2014**, *13*, 190–208.
70. Wegiel, J.; Kuchna, I.; Nowicki, K.; Imaki, H.; Wegiel, J.; Marchi, E.; Ma, S.Y.; Chauhan, A.; Chauhan, V.; Bobrowicz, T.W.; et al. The neuropathology of autism: Defects of neurogenesis and neuronal migration, and dysplastic changes. *Acta Neuropathol.* **2010**, *119*, 755–770. [CrossRef]
71. Hamonet, C.; Fredy, D.; Lefevre, J.H.; Bourgeois-Gironde, S.; Zeiton, J.-D. Brain injury unmasking Ehlers-Danlos syndromes after trauma: The fiber print. *Orphanet J. Rare Dis.* **2016**, *11*, 45. [CrossRef]
72. Chang, H.K.; Hsu, J.W.; Wu, J.C.; Huang, K.L.; Chang, H.C.; Bai, Y.M.; Chen, T.J.; Chen, M.H. Traumatic brain injury in early childhood and risk of attention-deficit/hyperactivity disorder and autism spectrum disorder: A nationwide longitudinal study. *J. Clin. Psychiatry* **2018**, *79*, 17m11857. [CrossRef]
73. Goldman, S.E.; Richdale, A.L.; Clemons, T.; Malow, B.A. Parental sleep concerns in autism spectrum disorders: Variations from childhood to adolescence. *J. Autism Dev. Disord.* **2012**, *42*, 531–538. [CrossRef]
74. Richdale, A.L.; Schreck, K.A. Sleep problems in autism spectrum disorders: Prevalence, nature, & possible biopsychosocial aetiologies. *Sleep Med. Rev.* **2009**, *13*, 403–411.
75. Domany, K.A.; Hantragool, S.; Smith, D.F.; Xu, Y.; Hossain, M.; Simakajornboon, N. Sleep disorders and their management in children with Ehlers-Danlos syndrome referred to sleep clinics. *J. Clin. Sleep Med.* **2018**, *14*, 623–629. [CrossRef] [PubMed]
76. Guilleminault, C.; Primeau, M.; Chiu, H.-Y.; Yuen, K.M.; Leger, D.; Metlaine, A. Sleep-disordered breathing in Ehlers-Danlos syndrome: A genetic model of OSA. *Chest* **2013**, *144*, 1503–1511. [CrossRef] [PubMed]
77. Gaisl, T.; Giunta, C.; Bratton, D.J.; Sutherland, K.; Schlatzer, C.; Sievi, N.; Franzen, D.; Cistulli, P.A.; Rohrbach, M.; Kohler, M. Obstructive sleep apnoea and quality of life in Ehlers-Danlos syndrome: A parallel cohort study. *Thorax* **2017**, *72*, 729–735. [CrossRef]

78. Elrod, M.G.; Nylund, C.M.; Susi, A.L.; Gorman, G.H.; Hisle-Gorman, E.; Rogers, D.J.; Erdie-Lalena, C. Prevalence of diagnosed sleep disorders and related diagnostic and surgical procedures in children with autism spectrum disorders. *J. Dev. Behav. Pediatrics* **2016**, *37*, 377–384. [CrossRef]
79. Fournier, K.A.; Hass, C.J.; Naik, S.K.; Lodha, N.; Cauraugh, J.H. Motor coordination in autism spectrum disorders: A synthesis and meta-analysis. *J. Autism Dev. Disord.* **2010**, *40*, 1227–1240. [CrossRef] [PubMed]
80. Harris, S.R. Early motor delays as diagnostic clues in autism spectrum disorder. *Eur. J. Pediatrics* **2017**, *176*, 1259–1262. [CrossRef] [PubMed]
81. Lloyd, M. Motor skills of toddlers with autism spectrum disorders. *Autism* **2013**, *17*, 133–146. [CrossRef]
82. Sumner, E.; Leonard, H.C.; Hill, E.L. Overlapping phenotypes in autism spectrum disorder and developmental coordination disorder: A cross-syndrome comparison of motor and social skills. *J. Autism Dev. Disord.* **2016**, *46*, 2609–2620. [CrossRef]
83. Kopp, S.; Beckung, E.; Gillberg, C. Developmental coordination disorder and other motor control problems in girls with autism spectrum disorder and/or attention-deficit/hyperactivity disorder. *Res. Dev. Disabil.* **2010**, *31*, 350–361. [CrossRef]
84. Mon-Williams, M.A.; Wann, J.P.; Pascal, E. Visual-proprioceptive mapping in children with developmental coordination disorder. *Dev. Med. Child Neurol.* **1999**, *41*, 247–254. [CrossRef] [PubMed]
85. Tseng, Y.T.; Tsai, C.L.; Chen, F.C.; Konczak, J. Wrist position sense acuity and its relation to motor dysfunction in children with developmental coordination disorder. *Neurosci. Lett.* **2018**, *674*, 106–111. [CrossRef] [PubMed]
86. Tseng, Y.T.; Tsai, C.L.; Chen, F.C.; Chen, F.C.; Konczak, J. Position sense dysfunction affects proximal and distal arm joints in children with developmental coordination disorder. *J. Mot. Behav.* **2019**, *51*, 49–58. [CrossRef]
87. Blanche, E.I.; Reinoso, G.; Chang, M.C.; Bodison, S. Proprioceptive processing difficulties among children with autism spectrum disorders and developmental disabilities. *Am. J. Occup. Ther.* **2012**, *66*, 621–624. [CrossRef] [PubMed]
88. Riquelme, I.; Hatem, S.M.; Montoya, P. Abnormal pressure pain, touch sensitivity, proprioception, and manual dexterity in children with autism spectrum disorders. *Neural Plast.* **2016**, *2016*, 1723401. [CrossRef] [PubMed]
89. Clayton, H.A.; Cressman, E.K.; Henriques, D.Y. Proprioceptive sensitivity in Ehlers-Danlos syndrome patients. *Exp. Brain Res.* **2013**, *230*, 311–321. [CrossRef]
90. Clayton, H.A.; Jones, S.A.; Henriques, D.Y. Proprioceptive precision is impaired in Ehlers-Danlos syndrome. *SpringerPlus* **2015**, *4*, 323. [CrossRef]
91. Chien, Y.L.; Chao, C.C.; Wu, S.W.; Hsueh, H.W.; Chiu, Y.N.; Tsai, W.C.; Gau, S.S.F.; Hsieh, S.T. Small fiber pathology in autism and clinical implications. *Neurology* **2020**. [CrossRef]
92. Silva, L.; Schalock, M. First skin biopsy reports in children with autism show loss of C-tactile fibers. *J. Neurol. Disord.* **2016**, *4*, 2. [CrossRef]
93. Skilling, S.R.; Harkness, D.H.; Larson, A.A. Experimental peripheral neuropathy decreases the dose of substance P required to increase excitatory amino acid release in the CSF of the rat spinal cord. *Neurosci. Lett.* **1992**, *139*, 92–96. [CrossRef]
94. Rombaut, L.; Scheper, M.; De Wandele, I.; De Vries, J.; Meeus, M.; Malfait, F.; Engelbert, R.; Calders, P. Chronic pain in patients with the hypermobility type of Ehlers-Danlos syndrome: Evidence for generalized hyperalgesia. *Clin. Rheumatol.* **2015**, *34*, 1121–1129. [CrossRef] [PubMed]
95. Cazzato, D.; Castori, M.; Lombardi, R.; Caravello, F.; Dalla Bella, E.; Petrucci, A.; Grammatico, P.; Dordoni, C.; Colombi, M.; Lauria, G. Small fiber neuropathy is a common feature of Ehlers-Danlos syndromes. *Neurology* **2016**, *87*, 155–159. [CrossRef] [PubMed]
96. Camerota, F.; Celletti, C.; Castori, M.; Grammatico, P.; Padua, L. Neuropathic pain is a common feature in Ehlers-Danlos syndrome. *J. Pain Symptom Manag.* **2011**, *41*, e2–e4. [CrossRef] [PubMed]
97. Granata, G.; Padua, L.; Celletti, C.; Castori, M.; Saraceni, V.M.; Camerota, F. Entrapment neuropathies and polyneuropathies in joint hypermobility syndrome/Ehlers-Danlos syndrome. *Clin. Neurophysiol.* **2013**, *124*, 1689–1694. [CrossRef] [PubMed]
98. Syx, D.; Miller, R.E.; Obeidat, A.M.; Tran, P.B.; Vroman, R.; Malfait, Z.; Miller, R.J.; Malfait, F.; Malfait, A.M. Pain-related behaviors and abnormal cutaneous innervation in a murine model of classical Ehlers-Danlos syndrome. *Pain* **2020**, *161*, 2274–2283. [CrossRef]

99. Minshew, N.J.; Hobson, J.A. Sensory sensitivities and performance on sensory perceptual tasks in high-functioning individuals with autism. *J. Autism Dev. Disord.* **2008**, *38*, 1485–1498. [CrossRef] [PubMed]
100. Fedorowski, A. Postural orthostatic tachycardia syndrome: Clinical presentation, aetiology and management. *J. Intern. Med.* **2019**, *285*, 352–366. [CrossRef]
101. Goswami, R.; Frances, M.F.; Steinback, C.D.; Shoemaker, J.K. Forebrain organization representing baroreceptor gating of somatosensory afferents within the cortical autonomic network. *J. Neurophysiol.* **2012**, *108*, 453–466. [CrossRef]
102. Stewart, J.M. Autonomic nervous system dysfunction in adolescents with postural orthostatic tachycardia syndrome and chronic fatigue syndrome is characterized by attenuated vagal baroreflex and potentiated sympathetic vasomotion. *Pediatric Res.* **2000**, *48*, 218–226. [CrossRef]
103. Henderson, F.C., Sr.; Austin, C.; Benzel, E.; Bolognese, P.; Ellenbogen, R.; Francomano, C.A.; Ireton, C.; Klinge, P.; Koby, M.; Long, M.; et al. Neurological and spinal manifestations of the Ehlers-Danlos syndromes. *Am. J. Med. Genet. Part C Semin. Med. Genet.* **2017**, *175*, 195–211. [CrossRef]
104. Jayarao, M.; Sohl, K.; Tanaka, T. Chiari malformation I and autism spectrum disorder: An underrecognized coexistence. *J. Neurosurg. Pediatrics* **2015**, *15*, 96–100. [CrossRef] [PubMed]
105. Kushki, A.; Drumm, E.; Mobarak, M.P.; Tanel, N.; Dupuis, A.; Chau, T.; Anagnostou, E. Investigating the autonomic nervous system response to anxiety in children with autism spectrum disorders. *PLoS ONE* **2013**, *8*, e59730. [CrossRef] [PubMed]
106. Vernetti, A.; Shic, F.; Boccanfuso, L.; Macari, S.; Kane-Grade, F.; Milgramm, A.; Hilton, E.; Heymann, P.; Goodwin, M.S.; Chawarska, K. Atypical emotional electrodermal activity in toddlers with autism spectrum disorder. *Autism Res.* **2020**, in press. [CrossRef] [PubMed]
107. Hirstein, W.; Iversen, P.; Ramachandran, V.S. Autonomic responses of autistic children to people and objects. *Proc. R. Soc. Lond. Ser. B Biol. Sci.* **2001**, *268*, 1883–1888. [CrossRef] [PubMed]
108. Bricout, V.A.; Pace, M.; Dumortier, L.; Favre-Juvin, A.; Guinot, M. Autonomic responses to head-up tilt test in children with autism spectrum disorders. *J. Abnorm. Child Psychol.* **2018**, *46*, 1121–1128. [CrossRef]
109. Anderson, C.J.; Colombo, J. Larger tonic pupil size in young children with autism spectrum disorder. *Dev. Psychobiol. J. Int. Soc. Dev. Psychobiol.* **2009**, *51*, 207–211. [CrossRef]
110. Zahn, T.P.; Rumsey, J.M.; Van Kammen, D.P. Autonomic nervous system activity in autistic, schizophrenic, and normal men: Effects of stimulus significance. *J. Abnorm. Psychol.* **1987**, *96*, 135. [CrossRef]
111. Harder, R.; Malow, B.A.; Goodpaster, R.L.; Igbal, F.; Halbower, A.; Goldman, S.E.; Fawkes, D.B.; Wang, L.; Shi, Y.; Baudenbacher, F.; et al. Heart rate variability during sleep in children with autism spectrum disorder. *Clin. Auton. Res.* **2016**, *26*, 423–432. [CrossRef]
112. O'Haire, M.E.; McKenzie, S.J.; Beck, A.M.; Slaughter, V. Animals may act as social buffers: Skin conductance arousal in children with autism spectrum disorder in a social context. *Dev. Psychobiol.* **2015**, *57*, 584–595. [CrossRef]
113. Tessier, M.P.; Pennestri, M.H.; Godbout, R. Heart rate variability of typically developing and autistic children and adults before, during and after sleep. *Int. J. Psychophysiol.* **2018**, *134*, 15–21. [CrossRef]
114. Guy, L.; Souders, M.; Bradstreet, L.; DeLussey, C.; Herrington, J.D. Brief report: Emotion regulation and respiratory sinus arrthythmia in autism spectrum disorder. *J. Autism Dev. Disord.* **2014**, *44*, 2614–2620. [CrossRef]
115. Ferguson, B.J.; Marler, S.; Altstein, L.L.; Batey Lee, E.; Akers, J.; Sohl, K.; McLaughlin, A.; Hartnett, K.; Kille, M.; Mazurek, M.; et al. Psychophysiological associations with gastrointestinal symptomatology in autism spectrum disorder. *Autism Res.* **2016**, *10*, 276–288. [CrossRef]
116. Sagar-Ouriaghli, I.; Lievesley, K.; Santosh, P.J. Propranolol for treating emotional, behavioural, autonomic dysregulation in children and adolescents with autism spectrum disorders. *J. Psychopharmacol.* **2018**, *32*, 641–653. [CrossRef] [PubMed]
117. Emin, O.; Esra, G.; Aysegül, D.; Ufuk, E.; Ayhan, S.; Rusen, D.M. Autonomic nervous system dysfunction and their relationship with disease severity in children with atopic asthma. *Respir. Physiol. Neurobiol.* **2012**, *183*, 206–210. [CrossRef] [PubMed]
118. Casanova, M.F.; Hensley, M.K.; Sokhadze, E.M.; El-Baz, A.S.; Wang, Y.; Li, X.; Sears, L. Effects of weekly low-frequency rTMS on autonomic measures in children with autism spectrum disorder. *Front. Hum. Neurosci.* **2014**, *8*, 851. [CrossRef]

119. Sokhadze, G.; Casanova, M.F.; Kelly, D.; Casanova, E.; Russell, B.; Sokhadze, E.M. Neuromodulation based on rTMS affects behavioral measures and autonomic nervous system activity in children with autism. *NeuroRegulation* **2017**, *4*, 65. [CrossRef]
120. De Wandele, I.; Calders, P.; Peersman, W.; Rimbaut, S.; De Backer, T.; Malfait, F.; De Paepe, A.; Rombaut, L. Autonomic symptom burden in the hypermobility type of Ehlers-Danlos syndrome: A comparative study with two other EDS types, fibromyalgia, and health controls. *Semin. Arthritis Rheum.* **2014**, *44*, 353–361. [CrossRef]
121. De Wandele, I.; Rombaut, L.; Leybaert, L.; Van de Borne, P.; De Backer, T.; Malfait, F.; De Paepe, A.; Calders, P. Dysautonomia and its underlying mechanisms in the hypermobility type of Ehlers-Danlos syndrome. *Semin. Arthritis Rheum.* **2014**, *44*, 93–100. [CrossRef]
122. Hakim, A.; O'Callaghan, C.; De Wandele, I.; Stiles, L.; Pocinki, A.; Rowe, P. Cardiovascular autonomic dysfunction in Ehlers-Danlos syndrome—Hypermobile type. *Am. J. Med. Genet. Part C Semin. Med. Genet.* **2017**, *175*, 168–174. [CrossRef]
123. Health Quality Ontario. Positional magnetic resonance imaging for people with Ehlers-Danlos syndrome or suspected craniovertebral or cervical spine abnormalities: An evidence-based analysis. *Ont. Health Technol. Assess. Ser.* **2015**, *15*, 1.
124. Onore, C.; Careaga, M.; Ashwood, P. The role of immune dysfunction in the pathophysiology of autism. *Brain Behav. Immun.* **2012**, *26*, 383–392. [CrossRef]
125. Ahmad, S.F.; Zoheir, K.M.; Ansari, M.A.; Nadeem, A.; Bakheet, S.A.; Al-Ayadhi, L.Y.; Alzahrani, M.Z.; Al-Shabanah, O.A.; Al-Harbi, M.M.; Attia, S.M. Dysregulation of Th1, Th2, Th17, and T regulatory cell-related transcription factor signaling in children with autism. *Mol. Neurobiol.* **2017**, *54*, 4390–4400. [CrossRef] [PubMed]
126. Jones, K.L.; Crown, L.A.; Yoshida, C.K.; Heuer, L.; Hansen, R.; Zerbo, O.; DeLorenze, G.N.; Kharrazi, M.; Yolken, R.; Ashwood, P.; et al. Autism with intellectual disability is associated with increased levels of maternal cytokines and chemokines during gestation. *Mol. Psychiatry* **2017**, *22*, 273–279. [CrossRef] [PubMed]
127. Smith, S.E.; Elliott, R.M.; Anderson, M.P. Maternal immune activation increases neonatal mouse cortex thickness and cell density. *J. Neuroimmune Pharmacol.* **2012**, *7*, 529–532. [CrossRef] [PubMed]
128. Gallagher, D.; Norman, A.A.; Woodard, C.L.; Yang, G.; Gauthier-Fisher, A.; Fujitani, M.; Vessey, J.P.; Cancino, G.I.; Sachewsky, N.; Woltjen, K. Transient maternal IL-6 mediates long-lasting changes in neural stem cell pools by deregulating an endogenous self-renewal pathway. *Cell Stem Cell* **2013**, *13*, 564–576. [CrossRef] [PubMed]
129. Ecker, C.; Ginestet, C.; Feng, Y.; Johnston, P.; Lombardo, M.V.; Lai, M.C.; Suckling, J.; Palaniyappan, L.; Daly, E.; Murphy, C.M.; et al. Brain surface anatomy in adults with autism: The relationship between surface area, cortical thickness, and autistic symptoms. *JAMA Psychiatry* **2013**, *70*, 59–70. [CrossRef] [PubMed]
130. Zielinski, B.A.; Prigge, M.B.; Nielsen, J.A.; Froehlich, A.L.; Abildskov, T.J.; Anderson, J.S.; Fletcher, P.T.; Zygmut, K.M.; Travers, B.G.; Lange, N.; et al. Longitudinal changes in cortical thickness in autism and typical development. *Brain* **2014**, *137*, 1799–1812. [CrossRef]
131. Seneviratne, S.L.; Maitland, A.; Afrin, L. Mast cell disorders in Ehlers-Danlos syndrome. *Am. J. Med. Genet. Part C Semin. Med. Genet.* **2017**, *175*, 226–236. [CrossRef]
132. Chang, A.R.; Vadas, P. Prevalence of symptoms of mast cell activation in patients with postural orthostatic tachycardia syndrome and hypermobile Ehlers-Danlos syndrome. *J. Allergy Clin. Immunol.* **2019**, *143*, AB182. [CrossRef]
133. Chiarelli, N.; Ritelli, M.; Zoppi, N.; Colombi, M. Cellular and molecular mechanisms in the pathogenesis of classical, vascular, and hypermobile Ehlers-Danlos syndromes. *Genes* **2019**, *10*, 609. [CrossRef]
134. Chou, D.H.; Lee, W.; McCulloch, C.A. TNF-alpha inactivation of collagen receptors: Implications for fibroblast function and fibrosis. *J. Immunol.* **1996**, *156*, 4354–4362. [PubMed]
135. Duncan, M.R.; Berman, B. Differential regulation of collagen, glycosaminoglycan, fibronectin, and collagenase activity production in cultured human adult dermal fibroblasts by interleukin 1-alpha and beta and tumor necrosis factor-alpha and beta. *J. Investig. Dermatol.* **1989**, *92*, 699–706. [CrossRef]
136. Winarni, T.I.; Chonchaiya, W.; Sumekar, T.A.; Ashwood, P.; Morales, G.M.; Tassone, F.; Nguyen, D.V.; Faradz, S.M.; Van de Water, J.; Cook, K.; et al. Immune-mediated disorders among women carriers of fragile X premutation alleles. *Am. J. Med. Genet. Part A* **2012**, *158*, 2473–2481. [CrossRef]

137. Careaga, M.; Rose, D.; Tassone, F.; Berman, R.F.; Hagerman, R.; Ashwood, P. Immune dysregulation as a cause of autoinflammation in fragile X premutation carriers: Link between *FMR1* CGG repeat number and decreased cytokine responses. *PLoS ONE* **2014**, *9*, e94475. [CrossRef] [PubMed]
138. Jalnapurkar, I.; Rafika, N.; Tassone, F.; Hagerman, R. Immune mediated disorders in women with a fragile X expansion and FXTAS. *Am. J. Med. Genet. Part A* **2015**, *167*, 190–197. [CrossRef] [PubMed]
139. Larsen, C.M.; Juul-Kristensen, B.; Lund, H.; Sogaard, K. Measurement properties of existing clinical assessment methods evaluating scapular positioning and function. A systematic review. *Physiother. Theory Pract.* **2014**, *30*, 453–482. [CrossRef]
140. Engelbert, R.H.H.; Juul-Kristensen, B.; Pacey, V.; de Wandele, I.; Smeenk, S.; Woinarosky, N.; Sabo, S.; Scheper, M.C.; Russek, L.; Simmonds, J.V. The evidence-based rationale for physical therapy treatment of children, adolescents, and adults diagnosed with joint hypermobility syndrome/hypermobile Ehlers Danlos syndrome. *Am. J. Med. Genet. Part C Semin. Med. Genet.* **2017**, *175*, 158–167. [CrossRef]
141. Ferrell, W.R.; Tennant, N.; Sturrock, R.D.; Ashton, L.; Creed, G.; Brydson, G.; Rafferty, D. Amelioration of symptoms by enhancement of proprioception in patients with joint hypermobility syndrome. *Arthritis Rheum.* **2004**, *50*, 3323–3328. [CrossRef]

Publisher's Note: MDPI stays neutral with regard to jurisdictional claims in published maps and institutional affiliations.

© 2020 by the authors. Licensee MDPI, Basel, Switzerland. This article is an open access article distributed under the terms and conditions of the Creative Commons Attribution (CC BY) license (http://creativecommons.org/licenses/by/4.0/).

Journal of *Personalized Medicine*

MDPI

Article

Evaluation of Chromosome Microarray Analysis in a Large Cohort of Females with Autism Spectrum Disorders: A Single Center Italian Study

Sara Calderoni [1,2,*,†], Ivana Ricca [3,†], Giulia Balboni [4], Romina Cagiano [1], Denise Cassandrini [3], Stefano Doccini [3], Angela Cosenza [1], Deborah Tolomeo [3,5], Raffaella Tancredi [1], Filippo Maria Santorelli [3] and Filippo Muratori [1,2]

1 Department of Developmental Neuroscience, IRCCS Fondazione Stella Maris, Viale del Tirreno 331, Calambrone, 56128 Pisa, Italy; romina.cagiano@fsm.unipi.it (R.C.); angela.cosenza@fsm.unipi.it (A.C.); r.tancredi@fsm.unipi.it (R.T.); f.muratori@fsm.unipi.it (F.M.)

2 Department of Clinical and Experimental Medicine, University of Pisa, Via Savi, 10, 56126 Pisa, Italy

3 Molecular Medicine, IRCCS Fondazione Stella Maris, via dei Giacinti 2, Calambrone, 56128 Pisa, Italy; ivana.ricca@fsm.unipi.it (I.R.); d.cassandrini@fsm.unipi.it (D.C.); s.doccini@fsm.unipi.it (S.D.); d.tolomeo@fsm.unipi.it (D.T.); f.santorelli@fsm.unipi.it (F.M.S.)

4 Department of Philosophy, Social and Human Sciences and Education, University of Perugia, Piazza G. Ermini 1, 06123 Perugia, Italy; giulia.balboni@unipg.it

5 Department of Neurosciences, Psychology, Drug Research and Child Health (NEUROFARBA), University of Florence, Viale Pieraccini, 6-50139 Florence, Italy

* Correspondence: sara.calderoni@fsm.unipi.it; Tel.: +39-050-886-200; Fax: +39-050-886-273

† These authors contributed equally to this work.

Received: 7 September 2020; Accepted: 21 September 2020; Published: 9 October 2020

Abstract: Autism spectrum disorders (ASD) encompass a heterogeneous group of neurodevelopmental disorders resulting from the complex interaction between genetic and environmental factors. Thanks to the chromosome microarray analysis (CMA) in clinical practice, the accurate identification and characterization of submicroscopic deletions/duplications (copy number variants, CNVs) associated with ASD was made possible. However, the widely acknowledged excess of males on the autism spectrum reflects on a paucity of CMA studies specifically focused on females with ASD (f-ASD). In this framework, we aim to evaluate the frequency of causative CNVs in a single-center cohort of idiopathic f-ASD. Among the 90 f-ASD analyzed, we found 20 patients with one or two potentially pathogenic CNVs, including those previously associated with ASD (located at 16*p*13.2 16*p*11.2, 15*q*11.2, and 22*q*11.21 regions). An exploratory genotype/phenotype analysis revealed that the f-ASD with causative CNVs had statistically significantly lower restrictive and repetitive behaviors than those without CNVs or with non-causative CNVs. Future work should focus on further understanding of f-ASD genetic underpinnings, taking advantage of next-generation sequencing technologies, with the ultimate goal of contributing to precision medicine in ASD.

Keywords: autism spectrum disorders; copy number variants; females; Array-Comparative Genomic Hybridization (Array-CGH)

1. Introduction

Autism spectrum disorders (ASD) are a heterogeneous group of neurodevelopmental pathologies characterized by early onset abnormalities in social communication and interaction, as well as atypically restricted and repetitive behaviors and interests [1]. Despite the exact pathogenesis of idiopathic ASD not yet being fully elucidated, recent evidences suggest an interaction between genetic liability and environmental influences in producing early alteration of brain development [2].

In particular, among environmental risk factors, several maternal factors (including age ≥ 35 years, chronic hypertension, preeclampsia, gestational hypertension, and overweight before or during pregnancy) were associated with ASD in an updated review of the literature [3]. Updated data on the prevalence of ASD in the US (Centers for Disease Control and Prevention, CDC [4]) identified 1 in 54 children as having ASD, while the estimated prevalence of ASD in Italian population is 1 in 87, according to a recent investigation [5].

Crucially, since the first descriptions of autism [6,7], a strong male bias in ASD prevalence has been consistently observed, which becomes even more pronounced in individuals without intellectual disability, according to data from the 80s [8,9]. More recent studies have challenged this assertion, suggesting that missed or wrong diagnoses of ASD females, especially of those with good intellectual and language abilities, contribute to the skewed sex ratio in ASD [10].

The exact mechanisms underlying male vulnerability or female protection in ASD remain complex and scarcely investigated. A multifactorial model has been proposed where a mixture of gene variants and environmental factors contribute to liability, possibly interacting with sex-specific pathways such as those related to hormones or immune function [11,12].

Genetic investigations in ASD revealed frequently sexually dimorphic results. For example, a greater number of de novo copy number variants (CNVs) [13–16] as well as a higher rate of de novo single nucleotide variants (SNVs) found in exome sequences [17,18] have been observed in females with ASD (f-ASD) than in male cases, especially non-sense and splice site [19,20]. Conversely, a more recent study pointed to sex-specific mutations, specifically on the X chromosome, that may contribute to male prevalence in ASD [21]. On the other hand, as far as sex differences in symptom profiles are concerned, some previous studies suggested different phenotypic features in females than in males with ASD [22] like lower IQ [23], more impaired social and/or communicative functioning [24], psychopathological problems [25] and milder restricted and repetitive behaviors [26–28]. However, this issue remains controversial [29–33]. Females with ASD displayed also a higher rate of co-occurring neurological conditions than ASD males, i.e., microcephaly, developmental regression in socialization, minor neurological and musculoskeletal deficits [34], and epilepsy [35], all pointing to sex differences in genetic backgrounds.

The advent of chromosome microarray analysis (CMA) in clinical practice [36] allows for fast detection and accurate characterization of submicroscopic deletions and duplications (CNVs) of genomic DNA associated with ASD [37,38]. Learning societies and ASD experts recommend CMA as part of the first-line evaluation for individuals with ASD [39–41]. However, CMA brings up a higher level of polymorphic genomic rearrangements and the process to attribute causality in complex conditions such as ASD is not easy and straightforward.

This study aims to investigate the frequency of causative CNVs in a single-center cross-sectional idiopathic f-ASD cohort to delineate possible genotype/phenotype associations.

2. Methods

We collected the clinical data of a group of 93 females referred consecutively to the Autism Spectrum Disorders Unit of our Children Neuropsychiatry Hospital between 2015 and 2016. The age at the last clinical evaluation ranged from 21 months to 17 years. All participants received a clinical diagnosis of ASD based on the criteria of the Diagnostic and Statistical Manual of Mental Disorders (DSM-5) [1]. All the patients were unrelated.

According to our ASD-screening protocol, neurometabolic conditions and hypoxic-ischemic injury were investigated. All participants were evaluated by an expert clinical geneticist in order to exclude recognizable monogenic syndromes. Prior to this study, each individual had also been tested for the expanded repeat sequences in 5′-UTR of the *FMR1* gene as previously reported [42].

Based on this screening, we excluded two females with a history of perinatal hypoxia and diffuse white matter disease detected on brain magnetic resonance imaging (MRI), and one patient with macrocephaly harboring a pathogenic mutation in *PTEN*. In a single case (patient P11) we analyzed

CNVs in spite of her presentation of a low-level somatic mosaicism for a fully-mutated/pre-mutated *FMR1* allele, because the patient's phenotype could not be fully explained by this genetic condition.

Hence, we tested 90 ASD female individuals for CNVs. Participants were classified as clinically affected by "essential" autism, based on the absence of major congenital abnormalities and major dysmorphism [43,44].

Cognitive evaluation was performed in 87 participants with specific cognitive scales based on the age and the language level. According to the age, children were tested respectively with the Griffiths Mental Development Scale—Revised (GMDS-R) [45], Wechsler Preschool and Primary Scale of Intelligence—third edition (WPPSI, III) [46] or Wechsler Intelligence Scale for Children—IV (WISC, IV) [47]. The evaluation of non-verbal females was performed using the Leiter International Performance Scale-Revised (Leiter-R) [48]. In three participants, the cognitive assessment was not performed because of scarce compliance due to severe autism symptoms.

Clinical assessment of expressive language skills defined females with a complete absence of language ($n = 27$) and a group of "verbal" f-ASD ($n = 63$).

The semi-structured Autism Diagnostic Observation Schedule second edition (ADOS-2) evaluation [49], which provides a measure of autism severity, was available in 67 participants. We recorded the score on the Social Affect (SA) and the Restricted and Repetitive Behaviors (RRB) domains for each proband. Since we used different ADOS modules according to the non-echolalic expressive language level of each patient at the time of the evaluation, we converted the global ADOS scores and the sub-scores of the SA and RRB domains in the corresponding Calibrated Severity Score (CSS) [50,51].

This study was approved by the Pediatric Ethic Committee of Tuscany Region (Italy), and was performed according to the Declaration of Helsinki and its later amendments or comparable ethical standards. All parents or legal representatives signed an informed consent form before the inclusion of their child in the study. The identities of all individuals were omitted.

3. Procedure

3.1. Genetic Analysis

CMA analyses were performed using the Agilent 8 × 60 K Microarray oligonucleotide platform with a median resolution of 100 Kbp, according to the manufacture's protocol (Agilent Technologies, Santa Clara, CA, USA). CNV coordinates refer to the Genome Reference Consortium Human Build 37 (GRCh37/hg19).

In each proband, CNVs were confirmed by quantitative polymerase chain reaction (qPCR). Segregation analyses in parental DNA (whenever available) were performed by qPCR. Polymorphic CNVs, based on Database of Genomic Variants data (DGV) [52]), were filtered out.

Non-polymorphic CNVs were classified as "causative" (C-CNVs) or "non-causative" (N-CNVs) according to the American College of Medical Genetics and Genomics (ACMG) guidelines [53]. We considered as "causative": (i) CNVs encompassing genomic regions or genes associated with ASD or with other neuropsychiatric conditions (i.e., intellectual disability, epilepsy and schizophrenia) in the Online Mendelian Inheritance in Man (OMIM) database [54]; (ii) CNVs containing "high confidence" ASD-genes reported in the Simons Foundation Autism Research Initiative (SFARI) Gene database [55] with a score < 3 or in the Autism Knowledge Base version 2.0 (Autism KB 2.0) database [56] with a score > 16; (iii) CNVs involving "candidate-genes" for ASD either reported in association with autism in literature, or listed in the aforementioned databases and with a SFARI Gene score ≥ 3 or an Autism KB score ≤ 16 (suggestive or "low confidence" candidate-genes). Conversely, CNVs were considered non-causative (N-CNVs) if they have never been associated with ASD or other neurodevelopmental disorders (NDDs). Patients who tested negative for CNVs were classified as "without CNVs" (w-CNVs).

To recognize significantly enriched functional modules, ASD-candidate genes encompassed by C-CNVs were evaluated by bioinformatics tools. A Core analysis run in the Variant Effects Analysis mode through the use of the Ingenuity Pathway Analysis (IPA) software [57] figured out cellular processes related to our gene dataset (21 genes). A functional network encompassing our ASD-candidate genes was generated. Bridging nodes were denoted evaluating both direct and indirect interactions with stringent level of confidence and only related to neurological diseases. Gene ontology (GO) categorization was carried out using ToppGene Suite [58]. The top three ontologies for Molecular Functions and Cellular Component were annotated and statistical significance of GO terms was reported as -log10 (p-value).

3.2. Statistical Analyses

We used a chi-square test to investigate the association between the CNVs subtype and the type of CNVs (duplication or deletion) and the pattern of inheritance (de novo or inherited, paternal or maternal). A Mann–Whitney test was used to verify if there were any differences in the CNVs burden of the different CNVs subtypes (excluding patient P23 who carried a whole X-chromosome duplication).

We also investigated the phenotype of the individuals with the different CNVs subtypes testing with the chi-square test the association between the CNVs subtype and cognitive (IQ $\leq$ 70 vs. >70) and language (non-verbal vs. verbal) levels. A Mann–Whitney test was used to ascertain that the groups with different CNVs subtype were matched on age and to verify if there were any differences in the CCS score obtained on the total ADOS and on its AS and RRB domains. In case of statistically significantly differences we compute for r score as effect size index. This was interpreted as negligible ($r < 0.10$), small ($0.10 \leq r < 0.30$), medium ($0.30 \leq r < 0.50$), or large ($r \geq 0.50$).

4. Results

4.1. Chromosome Microarray Analysis (CMA)

We performed CMA in 90 females affected by idiopathic ASD, detecting 35 CNVs (17 duplications and 18 deletions) in 29 (32.2%). Twenty-three participants had one CNV and six carried 2 imbalances. Sixty-one f-ASD were considered w-CNVs (67.8% of the whole group).

Out of 35 CNVs, 25 were classified C-CNVS (71.4%) and 10 N-CNVs (28.6%). In the whole group of 90 f-ASD, 20 patients harbored at least one possible disease-causing CNV (diagnostic yield 22.2%) (Figure 1).

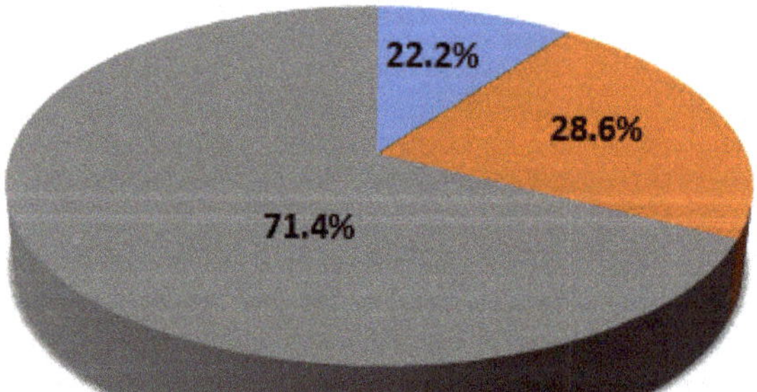

Figure 1. Graphical representation of chromosome microarray analysis (CMA) results in our group of 90 females affected by autism. In the pie chart is depicted the percentage of individuals with causative copy number variants (C-CNVs), non-causative copy number variants (N-CNVs) or without copy number variants (w-CNVs).

Table 1 illustrates the results of CMA investigations. There were not recurrent C-CNVs, with the exception of two unrelated subjects who harbored a 15q11-q13 microduplication. Ten CNVs involved genomic regions already associated with known contiguous gene-deletion/duplication syndromes associated with ASD or NDDs, 5 CNVs encompassed "high-confident" ASD-genes and ten involved genes reported in literature or in the SFARI Gene/Autism KB databases as possible candidates for autism.

The function and evidence of possible disease-association of the reported candidate-genes are summarized in Table 2. Bioinformatic analysis showed that 11 out of 21 of the reported disease-associated and candidate genes are involved in synaptic structure and transmission (*ADARB1, ASIC2, CADM2, DMD, GRIN2A, GRM7, NEDD4, NRXN1, PCDH15, PTPRD, TRPM2*) (Figure 2).

In 24 f-ASD, carrying 29 CNVs, we assessed a de novo origin in 8 and a paternal in 12, whereas CNVs were maternally-inherited in 9 patients. In 5 children we could not assess segregation because of lack of parental DNA. Table 3 shows the proportion of duplications and deletions and the mode of inheritance in relation to the different subtypes of CNVs. Overall, the rate of de novo CNV was 9.4%. All de novo CNVs involved known NDDs-associated genes/chromosomal regions. CNVs encompassing suggestive or "low confidence" ASD-genes were all inherited; 6 out 9 disrupted more than one NDD-gene or were associated with an additional C-CNV. Seven out of 9 maternally inherited vs. 6 out of 12 paternally inherited CNVs were causative.

Table 1. Chromosomal microarray (CMA) results in the 29 participants carrying at least one Copy Number Variant (CNV). For each participant with positive CMA results are reported the genomic location and breakpoints of each CNV, the CNV subtype (deletion or duplication), the size in base pairs, the inheritance status, the associated known genetic syndrome or Autism Spectrum Disorders (ASD) candidate genes involved in the rearrangement, and the CNV classification (causative or non-causative).

ID.	CNV Breakpoints	CNV Type	Size (bp)	Inheritance	Syndrome/Candidate Gene	CNV Class	Reference
P1	22q13.33 (50781138-51219009)	del	437,871	de novo	Phelan-McDermid syndrome	C	#MIM 606232
	Xp11.4 (38491539-38628756)	dup	137,217	mat	*TSPAN7*	C	#MIM 300210
P2	14q32.13 (94817951-94883978)	del	66,027	-	-	N	-
P3	16p13.3 (6881091-7070689)	del	189,598	mat	*RBFOX1*	C	[59]
	16p13.2 (9015110-10321593)	dup	1,306,483	de novo	*USP7, GRIN2A*	C	[60]
P4	21q22.3 (45822805-46530451)	dup	707,646	mat	*ADARB1, TRPM2, ITGB2, SUMO3*	C	[61]
P5	1q31.2 (191644543-191775583)	del	131,040	pat	-	N	-
P6	2q34.3 (214919902-215051057)	del	131,155	mat	-	N	-
P7	1q21.2 (147211160-147824207)	dup	613,047	pat	-	N	-
P8	17p11.2 (16822483-20193310)	del	3,370,827	de novo	Smith-Magenis syndrome	C	#MIM 182290
P9	15q21.3 (56283008-56384604)	del	101,596	mat	*NEDD4, RFX7*	C	[62]
P10	17q12 (34851537-36168104)	del	1,316,567	de novo	17q12 deletion syndrome	C	#MIM 614527
P11	10q21.1 (55616917-55791973)	del	175,056	mat	*PCDH15*	C	[63]
P12	4q34.1 (172930618-173074943)	dup	144,325	pat	-	N	-
	4q34.2 (176984739-177190235)	dup	205,496	pat	-	N	-
P13	17q12 (31953228-32922965)	dup	969,737	mat	*ACCN1, TMEM132E*	C	[64]
P14	3p12.1 (85615568-85672801)	del	57,233	pat	*CADM2*	C	[32]
	3p26.1 (7353126-7403750)	del	50,624	pat	*GRM7*	C	[65]
P15	7q31.1 (110954950-111202026)	del	247,076	pat	*IMMP2L*	C	[66]
P16	2q23.3 (153898093-154164672)	del	266,579	pat	-	N	-
P17	5q23.3 (129687092-130006500)	del	319,408	mat	-	N	-
P18	15q11.2q13.1 (23669701-28525460)	dup	4,825,759	-	15q11q13 duplication syndrome	C	#MIM 608636
P19	2p16.1p15 (58566616-61546442)	del	2,979,826	de novo	2p16.1p15 deletion syndrome	C	#MIM 612513
P20	16p11.2 (29673954-30197341)	dup	523,387	-	16p11.2 duplication syndrome	C	#MIM 614671
P21	15q11.2q13.1 (23669701-28525460)	dup	4,855,759	mat	15q11-q13 duplication syndrome	C	#MIM 608636
P22	9p24.1 (7800020-8528849)	dup	728,829	-	*PTPRD*	C	[61]
	Xp22.31 (6552712-8115153)	del	1,562,441	-	Xp22.31 deletion syndrome	C	[67]
P23	2p16.3 (48915312-48979903)	del	64,591	pat	-	N	-
P24	Xp22.33q28 (61529-155190083)	dup	155,128,554	de novo	47, XXX	C	[68]

Table 1. *Cont.*

ID.	CNV Breakpoints	CNV Type	Size (bp)	Inheritance	Syndrome/Candidate Gene	CNV Class	Reference
P25	Xp21.1 (31893344-32289012)	dup	395,668	de novo	*DMD*	C	[69]
P26	8q24.3 (146053353-146174033	dup	120,680	-	-	N	-
P27	2q12.2q12.3 (106929257-108403252)	dup	1,473,995	pat	*ST6GAL2*	C	[70]
P28	22q11.21 (20754422-21440514)	dup	686,092	pat	22q11.2 duplication syndrome	C	#MIM 608363
P29	2p16.2 (50909765-51083469)	del	173,704	pat	*NRXN1*	C	[71]
	Xp22.33 (581803-920279)	dup	338,476	de novo	*SHOX*	C	[72]

Pt: participant; CNV: copy number variant; bp: base pairs; del: deletion; dup: duplication; mat: maternal; pat: paternal; C: causative; N: non-causative.

Table 2. Function and evidences of disease-association of the reported candidate-genes encompassed in causative- Copy Number Variants (CNVs). The table reports evidences that supports the possible role in autism of the reported "high confidence" autism spectrum disorder (ASD) genes (genes with a Simons Foundation Autism Research Initiative SFARI Gene score < 3 or with an Autism KB 2.0 score > 16), and suggestive or "low confidence" candidate-genes (genes with a SFARI Gene score ≥ 3 or with an AutismKB 2.0 score ≤ 16). For each gene, genomic region, participant ID, function of the encoded protein and scores assigned in the SFARI Gene and AutismKB 2.0 databases are reported (NR: gene not reported in the database).

Gene	Genomic Region (Participant ID)	Protein Function	SFARI Gene/AutismKB 2.0
		"High confidence" ASD-genes	
USP7	16p13.2 (P3)	Ubiquitin-specific protease; regulates ubiquitination processes	2/4
GRIN2A	16p13.2 (P3)	Subunit 2A of the glutamate N-Methyl-D-Aspartate (NMDA) receptor	2/10
RBFOX1	16p13.3 (P3)	RNA-binding protein that regulates alternative splicing events	2/28
DMD	Xp21.1 (P25)	Component of the dystrophin-glycoprotein complex (DGC), which bridges the inner cytoskeleton and the extracellular matrix	S/28
SHOX	Xp22.33 (P29)	Belongs to the paired homeobox family, nuclear transcription factors involved in cell-cycle and growth regulation	2/2
NRXN1	2p16.2 (P29)	Cell adhesion molecule, form a complex with neuroligins at synapses in the central nervous system required for neurotransmission and involved in the formation of synaptic contacts.	1/68
		Suggestive or "low confidence" candidate ASD-genes	
TSPAN7	Xp11.4 (P1)	Member of the tetraspanin family, encodes a cell surface glycoprotein that complex with integrins. It may have a role in neurite outgrowth and Alpha-amino-3-hydroxy-5-methyl-4-isoxazolepropionate (AMPA) receptor trafficking	3/2
ITGB2	21q22.3 (P4)	Integrin B2, adhesion molecule implicated in synaptic pruning	NR/3

Table 2. *Cont.*

Gene	Genomic Region (Participant ID)	Protein Function	SFARI Gene/AutismKB 2.0
TRPM2	21q22.3 (P4)	Voltage-independent cation channel, mediates sodium and calcium ion influx in response to oxidative stress; modulates oxytocin release.	NR/11
ADARB1	21q22.3 (P4)	Protein involved in the editing of the RNA of glutamate, serotonin and Gamma-Aminobutyric Acid (GABA) receptors, and potassium voltage-gated channels.	5/1
SUMO3	21q22.3 (P4)	Involved in SUMOylation of proteins, a post-translational modification that modulates the activity of several neuronal transcription factors	NR/0
RFX7	15q21.3 (P9)	Transcription factor	NR/4
NEDD4	15q21.3 (P9)	Protein involved in the ubiquitin proteasome system. It plays a critical role in the ubiquitination and degradation of AMPA receptors, endocytic machinery components and Phosphatase and Tensin Homolog (PTEN) protein.	NR/4
PCDH15	10q21.1 (P11)	Member of the cadherin superfamily, membrane proteins that mediate cellular adhesion	3/16
ACCN1 (ASIC2)	17q12 (P13)	Non-voltage-dependent Na^+ channel; facilitates Acid-Sensing Ion Channel (ASIC) localization to synapses interacting with synaptic scaffolding proteins as Postsynaptic Density Protein 95 (PSD95)	NR/7
TMEM132E	17q12 (P13)	Neural adhesion molecule	NR/NR
CADM2	3p12.1 (P14)	Adhesion molecule involved in synapse organization, providing regulated trans-synaptic adhesion.	3/0
GRM7	3p26.1 (P14)	Metabotropic glutamate receptor mGluR7	3/12
IMMP2L	7q31.1 (P15)	Subunit of an inner mitochondrial membrane peptidase complex involved in processing of mitochondrial proteins	3/10
PTPRD	9p23p24 (P22)	Receptor protein tyrosine phosphatase, induces pre- and post-synaptic differentiation and regulates neurogenesis. Interacts with proteins involved in intellectual disability/ASD as IL1RAP and IL1RAPL1 and proteins of the mitogen-activated protein kinase (MEK)/extracellular signal-regulated kinase (ERK) pathway.	NR/7
ST6GAL2	2q12.3 (P27)	Encodes a sialyltransferase mostly expressed in embryonic and adult brain. CNVs were reported in autism studies.	NR/2

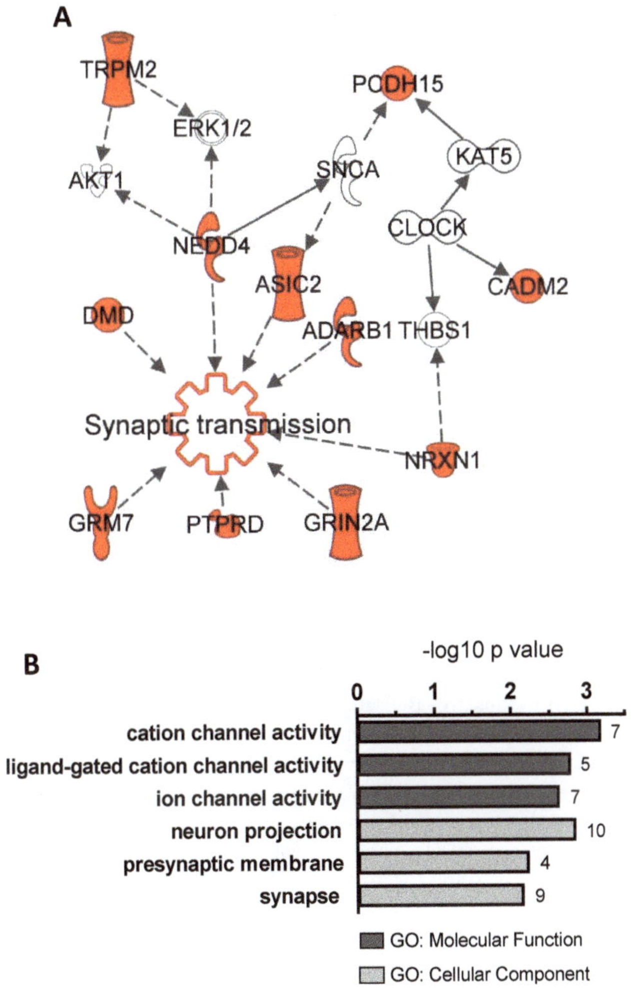

Figure 2. Bioinformatic analyses performed on ASD-candidate genes encompassed by C-CNVs. (**A**) A Core analysis run in Variant Effects Analysis mode using the Ingenuity Pathway Analysis software figured out cellular processes related to our gene dataset (21 genes) generating a functional network encompassing 11 genes (in red). *Synaptic transmission* resulted the most significant functional annotation (p-value 6.05×10^{-9}). Bridging nodes (in white) were denoted evaluating both direct and indirect interactions related only to neurological diseases and with stringent level of confidence (**B**). Gene ontology (GO) categorization was carried out using ToppGene Suite. Top three ontologies for *Molecular Function* (dark grey) and *Cellular Component* (light grey) were annotated; statistical significance of GO terms was reported as −log10 (p-value). The number of genes belonging to each category was reported on the right of each bar.

4.2. Phenotypic Characterization

Twenty-seven f-ASD had an absence of language whereas 63 were "verbal".

Cognitive evaluation was performed in 87 participants, being three participants unfit for psychometric testing. Forty-two of the tested individuals had IQ ≤ 70 and 45 had IQ ≥ 70.

The 67 participants tested with ADOS-2 had the following mean (SD) Total, SA and RRB ADOS CSS, respectively: 6.57 (2.36), 6.79 (2.34), and 7.22 (2.30).

Supplementary Table S1 recapitulates clinical data of the studied population.

Table 3. Proportion of deletions vs. duplications and pattern of inheritance of the reported CNVs according to their classification (causative vs. non-causative).

	Type of CNVs		Inheritance		
	Duplication (n = 17)	**Deletion (n = 18)**	**De novo (n = 8)**	**Paternal (n = 12)**	**Maternal (n = 9)**
C-CNVs (n = 25)	13/25 (52%)	12/25 (48%)	8/21 (38.1%)	6/21 (28.6%)	7/21 (33.3%)
N-CNVs (n = 10)	4/10 (40%)	6/10 (60%)	0/8 (0%)	6/8 (75%)	2/8 (25%)
Total	17/35 (48.6%)	18/35 (51.4%)	8/29 (27.6%)	12/29 (41.4%)	9/29 (31%)

Note: Inheritance was assessed in 29 out of 35 CNVs. C-CNVs = causative CNVs; N-CNVs = non-causative CNVs; n = number of CNVs for each group.

4.3. Statistical Analysis

We observed a statistically significant association between the heritage (de novo vs. maternal and paternal) and the subtypes of CNVs (C-CNVs vs. N-CNVs) ($Chi^2_{(1)} = 4.21$, $p = 0.04$). Indeed, all N-CNVs were transmitted and never arose de novo while all de novo CNVs were causative (38% of C-CNVs); 7 out of 9 (77.8%) C-CNVs were maternal and 6 out of 12 (50%) were paternal.

Whilst the type of genomic micro-rearrangement (deletion vs. duplication) was not statistically correlated to causative/non-causative definition ($Chi^2_{(1)} = 0.41$, $p = 0.52$), not considering CNVs associated with contiguous-gene syndromes, most of the breakpoints of causative duplications lie within at least one NDD-candidate gene (n = 6/8). C-CNVs had a CNVs burden value statistcal significantly higher than those of the N-CNVs subtypes (mean (SD) = 1.14 (1.43) vs. 0.19 (0.16); Mann-Whitney $U = 52.50$, $z = 2.56$, $p = 0.01$, $r = 0.49$).

Table 4 shows the age, the cognitive and linguistic level as well as the autism severity of the three groups of individuals according to different CNV subtypes (causative, non-causative and without CNVs).

To investigate whether there were significant differences in clinical features between groups, we regrouped participants with negative CMA results (N-CNVs and w-CNVs) and compared their characteristics with cases with C-CNVs. The two groups resulted matched for age [mean (SD) = 66.95 (38.55) vs. 56.74 (38.03); Mann–Whitney $U = 523.00$, $z = 1.72$, $p = 0.09$].

We found that there were no differences between the two groups on the cognitive level (IQ ≤ 70 vs. IQ > 70; $Chi^2_{(1)} = 0.47$, $p = 0.49$), language level (non-verbal vs. verbal; $Chi^2_{(1)} = 0.31$, $p = 0.58$), and on the CSS obtained on the total score and on the AS ADOS domain (Mann–Whitney $U = 262.50$, $z = 1.42$, $p = 0.16$; Mann–Whitney $U = 303.00$, $z = 0.77$, $p = 0.44$).

The relative frequencies of the phenotypic features were the following: in the group with C-CNVs, 55% (11/20) had IQ ≤ 70; 60% had a moderate-severe level of autism symptoms (9/15), 35% had absence of language (7/20); in the group with negative CMA, 46% (31/37) had IQ ≤ 70; 75% had a moderate-severe level of autism symptoms (47/62), 28% had absent language (20/70).

Conversely, we found that the f-ASD with C-CNVs had a statistically significantly lower CSS on the RRB ADOS domain that those without CNVs or with non-causative (mean (SD) = 6.08 (2.14) vs. 7.50 (2.27); Mann–Whitney $U = 197$, $z = 2.48$, $p = 0.01$, $r = 0.30$).

Table 4. Demographic features of participants grouped according to CMA results. For each group (with causative and non-causative CNVs, or without CNVs) are reported the mean age at the last examination (in months), the rate of patients with a IQ level > 70 vs. ≤70, the rate of verbal vs. non-verbal patients, and the mean calibrated severity scores (CSS) of the global Autism Diagnostic Observation Schedule (ADOS) scores and the sub-scores of the Social Affect (SA) and Restricted and Repetitive Behaviors (RRB) domains. The language level was assessed in all 90 participants, the IQ level and the ADOS scores were available for 87 and 67 of the 90 individuals, respectively.

	C-CNVs (n = 20)	N-CNVs (n = 9)	w-CNVs (n = 61)
Mean age at the last examination in months (SD)	66.95 (38.55)	47.11 (15.57)	58.16 (40.19)
IQ > 70	9/20 (45%)	4/8 (50%)	32/59 (54.2%)
IQ ≤ 70	11/20 (55%)	4/8 (50%)	27/59 (45.8%)
Verbal	13/20 (65%)	5/9 (55.6%)	45/61 (73.7%)
Non-verbal	7/20 (35%)	4/9 (44.4%)	16/61 (26.3%)
Mean ADOS-CSS:	-	-	-
Mean SA-CSS (SD)	6.38 (2.26)	7.50 (1.64)	6.81 (2.45)
Mean RRB-CSS (SD)	6.08 (2.14)	5.50 (3.83)	7.75 (1.92)
Mean Global-CSS (SD)	5.69 (2.25)	6.83 (2.64)	6.77 (2.35)

C-CNVs = participants with causative CNVs; N-CNVs = participants with non-causative CNVs; w-CNVs = participants without; n = number of patients for each group; SD = standard deviation.

5. Discussion

Although a recent meta-analysis and multidisciplinary consensus statement proposes exome sequencing at the beginning of the evaluation of unexplained neurodevelopmental disorders [73], CMA is still the recommended first-tier genetic analysis in the evaluation of ASD subjects [40,74].

In the last few years, investigations of large cohorts of ASD individuals [13,37,75] have identified a high burden of CNVs with rare C-CNVs being found in 5–10% of idiopathic ASD [76]. However, these data are often affected by gender-bias due to the high M/F ratio in the vast majority of the studies and even more recent investigations addressing type and frequency of C-CNVs did not allow—with few exceptions—for separate gender examinations due to relatively small sample size [77–80].

Herein, we focused exclusively on a cohort of f-ASD and we found clinically significant CNVs in about 22% of patients. Few investigations have considered CNVs and clinical features in f-ASD in comparison with ASD males. In one study, large CNVs (>400 kb) were more frequent in f-ASD than in males (29% vs. 16%), and this difference was even higher (F/M 3:1) if analyses were limited to regions containing genes involved in NDDs [81]. In a similar vein, Levy and colleagues (2011) [13] detected that f-ASD have a high frequency of de novo CNVs (11.7% vs. 7.4% in males), and Sanders et al. (2015) [15] identified a significant difference in the rate of de novo CNVs between boys (5.3%) and girls (8.7%). Our numbers in an only girl cross-sectional, monocentric study denote a similar sex effect with a high diagnostic yield and a 9.4% occurrence of de novo variants.

All de novo CNVs involved known NDDs-associated chromosomal regions whereas CNVs encompassing suggestive or "low confidence" ASD-genes were all inherited and mostly disrupting more than one NDD-gene or associated with an additional C-CNV. Among C-CNVs, there was an excess of maternally-inherited potentially pathogenic CNVs. These findings support the "two-hit model" suggested in previous studies in which the compound effect of a small number of rare variants may contribute to phenotypic heterogeneity of ASD [82].

While literature in the ASD field reported an excess of clinically-significant deletions, we did not find a correlation between the type of genomic rearrangement and causative/non causative definition. Haploinsufficiency for genes within a deletion is a well-recognized cause of genetic disease. Conversely, interpreting the phenotypic consequences of microduplications is often challenging because the pathogenicity of most duplications cannot be explained by triplosensitivity. Sequencing the breakpoints of 119 duplications, Newman et al. (2015) demonstrated that, rather than an extra copy effect, the phenotype of microduplications can be related to the misregulation of genes that span the breakpoints, through loss-of-function mechanisms due to altered transcription or translation or to the creation of fusion proteins with unknown functions [83]. In our f-ASD cohort, most of the causative non-syndromic duplications breakpoints disrupted at least one NDD-candidate gene, hence we can suppose that the pathogenic phenotype could be caused by similar mechanisms.

Unlike previous literature results [78], we did not find any association between C-CNVs and IQ or language deficits. Analyzing the phenotypic features of females with C-CNVs versus those with negative CMA results, we only observed statistically significantly lower scores on the restricted repetitive behaviors (RRB) ADOS domain in f-ASD with clinically significant variants. Recently, Barone et al. reported more severe autistic symptoms in individuals with C-CNVs [79]. The discrepancies with our data could reflect the diverse characteristics of the studied population, indeed several studies suggested a sex effect on RRB scores, which are reported to be repeatedly lower in female than in male subgroups [28,84–86]. Crucially, several lines of evidence suggest that social-communication (SC) and RRB symptom domains are underpinned by different genetic mechanisms. For instance, a recent genome-wide association study demonstrated that the RRB trait "systemizing" is heritable and genetically correlated with autism in the general population and that the SC and RRB domains in autistic subjects show low shared genetics [87]. In particular, the contribution of genetic factors to the RRB domain is sustained by their significative presence on both parents [88] and siblings [89] of probands with ASD. Overall, the impact of C-CNVs on ASD symptoms is still unclear and a recent work highlighted the contribution of environmental factors (i.e., maternal infections during pregnancy) on RRB severity in individuals with CNVs [90]. We can only speculate that we registered lower RRB scores in our f-ASD with positive CMA results because this sample represents the mild-end of a genomic "simple" disorder, while those girls with negative results could reflect the group of f-ASD with "complex" multifactorial etiology, as the largest portion of idiopathic autistic males.

With the exception of two subjects with a 15q11-q13 microduplication, no overlapping CNVs were detected, confirming the high genetic heterogeneity of ASD. Fifteen CNVs involved ASD/NDDs-associated genes or genomic regions already identified, whereas 10 CNVs encompassed genes reported as possible candidates for ASD in literature or in ASD databases (Tables 1 and 2). The contribution of each CNV to the phenotype of our f-ASD patients is discussed in the Supplementary File S1. Out of this list, some cases appear worth discussing.

The known contiguous-gene deletion/duplication syndromes detected in our cases were associated with a diagnosis of "idiopathic" ASD because these patients did not display any of the additional non-neurodevelopmental features specific of these syndromes, as dysmorphisms or congenital defects which can be seen in Smith-Magenis (P8), 17q12 microdeletion (P10), 2p15p16 deletion (P19), 22q11 duplication (P28) and SHOX duplication (P29) syndromes. These patients could represent the mild-end of the phenotypic spectrum of these genomic disorders, due to the "NDDs-protective effect" reported in females [16].

In some cases, reverse phenotyping allowed the investigation and prevention of important comorbidities, as in P25, who carries a de novo partial duplication of the *DMD* gene, which in females could manifest with muscle weakness and cardiomyopathy, and in P20, who carries a 16p11.2 duplication widely reported in ASD studies which is associated with the risk of developing psychotic symptoms [91].

Among clinically relevant rearrangements, aneuploidy was identified in a single subject, who presented an X chromosome trisomy (47, XXX). Interestingly, data in the literature did not report a greater risk for autism in X chromosome trisomy [92], even if difficulties in social functioning and, more broadly, an increased vulnerability for autistic traits are described [68].

The de novo 16p13 duplication detected in one patient (P3) involves partially *UPS7*. Variants affecting this gene were recently reported in 23 individuals with syndromic Developmental Delay/Intellectual Disability [93], and about half of reported subjects had ASD. P3 presents mild motor developmental delay, absent speech, behavioral anomalies and ASD, suggesting that *USP7* haploinsufficiency should be suspected in a case of ASD with absence of speech and behavioral disorders. CNVs detected in P3 spans also *GRIN2A* and *RBFOX1*, so we cannot exclude a possible additional role of these genes in the phenotype of the patient.

The deletions found in P11, P14 and P15 reinforce the evidence of a possible contribution of *PCDH15*, *GRM7*, *CADM2* and *IMMP2L* genes to ASD susceptibility.

Finally, five CNVs spanned some "low-confidence" ASD-genes, which can be investigated in future studies (i.e., *TRPM2*, *ADARB1*, *RFX7*, *NEDD4*, *ASIC2*, *PTPRD*, *ST6GAL2*).

When new and old genes pinpointed by CMA studies were combined in functional modules using IPA and ToppGene Suite, we observed an enrichment in genes involved in synaptic function and transmission, which are well-established biological processes involved in autism and NDDs [94].

In conclusion, this study provides a representative picture of the spectrum of CNV in f-ASD investigated in a clinical setting. As expected, no specific CNVs have been found to be required for developing ASD, supporting the heterogeneity of affected molecular pathways. However, genes in the C-CNVs of our sample of f-ASD code mainly for proteins that could be grouped in two different functional systems: synaptic function/structure, and mRNA/protein processing. Of note, environmental exposures during specific windows of vulnerabilities in prenatal and perinatal life critically interact with genetic susceptibility contributing to ASD pathogenesis [95]. Our study suggests that females with idiopathic ASD have a high rate of pathogenic CNVs encompassing both known and new candidate ASD genes. Hence, studies on large samples of f-ASD carefully assessed from a clinical point of view could help in unraveling the genetic determinants of autism. Moreover, f-ASD with normal-array comparative genomic hybridization analysis could benefit from whole exome or genome sequencing [96], paving the way for the implementation of personalized treatments based on genetic findings.

Supplementary Materials: The following are available online at http://www.mdpi.com/2075-4426/10/4/160/s1, Table S1: Phenotipic characteristics of participants; Supplementary File S1: Contribution of each CNV to the phenotype of f-ASD patients.

Author Contributions: Conceptualization of the article, S.C., I.R., G.B., F.M.S., F.M.; Major contributors in writing the manuscript, S.C., I.R.; Sample collection and clinical characterization of patients, A.C., R.T.; Data Acquisition, R.C., D.T.; Statistical Analyses, G.B.; Genetic Analyses, D.C., S.D.; Contributed to review and editing the manuscript, F.M.S., F.M. All authors have read and agreed to the published version of the manuscript.

Funding: This work has been partially supported by grant from the IRCCS Fondazione Stella Maris (Ricerca Corrente, and the "5 × 1000" voluntary contributions, Italian Ministry of Health). S.C. was partially funded by AIMS-2-Trials.

Acknowledgments: We gratefully acknowledge all the subjects who have participated in the study.

Conflicts of Interest: The authors declare that they have no conflict of interest.

Ethical Statement: The study was conducted in accordance with the Declaration of Helsinki, and the protocol was approved by the Pediatric Ethic Committee of Tuscany Region.

References

1. American Psychiatric Association. *Diagnostic and Statistical Manual of Mental Disorders (DSM-5®)*; American Psychiatric Publication: Washington, DC, USA, 2013.
2. Muhle, R.A.; Reed, H.E.; Stratigos, K.A.; Weele, J.V.-V. The Emerging Clinical Neuroscience of Autism Spectrum Disorder: A Review. *JAMA Psychiatry* **2018**, *75*, 514–523. [CrossRef]
3. Kim, J.Y.; Son, M.J.; Son, C.Y.; Radua, J.; Eisenhut, M.; Gressier, F.; Koyanagi, A.; Carvalho, A.F.; Stubbs, B.; Solmi, M.; et al. Environmental risk factors and biomarkers for autism spectrum disorder: An umbrella review of the evidence. *Lancet Psychiatry* **2019**, *6*, 590–600. [CrossRef]
4. Maenner, M.J.; Shaw, K.A.; Baio, J.; Washington, A.; Patrick, M.; DiRienzo, M.; Christensen, D.L.; Wiggins, L.D.; Pettygrove, S.; Andrews, J.G.; et al. Prevalence of Autism Spectrum Disorder among Children Aged 8 Years—Autism and Developmental Disabilities Monitoring Network, 11 Sites, United States, 2016. *MMWR Surveill. Summ.* **2020**, *69*, 1–12. [CrossRef]

5. Narzisi, A.; Posada, M.; Barbieri, F.; Chericoni, N.; Ciuffolini, D.; Pinzino, M.; Romano, R.; Scattoni, M.L.; Tancredi, R.; Calderoni, S.; et al. Prevalence of Autism Spectrum Disorder in a large Italian catchment area: A school-based population study within the ASDEU project. *Epidemiol. Psychiatr. Sci.* **2018**, *29*, e5. [CrossRef]
6. Kanner, L. Autistic disturbances of affective contact. *Nerv. Child* **1943**, *2*, 217–250.
7. Asperger, H. Die "Autistischen Psychopathen" im Kindesalter. *Arch. Psychiatr. Nervenkr.* **1944**, *117*, 76–136. [CrossRef]
8. Wing, L. Sex ratios in early childhood autism and related conditions. *Psychiatry Res.* **1981**, *5*, 129–137. [CrossRef]
9. Lord, C.; Schopler, E. Neurobiological Implications of Sex Differences in Autism. In *Neurobiological Issues in Autism*; Schopler, E., Mesibov, G., Eds.; Plenum Press: New York, NY, USA, 1987; pp. 191–211.
10. Loomes, R.; Hull, L.; Mandy, W.P.L. What Is the Male-to-Female Ratio in Autism Spectrum Disorder? A Systematic Review and Meta-Analysis. *J. Am. Acad. Child Adolesc. Psychiatry* **2017**, *56*, 466–474. [CrossRef]
11. McCarthy, M.M.; Wright, C.L. Convergence of Sex Differences and the Neuroimmune System in Autism Spectrum Disorder. *Biol. Psychiatry* **2017**, *81*, 402–410. [CrossRef] [PubMed]
12. Werling, D.M.; Parikshak, N.N.; Geschwind, D.H. Gene expression in human brain implicates sexually dimorphic pathways in autism spectrum disorders. *Nat. Commun.* **2016**, *7*, 10717. [CrossRef] [PubMed]
13. Levy, D.; Ronemus, M.; Yamrom, B.; Lee, Y.; Leotta, A.; Kendall, J.; Marks, S.; Lakshmi, B.; Pai, D.; Ye, K.; et al. Rare de novo and transmitted copy-number variation in autistic spectrum disorders. *Neuron* **2011**, *70*, 886–897. [CrossRef] [PubMed]
14. Sanders, S.J.; Ercan-Sencicek, A.G.; Hus, V.; Luo, R.; Murtha, M.T.; Moreno-De-Luca, D.; Chu, S.H.; Moreau, M.P.; Gupta, A.R.; Thomson, S.A.; et al. Multiple recurrent de novo CNVs, including duplications of the 7q11.23 Williams syndrome region, are strongly associated with autism. *Neuron* **2011**, *70*, 863–885. [CrossRef]
15. Sanders, S.J.; He, X.; Willsey, A.J.; Ercan-Sencicek, A.G.; Samocha, K.E.; Cicek, A.E.; Murtha, M.T.; Bal, V.H.; Bishop, S.L.; Dong, S.; et al. Insights into Autism Spectrum Disorder Genomic Architecture and Biology from 71 Risk Loci. *Neuron* **2015**, *87*, 1215–1233. [CrossRef]
16. Desachy, G.; Croen, L.A.; Torres, A.R.; Kharrazi, M.; Delorenze, G.N.; Windham, G.C.; Yoshida, C.K.; Weiss, L.A. Increased female autosomal burden of rare copy number variants in human populations and in autism families. *Mol. Psychiatry* **2015**, *20*, 170–175. [CrossRef] [PubMed]
17. Neale, B.M.; Kou, Y.; Liu, L.; Ma'ayan, A.; Samocha, K.E.; Sabo, A.; Lin, C.-F.; Stevens, C.; Wang, L.-S.; Makarov, V.; et al. Patterns and rates of exonic de novo mutations in autism spectrum disorders. *Nature* **2012**, *485*, 242–245. [CrossRef] [PubMed]
18. O'Roak, B.J.; Vives, L.; Girirajan, S.; Karakoc, E.; Krumm, N.; Coe, B.P.; Levy, R.; Ko, A.; Lee, C.; Smith, J.D.; et al. Sporadic autism exomes reveal a highly interconnected protein network of de novo mutations. *Nature* **2012**, *485*, 246–250. [CrossRef] [PubMed]
19. Sanders, S.J.; Murtha, M.T.; Gupta, A.R.; Murdoch, J.D.; Raubeson, M.J.; Willsey, A.J.; Ercan-Sencicek, A.G.; DiLullo, N.M.; Parikshak, N.N.; Stein, J.L.; et al. De novo mutations revealed by whole-exome sequencing are strongly associated with autism. *Nature* **2012**, *485*, 237–241. [CrossRef]
20. Iossifov, I.; Ronemus, M.; Levy, D.; Wang, Z.; Hakker, I.; Rosenbaum, J.; Yamrom, B.; Lee, Y.-H.; Narzisi, G.; Leotta, A.; et al. De novo gene disruptions in children on the autistic spectrum. *Neuron* **2012**, *74*, 285–299. [CrossRef]
21. Mitra, I.; Tsang, K.; Ladd-Acosta, C.; Croen, L.A.; Aldinger, K.A.; Hendren, R.L.; Traglia, M.; Lavillaureix, A.; Zaitlen, N.; Oldham, M.C.; et al. Pleiotropic Mechanisms Indicated for Sex Differences in Autism. *PLoS Genet.* **2016**, *12*, e1006425. [CrossRef]
22. Van Wijngaarden-Cremers, P.J.M.; van Eeten, E.; Groen, W.B.; Van Deurzen, P.A.; Oosterling, I.J.; Van der Gaag, R.J. Gender and age differences in the core triad of impairments in autism spectrum disorders: A systematic review and meta-analysis. *J. Autism Dev. Disord.* **2014**, *44*, 627–635. [CrossRef]
23. Banach, R.; Thompson, A.; Szatmari, P.; Goldberg, J.; Tuff, L.; Zwaigenbaum, L.; Mahoney, W. Brief Report: Relationship between non-verbal IQ and gender in autism. *J. Autism Dev. Disord.* **2009**, *39*, 188–193. [CrossRef]
24. Carter, A.S.; Black, D.O.; Tewani, S.; Connolly, C.E.; Kadlec, M.B.; Tager-Flusberg, H. Sex differences in toddlers with autism spectrum disorders. *J. Autism Dev. Disord.* **2007**, *37*, 86–97. [CrossRef] [PubMed]

25. Holtmann, M.; Bölte, S.; Poustka, F. Autism spectrum disorders: Sex differences in autistic behaviour domains and coexisting psychopathology. *Dev. Med. Child Neurol.* **2007**, *49*, 361–366. [CrossRef] [PubMed]
26. Duvekot, J.; van der Ende, J.; Verhulst, F.C.; Slappendel, G.; van Daalen, E.; Maras, A.; Greaves-Lord, K. Factors influencing the probability of a diagnosis of autism spectrum disorder in girls versus boys. *Autism* **2017**, *21*, 646–658. [CrossRef]
27. Hartley, S.L.; Sikora, D.M. Sex differences in autism spectrum disorder: An examination of developmental functioning, autistic symptoms, and coexisting behavior problems in toddlers. *J. Autism Dev. Disord.* **2009**, *39*, 1715–1722. [CrossRef]
28. Tillmann, J.; Ashwood, K.; Absoud, M.; Bölte, S.; Bonnet-Brilhault, F.; Buitelaar, J.K.; Calderoni, S.; Calvo, R.; Canal-Bedia, R.; Canitano, R.; et al. Evaluating Sex and Age Differences in ADI-R and ADOS Scores in a Large European Multi-site Sample of Individuals with Autism Spectrum Disorder. *J. Autism Dev. Disord.* **2018**, *48*, 2490–2505. [CrossRef] [PubMed]
29. Andersson, G.W.; Gillberg, C.; Miniscalco, C. Pre-school children with suspected autism spectrum disorders: Do girls and boys have the same profiles? *Res. Dev. Disabil.* **2013**, *34*, 413–422. [CrossRef]
30. Postorino, V.; Fatta, L.M.; De Peppo, L.; Giovagnoli, G.; Armando, M.; Vicari, S.; Mazzone, L. Longitudinal comparison between male and female preschool children with autism spectrum disorder. *J. Autism Dev. Disord.* **2015**, *45*, 2046–2055. [CrossRef] [PubMed]
31. Messinger, D.S.; Young, G.S.; Webb, S.J.; Ozonoff, S.; Bryson, S.E.; Carter, A.; Carver, L.; Charman, T.; Chawarska, K.; Curtin, S.; et al. Early sex differences are not autism-specific: A Baby Siblings Research Consortium (BSRC) study. *Mol. Autism* **2015**, *6*, 32. [CrossRef]
32. Casey, J.P.; Magalhaes, T.; Conroy, J.M.; Regan, R.; Shah, N.; Anney, R.; Shields, D.C.; Abrahams, B.S.; Almeida, J.; Bacchelli, E.; et al. A novel approach of homozygous haplotype sharing identifies candidate genes in autism spectrum disorder. *Hum. Genet.* **2012**, *131*, 565–579. [CrossRef]
33. Zwaigenbaum, L.; Bryson, S.E.; Szatmari, P.; Brian, J.; Smith, I.M.; Roberts, W.; Vaillancourt, T.; Roncadin, C. Sex differences in children with autism spectrum disorder identified within a high-risk infant cohort. *J. Autism Dev. Disord.* **2012**, *42*, 2585–2596. [CrossRef] [PubMed]
34. Ben-Itzchak, E.; Ben-Shachar, S.; Zachor, D.A. Specific neurological phenotypes in autism spectrum disorders are associated with sex representation. *Autism Res.* **2013**, *6*, 596–604. [CrossRef]
35. Amiet, C.; Gourfinkel-An, I.; Bouzamondo, A.; Tordjman, S.; Baulac, M.; Lechat, P.; Mottron, L.; Cohen, D. Epilepsy in autism is associated with intellectual disability and gender: Evidence from a meta-analysis. *Biol. Psychiatry* **2008**, *64*, 577–582. [CrossRef] [PubMed]
36. Cheung, S.W.; Shaw, C.A.; Yu, W.; Li, J.; Ou, Z.; Patel, A.; Yatsenko, S.A.; Cooper, M.L.; Furman, P.; Stankiewicz, P.; et al. Development and validation of a CGH microarray for clinical cytogenetic diagnosis. *Genet. Med.* **2005**, *7*, 422–432. [CrossRef]
37. Sebat, J.; Lakshmi, B.; Malhotra, D.; Troge, J.; Lese-Martin, C.; Walsh, T.; Yamrom, B.; Yoon, S.; Krasnitz, A.; Kendall, J.; et al. Strong association of de novo copy number mutations with autism. *Science* **2007**, *316*, 445–449. [CrossRef]
38. Baio, J.; Wiggins, L.; Christensen, D.L.; Maenner, M.J.; Daniels, J.; Warren, Z.; Kurzius-Spencer, M.; Zahorodny, W.; Rosenberg, C.R.; White, T.; et al. Prevalence of Autism Spectrum Disorder among Children Aged 8 Years—Autism and Developmental Disabilities Monitoring Network, 11 Sites, United States, 2014. *MMWR Surveill. Summ.* **2018**, *67*, 1–23. [CrossRef] [PubMed]
39. Committee on Bioethics, Committee on Genetics, and the American College of Medical Genetics and Genomics Social, Ethical, and Legal Issues Committee. Ethical and Policy Issues in Genetic Testing and Screening of Children. *Pediatrics* **2013**, *131*, 620–622. [CrossRef]
40. Manning, M.; Hudgins, L. Professional Practice and Guidelines Committee Array-based technology and recommendations for utilization in medical genetics practice for detection of chromosomal abnormalities. *Genet. Med.* **2010**, *12*, 742–745. [CrossRef]
41. Volkmar, F.; Siegel, M.; Woodbury-Smith, M.; King, B.; McCracken, J.; State, M.; American Academy of Child and Adolescent Psychiatry (AACAP) Committee on Quality Issues (CQI). Practice parameter for the assessment and treatment of children and adolescents with autism spectrum disorder. *J. Am. Acad. Child Adolesc. Psychiatry* **2014**, *53*, 237–257. [CrossRef]
42. Cannon, B.; Pan, C.; Chen, L.; Hadd, A.G.; Russell, R. A dual-mode single-molecule fluorescence assay for the detection of expanded CGG repeats in Fragile X syndrome. *Mol. Biotechnol.* **2013**, *53*, 19–28. [CrossRef]

43. Tammimies, K.; Marshall, C.R.; Walker, S.; Kaur, G.; Thiruvahindrapuram, B.; Lionel, A.C.; Yuen, R.K.C.; Uddin, M.; Roberts, W.; Weksberg, R.; et al. Molecular Diagnostic Yield of Chromosomal Microarray Analysis and Whole-Exome Sequencing in Children With Autism Spectrum Disorder. *JAMA* **2015**, *314*, 895–903. [CrossRef]
44. Miles, J.H.; Takahashi, T.N.; Bagby, S.; Sahota, P.K.; Vaslow, D.F.; Wang, C.H.; Hillman, R.E.; Farmer, J.E. Essential versus complex autism: Definition of fundamental prognostic subtypes. *Am. J. Med. Genet. Part A* **2005**, *135*, 171–180. [CrossRef]
45. Griffiths, R. *The Griffiths Mental Developmental Scales, Revised. Henley: Association for Research in Infant and Child Development*; Test Agency: Oxford, UK, 1996.
46. Wechsler, D. *WPPSI-III Wechsler Preschool and Primary Scale of Intelligence—III. Adattamento Italiano a cura di G. Sannio Fancello e C. Cianchetti*; Giunti O.S.: Firenze, Italy, 2008.
47. Wechsler, D. *Wechsler Intelligence Scale for Children—Fourth Edition (WISC-IV)*; The Psychological Corporation: San Antonio, TX, USA, 2003.
48. Roid, G.H.; Miller, L.J. *The Leiter International Performance Scale-Revised Edition*; Psychological Assessment Resources: Lutz, FL, USA, 1997.
49. Lord, C.; Rutter, M.; DiLavore, P.C.; Risi, S.; Gotham, K.; Bishop, S. *ADOS-2 Autism Diagnostic Observation Schedule*, 2nd ed.; Western Psychological Services: Torrance, CA, USA, 2012.
50. Gotham, K.; Pickles, A.; Lord, C. Standardizing ADOS scores for a measure of severity in autism spectrum disorders. *J. Autism Dev. Disord.* **2009**, *39*, 693–705. [CrossRef]
51. Esler, A.N.; Bal, V.H.; Guthrie, W.; Wetherby, A.; Weismer, S.E.; Lord, C. The Autism Diagnostic Observation Schedule, Toddler Module: Standardized Severity Scores. *J. Autism Dev. Disord.* **2015**, *45*, 2704–2720. [CrossRef] [PubMed]
52. Database of Genomic Variants (DGV). Available online: http://dgv.tcag.ca/dgv/app/home (accessed on 26 July 2020).
53. Kearney, H.M.; Thorland, E.C.; Brown, K.K.; Quintero-Rivera, F.; South, S.T.; Working Group of the American College of Medical Genetics Laboratory Quality Assurance Committee. American College of Medical Genetics standards and guidelines for interpretation and reporting of postnatal constitutional copy number variants. *Genet. Med.* **2011**, *13*, 680–685. [CrossRef] [PubMed]
54. Online Mendelian Inheritance in Man (OMIM) Database. Available online: https://www.omim.org (accessed on 26 July 2020).
55. Simons Foundation Autism Research Initiative (SFARI). Gene Database. Available online: https://gene.sfari.org/database/human-gene (accessed on 26 July 2020).
56. Autism KnowledgeBase Version 2.0 (Autism KB 2.0). Database. Available online: http://db.cbi.pku.edu.cn/autismkb_v2/index.php (accessed on 26 July 2020).
57. Krämer, A.; Green, J.; Pollard, J.; Tugendreich, S. Causal analysis approaches in Ingenuity Pathway Analysis. *Bioinformatics* **2014**, *30*, 523–530. [CrossRef] [PubMed]
58. ToppGene Suite. Available online: https://toppgene.cchmc.org (accessed on 31 August 2020).
59. Lal, D.; Pernhorst, K.; Klein, K.M.; Reif, P.; Tozzi, R.; Toliat, M.R.; Winterer, G.; Neubauer, B.; Nürnberg, P.; Rosenow, F.; et al. Extending the phenotypic spectrum of RBFOX1 deletions: Sporadic focal epilepsy. *Epilepsia* **2015**, *56*, e129–e133. [CrossRef] [PubMed]
60. Ciaccio, C.; Tucci, A.; Scuvera, G.; Estienne, M.; Esposito, S.; Milani, D. 16p13 microduplication without CREBBP involvement: Moving toward a phenotype delineation. *Eur. J. Med. Genet.* **2017**, *60*, 159–162. [CrossRef] [PubMed]
61. Gai, X.; Xie, H.M.; Perin, J.C.; Takahashi, N.; Murphy, K.; Wenocur, A.S.; D'Arcy, M.; O'Hara, R.J.; Goldmuntz, E.; Grice, D.E.; et al. Rare structural variation of synapse and neurotransmission genes in autism. *Mol. Psychiatry* **2012**, *17*, 402–411. [CrossRef] [PubMed]
62. Drinjakovic, J.; Jung, H.; Campbell, D.S.; Strochlic, L.; Dwivedy, A.; Holt, C.E. E3 ligase Nedd4 promotes axon branching by downregulating PTEN. *Neuron* **2010**, *65*, 341–357. [CrossRef] [PubMed]
63. Ishizuka, K.; Kimura, H.; Wang, C.; Xing, J.; Kushima, I.; Arioka, Y.; Oya-Ito, T.; Uno, Y.; Okada, T.; Mori, D.; et al. Investigation of Rare Single-Nucleotide PCDH15 Variants in Schizophrenia and Autism Spectrum Disorders. *PLoS ONE* **2016**, *11*, e0153224. [CrossRef] [PubMed]
64. Stone, J.L.; Merriman, B.; Cantor, R.M.; Geschwind, D.H.; Nelson, S.F. High density SNP association study of a major autism linkage region on chromosome 17. *Hum. Mol. Genet.* **2007**, *16*, 704–715. [CrossRef] [PubMed]

65. Yang, Y.; Pan, C. Role of metabotropic glutamate receptor 7 in autism spectrum disorders: A pilot study. *Life Sci.* **2013**, *92*, 149–153. [CrossRef] [PubMed]
66. Baldan, F.; Gnan, C.; Franzoni, A.; Ferino, L.; Allegri, L.; Passon, N.; Damante, G. Genomic Deletion Involving the IMMP2L Gene in Two Cases of Autism Spectrum Disorder. *Cytogenet. Genome Res.* **2018**, *154*, 196–200. [CrossRef]
67. Ben Khelifa, H.; Soyah, N.; Ben-Abdallah-Bouhjar, I.; Gritly, R.; Sanlaville, D.; Elghezal, H.; Saad, A.; Mougou-Zerelli, S. Xp22.3 interstitial deletion: A recognizable chromosomal abnormality encompassing VCX3A and STS genes in a patient with X-linked ichthyosis and mental retardation. *Gene* **2013**, *527*, 578–583. [CrossRef]
68. Van Rijn, S.; Stockmann, L.; Borghgraef, M.; Bruining, H.; van Ravenswaaij-Arts, C.; Govaerts, L.; Hansson, K.; Swaab, H. The social behavioral phenotype in boys and girls with an extra X chromosome (Klinefelter syndrome and Trisomy X): A comparison with autism spectrum disorder. *J. Autism Dev. Disord.* **2014**, *44*, 310–320. [CrossRef]
69. Taylor, P.J.; Betts, G.A.; Maroulis, S.; Gilissen, C.; Pedersen, R.L.; Mowat, D.R.; Johnston, H.M.; Buckley, M.F. Dystrophin gene mutation location and the risk of cognitive impairment in Duchenne muscular dystrophy. *PLoS ONE* **2010**, *5*, e8803. [CrossRef]
70. Guo, H.; Peng, Y.; Hu, Z.; Li, Y.; Xun, G.; Ou, J.; Sun, L.; Xiong, Z.; Liu, Y.; Wang, T.; et al. Genome-wide copy number variation analysis in a Chinese autism spectrum disorder cohort. *Sci. Rep.* **2017**, *7*, 44155. [CrossRef]
71. Dabell, M.P.; Rosenfeld, J.A.; Bader, P.; Escobar, L.F.; El-Khechen, D.; Vallee, S.E.; Dinulos, M.B.P.; Curry, C.; Fisher, J.; Tervo, R.; et al. Investigation of NRXN1 deletions: Clinical and molecular characterization. *Am. J. Med. Genet. Part A* **2013**, *161A*, 717–731. [CrossRef]
72. Tropeano, M.; Howley, D.; Gazzellone, M.J.; Wilson, C.E.; Ahn, J.W.; Stavropoulos, D.J.; Murphy, C.M.; Eis, P.S.; Hatchwell, E.; Dobson, R.J.B.; et al. Microduplications at the pseudoautosomal SHOX locus in autism spectrum disorders and related neurodevelopmental conditions. *J. Med. Genet.* **2016**, *53*, 536–547. [CrossRef]
73. Srivastava, S.; Love-Nichols, J.A.; Dies, K.A.; Ledbetter, D.H.; Martin, C.L.; Chung, W.K.; Firth, H.V.; Frazier, T.; Hansen, R.L.; Prock, L.; et al. Meta-analysis and multidisciplinary consensus statement: Exome sequencing is a first-tier clinical diagnostic test for individuals with neurodevelopmental disorders. *Genet. Med.* **2019**, *21*, 2413–2421. [CrossRef] [PubMed]
74. Schaefer, G.B.; Mendelsohn, N.J. Professional Practice and Guidelines Committee Clinical genetics evaluation in identifying the etiology of autism spectrum disorders: 2013 guideline revisions. *Genet. Med.* **2013**, *15*, 399–407. [CrossRef] [PubMed]
75. Pinto, D.; Delaby, E.; Merico, D.; Barbosa, M.; Merikangas, A.; Klei, L.; Thiruvahindrapuram, B.; Xu, X.; Ziman, R.; Wang, Z.; et al. Convergence of genes and cellular pathways dysregulated in autism spectrum disorders. *Am. J. Hum. Genet.* **2014**, *94*, 677–694. [CrossRef] [PubMed]
76. Devlin, B.; Scherer, S.W. Genetic architecture in autism spectrum disorder. *Curr. Opin. Genet. Dev.* **2012**, *22*, 229–237. [CrossRef]
77. Chen, C.-H.; Chen, H.-I.; Chien, W.-H.; Li, L.-H.; Wu, Y.-Y.; Chiu, Y.-N.; Tsai, W.-C.; Gau, S.S.-F. High resolution analysis of rare copy number variants in patients with autism spectrum disorder from Taiwan. *Sci. Rep.* **2017**, *7*, 11919. [CrossRef]
78. Napoli, E.; Russo, S.; Casula, L.; Alesi, V.; Amendola, F.A.; Angioni, A.; Novelli, A.; Valeri, G.; Menghini, D.; Vicari, S. Array-CGH Analysis in a Cohort of Phenotypically Well-Characterized Individuals with "Essential" Autism Spectrum Disorders. *J. Autism Dev. Disord.* **2018**, *48*, 442–449. [CrossRef]
79. Barone, R.; Gulisano, M.; Amore, R.; Domini, C.; Milana, M.C.; Giglio, S.; Madia, F.; Mattina, T.; Casabona, A.; Fichera, M.; et al. Clinical correlates in children with autism spectrum disorder and CNVs: Systematic investigation in a clinical setting. *Int. J. Dev. Neurosci.* **2020**, *80*, 276–286. [CrossRef]
80. Bacchelli, E.; Cameli, C.; Viggiano, M.; Igliozzi, R.; Mancini, A.; Tancredi, R.; Battaglia, A.; Maestrini, E. An integrated analysis of rare CNV and exome variation in Autism Spectrum Disorder using the Infinium PsychArray. *Sci. Rep.* **2020**, *10*, 3198. [CrossRef]
81. Jacquemont, S.; Coe, B.P.; Hersch, M.; Duyzend, M.H.; Krumm, N.; Bergmann, S.; Beckmann, J.S.; Rosenfeld, J.A.; Eichler, E.E. A higher mutational burden in females supports a "female protective model" in neurodevelopmental disorders. *Am. J. Hum. Genet.* **2014**, *94*, 415–425. [CrossRef]

82. Girirajan, S.; Rosenfeld, J.A.; Coe, B.P.; Parikh, S.; Friedman, N.; Goldstein, A.; Filipink, R.A.; McConnell, J.S.; Angle, B.; Meschino, W.S.; et al. Phenotypic heterogeneity of genomic disorders and rare copy-number variants. *N. Engl. J. Med.* **2012**, *367*, 1321–1331. [CrossRef]
83. Newman, S.; Hermetz, K.E.; Weckselblatt, B.; Rudd, M.K. Next-generation sequencing of duplication CNVs reveals that most are tandem and some create fusion genes at breakpoints. *Am. J. Hum. Genet.* **2015**, *96*, 208–220. [CrossRef] [PubMed]
84. Rubenstein, E.; Wiggins, L.D.; Lee, L.-C. A Review of the Differences in Developmental, Psychiatric, and Medical Endophenotypes Between Males and Females with Autism Spectrum Disorder. *J. Dev. Phys. Disabil.* **2015**, *27*, 119–139. [CrossRef] [PubMed]
85. Charman, T.; Loth, E.; Tillmann, J.; Crawley, D.; Wooldridge, C.; Goyard, D.; Ahmad, J.; Auyeung, B.; Ambrosino, S.; Banaschewski, T.; et al. The EU-AIMS Longitudinal European Autism Project (LEAP): Clinical characterisation. *Mol. Autism* **2017**, *8*, 27. [CrossRef] [PubMed]
86. Knutsen, J.; Crossman, M.; Perrin, J.; Shui, A.; Kuhlthau, K. Sex differences in restricted repetitive behaviors and interests in children with autism spectrum disorder: An Autism Treatment Network study. *Autism* **2019**, *23*, 858–868. [CrossRef]
87. Warrier, V.; Toro, R.; Won, H.; Leblond, C.S.; Cliquet, F.; Delorme, R.; De Witte, W.; Bralten, J.; Chakrabarti, B.; Børglum, A.D.; et al. Social and non-social autism symptoms and trait domains are genetically dissociable. *Commun. Biol.* **2019**, *2*, 328. [CrossRef]
88. Uljarević, M.; Evans, D.W.; Alvares, G.A.; Whitehouse, A.J.O. Short report: Relationship between restricted and repetitive behaviours in children with autism spectrum disorder and their parents. *Mol. Autism* **2016**, *7*, 29. [CrossRef]
89. Szatmari, P.; Liu, X.-Q.; Goldberg, J.; Zwaigenbaum, L.; Paterson, A.D.; Woodbury-Smith, M.; Georgiades, S.; Duku, E.; Thompson, A. Sex differences in repetitive stereotyped behaviors in autism: Implications for genetic liability. *Am. J. Med. Genet. Part B Neuropsychiatr. Genet.* **2012**, *159B*, 5–12. [CrossRef]
90. Mazina, V.; Gerdts, J.; Trinh, S.; Ankenman, K.; Ward, T.; Dennis, M.Y.; Girirajan, S.; Eichler, E.E.; Bernier, R. Epigenetics of autism-related impairment: Copy number variation and maternal infection. *J. Dev. Behav. Pediatr.* **2015**, *36*, 61–67. [CrossRef]
91. Niarchou, M.; Chawner, S.J.R.A.; Doherty, J.L.; Maillard, A.M.; Jacquemont, S.; Chung, W.K.; Green-Snyder, L.; Bernier, R.A.; Goin-Kochel, R.P.; Hanson, E.; et al. Psychiatric disorders in children with 16p11.2 deletion and duplication. *Transl. Psychiatry* **2019**, *9*, 8. [CrossRef]
92. Bishop, D.V.M.; Jacobs, P.A.; Lachlan, K.; Wellesley, D.; Barnicoat, A.; Boyd, P.A.; Fryer, A.; Middlemiss, P.; Smithson, S.; Metcalfe, K.; et al. Autism, language and communication in children with sex chromosome trisomies. *Arch. Dis. Child.* **2011**, *96*, 954–959. [CrossRef]
93. Fountain, M.D.; Oleson, D.S.; Rech, M.E.; Segebrecht, L.; Hunter, J.V.; McCarthy, J.M.; Lupo, P.J.; Holtgrewe, M.; Moran, R.; Rosenfeld, J.A.; et al. Pathogenic variants in USP7 cause a neurodevelopmental disorder with speech delays, altered behavior, and neurologic anomalies. *Genet. Med.* **2019**, *21*, 1797–1807. [CrossRef] [PubMed]
94. Moyses-Oliveira, M.; Yadav, R.; Erdin, S.; Talkowski, M.E. New gene discoveries highlight functional convergence in autism and related neurodevelopmental disorders. *Curr. Opin. Genet. Dev.* **2020**, *65*, 195–206. [CrossRef] [PubMed]
95. Cheroni, C.; Caporale, N.; Testa, G. Autism spectrum disorder at the crossroad between genes and environment: Contributions, convergences, and interactions in ASD developmental pathophysiology. *Mol. Autism.* **2020**, *11*, 69. [CrossRef] [PubMed]
96. Bourgeron, T. From the genetic architecture to synaptic plasticity in autism spectrum disorder. *Nat. Rev. Neurosci.* **2015**, *16*, 551–563. [CrossRef]

© 2020 by the authors. Licensee MDPI, Basel, Switzerland. This article is an open access article distributed under the terms and conditions of the Creative Commons Attribution (CC BY) license (http://creativecommons.org/licenses/by/4.0/).

Journal of *Personalized Medicine*

MDPI

Article

Locked-in Intact Functional Networks in Children with Autism Spectrum Disorder: A Case-Control Study

Andrew R. Pines [1], Bethany Sussman [2], Sarah N. Wyckoff [2], Patrick J. McCarty [3], Raymond Bunch [4], Richard E. Frye [5,*] and Varina L. Boerwinkle [2]

1 Mayo Clinic Alix School of Medicine, 13400 E Shea Blvd, Scottsdale, AZ 85259, USA; pines.andrew@mayo.edu
2 Division of Neurology, Barrow Neurological Institute at Phoenix Children's Hospital, 1919 E. Thomas Rd, Ambulatory Building, Phoenix, AZ 85016, USA; bsussman@phoenixchildrens.com (B.S.); swyckoff@phoenixchildrens.com (S.N.W.); vboerwinkle@phoenixchildrens.com (V.L.B.)
3 Section on Neurodevelopmental Disorders, Division of Neurology, Barrow Neurological Institute at Phoenix Children's Hospital, 1919 E. Thomas Rd, Ambulatory Building, Phoenix, AZ 85016, USA; pmccarty@phoenixchildrens.com
4 Division of Psychiatry, Barrow Neurological Institute at Phoenix Children's Hospital, 1919 E. Thomas Rd, Ambulatory Building, Phoenix, AZ 85016, USA; rbunch@phoenixchildrens.com
5 Department of Child Health, University of Arizona College of Medicine–Phoenix, Phoenix, AZ 85004, USA
* Correspondence: rfrye@phoenixchildrens.com; Tel.: +1-602-933-0970

Abstract: Resting-state functional magnetic resonance imaging (rs-fMRI) has the potential to investigate abnormalities in brain network structure and connectivity on an individual level in neurodevelopmental disorders, such as autism spectrum disorder (ASD), paving the way toward using this technology for a personalized, precision medicine approach to diagnosis and treatment. Using a case-control design, we compared five patients with severe regressive-type ASD to five patients with temporal lobe epilepsy (TLE) to examine the association between brain network characteristics and diagnosis. All children with ASD and TLE demonstrated intact motor, language, and frontoparietal (FP) networks. However, aberrant networks not usually seen in the typical brain were also found. These aberrant networks were located in the motor (40%), language (80%), and FP (100%) regions in children with ASD, while children with TLE only presented with aberrant networks in the motor (40%) and language (20%) regions, in addition to identified seizure onset zones. Fisher's exact test indicated a significant relationship between aberrant FP networks and diagnosis ($p = 0.008$), with ASD and atypical FP networks co-occurring more frequently than expected by chance. Despite severe cognitive delays, children with regressive-type ASD may demonstrate intact typical cortical network activation despite an inability to use these cognitive facilities. The functions of these intact cognitive networks may not be fully expressed, potentially because aberrant networks interfere with their long-range signaling, thus creating a unique "locked-in network" syndrome.

Keywords: autism spectrum disorder; locked-in network syndrome; resting-state functional magnetic resonance imaging; temporal lobe epilepsy

Citation: Pines, A.R.; Sussman, B.; Wyckoff, S.N.; McCarty, P.J.; Bunch, R.; Frye, R.E.; Boerwinkle, V.L. Locked-In Intact Functional Networks in Children with Autism Spectrum Disorder: A Case-Control Study. *J. Pers. Med.* **2021**, *11*, 854. https://doi.org/10.3390/jpm11090854

Academic Editor: Chiara Villa

Received: 22 June 2021
Accepted: 25 August 2021
Published: 28 August 2021

Publisher's Note: MDPI stays neutral with regard to jurisdictional claims in published maps and institutional affiliations.

Copyright: © 2021 by the authors. Licensee MDPI, Basel, Switzerland. This article is an open access article distributed under the terms and conditions of the Creative Commons Attribution (CC BY) license (https://creativecommons.org/licenses/by/4.0/).

1. Introduction

Autism spectrum disorder (ASD) has a prevalence of 1 in 54 children in the United States and is characterized by deficits in social communication and interaction, and restricted and repetitive behaviors [1]. The neurological basis of ASD remains elusive in this highly heterogenous population. Resting-state functional magnetic resonance imaging (rs-fMRI) is a promising tool that has been used to analyze neural networks in patients with neurodevelopmental and neurological disorders. A review of prior group-level rs-fMRI investigations suggests hypo-, hyper-, and mixed-connectivity patterns among individuals with ASD, with contradictory findings attributed to differences in age, sex, comorbidities, and/or variations in the rs-fMRI scanning and analysis procedures [2]. Other researchers demonstrated that traditional case-control methods that assume homogeneity within clinical populations lead to a loss of subject-specific features of ASD at the group level and disguise the interindividual variation crucial for precision medicine [3].

To investigate these inconsistencies, a large-scale database replication study that characterized and evaluated connectivity patterns was conducted. The study reports evidence of reproducible ASD-associated functional hyper- and hypo- connectivity linked to clinical symptoms [4]. The authors reported that overall global connectivity was preserved in individuals with ASD, and hyperconnectivity patterns observed in the parietal and prefrontal regions were associated with the severity of deficits in communication and adaptive behavior. Furthermore, they suggested that the connectivity findings support the idea that individuals with ASD are unable to engage or disengage specific networks to the same degree as healthy, typically developing controls. If network engagement capacity is a key mechanism of ASD, then individual-based analysis may elucidate the network engagement potential and allow a better understanding of the clinical heterogeneity of ASD [5].

To address these knowledge gaps in ASD, we used a data-driven rs-fMRI whole-brain-network analysis to identify individual network pathology [6,7], similar to our work in epilepsy [8–10]. Independent component analysis (ICA) of rs-fMRI allows for the characterization and visualization of individual resting-state networks (RSNs), both typical and atypical [11–14]. In epilepsy, we utilize this method clinically to both identify the aberrant RSNs associated with seizure foci and to visualize intact cognitive RSNs. This allows the confirmation of intact cognitive networks and provides information regarding the proximity of intact cognitive networks to aberrant networks [15].

Similarly, in individuals with ASD, we may use rs-fMRI clinically to visualize network patterns in relation to the patient's clinical phenotype. One feature that differentiates individuals with ASD from those with brain injury is that individuals with ASD can have normal or extraordinary skills despite their disability, and some children with ASD can make substantial improvement with therapies, losing many, if not most, of their ASD symptoms. One of the most enigmatic subsets of ASD includes those that undergo neurodevelopmental regression, suddenly losing normal skills and rapidly developing the ASD phenotype. This suggests that the brains of some individuals with ASD have the capacity to support typical cognitive networks, at least at some time in their life, but may be unable to express these cognitive networks. For children with epilepsy, aberrant networks resulting from ongoing subclinical interictal discharges originating from the seizure onset zone (SOZ) can interfere with the function of typical cognitive brain networks, disrupting their ability to function optimally.

Thus, on the basis of the existing literature and our clinical observations, we hypothesized that some children with ASD may have intact cognitive networks identified on the individual level that are not fully realized, similar to children with epilepsy, perhaps because aberrant networks interfere with their function. However, unlike in children with epilepsy, we hypothesized that these aberrant networks are not localized to a SOZ. To investigate this possibility, subject-level ICA of rs-fMRI was used to identify and characterize the RSNs of children with regressive-type ASD and temporal lobe epilepsy (TLE). The unique relationship between patient and network characteristics was examined.

2. Materials and Methods

Using a case-control design, this study examined an age- and sex-matched cohort of children severely affected with regressive-type ASD, and a cohort of children with TLE without ASD. A 2017 meta-analysis reported an ASD pooled prevalence of 6.3% in patients with epilepsy, with a 41.9% risk of ASD in patients with focal seizures (TLE) [16]. Thus, a pathological control group was selected to distinguish ASD-specific atypical rs-fMRI biomarkers from known TLE-specific markers given the increased comorbidity of these conditions. For the ASD cohort, children with regressive-type ASD were chosen since these children had documented normal development early in life, suggesting that their brain could previously support normal cognitive networks. ASD was diagnosed using the Diagnostic Statistical Manual of Mental Disorders (5th ed., DSM-5).

The study sample size was limited due to rs-fMRI data availability for this patient population. Five patients with regressive-type ASD who were not making sufficient progress with standard therapy and five patients with TLE undergoing pre-surgical planning for epilepsy surgery underwent clinically indicated rs-fMRI at Phoenix Children's Hospital (PCH) between November 2018 and December 2020. The patient cohorts were age- and sex-matched. The PCH Institutional Review Board approved the study, and caretakers provided informed consent to authorize secondary analysis of the rs-fMRI data and review of the medical records.

2.1. Resting-State MRI

The rs-fMRI images were acquired and analyzed per prior reported standards [15]. Acquisition was from a 3 T MRI scanner (Ingenuity; Philips Medical Systems, Best, The Netherlands) with a 32-channel head coil. Patients received conscious sedation by propofol, per hospital clinical standards. Acquisition of rs-fMRI consisted of two 10-min runs totaling 20 min. Parameters were 2000 millisecond repetition time (TR), 30 millisecond echo time (TE), 80×80 matrix size, 80° flip angle, 46 slices, 3.4 mm slice thickness with no gap, 3×3 mm in-plane resolution, interleaved acquisition, and 600 total volumes. For anatomical reference, a T1-weighted turbo field-echo whole-brain sequence was obtained with TR 9 milliseconds, TE 4 milliseconds, flip angle 80°, slice thickness 0.9 mm, and an in-plane resolution of 0.9×0.9 mm.

2.2. Independent Component Analysis Approach

ICA is driven by empirical data rather than a priori information. Briefly, rs-fMRI voxels are grouped together into components according to similarity of blood oxygen level dependent (BOLD) signal oscillation [6,7]. The resulting independent components (ICs) are independently fluctuating clusters of brain activity or sources of noise that require expert review and interpretation [17]. ICA procedures were completed via the Multivariate Exploratory Linear Optimized Decomposition into Independent Components (MELODIC) tool [7]. The following standard preprocessing steps were applied: (1) deletion of the first five volumes to remove T1 saturation effects, (2) high-pass filtering at 100 s, (3) inter-leaved slice time correction, (4) no spatial smoothing, and (5) motion correction with MCLFIRT [18], with non-brain structures removed. Individual functional scans were registered to the patient's corresponding anatomical scan using linear registration [19], and optimized using boundary-based registration [20]. All participants had <1 mm head-motion displacement in any direction. As ICA was applied in the subject space, no standardized templates or spatial normalization procedures was performed. The total number of detected ICs was determined for each patient from established automated dimensionality estimates using a Bayesian approach, and an ICA threshold ($p < 0.05$) for IC detection was set by the standard local false discovery rate [6].

2.3. Component Categorization

IC categorization followed the working paradigm previously published [15], separating patient ICs into four categories—noise, typical RSNs, SOZ, and atypical (aberrant) networks—using criteria modified from established norms [11–15,21]. Noise components arise from respirations, cerebrospinal fluid movement, and tissue–fluid junctions. A component was determined to be noise if: it was not primarily located in grey matter; it varied significantly in coordination with physiological cycles (i.e., respiratory-related frequency range, 0.1–0.5 Hz; cardiac-related, 0.6–1.2 Hz; regular but fast oscillation pattern); or it was in a spatial distribution consistent with a machine-generated artifact [11,12]. Components determined to be neural networks were categorized as either typical RSNs, SOZs, or atypical (aberrant) networks. Typical RSNs were determined by visually comparing spatial features to established RSNs (e.g., motor, language, and frontoparietal), and comparing temporal features of frequency and frequency power spectra with a known low-frequency, regular, slow-oscillating time course, and low-frequency power-spectra features of RSN norms [12–14]. SOZs were distinguished by a spatial pattern (more asymmetrically unilateral than expected, alternating localized activation-deactivation patterns of gray matter, and with a tapered tail from the cortex extending toward the ventricles) not conforming with noise or typical RSNs, an irregular time course, or containing a frequency >0.4 Hz [15]. Aberrant networks were distinguished by spatial locations that may overlap with known RSN, but do not conform to the RSN spatial pattern, noise, or SOZ criteria, having a regular sinusoidal oscillation pattern that is overlaid with irregular faster frequency, and having an atypical BOLD oscillation frequency >0.039 Hz [13–15]. rs-fMRI data were interpreted by an rs-fMRI specialist (senior author), wherein typical RSNs were operationally defined as those meeting the spatial and temporal criteria above by expert visual inspection, as in prior publications [12,15].

2.4. Statistical Analysis

Categorical variables (e.g., typical RSN: present, absent; aberrant (non-SOZ) network: present, absent) were generated for the motor, language, and frontoparietal networks for each patient. Due to the small sample size, a two-tailed Fisher's exact test was used to examine the significance of the association between the two factors in the contingency tables. Since, for each set of tests, we compared three cortical regions, requiring three statistical tests, the Bonferroni correction for inflated alpha was used to set the significance threshold at $p <= 0.017$ (0.5/3). An independent-samples t-test (two-tailed, $p < 0.05$) was used for the analysis of continuous variables.

3. Results

Figure 1 visually summarizes the clinical characteristics and typical and aberrant rs-fMRI ICA-based networks for children with ASD. Figure 2 demonstrates a detailed example of typical RSNs and aberrant networks for a single ASD case (Patient 1). A narrative summary of the clinical and network features is presented below for all patients, followed by a statistical analysis of patient characteristics and resting-state networks.

3.1. Patient Summaries of ASD Patients

3.1.1. Patient 1

A 7-year-old (yo) male progressively lost social interactions and eye contact from 9 to 15 months of age. At the time of rs-fMRI, he was diagnosed with ASD, cognitive delay, severe language impairment (LI), and developmental coordination disorder (DCD). Despite these deficits, frontoparietal (FP), language, and motor RSNs were intact. Aberrant networks were found over sensory, FP, and contralateral non-dominant language regions (Figure 2).

3.1.2. Patient 2

A 4 yo female suddenly lost normal speech, social, language, cognitive, and motor abilities at 3.5 yo. At the time of rs-fMRI, she was diagnosed with ASD, borderline intellectual disability (ID), severe LI, and delayed visual-motor skills. Despite these deficits, FP, language, and motor RSNs were normal. Aberrant networks were found over the right FP, bilateral temporal, and opercular regions.

3.1.3. Patient 3

A 16 yo female lost social skills and ceased making eye contact with others at 3 yo. At the time of rs-fMRI, she was diagnosed with ASD, ID, severe LI, and DCD. Despite these deficits, FP, language, and motor RSNs were detected. Aberrant networks were found over the left FP-temporal regions.

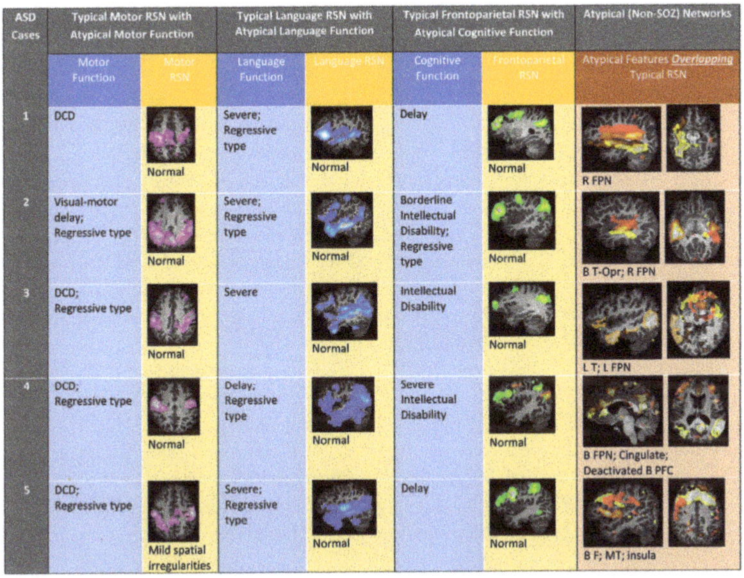
ASD Cases
Typical Motor RSN with Atypical Motor Function
Typical Language RSN with Atypical Language Function
Typical Frontoparietal RSN with Atypical Cognitive Function
Atypical (Non-SOZ) Networks
Motor Function
Motor RSN
Language Function
Language RSN
Cognitive Function
Frontoparietal RSN
Atypical Features Overlapping Typical RSN
1
DCD
Normal
Severe; Regressive type
Normal
Delay
Normal
R FPN
2
Visual-motor delay; Regressive type
Normal
Severe; Regressive type
Normal
Borderline Intellectual Disabilty; Regressive type
Normal
B T-Opr; R FPN
3
DCD; Regressive type
Normal
Severe
Normal
Intellectual Disability
Normal
L T; L FPN
4
DCD; Regressive type
Normal
Delay; Regressive type
Normal
Severe Intellectual Disability
Normal
B FPN; Cingulate; Deactivated B PFC
5
DCD; Regressive type
Mild spatial irregularities
Severe; Regressive type
Normal
Delay
Normal
B F; MT; insula

Figure 1. Comparison of clinical and rs-fMRI findings in ASD patients. Columns 1–3: ASD patient typical motor, language, and frontoparietal network images and interpretation with corresponding discordant phenotypic clinical impairments. Column 4: ASD participant atypical (aberrant) network (non-SOZ, overlapping typical RSN) images. B, bilateral; DCD, developmental coordination disorder; F, frontal; FPN, frontoparietal network; L, left; MT, mesial temporal; Opr, operculum; R, right; RSN, resting state network; vmPFC, ventromedial prefrontal cortex.

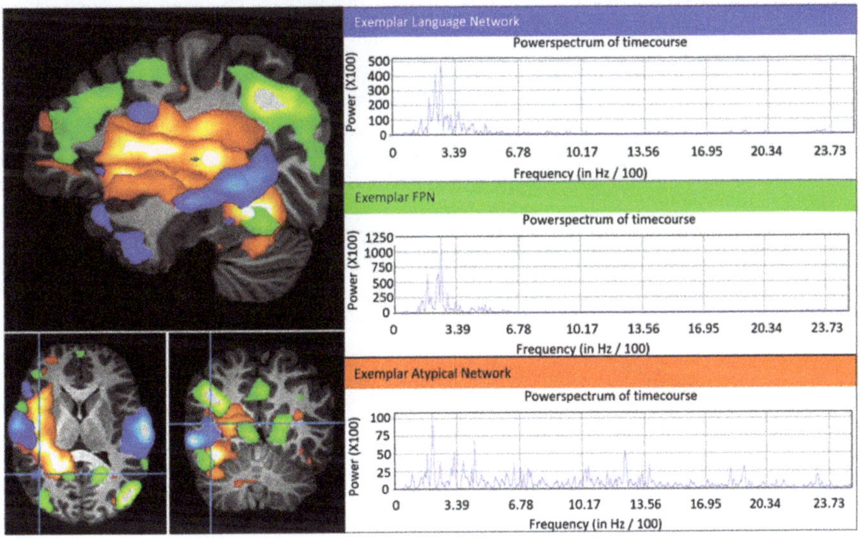

Figure 2. Example of right-sided language, frontoparietal, and aberrant networks in ASD Patient 1. Image shown is the sagittal, axial, and coronal T1-weighted MRI of Patient 1 with overlayed language (blue), frontoparietal (green), and aberrant (red) networks. Plotted are the respective network blood oxygen dependent signal (BOLD) power versus frequency (Hz/100), wherein typical is less than 6 Hz/100. The frontoparietal and language network spatial distribution and the BOLD power spectrum are typical, whereas the atypical networks have abnormal spatial and widely distributed power spectra.

3.1.4. Patient 4

A 12 yo male lost language skills (from saying short sentences to saying only single words) and motor skills (ceased walking and performing fine motor skills) at 2.5 yo. He regained some language and motor skills at 5 yo and began to walk again, but he did not regain fine motor skills. At the time of rs-fMRI, he was diagnosed with ASD, severe ID, moderate LI, DCD, and epilepsy. Despite these deficits, FP, motor and bilaterally-dominant language RSNs were intact. Bilateral language dominance is a relatively mild atypical feature found in children with epilepsy and dominate-sided language region network pathology [22]. Aberrant networks were found over the FP and language regions. The network pathology is consistent with children with drug-resistant epilepsy [8,15] which, in comparison to other aberrant networks discussed, has markedly erratic, high-frequency BOLD time courses and generalized spatial distribution of the cingulate, lateral temporal, and bilateral frontal regions.

3.1.5. Patient 5

A 12 yo male lost language (from knowing 10 words to non-verbal) and motor skills (normal development to stereotypic movements) at 2 yo. At the time of the rs-fMRI, he was diagnosed with ASD, global developmental delay, severe LI, and DCD. Despite these deficits, FP, motor, and bilateral language RSNs were intact. Aberrant networks were localized to the FP, insular, and mesial temporal regions.

3.2. Patient Summaries of TLE Patients (Controls)

3.2.1. Patient 6

A 15 yo female was diagnosed with intractable localization-related symptomatic epilepsy without status epilepticus after unprovoked complex partial seizures at 10 yo. The seizure focus was associated with an inferior temporal lobe encephalocele. Medical and developmental history was otherwise normal. The expected whole-brain network profiles were well-detected, including the motor, language, and FP networks. The SOZ was detected in the right temporal and right frontal regions. Non-SOZ aberrant networks were detected in the hand-arm motor areas.

3.2.2. Patient 7

An 11 yo female was diagnosed with intractable epilepsy without status epilepticus after complex partial seizures at 10 yo. The seizure focus was associated with a left temporal lobe tumor. Early medical history was notable for appendectomy. Early developmental language milestones were delayed. Expected whole-brain network profiles were well-detected, including the motor, language, and FP networks. The SOZ was detected in the anterior half of the anterior temporal lobe. Non-SOZ aberrant network features were detected in the facial motor and language areas.

3.2.3. Patient 8

A 4 yo male had a history of complex febrile seizures starting at 20 months of age. The patient presented with typical motor and cognitive developmental milestones but had a diagnosis of expressive language disorder with poor articulation. Overall, the expected whole-brain network profiles were well-detected, including the motor, language, and FP networks. The SOZ was detected in the left mesial-anterior temporal regions (language). No non-SOZ aberrant networks were detected.

3.2.4. Patient 9

A 9 yo male was diagnosed with intractable absence epilepsy without status epilepticus at 7 yo. Medical and developmental history was normal. The expected whole-brain network profiles were well-detected, including the motor, language, and FP networks. The SOZ was detected in the left mesial-temporal region. No non-SOZ aberrant networks were detected.

3.2.5. Patient 10

A 13 yo male was diagnosed with intractable localization-related idiopathic epilepsy without status epilepticus at 12 yo. Medical and developmental history was normal. The expected whole-brain network profiles were well-detected, including the motor, language, and FP networks. The SOZ was detected in the right and left mesial-temporal regions. No non-SOZ aberrant networks were detected.

3.3. Statistical Analysis

Table 1 presents the clinical characteristics and rs-fMRI ICA-based network characteristics and the corresponding Fisher's exact tests' statistics.

Table 1. Clinical and resting-state network characteristics. Fisher's exact test (two-tailed) was used to test the difference in frequencies. Significant p values ($p < 0.017$) are indicated in bold and italics.

Characteristic/Network	Participants with ASD ($n = 5$)	Participants with TLE ($n = 5$)	Fisher Exact Test p-Value
Clinical Characteristics			
Motor Dysfunction	100% (5)	0% (0)	***0.008***
Language Dysfunction	100% (5)	40% (2)	0.167
Cognitive Dysfunction	100% (5)	0% (0)	***0.008***
Typical Resting-State Networks			
Motor Network	100% (5)	100% (5)	1.000
Language Network	100% (5)	100% (5)	1.000
Frontoparietal Network	100% (5)	100% (5)	1.000
Aberrant Resting-State Networks			
Motor Network	40% (2)	40% (2)	1.000
Language Network	80% (4)	20% (1)	0.167
Frontoparietal Network	100% (5)	0% (0)	***0.008***

3.3.1. Clinical Characteristics

Children with ASD were between 4 and 16 yo ($M = 10.66$, $SD = 4.71$) and predominantly male (60%). Similarly, children with TLE were between 4 and 15 yo ($M = 10.98$, $SD = 4.57$) and predominantly male (60%). There were no significant differences in age ($t(8) = 3.4$, $p = 0.916$) or sex (Fisher's exact test, $p = 1.0$) between the children with ASD and TLE.

All children with ASD presented with clinically significant motor (100%), language (100%), and cognitive (100%) dysfunction, while children with TLE only presented with language dysfunction (40%) in addition to the epilepsy-related symptoms. Fisher's exact test (two-tailed) indicated a significant relationship between motor and cognitive dysfunction and ASD diagnosis (Table 1).

3.3.2. rs-fMRI Networks

ICA of rs-fMRI data yielded 91, 119, 49, 48, 58, 66, 105, 96, 95, and 111 ICs for patients 1–10, respectively. There was no significant difference (t (8) = 2.3, $p = 0.212$) in the mean number of ICs generated from subject-level ICA of rs-fMRI for the children with ASD ($M = 73$, $SD = 31.09$) and children with TLE ($M = 94.6$, $SD = 17.3$).

There was no significant association between typical networks and diagnosis, as all children with ASD and TLE presented with intact motor, language, and FP RSNs (Table 1). Children with ASD presented with non-SOZ aberrant motor (40%), language (80%), and FP (100%) networks, while children with TLE only presented with non-SOZ aberrant motor (40%) and language (20%) networks in addition to the identified SOZs. Thus, children with ASD were significantly more likely to manifest aberrant FP networks (Table 1).

3.3.3. Aberrant rs-fMRI Networks and Clinical Symptomatology

The relationship between network characteristics and clinical dysfunction was assessed using the full study cohort (n = 10). There was a significant relationship between atypical (non-SOZ) FP networks and cognitive dysfunction (Table 2). Specifically, clinically significant cognitive dysfunction was documented in 100% of the children with detected atypical FP networks, while cognitive dysfunction was not reported (0%) in children without atypical (non-SOZ) FP networks.

Table 2. Relationship between clinical symptomatology and presence of aberrant resting-state network. Fisher's exact test (two-tailed) was used to test the difference in frequencies. Significant p values ($p < 0.017$) are indicated in bold and italics.

Aberrant Network	Clinical Dysfunction Subserved by Network	No Clinical Dysfunction Subserved by Network	Fisher's Exact Test *p*-Value
Motor Dysfunction	100% (5)	0% (0)	1.000
Language Dysfunction	100% (5)	40% (2)	0.167
Frontoparietal Network	100% (5)	0% (0)	***0.008***

4. Discussion

For the first time, we demonstrate that children with regressive-type ASD have intact motor, language, and FP neural networks with relatively typical spatial and temporal features, despite having moderate to severe disability in the skills typically subserved by these networks. The finding of overall preserved connectivity is consistent with prior ASD research [4,23]. Interestingly, the case sample only included children with regressive-type ASD, suggesting that these intact typical cognitive networks did subserve their normal expression prior to the regression. Furthermore, the rs-fMRI ICA data-driven approach extracts typical and atypical neural circuitry on an individual basis, demonstrating that multiple widespread aberrant neural networks characterize regressive-type ASD. Given that typical RSNs are intact but not well-expressed, we think that the atypical aberrant networks disrupt the fidelity of signaling within these long-range typical RSNs, essentially creating a locked-in network syndrome.

The ASD participants were found to have typical RSNs and additional broad aberrant networks. In comparison, the TLE controls had fewer aberrant networks beyond those localized to regions disrupted by seizure activity (SOZ). The aberrant networks found in ASD patients were not orthogonal to any canonical network, and this finding, in addition to their spatial location, may provide hints to the pathophysiology of ASD symptoms. In these patients, aberrant networks traversing regions associated with the FP network could interfere with the fidelity of signals of typical RSNs as they are communicated between distal regions. Higher-order networks typically integrate into other brain networks at around 18–24 months [24,25], which is around the same time children with ASD begin to show core symptoms and regression may occur [26]. According to our theory, interference from aberrant networks could impair the acquisition of cognitive inhibitory control [27], social skills, and other complex behavior. We think that interference from aberrant networks hinders communication and the optimal functioning of long-range typical RSNs, essentially creating a locked-in network effect. Alternatively, or complementarily, aberrant networks could inappropriately activate cortical areas. For example, aberrant networks traversing the somatosensory area, as in Patient 1, may be a biomarker of the expressed sensory symptoms.

Interventions that inhibit atypical networks could effectively "unlock" the intact RSNs, leading to symptomatic recovery. Recovery from locked-in syndrome, with compromised capacity to demonstrate consciousness yet intact supratentorial network function on rs-fMRI, was reported [28]. The patients presented in this study were all refractory to standard treatments, such as behavioral and speech therapy. Potentially, other network-targeted treatments, including those used in epilepsy, such as surgical and neuromodulatory treatments, could improve recovery rates of these patients [9,28,29].

This study has several limitations. The small sample size limits the generalizability of our results. It is also possible that the aberrant networks seen on imaging are an epiphenomenon and do not affect ASD symptoms. However, a recent large study found differences in the FP network regions between individuals with ASD and typically developing controls [4], thus supporting the notion that these aberrant networks interfere with typical RSNs. It is also possible that the aberrant networks reflect activity that does not interact with RSNs in an awake brain as our patients were sedated during scanning. However, such findings are not reported in neurotypical individuals studied under low-dose conscious sedation [30–32]. Further studies will be needed to correlate the presence or absence of aberrant networks and their characteristics, such as location, with detailed measures of cognitive and language function, as well as ASD symptomology, in larger cohorts. Unfortunately, with the current sample size, such analysis would not be valid. Thus, we look forward to larger studies in the future.

5. Conclusions

From these data, we propose that analyzing individual patients may provide evidence that ASD symptoms may correlate with aberrant networks that interfere with the maturation of typical RSNs, effectively creating a locked-in network syndrome. Further, we propose that it may be clinically useful to perform rs-fMRI on select patients with ASD. We believe this case series warrants larger systematic studies of ASD patients with rs-fMRI before and after typical treatment. rs-fMRI could help personalize treatment strategies by categorizing a patient's aberrant networks based on treatment response and symptom profile. In this way, rs-fMRI can act as an integrative tool to support a personalized precision medicine approach to ASD diagnosis and treatment.

6. Patents

Nothing to report.

Author Contributions: Conceptualization, A.R.P., B.S., P.J.M., R.B., R.E.F., and V.L.B.; methodology, V.L.B.; formal analysis, B.S., S.N.W., R.E.F., and V.L.B.; data curation, A.R.P., B.S., P.J.M., R.E.F., and V.L.B.; writing—original draft preparation, A.R.P., B.S., P.J.M., R.E.F., and V.L.B.; writing—review and editing, A.R.P., B.S., P.J.M., S.N.W., R.E.F., and V.L.B.; visualization, A.R.P., B.S., P.J.M., R.E.F., and V.L.B. All authors have read and agreed to the published version of the manuscript.

Funding: This research received no external funding.

Institutional Review Board Statement: The study was conducted according to the guidelines of the Declaration of Helsinki and approved by the Institutional Review Board of Phoenix Children's Hospital, Phoenix, AZ, USA.

Informed Consent Statement: Informed consent was obtained from the parents of all participants involved in the study.

Data Availability Statement: Data are available upon request.

Acknowledgments: We would like to thank the patients and families who volunteered their time to be part of our research program.

Conflicts of Interest: The authors declare no conflict of interest.

References

1. Maenner, M.J.; Shaw, K.A.; Baio, J.; Washington, A.; Patrick, M.; DiRienzo, M.; Christensen, D.L.; Wiggins, L.D.; Pettygrove, S.; Andrews, J.G.; et al. Prevalence of Autism Spectrum Disorder Among Children Aged 8 Years-Autism and Developmental Disabilities Monitoring Network, 11 Sites, United States, 2016. *MMWR Surveill. Summ.* **2020**, *69*, 1–12. [CrossRef]
2. Hull, J.V.; Dokovna, L.B.; Jacokes, Z.J.; Torgerson, C.M.; Irimia, A.; Van Horn, J.D. Resting-State Functional Connectivity in Autism Spectrum Disorders: A Review. *Front. Psychiatry* **2016**, *7*, 205. [CrossRef] [PubMed]

3. Zabihi, M.; Oldehinkel, M.; Wolfers, T.; Frouin, V.; Goyard, D.; Loth, E.; Charman, T.; Tillmann, J.; Banaschewski, T.; Dumas, G.; et al. Dissecting the Heterogeneous Cortical Anatomy of Autism Spectrum Disorder Using Normative Models. *Biol. Psychiatry Cogn. Neurosci. Neuroimaging* **2019**, *4*, 567–578. [CrossRef] [PubMed]
4. Holiga, S.; Hipp, J.F.; Chatham, C.H.; Garces, P.; Spooren, W.; D'Ardhuy, X.L.; Bertolino, A.; Bouquet, C.; Buitelaar, J.K.; Bours, C.; et al. Patients with autism spectrum disorders display reproducible functional connectivity alterations. *Sci. Transl. Med.* **2019**, *11*. [CrossRef] [PubMed]
5. Marek, S.; Dosenbach, N.U.F. The frontoparietal network: Function, electrophysiology, and importance of individual precision mapping. *Dialogues Clin. Neurosci.* **2018**, *20*, 133–140.
6. Beckmann, C.F.; DeLuca, M.; Devlin, J.T.; Smith, S.M. Investigations into resting-state connectivity using independent component analysis. *Philos. Trans. R. Soc. Lond. B Biol. Sci.* **2005**, *360*, 1001–1013. [CrossRef]
7. Beckmann, C.F.; Smith, S.M. Probabilistic independent component analysis for functional magnetic resonance imaging. *IEEE Trans. Med. Imaging* **2004**, *23*, 137–152. [CrossRef]
8. Boerwinkle, V.L.; Cediel, E.G.; Mirea, L.; Williams, K.; Kerrigan, J.F.; Lam, S.; Raskin, J.S.; Desai, V.R.; Wilfong, A.A.; Adelson, P.D.; et al. Network-targeted approach and postoperative resting-state functional magnetic resonance imaging are associated with seizure outcome. *Ann. Neurol.* **2019**, *86*, 344–356. [CrossRef]
9. Boerwinkle, V.L.; Mirea, L.; Gaillard, W.D.; Sussman, B.L.; Larocque, D.; Bonnell, A.; Ronecker, J.S.; Troester, M.M.; Kerrigan, J.F.; Foldes, S.T.; et al. Resting-state functional MRI connectivity impact on epilepsy surgery plan and surgical candidacy: Prospective clinical work. *J. Neurosurg. Pediatr.* **2020**, 1–8. [CrossRef]
10. Boerwinkle, V.L.; Wilfong, A.A.; Curry, D.J. Resting-state functional connectivity by independent component analysis-based markers corresponds to areas of initial seizure propagation established by prior modalities from the hypothalamus. *Brain Connect.* **2016**, *6*, 642–651. [CrossRef]
11. Beckmann, C.F.; Noble, J.A.; Smith, S.M. Artefact detection in FMRI data using independent component analysis. *NeuroImage* **2000**, *11*, S614. [CrossRef]
12. Griffanti, L.; Douaud, G.; Bijsterbosch, J.; Evangelisti, S.; Alfaro-Almagro, F.; Glasser, M.F.; Duff, E.P.; Fitzgibbon, S.; Westphal, R.; Carone, D.; et al. Hand classification of fMRI ICA noise components. *Neuroimage* **2017**, *154*, 188–205. [CrossRef]
13. Damoiseaux, J.S.; Rombouts, S.A.; Barkhof, F.; Scheltens, P.; Stam, C.J.; Smith, S.M.; Beckmann, C.F. Consistent resting-state networks across healthy subjects. *Proc. Natl. Acad. Sci. USA* **2006**, *103*, 13848–13853. [CrossRef]
14. Smith, S.M.; Fox, P.T.; Miller, K.L.; Glahn, D.C.; Fox, P.M.; Mackay, C.E.; Filippini, N.; Watkins, K.E.; Toro, R.; Laird, A.R.; et al. Correspondence of the brain's functional architecture during activation and rest. *Proc. Natl. Acad. Sci. USA* **2009**, *106*, 13040–13045. [CrossRef] [PubMed]
15. Boerwinkle, V.L.; Mohanty, D.; Foldes, S.T.; Guffey, D.; Minard, C.G.; Vedantam, A.; Raskin, J.S.; Lam, S.; Bond, M.; Mirea, L.; et al. Correlating Resting-State Functional Magnetic Resonance Imaging Connectivity by Independent Component Analysis-Based Epileptogenic Zones with Intracranial Electroencephalogram Localized Seizure Onset Zones and Surgical Outcomes in Prospective Pediatric Intractable Epilepsy Study. *Brain Connect.* **2017**, *7*, 424–442. [CrossRef]
16. Strasser, L.; Downes, M.; Kung, J.; Cross, J.H.; De Haan, M. Prevalence and risk factors for autism spectrum disorder in epilepsy: A systematic review and meta-analysis. *Dev. Med. Child. Neurol.* **2018**, *60*, 19–29. [CrossRef] [PubMed]
17. De Martino, F.; Gentile, F.; Esposito, F.; Balsi, M.; Di Salle, F.; Goebel, R.; Formisano, E. Classification of fMRI independent components using IC-fingerprints and support vector machine classifiers. *Neuroimage* **2007**, *34*, 177–194. [CrossRef] [PubMed]
18. Jenkinson, M.; Bannister, P.; Brady, M.; Smith, S. Improved optimization for the robust and accurate linear registration and motion correction of brain images. *Neuroimage* **2002**, *17*, 825–841. [CrossRef] [PubMed]
19. Jenkinson, M.; Smith, S. A global optimisation method for robust affine registration of brain images. *Med. Image Anal.* **2001**, *5*, 143–156. [CrossRef]
20. Greve, D.N.; Fischl, B. Accurate and robust brain image alignment using boundary-based registration. *Neuroimage* **2009**, *48*, 63–72. [CrossRef]
21. Pruim, R.H.R.; Mennes, M.; van Rooij, D.; Llera, A.; Buitelaar, J.K.; Beckmann, C.F. ICA-AROMA: A robust ICA-based strategy for removing motion artifacts from fMRI data. *Neuroimage* **2015**, *112*, 267–277. [CrossRef]
22. Desai, V.R.; Vedantam, A.; Lam, S.K.; Mirea, L.; Foldes, S.T.; Curry, D.J.; Adelson, P.D.; Wilfong, A.A.; Boerwinkle, V.L. Language lateralization with resting-state and task-based functional MRI in pediatric epilepsy. *J. Neurosurg. Pediatr.* **2018**, *23*, 171–177. [CrossRef]
23. Hahamy, A.; Behrmann, M.; Malach, R. The idiosyncratic brain: Distortion of spontaneous connectivity patterns in autism spectrum disorder. *Nat. Neurosci.* **2015**, *18*, 302–309. [CrossRef] [PubMed]
24. Gao, W.; Alcauter, S.; Smith, J.K.; Gilmore, J.H.; Lin, W. Development of human brain cortical network architecture during infancy. *Brain Struct. Funct.* **2015**, *220*, 1173–1186. [CrossRef] [PubMed]
25. Fransson, P.; Aden, U.; Blennow, M.; Lagercrantz, H. The functional architecture of the infant brain as revealed by resting-state fMRI. *Cereb. Cortex* **2011**, *21*, 145–154. [CrossRef] [PubMed]
26. Bright Futures Steering Committee; Medical Home Initiatives for Children with Special Needs Project Advisory Committee. Identifying infants and young children with developmental disorders in the medical home: An algorithm for developmental surveillance and screening. *Pediatrics* **2006**, *118*, 405–420. [CrossRef]

27. Marek, S.; Hwang, K.; Foran, W.; Hallquist, M.N.; Luna, B. The Contribution of Network Organization and Integration to the Development of Cognitive Control. *PLoS Biol.* **2015**, *13*, e1002328. [CrossRef]
28. Boerwinkle, V.L.; Torrisi, S.J.; Foldes, S.T.; Marku, I.; Ranjan, M.; Wilfong, A.A.; Adelson, P.D. Resting-state fMRI in disorders of consciousness to facilitate early therapeutic intervention. *Neurol. Clin. Pract.* **2019**, *9*, e33–e35. [CrossRef] [PubMed]
29. Boerwinkle, V.L.; Foldes, S.T.; Torrisi, S.J.; Temkit, H.; Gaillard, W.D.; Kerrigan, J.F.; Desai, V.R.; Raskin, J.S.; Vedantam, A.; Jarrar, R.; et al. Subcentimeter epilepsy surgery targets by resting state functional magnetic resonance imaging can improve outcomes in hypothalamic hamartoma. *Epilepsia* **2018**, *59*, 2284–2295. [CrossRef]
30. Golkowski, D.; Larroque, S.K.; Vanhaudenhuyse, A.; Plenevaux, A.; Boly, M.; Di Perri, C.; Ranft, A.; Schneider, G.; Laureys, S.; Jordan, D.; et al. Changes in Whole Brain Dynamics and Connectivity Patterns during Sevoflurane- and Propofol-induced Unconsciousness Identified by Functional Magnetic Resonance Imaging. *Anesthesiology* **2019**, *130*, 898–911. [CrossRef]
31. Hudetz, A.G. General anesthesia and human brain connectivity. *Brain Connect.* **2012**, *2*, 291–302. [CrossRef] [PubMed]
32. Kirsch, M.; Guldenmund, P.; Ali Bahri, M.; Demertzi, A.; Baquero, K.; Heine, L.; Charland-Verville, V.; Vanhaudenhuyse, A.; Bruno, M.A.; Gosseries, O.; et al. Sedation of Patients With Disorders of Consciousness During Neuroimaging: Effects on Resting State Functional Brain Connectivity. *Anesth. Analg.* **2017**, *124*, 588–598. [CrossRef] [PubMed]

Journal of *Personalized Medicine*

Case Report

Resting State Functional Magnetic Resonance Imaging Elucidates Neurotransmitter Deficiency in Autism Spectrum Disorder

Patrick J. McCarty [1], Andrew R. Pines [2], Bethany L. Sussman [3], Sarah N. Wyckoff [3], Amanda Jensen [1], Raymond Bunch [4], Varina L. Boerwinkle [3] and Richard E. Frye [1,*]

1 Division of Neurology, Section on Neurodevelopmental Disorders, Barrow Neurological Institute at Phoenix Children's Hospital, 1919 E. Thomas Rd., Ambulatory Building, Phoenix, AZ 85016, USA; pmccarty@phoenixchildrens.com (P.J.M.); ajensen1@phoenixchildrens.com (A.J.)
2 Mayo Clinic Alix School of Medicine, 13400 E Shea Blvd, Scottsdale, AZ 85259, USA; pines.andrew@mayo.edu
3 Division of Neurology, Barrow Neurological Institute at Phoenix Children's Hospital, 1919 E. Thomas Rd., Ambulatory Building, Phoenix, AZ 85016, USA; bsussman@phoenixchildrens.com (B.L.S.); swyckoff@phoenixchildrens.com (S.N.W.); vboerwinkle@phoenixchildrens.com (V.L.B.)
4 Division of Psychiatry, Barrow Neurological Institute at Phoenix Children's Hospital, 1919 E. Thomas Rd., Ambulatory Building, Phoenix, AZ 85016, USA; rbunch@phoenixchildrens.com
* Correspondence: rfrye@phoenixchildrens.com; Tel.: +1-602-933-0970

Abstract: Resting-state functional magnetic resonance imaging provides dynamic insight into the functional organization of the brains' intrinsic activity at rest. The emergence of resting-state functional magnetic resonance imaging in both the clinical and research settings may be attributed to recent advancements in statistical techniques, non-invasiveness and enhanced spatiotemporal resolution compared to other neuroimaging modalities, and the capability to identify and characterize deep brain structures and networks. In this report we describe a 16-year-old female patient with autism spectrum disorder who underwent resting-state functional magnetic resonance imaging due to late regression. Imaging revealed deactivated networks in deep brain structures involved in monoamine synthesis. Monoamine neurotransmitter deficits were confirmed by cerebrospinal fluid analysis. This case suggests that resting-state functional magnetic resonance imaging may have clinical utility as a non-invasive biomarker of central nervous system neurochemical alterations by measuring the function of neurotransmitter-driven networks. Use of this technology can accelerate and increase the accuracy of selecting appropriate therapeutic agents for patients with neurological and neurodevelopmental disorders.

Keywords: monoamine neurotransmitters; neurotransmitter deficiency; resting-state functional magnetic resonance imaging

Citation: McCarty, P.J.; Pines, A.R.; Sussman, B.L.; Wyckoff, S.N.; Jensen, A.; Bunch, R.; Boerwinkle, V.L.; Frye, R.E. Resting State Functional Magnetic Resonance Imaging Elucidates Neurotransmitter Deficiency in Autism Spectrum Disorder. *J. Pers. Med.* **2021**, *11*, 969. https://doi.org/10.3390/jpm11100969

Academic Editor: Mayra Paolillo

Received: 12 July 2021
Accepted: 27 September 2021
Published: 28 September 2021

Publisher's Note: MDPI stays neutral with regard to jurisdictional claims in published maps and institutional affiliations.

Copyright: © 2021 by the authors. Licensee MDPI, Basel, Switzerland. This article is an open access article distributed under the terms and conditions of the Creative Commons Attribution (CC BY) license (https://creativecommons.org/licenses/by/4.0/).

1. Introduction

Neurotransmitters are essential for normal brain development and function. Many neurological, neurodevelopmental, and psychiatric disorders have been shown to be associated with alterations in neurotransmitter function and neurotransmitter concentrations in the brain.

Autism spectrum disorder (ASD) is a very heterogenous neurodevelopmental disorder, primarily due to the fact that its diagnosis is based on behavioral observations which do not, at this time, have a precise neurological underpinning, although many brain systems have been implicated in driving ASD behavior. In fact, it has been proposed that ASD may have numerous underlying causes [1], leading to the optimal treatment of this disorder being difficult to determine without a cumbersome trial and error process [2]. Many different neurochemical alterations have been implicated in ASD. Cortical circuitry is believed to demonstrate an excitatory-inhibitory imbalance, implicating imbalances in the major cortical excitatory neurotransmitter glutamate and the major inhibitory neurotransmitter gamma-aminobutyric acid (GABA), as well as defects in GABAergic interneuron transmission and function [3]. Oxytocin, a key neurotransmitter believed to be involved in social motivation and bonding, has also been implicated in ASD and is undergoing intense study [4]. Finally, abnormalities in monoamine neurotransmitters including dopamine, norepinephrine and serotonin, which are sometimes caused by defects in biosynthesis due to deficiencies in the critical cofactors pyridoxal-5-phosphate [3], tetrahydrobiopterin [5] and/or folate [6], are associated with ASD.

Identifying abnormalities in monoamine neurotransmitters are particularly important as medication used to modulate dopamine, norepinephrine and serotonin are not only well developed but also actively studied in ASD [2]. However, as previously mentioned, ASD, like many neurodevelopmental and psychiatric disorders, is very heterogenous. Thus, much of the research does not always translate well into clinical practice because the research findings may represent a subgroup of patients, while clinical treatment aims to address the abnormality of the specific patient who may or may not be one identified in a specific subgroup. For example, although defects in the serotonin system have been implicated in ASD, simply treating the general ASD population with common medication to improve serotonergic neurotransmission does not appear to be effective and may even cause more harm than good in select individuals [7]. Thus, precision medicine has developed to assist in identifying biomarkers which can further guide a more personalized treatment approach.

The timely and accurate detection of neurotransmitter deficits can lead to impactful treatments for many neurological and neurodevelopmental disorders [8]. Current modalities with the capacity to detect alterations in neurotransmitters, such as positron emissions tomography (PET) and magnetic resonance spectroscopy (MRS), are limited in their spatial resolution and sensitivity to pertinent neurotransmitters, respectively [9]. Analysis of cerebrospinal fluid (CSF) neurotransmitter metabolites via lumbar puncture (LP) is the current standard screening method for suspected neurotransmitter deficits but is not without invasive procedural risks [10]. Hence, pharmacotherapies for suspected neurotransmitter deficits may be prescribed empirically in the absence of confirmatory testing. Therefore, a low-risk and clinically feasible screening biomarker of neurotransmitter deficits is needed to determine who may benefit from confirmatory LP.

The spatial distribution of neurotransmitter-associated brain networks is well established [11]. These networks and their cortical and subcortical spatiotemporal alterations can be detected by resting state functional magnetic resonance imaging (rs-fMRI) [11]. rs-fMRI has clinical applications in the evaluation of epilepsy [12–14] and other disorders [8,15]. Furthermore, rs-fMRI has been validated against other measures including intracranial electroencephalography (iEEG) [12] and task-based functional MRI in children [16]. Due to their widespread and targeted projections to spatially distant brain regions, these neurotransmitter systems can rapidly alter cortical network activity. For example, pharmacologic depletion of the dopaminergic system increases node-specific hemodynamic signal variability and decreases functional connectivity, suggesting that this system is important for the functional integration and stability of specific brain regions within large-scale networks. Thus, dysregulation of one or more of these neurotransmitter systems can produce broader network-level effects which can influence higher cognitive functions [17,18]. In the current case, rs-fMRI-detected network patterns revealed atypical deactivation of deep brain structures involved in monoamine synthesis, which was subsequently confirmed by analysis of CSF neurotransmitter metabolites.

2. Materials and Methods

rs-fMRI were acquired and analyzed as previously reported [12]. Acquisition was from a 3T MRI scanner (Ingenuity; Philips Medical Systems, Best, the Netherlands) with a 32-channel head coil at Phoenix Children's Hospital. Acquisition consisted of two 10 min runs totaling 20 min. Parameters were 2000 millisecond repetition time (TR),

30 millisecond echo time (TE), 80 × 80 matrix size, 80-degree flip angle, 46 slices, 3.4 mm slice thickness with no gap, 3 × 3 mm in-plane resolution, interleaved acquisition, and 600 total volumes. For anatomical reference, a T1-weighted turbo field-echo whole-brain sequence was obtained with TR 9 milliseconds, TW 4 milliseconds, flip angle 80 degrees, slice thickness 0.9 mm, and in-plane resolution 0.9 × 0.9 mm. The Multivariate Exploratory Linear Optimized Decomposition into Independent Components (MELODIC) tool was used for characterization and visualization of individual resting state networks (RSNs), both typical and atypical, as previously reported [12].

3. Results

This case describes a 16-year-old female with a complicated medical history including developmental delay subtype of autism spectrum disorder (ASD), intellectual disability, severe hypotonia, developmental coordination disorder, mixed receptive-expressive language disorder, mitochondrial disease, immune dysfunction with a functional antibody deficiency, and irritable bowel syndrome with alternating diarrhea and constipation. She was born as a product of an in vitro fertilization triplet pregnancy requiring cerclage and terbutaline starting a 17-week gestation. She was born triple B at 34 weeks gestation by cesarean section. Her neonatal course was rather benign except for her prematurity, only requiring oxygen for 24 h and being discharged at day of life 17. She was born with a ventricular septal defect which closed spontaneously. Her triple sisters have a history of speech delay but have performed well academically. There is a history of depression and migraines on the maternal side of the family and thyroid disease and attention deficit hyperactivity disorder on the paternal side of the family.

At 2 years of age, she was diagnosed with global developmental delay and was diagnosed with ASD at 3 $\frac{1}{2}$ years of age. She did not have any clear regression early in life but said several words in grade school but gradually lost expressive language, currently using word-like sounds and augmentative communication device to express herself. She can read some words and understand others and she is able to follow one and two step commands.

At about 12 years of age, anorexia developed with a loss of 25 lbs. In approximately 6 months self-injurious behavior started with knee banging and hitting hips to the point of bruising. Tic-like hand movements and ritualistic checking soon started. Workup for Pediatric Autoimmune Neuropsychiatric Disorder Associated with Streptococcus revelated elevated Streptococcus titers. Treatment with Augmentin, herbs and seven rounds of intravenous immunoglobulin improved the self-injurious behavior and tics-like movements and resulted in normalization of weight, but the severe repetitive behaviors continued. This deterioration was not associated with a clear clinical illness or seizures. She did manifest two brief staring episodes during this time, but an electroencephalograph was negative.

Her symptoms continued to progress. She progressively became more fatigued and stopped engaging in sports she enjoyed such as trampoline and swimming. She became more withdrawn with less family interactions and started to perseverate on YouTube videos. She developed chronic constipation requiring repeated cleanout. She developed period pain, including abdominal pain, headaches and leg cramps. Because of her continued deterioration she was referred to our center for further workup. Metabolic testing demonstrated laboratory values suspicious for mitochondrial disease and buccal enzymology (MITO-SWAB Religen, Plymouth Meeting, PA, USA), confirmed multiple complex deficiencies. Whole exome sequencing (Lineagen, Salt Lake City, UT, USA) demonstrated carrier status for a mutation in EIF3F (c.694T > G, p.Phe232Val) related to autosomal recessive EIF3F-related intellectual disability. She also underwent rs-fMRI due to late regression in cognitive abilities and worsening aberrant behavior.

Her rs-fMRI revealed aberrant and strongly deactivated networks localized to the brainstem and other subcortical structures involved in monoamine synthesis (Figure 1A). Additional aberrant networks extended over multiple bilateral regions including the ventromedial prefrontal cortex (vmPFC), the left fronto-temporo-parietal, and occipital networks with deactivation patterns localized to language and cognition-related regions (Figure 1B). Despite her deficits, she had typical frontoparietal (FP), language, and motor RSNs (Figure 1C). Suspicion for neurotransmitter deficiency was triggered given her history of prior severe late regression without known brain insult in the presence of aberrant deactivation patterns between the brain stem and vmPFC with a similar spatial distribution as the monoaminergic networks. Examples of typical rs-fMRI networks localized to the subcortical and brainstem networks (Figure 2A), vmPFC (Figure 2B), and language networks (Figure 2C) are provided for a case-control.

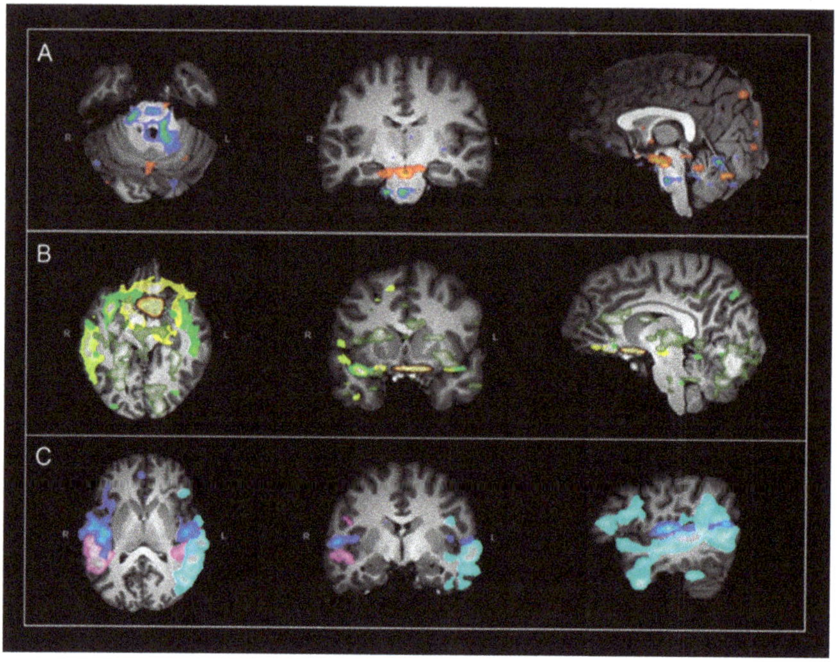

Figure 1. Select rs-fMRI networks in 16-year-old patient with ASD (case study). All images are in radiological orientation. The indicated networks are overlaid on T1-weighted images in axial, coronal, and sagittal views. (**A**) Evidence of atypical and strongly deactivated subcortical and brainstem networks in similar anatomic spatial distribution as the monoaminergic networks; (**B**) Additional atypical networks extending over multiple bilateral regions including vmPFC, FP, temporal, and occipital regions; (**C**) Normal language networks with bilateral presence of typical connectivity between receptive and expressive regions. Row A, blue color denotes BOLD deactivation, red color denotes BOLD activation. Rows B and C, each color denotes a separate network. Abbreviations: rs-fMRI = resting state functional magnetic imaging; vmPFC = ventromedial prefrontal cortex; FP = fronto-parietal.

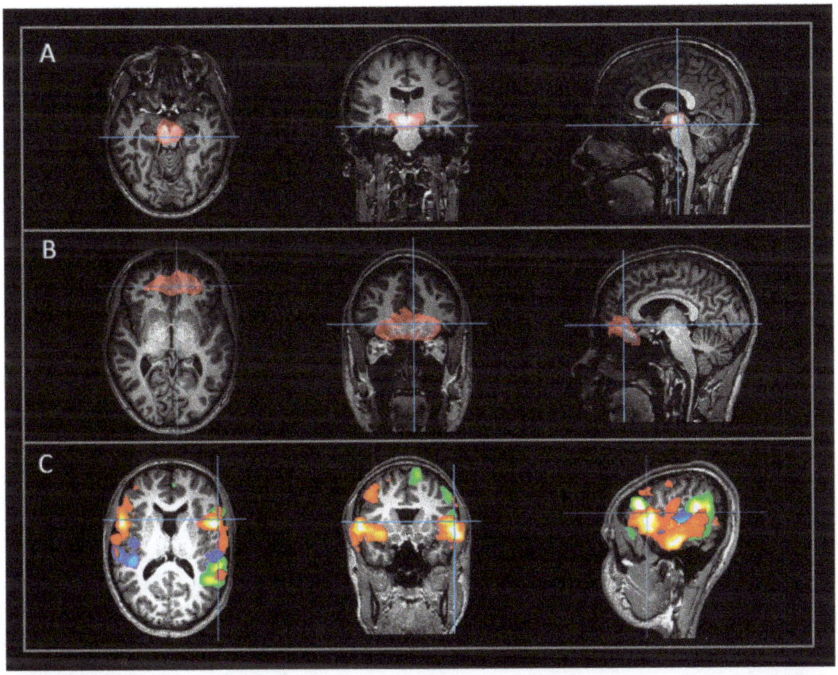

Figure 2. Select rs-fMRI networks in patient (case–control) evaluated for possible seizure focus (not detected, otherwise typical networks). All images are in radiological orientation. The indicated networks are overlaid on T1-weighted images in axial, coronal, and sagittal views. (**A**) Example of typical subcortical and brainstem networks; (**B**) Additional examples of typical networks extending over bilateral vmPFC region; (**C**) Typical language networks. Rows A and B, red color denotes BOLD activation. Row C, each color denotes a separate language network. Abbreviations: rs-fMRI = resting state functional magnetic imaging; vmPFC = ventromedial prefrontal cortex.

LP was performed to measure CSF neurotransmitter metabolites and rule out other neurometabolic disorders. Results (Table 1) were remarkable for decreased concentrations of 5-hydroxyindolacetic acid (58 nmol/L, reference range: 67–140 nmol/L) and homovanillic acid (117 nmol/L, reference range: 145–324 nmol/L), indicating decreased serotonin and dopamine synthesis, respectively. Pyridoxal 5′-phosphate (P5P), a required cofactor in the biosynthesis of serotonin and dopamine, was elevated at 82 nmol/L (reference range: 10–37 nmol/L). 3-O-methyldopa (18 nmol/L), 5-methyltetrahydrofolate (101 nmol/L), neopterin (12 nmol/L), tetrahydrobiopterin (16 nmol/L), and all amino acids were within reference ranges.

Table 1. Results of CSF metabolite analysis. * Abnormal results. WNL: Within normal limits.

Test	Result	Reference Rnge
5-Hydroxyindoleacetic acid	58 *	67–140 nmol/L
Homovanillic acid	117 *	145–324 nmol/L
3-O-Methyldopa	18	<100 nmol/L
5 -Methyltetrahydrofolate	101	40–120 nmol/L
Neopterin	12	8–28 nmol/L
Tetrahydrobiopterin	16	10–30 nmol/L
Pyridoxal 5 Phosphate	82 *	10–37 nmol/L
Amino Acids	WNL	-
Succinyladenosine	1.8	0.74–4.92 umol/L

4. Discussion

We present a rare and unique case of neurotransmitter deficiency initially identified by objective evidence on rs-fMRI. Whole exome sequencing did not reveal a known inborn error of metabolism to account for this finding. Thus, the presumed underlying pathophysiology of her monoamine deficiency is acquired neuronal injury secondary to mitochondrial disease-mediated neurodegeneration. Workup of the origin of the mitochondrial disease is ongoing at this time.

Regional cerebral blood flow is temporally and spatially regulated by a process known as neurovascular coupling which involves the coordinated action of neurons and vascular cells to meet the high metabolic demand of the brain [19,20]. A decrease in monoamine neurotransmitters may cause reduced neurotransmission, resulting in deactivated network activity and a corresponding reduction in spatial oxygen utilization that can be observed on rs-fMRI as atypical blood-oxygen-level-dependent (BOLD) signals. Simultaneous acquisition of PET and rs-fMRI highlights the association between hemodynamic changes and neurotransmitter receptor density in relation to functional network organization, supporting the contribution of neurotransmitter systems to BOLD signal alterations [21,22].

While neurotransmitter systems and their association with large-scale brain networks are understood, and rs-fMRI has shown sensitivity to locations in the basilar brain regions [23,24], future work establishing the sensitivity and specificity of rs-fMRI biomarkers of neurotransmitter dysfunction is needed. Neurovascular coupling may differ between neurotransmitter systems due to intrinsic differences in mechanisms of neurotransmitter release, uptake, or transport, as well as release of small vasoactive molecules during these processes, like that reported between glutamate and dopamine [22]. Additionally, the dopaminergic modulation of prefrontal cortex NMDA receptor activity appears to be associated with the NMDA receptor co-agonist D-serine [25], suggesting a dynamic relationship between multiple neurotransmitter systems and other molecules that could further influence neurovascular coupling. The case herein likely has a relatively extreme clinical phenotype of severe regression, allowing for contextual interpretation of the atypical monoamine network patterns to inform the decision for invasive CSF confirmation with LP.

In addition to atypical subcortical and brainstem network patterns, this patient also had relatively deactivated language and cognition-related networks, commensurate with severe developmental regression. In children with ASD, there is evidence of atypical default mode network (DMN) connectivity profiles consisting of both hyper- and hypoconnectivity between specific nodes of the DMN as well as cross-network connectivity between the DMN and other large-scale brain networks, suggesting impaired functional intra- and inter-network integration in children with ASD [26]. Decreased or otherwise dysregulated neurotransmission secondary to neurotransmitter dysfunction may influence the existing network pathology resulting in such widespread network effect seen in the present case, as the monoaminergic deep brain structures are functionally integrated with broader networks such as the DMN [11]. Supportively, other monoamine disorders, such as chronic major depressive disorder (MDD), also demonstrate disease chronicity-associated BOLD signal reductions within the broader DMN [27], supporting the contribution of dysregulated neurotransmitter systems to large-scale networks over time. Thus, there may be a certain threshold of sustained neurotransmitter dysfunction that yields the relatively extreme network pattern we see in this case.

It is also possible that rs-fMRI may be useful as a biomarker of therapeutic effect, like that found in MDD with pharmacotherapy, wherein rs-fMRI showed an increase in functional connectivity within the DMN for patients with remitted MDD [27]. In patients with treatment-naïve MDD, rs-fMRI has been used to define biomarkers of depression subtypes and the differential response to various treatment modalities [28], which could greatly reduce the time and resources needed to identify the most appropriate and efficacious course of treatment. Additionally, characterization of DMN connectivity between specific nodes may correspond to clinical phenotype, wherein posterior cingulate cortex hyper-connectivity predicted social communication deficits in children with ASD [26], ultimately allowing for more targeted and personalized therapeutic interventions. Thus, rs-fMRI is being increasingly used in many different translational research initiatives, each with important clinical applications.

5. Conclusions

Numerous neurochemical alterations have been reported in individuals with ASD. Neurotransmitter systems play a crucial role in the overall functional relationship of large-scale networks and ostensibly impact the integration and modulation of these networks during development and beyond. rs-fMRI can be used to detect both typical and atypical RSNs, which can provide invaluable insight into the clinical implications of the neurochemical alterations associated with ASD. With continued research, rs-fMRI may soon emerge as a powerful tool in the diagnosis and management of various encephalopathies by characterizing biomarkers of neurotransmitter-driven network pathology, thus aiding in earlier detection of disease, and permitting the monitoring of response to treatment.

6. Patents

Nothing to report.

Author Contributions: Conceptualization, P.J.M., A.R.P., B.L.S., S.N.W., R.B., V.L.B. and R.E.F.; methodology, V.L.B.; formal analysis, B.L.S. and V.L.B.; data curation, P.J.M., A.R.P., B.L.S., V.L.B. and R.E.F. writing—original draft preparation, P.J.M., A.R.P., B.L.S., V.L.B. and R.E.F.; writing—review and editing, A.J., P.J.M., A.R.P., B.L.S., S.N.W., R.E.F. and V.L.B.; visualization, A.J., S.N.W., P.J.M., A.R.P., B.L.S., R.E.F. and V.L.B. All authors have read and agreed to the published version of the manuscript.

Funding: This research received no external funding.

Institutional Review Board Statement: The study was conducted according to the guidelines of the Declaration of Helsinki and approved by the Institutional Review Board of Phoenix Children's Hospital, Phoenix, AZ, USA.

Informed Consent Statement: Informed consent was obtained from the parents of all participants involved in the study.

Data Availability Statement: Data are available upon request.

Acknowledgments: We would like to thank the patients and families who volunteered their time to be part of our research program.

Conflicts of Interest: The authors declare no conflict of interest.

References

1. Rossignol, D.A.; Frye, R.E. A review of research trends in physiological abnormalities in autism spectrum disorders: Immune dysregulation, inflammation, oxidative stress, mitochondrial dysfunction and environmental toxicant exposures. *Mol. Psychiatry* **2012**, *17*, 389–401. [CrossRef] [PubMed]
2. Frye, R.E.; Rossignol, D.A. Identification and Treatment of Pathophysiological Comorbidities of Autism Spectrum Disorder to Achieve Optimal Outcomes. *Clin. Med. Insights Pediatr.* **2016**, *10*, 43–56. [CrossRef] [PubMed]
3. Frye, R.E.; Casanova, M.F.; Fatemi, S.H.; Folsom, T.D.; Reutiman, T.J.; Brown, G.L.; Edelson, S.M.; Slattery, J.C.; Adams, J.B. Neuropathological Mechanisms of Seizures in Autism Spectrum Disorder. *Front. Neurosci.* **2016**, *10*, 192. [CrossRef] [PubMed]
4. Frye, R.E. Social Skills Deficits in Autism Spectrum Disorder: Potential Biological Origins and Progress in Developing Therapeutic Agents. *CNS Drugs* **2018**, *32*, 713–734. [CrossRef]
5. Frye, R.E.; Huffman, L.C.; Elliott, G.R. Tetrahydrobiopterin as a novel therapeutic intervention for autism. *Neurotherapeutics* **2010**, *7*, 241–249. [CrossRef]
6. Frye, R.E.; Slattery, J.C.; Quadros, E.V. Folate metabolism abnormalities in autism: Potential biomarkers. *Biomark. Med.* **2017**, *11*, 687–699. [CrossRef]
7. Williams, K.; Brignell, A.; Randall, M.; Silove, N.; Hazell, P. Selective serotonin reuptake inhibitors (SSRIs) for autism spectrum disorders (ASD). *Cochrane Database Syst. Rev.* **2013**. [CrossRef]
8. Brennenstuhl, H.; Jung-Klawitter, S.; Assmann, B.; Opladen, T. Inherited Disorders of Neurotransmitters: Classification and Practical Approaches for Diagnosis and Treatment. *Neuropediatrics* **2019**, *50*, 2–14. [CrossRef]

9. Jauhar, S.; McCutcheon, R.; Borgan, F.; Veronese, M.; Nour, M.; Pepper, F.; Rogdaki, M.; Stone, J.; Egerton, A.; Turkheimer, F.; et al. The relationship between cortical glutamate and striatal dopamine in first-episode psychosis: A cross-sectional multimodal PET and magnetic resonance spectroscopy imaging study. *Lancet Psychiatry* **2018**, *5*, 816–823. [CrossRef]
10. Wright, B.L.; Lai, J.T.; Sinclair, A.J. Cerebrospinal fluid and lumbar puncture: A practical review. *J. Neurol.* **2012**, *259*, 1530–1545. [CrossRef] [PubMed]
11. Conio, B.; Martino, M.; Magioncalda, P.; Escelsior, A.; Inglese, M.; Amore, M.; Northoff, G. Opposite effects of dopamine and serotonin on resting-state networks: Review and implications for psychiatric disorders. *Mol. Psychiatry* **2020**, *25*, 82–93. [CrossRef]
12. Boerwinkle, V.L.; Mohanty, D.; Foldes, S.T.; Guffey, D.; Minard, C.G.; Vedantam, A.; Raskin, J.S.; Lam, S.; Bond, M.; Mirea, L.; et al. Correlating Resting-State Functional Magnetic Resonance Imaging Connectivity by Independent Component Analysis-Based Epileptogenic Zones with Intracranial Electroencephalogram Localized Seizure Onset Zones and Surgical Outcomes in Prospective Pediatric Intractable Epilepsy Study. *Brain Connect.* **2017**, *7*, 424–442. [CrossRef]
13. Boerwinkle, V.L.; Cediel, E.G.; Mirea, L.; Williams, K.; Kerrigan, J.F.; Lam, S.; Raskin, J.S.; Desai, V.R.; Wilfong, A.A.; Adelson, P.D.; et al. Network Targeted Approach and Postoperative Resting State Functional MRI are Associated with Seizure Outcome. *Ann. Neurol.* **2019**, *86*, 344–356. [CrossRef]
14. Boerwinkle, V.L.; Mirea, L.; Gaillard, W.D.; Sussman, B.L.; Larocque, D.; Bonnell, A.; Ronecker, J.S.; Troester, M.M.; Kerrigan, J.F.; Foldes, S.T.; et al. Resting-state functional MRI connectivity impact on epilepsy surgery plan and surgical candidacy: Prospective clinical work. *J. Neurosurg. Pediatr.* **2020**, *25*, 574–581. [CrossRef]
15. Boerwinkle, V.L.; Torrisi, S.J.; Foldes, S.T.; Marku, I.; Ranjan, M.; Wilfong, A.A.; Adelson, P.D. Resting-state fMRI in disorders of consciousness to facilitate early therapeutic intervention. *Neurol. Clin. Pract.* **2019**, *9*, e33–e35. [CrossRef]
16. Desai, V.R.; Vedantam, A.; Lam, S.K.; Mirea, L.; Foldes, S.T.; Curry, D.J.; Adelson, P.D.; Wilfong, A.A.; Boerwinkle, V.L. Language lateralization with resting-state and task-based functional MRI in pediatric epilepsy. *J. Neurosurg. Pediatr.* **2018**, *23*, 171–177. [CrossRef]
17. Hermans, E.J.; van Marle, H.J.; Ossewaarde, L.; Henckens, M.J.; Qin, S.; van Kesteren, M.T.; Schoots, V.C.; Cousijn, H.; Rijpkema, M.; Oostenveld, R.; et al. Stress-related noradrenergic activity prompts large-scale neural network reconfiguration. *Science* **2011**, *334*, 1151–1153. [CrossRef]
18. Shafiei, G.; Zeighami, Y.; Clark, C.A.; Coull, J.T.; Nagano-Saito, A.; Leyton, M.; Dagher, A.; Misic, B. Dopamine Signaling Modulates the Stability and Integration of Intrinsic Brain Networks. *Cereb. Cortex* **2019**, *29*, 397–409. [CrossRef] [PubMed]
19. Iadecola, C. The Neurovascular Unit Coming of Age: A Journey through Neurovascular Coupling in Health and Disease. *Neuron* **2017**, *96*, 17–42. [CrossRef]
20. Caffrey, T.M.; Button, E.B.; Robert, J. Toward three dimensional in vitro models to study neurovascular unit functions in health and disease. *Neural Regen. Res.* **2021**, *16*, 2132–2140. [CrossRef]
21. Ceccarini, J.; Liu, H.; Van Laere, K.; Morris, E.D.; Sander, C.Y. Methods for Quantifying Neurotransmitter Dynamics in the Living Brain With PET Imaging. *Front. Physiol.* **2020**, *11*, 792. [CrossRef] [PubMed]
22. Bruinsma, T.J.; Sarma, V.V.; Oh, Y.; Jang, D.P.; Chang, S.Y.; Worrell, G.A.; Lowe, V.J.; Jo, H.J.; Min, H.K. The Relationship between Dopamine Neurotransmitter Dynamics and the Blood-Oxygen-Level-Dependent (BOLD) Signal: A Review of Pharmacological Functional Magnetic Resonance Imaging. *Front. Neurosci.* **2018**, *12*, 238. [CrossRef] [PubMed]
23. Boerwinkle, V.L.; Foldes, S.T.; Torrisi, S.J.; Temkit, H.; Gaillard, W.D.; Kerrigan, J.F.; Desai, V.R.; Raskin, J.S.; Vedantam, A.; Jarrar, R.; et al. Subcentimeter epilepsy surgery targets by resting state functional magnetic resonance imaging can improve outcomes in hypothalamic hamartoma. *Epilepsia* **2018**, *59*, 2284–2295. [CrossRef]
24. Boerwinkle, V.L.; Wilfong, A.A.; Curry, D.J. Resting-state functional connectivity by independent component analysis-based markers corresponds to areas of initial seizure propagation established by prior modalities from the hypothalamus. *Brain Connect.* **2016**, *6*, 642–651. [CrossRef] [PubMed]
25. Dallérac, G.; Li, X.; Lecouflet, P.; Morisot, N.; Sacchi, S.; Asselot, R.; Pham, T.H.; Potier, B.; Watson, D.J.G.; Schmidt, S.; et al. Dopaminergic neuromodulation of prefrontal cortex activity requires the NMDA receptor coagonist d-serine. *Proc. Natl. Acad. Sci. USA* **2021**, *118*, e2023750118. [CrossRef] [PubMed]
26. Padmanabhan, A.; Lynch, C.J.; Schaer, M.; Menon, V. The Default Mode Network in Autism. *Biol. Psychiatry Cogn. Neurosci. Neuroimaging* **2017**, *2*, 476–486. [CrossRef] [PubMed]
27. Zhuo, C.; Li, G.; Lin, X.; Jiang, D.; Xu, Y.; Tian, H.; Wang, W.; Song, X. The rise and fall of MRI studies in major depressive disorder. *Transl. Psychiatry* **2019**, *9*, 335. [CrossRef] [PubMed]
28. Dunlop, B.W.; Rajendra, J.K.; Craighead, W.E.; Kelley, M.E.; McGrath, C.L.; Choi, K.S.; Kinkead, B.; Nemeroff, C.B.; Mayberg, H.S. Functional Connectivity of the Subcallosal Cingulate Cortex And Differential Outcomes to Treatment With Cognitive-Behavioral Therapy or Antidepressant Medication for Major Depressive Disorder. *Am. J. Psychiatry* **2017**, *174*, 533–545. [CrossRef]

Journal of
Personalized Medicine

MDPI

Article

Multivariate Analysis of Fecal Metabolites from Children with Autism Spectrum Disorder and Gastrointestinal Symptoms before and after Microbiota Transfer Therapy

Fatir Qureshi [1,2], James Adams [3], Kathryn Hanagan [4], Dae-Wook Kang [5,†], Rosa Krajmalnik-Brown [5,6,7] and Juergen Hahn [1,2,8,*]

1 Biomedical Engineering, Rensselaer Polytechnic Institute, Troy, NY 12180, USA; quresf2@rpi.edu
2 Center for Biotechnology and Interdisciplinary Studies, Rensselaer Polytechnic Institute, Troy, NY 12180, USA
3 School for Engineering of Matter, Transport, and Energy, Arizona State University, Tempe, AZ 85287, USA; Jim.Adams@asu.edu
4 Department of Computer Science, Purdue University, West Lafayette, IN 47907, USA; khanagan@purdue.edu
5 Biodesign Swette Center for Environmental Biotechnology, Arizona State University, Tempe, AZ 85287, USA; DaeWook.Kang@utoledo.edu (D.-W.K.); Dr.Rosy@asu.edu (R.K.-B.)
6 Biodesign Center for Health through Microbiome, Arizona State University, Tempe, AZ 85287, USA
7 School of Sustainable Engineering and the Built Environment, Arizona State University, Tempe, AZ 85281, USA
8 Department of Chemical and Biological Engineering, Rensselaer Polytechnic Institute, Troy, NY 12180, USA
* Correspondence: hahnj@rpi.edu; Tel.: +1-(518)-276-2138; Fax: +1-(518)-276-3035
† Current address: Department of Civil and Environmental Engineering, The University of Toledo, Toledo, OH 43606, USA.

Received: 18 August 2020; Accepted: 25 September 2020; Published: 2 October 2020

Abstract: Fecal microbiota transplant (FMT) holds significant promise for patients with Autism Spectrum Disorder (ASD) and gastrointestinal (GI) symptoms. Prior work has demonstrated that plasma metabolite profiles of children with ASD become more similar to those of their typically developing (TD) peers following this treatment. This work measures the concentration of 669 biochemical compounds in feces of a cohort of 18 ASD and 20 TD children using ultrahigh performance liquid chromatography-tandem mass spectroscopy. Subsequent measurements were taken from the ASD cohort over the course of 10-week Microbiota Transfer Therapy (MTT) and 8 weeks after completion of this treatment. Univariate and multivariate statistical analysis techniques were used to characterize differences in metabolites before, during, and after treatment. Using Fisher Discriminant Analysis (FDA), it was possible to attain multivariate metabolite models capable of achieving a sensitivity of 94% and a specificity of 95% after cross-validation. Observations made following MTT indicate that the fecal metabolite profiles become more like those of the TD cohort. There was an 82–88% decrease in the median difference of the ASD and TD group for the panel metabolites, and among the top fifty most discriminating individual metabolites, 96% report more comparable values following treatment. Thus, these findings are similar, although less pronounced, as those determined using plasma metabolites.

Keywords: fecal metabolites; ASD; microbiome; gastrointestinal symptoms; Fisher Discriminant Analysis

1. Introduction

Autism spectrum disorder (ASD) encompasses a large group of early onset neurological conditions that result in impairments in social behavior and communication, which are estimated to affect 1 in 54 children under the age of eight in the United States [1]. Despite this high rate of occurrence, the understanding of the pathophysiology of ASD is still poor, and it is believed that at least in some cases ASD begins prenatally as a result of complex interactions between environmental and genetic factors [2,3]. Although diagnosis of this disorder is only made through behavioral evaluations, many systems of the body are strongly affected by this condition. A diverse range of physiological mechanisms have been observed to be perturbed in ASD including the immune, endocrine, and gastrointestinal (GI) systems [4,5]. Notably, the prevalence of GI symptoms co-occurring with ASD (~46%) lends significant credence to investigating the relationship of ASD to the GI system [6].

In recent years, there have been growing efforts to study the effect of the microbiome on the Gut-Brain Axis in the context of ASD etiology. Some studies have shown that the gut microbiome of individuals with GI issues varies significantly from those without such complications [7–9]. However, the microbiota of individuals with ASD without the presence of GI issues have also consistently been found to be distinct from their typically developing (TD) peers [10,11]. Certain genera such as Prevotella and Coprococcus have been shown to be significantly less prevalent in the gut of children with ASD [12,13]. Furthermore, it has been proposed that the microbiota differences in children with ASD give rise to metabolomic differences that can be quantitatively evaluated to distinguish them from their TD peers [14,15].

Some previous work involving fecal metabolites identified isopropanol, p-cresol, acetyl-carnitine, free carnitine and neurotransmitters-gamma-Aminobutyrate (GABA) as metabolites that have significantly different concentrations between the ASD and TD cohorts [14,16,17]. There have also been mixed results regarding the fecal concentrations of short chain fatty acids. While some studies show that the fecal concentration of acetic, propionic and butyric acids were higher in children with ASD [18–20], other investigations found that the concentration of these short chain fatty acids were lower or comparable to their TD peers [21–23].

As the role of the microbiome in ASD is being in more detail, the question is raised as to whether using fecal microbiota transplant (FMT) can mitigate the severity of GI and other symptoms of ASD. In one notable study, offspring of germ-free mice subject to microbiome transfer from individuals with ASD exhibited more ASD-like behaviors and produced different metabolome profiles when compared to offspring of germ-free mice subject to microbiome transfer from TD controls [24]. The use of FMT has shown considerable potential in its capability to alleviate not only symptoms associated with GI complications, but also in some cases to reduce the severity of certain behavioral symptoms in children with ASD. For example, Kang et al. demonstrated in an open-label study that through a modified FMT (called, Microbiota Transfer Therapy (MTT)), there was an 80% reduction in GI symptoms and a 24% initial reduction in core ASD symptoms, with greater improvement in ASD symptoms at a two-year follow-up [25,26]. Probiotic intervention has also shown potential to have a positive influence on ameliorating both behavioral and GI symptoms in individuals with ASD [27,28].

Past work in analyzing metabolites prior and subsequent to MTT therapy have also yielded promising results. Children with ASD who underwent MTT presented changes in their plasma metabolite profiles to resemble more closely those of their typically developing peers [29,30]. The work presented in this paper builds on the analysis of this same study [25], but focuses on fecal metabolites instead of plasma metabolites. Univariate assessment of the fecal metabolites examined in this study have previously shown limited capability for differentiating between ASD and TD cohorts when corrected for multiple hypotheses [30]. Thus, here we explored the use of multivariate techniques to detect underlying relationships that may have been otherwise missed.

2. Materials and Methods

2.1. Study Design

The purpose of this study was to examine the differences in gut metabolites between children with ASD and GI problems vs. typically developing children without GI problems, and determine the effects of gut microbiota transfer therapy on the fecal metabolites of the ASD group. The study involved 38 children, aged 7–16 years, 18 of these professionally diagnosed with ASD by a healthcare provider (verified with the Autism Diagnostic Interview-Revised) and 20 determined to be typically developing. The participants with ASD were required to have moderate to severe GI problems, and the range of GI issues included constipation, diarrhea, and alternating diarrhea/constipation. GI symptoms were assessed biweekly with the Gastrointestinal Severity Rating Scale (GSRS) and daily with a Daily Stool Record using the Bristol Stool Form scale [25]. The study consisted of 2 weeks of antibiotic therapy, 1 day of bowel cleans, and a high major initial dose and 7–8 weeks of lower maintenance doses of FMT treatment followed by evaluation at 8 weeks post treatment. The TD group did not undergo MTT, but instead was used as a comparison group whose measurements were taken at the same time as the ASD group before treatment. The MTT experimental protocol and details of the study population are outlined in Kang et al. [25].

The pre-treatment protocol consisted of two weeks of oral vancomycin, which is a broad spectrum non-absorbable antibiotic. This treatment was intended to reduce pathogenic bacteria and prime the GI system for MTT. The dose of vancomycin administered was individualized to the weight of each participant at 40 mg/kg, with a maximum dose of 2 g [25]. Participants were then subjected to one day of fasting and a bowel cleanser (MoviPrep) in order to remove the vancomycin and further reduce levels of intestinal bacteria. Standardized Human Gut Microbiota (SHGM) consisted of a full spectrum of highly purified microbiota from healthy, carefully screened donors. The ASD cohort was split into two groups, each one following a different initial high dose (2.5×10^{12} cells/day) SHGM treatment. One MTT treatment consisted of a single dose administered rectally ($n = 6$) while the other involved doses administered orally on two days ($n = 12$). Both techniques were followed by a lower concentration SHGM maintenance dosage (around 2.5×10^9 cells) given orally, with treatment ending 8 weeks after the initial high dose [25]. However, the protocol differed slightly for both groups of ASD children as those that received SHGM rectally waited for one week prior to beginning low dose SHGM.

2.2. Metabolite Measurements

Once the study had concluded, aliquots of the fecal samples were shipped overnight on dry ice to Metabolon (Durham, NC, USA). Both the control and autism samples were blinded and randomized prior to being shipped. Metabolon utilized ultrahigh performance liquid chromatography-tandem mass spectroscopy (UHPLC-MS/MS) instruments for obtaining metabolomic information on 669 metabolites. A detailed overview regarding this protocol can be found in Long et al. [31]. By using this technique, it is possible to determine a signal intensity corresponding to a metabolite's presence in a sample. Subsequently, the signal intensity is used to derive the relative abundance of each metabolite. For this objective, peak area integration using the area under the curve was utilized. In the case of missing values, imputation was performed by taking the lowest value of each compound measurement divided by the square root of 2.

Fecal samples were taken at four time points from the participants with ASD (Figure 1). Parents were instructed to freeze these sample immediately after collection for up to 3 days, and the samples were then transported to Arizona State University on dry ice where they were stored in a −80 °C freezer. Initial fecal samples were collected from all participants at Week 0. Samples were also taken from ASD participants at the Week 3 mark from the beginning of the treatment (after about five days of microbiota transplant) and at the end of MTT treatment (Week 10). The ASD group was sampled again 8 weeks after administration of SHGM ceased (Week 18). In total, 18 ASD participants collected samples at all time points aside from Week 3, where only 17 samples were collected. The TD group received no treatment and 20 were sampled at the beginning (Week 0).

2.3. Statistical Analysis

The data collected for each of the metabolites underwent various forms of statistical analysis to assess differences between the ASD + GI and TD cohort. By comparing the differences observed for metabolites before and after MTT, it might be possible to gain some understanding of the role that this therapy could play in altering metabolic processes. Both univariate and multivariate techniques were used in this regard, and the implementation of the analysis routines was done in MATLAB.

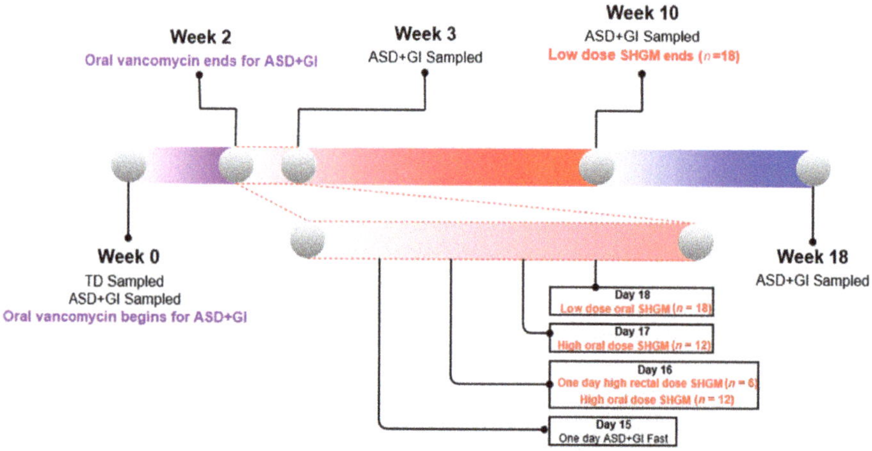

Figure 1. Timeline for the experimental protocol, which can be divided into three main phases. From Week 0 to Week 3, the Autism Spectrum Disorder (ASD) cohort is primed for Microbiota Transfer Therapy (MTT). From Week 3 to Week 10 the ASD cohort receives low dose fecal microbiota (FM) or is prepared for low dose FM, and finally from Week 10 to Week 18 no treatment is given to the individuals. A closeup is provided of Week 2–3 as this is when Standardized Human Gut Microbiota (SHGM) is initialized.

2.3.1. Preprocessing

In order to ensure continuous distribution of values across all participants, metabolites with too many values below the detection limit at their initial stool sample (Week 0) were removed. The detection limit for a metabolite was determined to be the minimum value recorded for that metabolite. If less than 40% of all measurements were above the detection limit, the metabolite was removed from subsequent analysis. This step accounted for the possibility that a measurement could be almost entirely below the detection limit in one cohort, while simultaneously being above the limit in the other cohort. The remaining metabolites were then normalized such that for each metabolite the median value was 1.0 in the Week 0 TD cohort.

2.3.2. Univariate Analysis

Univariate analysis identifies metabolites that are differentially expressed between the ASD and TD cohorts. Using this information, it is possible to examine common correlations and relationships across different measurement quantities. In turn, this has the potential to identify underlying mechanisms of ASD etiology as well as provide guidance for the development of a multivariate model that can more accurately distinguish between both groups. As there are 669 metabolites under investigation, there is significant concern related to overfitting of statistical models if many or all these measurements are used to develop a multivariate model. By reducing the number of measurements to a smaller subset, it is possible to alleviate some of the concerns related to overfitting.

Metabolites were individually analyzed for their ability to classify between the ASD and TD cohorts at their Week 0 measurements. The area under the receiver operator curve (AUROC) served as an assessment of the potential of a metabolite to distinguish between ASD and TD groups. This metric is defined as the false positive rate against the false negative rate at different ASD/TD classification thresholds. An AUROC of 1.0 indicates the capacity for perfect separation, while an AUROC of 0.5

indicates that there is no ability to distinguish between the groups. Metabolites with an AUROC value above 0.6 were selected as candidates for use in multivariate analysis in this work.

Univariate analysis techniques evaluated whether significant changes had occurred among the metabolites between the beginning and end of the study for the ASD cohort. For this purpose, the metabolite measurements at Week 0 and Week 18 were compared using a parametric or non-parametric test, depending upon their distribution. An Anderson-Darling test for normality was used at both time points to determine the distribution of each set of measurements. Subsequently, either a Wilcoxon signed-rank test or a paired t-test was performed on the ASD group, comparing measurements from Week 0 to Week 18. A relatively normal distribution employs the parametric paired t-test; otherwise, the non-parametric Wilcoxon signed-rank test is used. The resulting p-value indicates how significantly the concentration of the metabolite changed for the cohort over the course of the study.

As there were a considerable number of quantities measured per study participant, it was imperative that multiple hypothesis correction tests were utilized. Subsequently, a false discovery rate (FDR) for each individual metabolite was computed using leave-n-out (n = 1, 2, 3) cross validation (see Table A1). Leave-n-out is an iterative process and involves removing n individual data points from the total dataset and rerunning the univariate analysis on this subset. This procedure is repeated so that all possible combinations with n removed individuals are assessed. The FDR is calculated as the proportion of univariate results that were not deemed significant.

2.3.3. Multivariate Analysis

Fisher discriminant analysis (FDA), metabolites that had been identified as having an AUROC value above 0.6 were used to develop a multivariate model for distinguishing between the ASD and TD cohorts. FDA is a dimensionality reduction technique that seeks to separate classes of data by determining a projection where such separation is maximized [32]. This is achieved by maximizing the ratio between the between-class variability S_B and the within-class variability S_W for a weight vector $\boldsymbol{W}$.

$$J(W) = \frac{W^T S_B W}{W^T\, S_W\, W}$$

In the case of K classes with n number of samples and m measurements, S_B is defined as follows, where $\overline{x}$ denotes the global mean, $\overline{x}_k$ denotes the local class mean, and n_k is the number of samples within class k:

$$S_B = \sum_{k=1}^{K} n_k(\overline{x}_k - \overline{x})(\overline{x}_k - \overline{x})^T$$

In contrast, the within-class covariance matrix S_W is defined as the following, where x_i corresponds to an individual sample:

$$S_W = \sum_{k=1}^{K} n_k \sum_{i \in k} (\overline{x}_i - \overline{x}_k)(\overline{x}_i - \overline{x}_k)^T$$

Thus, FDA simultaneously maximizes the scatter between classes and minimizes the scatter within each class to find k-1 vectors that maximize the objective function. Subsequently, the eigenvector corresponding to the k-1 largest eigenvalue of $S_B S_W$ corresponds to the optimum weight vector.

For this dataset, the objective of FDA is to separate the ASD and TD cohorts with a combination of metabolites. The initial stool samples (Week 0) were used to develop these models, so that the model classifies individuals before any treatment.

The previously mentioned preprocessing and univariate analysis steps were performed to reduce the set of metabolites considered for FDA. An FDA model could potentially be created with all 669 metabolites, but this model would likely overfit the data. To account for this, only metabolites that passed the preprocessing step and achieved a univariate AUROC of over 0.6 remained in consideration. This resulted in 165 metabolites under further investigation.

An exhaustive search was performed through all possible combinations of 2, 3, or 4 metabolites of the reduced set of 165 metabolites to determine the models which best separate the ASD and TD groups at Week 0. The AUROC was used here as well, measuring how well the multivariate models classify the two groups. Using kernel density estimation, the probability density function of each model was computed. Iterating through all combinations, the models were assessed, and the combination of metabolites was determined for each number of variables. For each number of metabolites, the 1000 models that had achieved the highest possible AUROC were recorded. To derive the five-metabolite models, all 1000 four metabolite models that had achieved the highest AUROC were augmented with each of the remaining 161 metabolites that had an AUROC greater than 0.6. The top 1000 five metabolite models that had the highest AUROC were then subjected to leave-one-out cross validation.

2.4. Cross-Validation

Leave-one-out cross-validation was performed on the optimal FDA models to evaluate robustness and statistical independence. Cross-validation ensures that, rather than merely fitting a model to presented data, the model obtained is also capable of classifying new data. Although cross-validation generally has a lower accuracy than what is computed just by fitting a model to data, the cross-validation accuracy will better reflect generalizability to new data sets, i.e., data not used for developing a classifier. Leave-one-out cross-validation proceeds iteratively, as a single individual's data is removed from the total dataset, then an FDA model is computed with measurements from the remaining individuals [33]. The measurements from the removed individual are now used as a test case to determine if the model prediction regarding classification is correct. This process is repeated for measurements from each of the individuals in the dataset: their data are removed, a model is developed with the remaining data, then they are classified with this model, until the data for each individual has been removed once. A confusion matrix is computed which includes the true positive rate (TPR), or sensitivity, and the true negative rate (TNR), or specificity. Additionally, for each model, the Type II (false negative) error β was modulated between 0.01, 0.05, 0.1, and 0.2 during cross-validation. The Type II error determined the threshold value for separating the two groups. By alternating the values of β, it was possible to evaluate the cross-validated performances along different positions of the ASD distribution. Lowering β meant raising the Type I error while lowering the Type II error and the converse also holds true. Thus, each of the four models (2, 3, 4, or 5 metabolites) had cross-validation performed four times, with corresponding computation of TPRs and TNRs.

2.5. Model Evaluation

The models obtained after cross validating at different thresholds for data collected at Week 0 were used to make predictions about the ASD group at the other MTT time points. Specifically, measurements at Week 3, Week 10 and Week 18 were used to monitor the change in classification performance over the course of the MTT protocol. Data from these time points were rescaled with respect to the TD Week 0 median and standard deviation. The probability density functions were compared between the time points, and the discriminate scores for each model as well as of their constituent metabolites were determined. Changes resulting from MTT were quantified using the Type II error, with respect to the threshold associated with the probability density function (PDF) of the ASD + GI cohort's discriminant scores at each time point. Thus, both univariate assessments were performed as well as the total assessment of the multivariate models' discriminant score. Additionally, correlation analysis between significant metabolite pairs was performed to determine possible underlying relationships.

3. Results

3.1. Univariate Analysis

In total, there were 669 fecal metabolites that were measured in the study. Through the preprocessing step, 86 metabolites were determined not to have the prerequisite number of observations above the detection limit for further analysis. In order to classify ASD and TD cohorts at their Week 0 measurements, the area under the AUROC was used as an assessment of the potential of a metabolite to distinguish between ASD and TD groups. The remaining 583 metabolites were ranked according to their univariate AUROC, and 165 metabolites with an AUROC of at least 0.6 were identified. No single metabolite perfectly separated the cohorts (which would correspond to an AUROC = 1.0), as the metabolite with the highest AUROC, carnitine, achieved a value of 0.77 (Table 1).

Using the 165 metabolites with an AUROC greater than 0.6, additional univariate testing was performed to assess the degree to which measurements shifted following MTT. ASD metabolite samples measured at Week 0 were compared to their values following MTT at Week 18 using either a paired t-test or a Wilcoxon signed-rank test depending upon the distribution determined for the data via the Anderson-Darling normality test. It was found that 10.9% of the metabolites significantly changed ($p < 0.05$) following the MTT therapy when comparing the ASD group before and after treatment (see Table A1). The metabolites that had a threshold AUROC value of 0.6 were subsequently used for model discovery for the 2-, 3-, 4- and 5- metabolite models.

3.2. FDA Models

The FDA models with the greatest AUROC values for each number of constituent metabolites are listed in Table 2. The probability density function (PDF) of discriminant scores for the 2-, 3-, 4-, and 5-metabolite models that achieved the highest accuracy following cross validation are shown in Figure 2. There were two distinct models that were identified, using five separate metabolites, as having achieved the same accuracy after cross-validation. With the exception of one metabolite which differed between them (Adenosine and Indole), the constituents of these panels are identical. These two metabolite models are both shown in Table 2 and will be referred to as OFM-A and OFM-I, optimized fecal model-adenosine and optimized fecal model-indole, respectively (OFM-I/A). For all optimized metabolite panels, the TPR and TNR values for each are presented when the β value was modulated. The 5-metabolite models had higher AUROCs than the 2-, 3-, and 4-metabolite models, so they are the focus of the following analysis, due to their higher accuracy (0.95 specificity and 0.94 sensitivity). Modulating β revealed that the optimal cut-offs between the ASD and TD distributions for the OFM-I and OFM-A models was $\beta = 0.05$ for both the OFM-A and OFM-I.

For the 1000 best models with five metabolites, the AUROC ranged from 0.97 to 1.00 which are high values. The reason for using the 1000 best models is that there are not only one or two best models as judged by AUROC alone. Each of these models was subjected to cross validation, with OFM-I/A being derived from those that achieved the highest accuracy. The metabolites ultimately utilized for the development of a five-component model were all found to be in the top quartile of prevalence in the 1000 top models (Figure 3). Notably, among the top fecal metabolite models, adenosine and hydroxyproline appeared in 36.3% and 62.4% of models, respectively. Only three metabolites were present in more than 25% of the top 1000 models that were not among those included in the OFM-I/A panels. These metabolites were Adenine, 2-aminobutyrate and 1,7-dimethylurate (corresponding to the 5th, 57th, and 86th highest AUROC rank, respectively).

Table 1. The top 50 fecal metabolites (area under the receiver operator curve (AUROC) ≥ 0.66) distinguishing between ASD and typically developing (TD) groups at baseline ranked by univariate AUROC with at least 40% values above the detection limit (15 measurements). The AUROC at Week 18 is also provided. The entire list of top 165 metabolites is not shown due to space constraints (see Table A1). Either a Wilcoxon signed-rank test or a paired t-test was performed on the ASD group, comparing measurements from Week 0 to Week 18 for each of the metabolites. The *p*-value of those metabolites that significantly changed after MTT (p-value < 0.05) are presented. The primary associated sub-pathway for each metabolite is also provided [34].

Metabolite Rank	Metabolite	AUROC Week 0	AUROC Week 18	Pre/Post MTT *p*-Value	Associated Sub-Pathway
1	Carnitine	0.77	0.68		Carnitine Metabolism
2	Sphingosine	0.75	0.58		Sphingolipid Metabolism
3	2′-deoxyadenosine	0.75	0.59	0.02	Purine Metabolism, Adenine containing
4	Indole	0.74	0.72		Tryptophan Metabolism
5	Adenine	0.74	0.81		Purine Metabolism, Adenine containing
6	*N*-stearoyl-sphingosine (d18:1/18:0)	0.73	0.61		Sphingolipid Metabolism
7	Imidazole Propionate	0.71	0.64		Histidine Metabolism
8	10-nonadecenoate (19:1n9)	0.71	0.59	0.01	Long Chain Fatty Acid
9	p-cresol sulfate	0.71	0.53		Phenylalanine and Tyrosine Metabolism
10	Cystathionine	0.71	0.65		Methionine, Cysteine, SAM and Taurine Metabolism
11	5alpha-androstan-3beta,17alpha-diol monosulfate (1)	0.71	0.63	0.01	Steroid
12	3-(3-hydroxyphenyl)propionate	0.71	0.66		Phenylalanine and Tyrosine Metabolism
13	1-(1-enyl-oleoyl)-GPE (P-18:1)	0.71	0.87		Lysoplasmalogen
14	Deoxy-carnitine	0.71	0.58		Carnitine Metabolism
15	Gamma-glutamyl-histidine	0.71	0.68		Gamma-glutamyl Amino Acid
16	Diaminopimelate	0.70	0.62		Food Component/Plant
17	Tyramine O-sulfate	0.70	0.70		Phenylalanine and Tyrosine Metabolism
18	Gulonate	0.70	0.53		Ascorbate and Aldarate Metabolism
19	gamma-tocotrienol	0.70	0.62		Tocopherol Metabolism
20	4-hydroxyphenylacetate	0.70	0.56		Phenylalanine and Tyrosine Metabolism
21	Delta-tocopherol	0.70	0.53		Tocopherol Metabolism
22	Phenethylamine	0.69	0.55		Phenylalanine and Tyrosine Metabolism
23	Propionyl-glycine (C3)	0.69	0.61		Sphingolipid Metabolism

Table 1. *Cont.*

Metabolite Rank	Metabolite	AUROC Week 0	AUROC Week 18	Pre/Post MTT *p*-Value	Associated Sub-Pathway
24	*N*-acetyl-sphingosine	0.69	0.63		Sphingolipid Metabolism
25	Betaine	0.69	0.60		Glycine, Serine and Threonine Metabolism
26	Adenosine	0.69	0.65		Purine Metabolism, Adenine containing
27	Ornithine	0.68	0.51		Urea cycle; Arginine and Proline Metabolism
28	*N*-palmitoyl-sphingosine (d18:1/16:0)	0.68	0.54	0.03	Sphingolipid Metabolism
29	Galactonate	0.68	0.67		Fructose, Mannose and Galactose Metabolism
30	N1-Methyl-2-pyridone-5-carboxamide	0.68	0.74		Nicotinate and Nicotinamide Metabolism
31	1-palmitoylglycerol (16:0)	0.68	0.54		Monoacylglycerol
32	Phosphocholine	0.67	0.59		Phospholipid Metabolism
33	Theobromine	0.67	0.62	0.02	Xanthine Metabolism
34	3,5-dihydroxybenzoic acid	0.67	0.60		Food Component/Plant
35	Hydroxyproline	0.67	0.56		Urea cycle; Arginine and Proline Metabolism
36	L-urobilin	0.67	0.60	0.02	Hemoglobin and Porphyrin Metabolism
37	carboxyethyl-GABA	0.67	0.55		Glutamate Metabolism
38	oxalate (ethane-dioate)	0.67	0.53		Ascorbate and Aldarate Metabolism
39	Palmitoyl-carnitine (C16)	0.67	0.53		Fatty Acid Metabolism(Acyl Carnitine)
40	Copro-stanol	0.67	0.60		Sterol
41	Saccharopine	0.66	0.57		Lysine Metabolism
42	5-hydroxylysine	0.66	0.53		Lysine Metabolism
43	Stearoyl-carnitine (C18)	0.66	0.58		Fatty Acid Metabolism(Acyl Carnitine)
44	Biliverdin	0.66	0.60		Hemoglobin and Porphyrin Metabolism
45	3-(4-hydroxyphenyl)lactate (HPLA)	0.66	0.59		Phenylalanine and Tyrosine Metabolism
46	Carnosine	0.66	0.57		Dipeptide Derivative
47	10-hydroxystearate	0.66	0.64	0.01	Fatty Acid, Monohydroxy
48	Pentadecanoate (15:0)	0.66	0.55		Long Chain Fatty Acid
49	Hexadecanedioate (C16)	0.66	0.60		Fatty Acid, Dicarboxylate
50	Sphinganine	0.66	0.54		Sphingolipid Metabolism

Table 2. Fitting and cross-validation results for the best combinations of two, three, four, and five metabolites used as part of Fisher Discriminant Analysis (FDA). The cross-validated true positive rate (TPR) and true negative rate (TNR) are shown for classification thresholds associated with different values of β calculated from the fitted probability density functions (PDFs). The results for two distinct 5-metabolite models are presented as they were able to achieve the same accuracy following cross-validation. The notable TPRs and TNRs are highlighted for the 5-metabolite models.

Number of Metabolites	Metabolite Combination	Fitted AUROC	Cross-Validated Results		
			β	TPR	TNR
2	Carnitine 2′deoxyadenosine	0.88	0.01 0.05 0.10 0.20	1.00 1.00 1.00 0.89	0.20 0.35 0.50 0.75
3	Adenosine theobromine hydroxyproline	0.93	0.01 0.05 0.10 0.20	1.00 0.94 0.94 0.72	0.30 0.55 0.75 0.85
4	indole 1-(1-enyl-oleoyl)-GPE (P-18:1) Hydroxyproline Carnosine	0.98	0.01 0.05 0.10 0.20	0.94 0.89 0.83 0.83	0.35 0.60 0.60 0.80
5	Imidazole Propionate Hydroxyproline Theobromine 2-hydroxy-3-methylvalerate Adenosine	1.00	0.01 0.05 0.10 0.20	1.00 0.94 0.89 0.78	0.85 0.95 0.95 0.95
5	Imidazole Propionate Hydroxyproline Theobromine 2-hydroxy-3-methylvalerate Indole	1.00	0.01 0.05 0.10 0.20	1.00 0.94 0.89 0.78	0.85 0.95 0.95 0.95

3.3. *Correlation Analysis*

Correlation analysis was performed on the OFM metabolites as these were the ones that had been identified as being able to distinguish between the ASD and TD cohorts with the highest accuracy after cross-validation. It can be observed that many of the top 50 metabolites (AUROC ≥ 0.66) were significantly correlated with the OFM metabolites (Table 3). In contrast, the individual OFM metabolites for both models had little to no correlation with each other, apart from hydroxyproline with adenosine and 2-hydroxy-3-methylvalerate; these findings were expected since, if individual OFM metabolites were highly correlated with each other, then they would not be useful in the model due to their correlation.

3.4. *Assessing Effects of MTT*

Univariate assessment of the top 50 metabolites as ranked by AUROC demonstrated that 14% of these 50 metabolites showed significant differences in their Week 0 and Week 18 ASD measurements and that 47 of these 50 metabolites achieved a lower AUROC eight weeks following treatment (Table 1). In addition to classification at baseline, the multivariate models developed can be used to observe changes in fecal metabolome composition over the course of the study. Most metabolites in the OFM-I and OFM-A models changed significantly after MTT and have values closer to the TD group after MTT (see Table 4). The average difference between the median of the five metabolites for TD group at Week 0 and the ASD measurements at Week 18 compared to measurements at Week 0 diminished by 88% and 82% for the OFM-I and OFM-A models (see Table 4), so the ASD group became much more similar to the TD group.

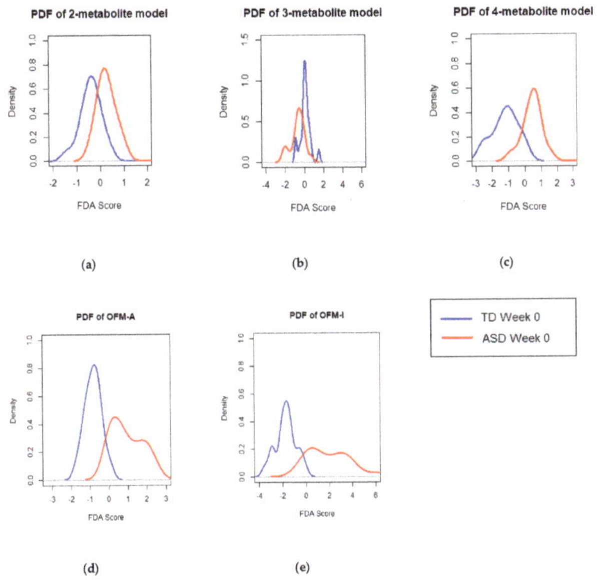

Figure 2. PDFs of ASD and TD discriminant scores at Week 0. The probability density function of the FDA score provides a visualization of a model's ability to distinguish between the ASD and TD cohorts. The (**a**) two-metabolite model has most of its FDA scores highly concentrated near the region where thresholds would be applied. The (**b**) three-metabolite model is not as highly concentrated, but there is a significant amount of overlap between the scores of the ASD and TD participants, which is visible in both plots. The four (**c**) and five (**d**,**e**) metabolite models better separated the cohorts, with little overlap in the discriminant scores of the ASD and TD groups.

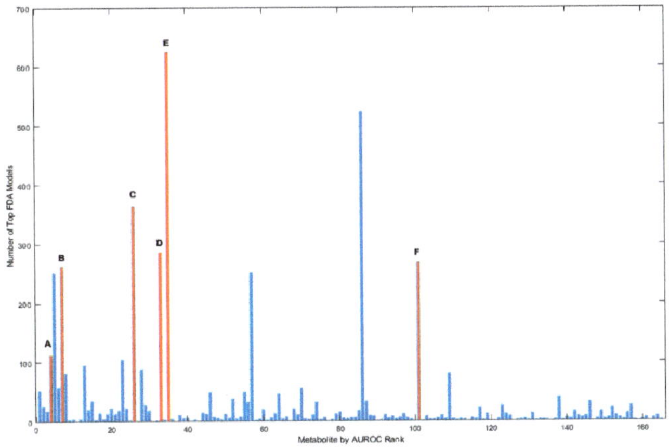

Figure 3. Frequency of appearance of each of the metabolites with AUROC > 0.6 in the top 1000 five-metabolite Fisher discriminant analysis (FDA) models. The metabolites are ranked from highest to lowest area under the receiver operating characteristic curve (AUROC) as shown in Table 1. The metabolites included in the FDA models which achieved maximal separation following cross-validation are shown in red: (A) indole (B) imidazole Propionate (C) adenosine (D) theobromine (E) hydroxyproline, (F) 2-hydroxy-3-methylvalerate.

Table 3. The correlation coefficients between the optimized fecal model-indole/adenosine (OFM-I/A) metabolites and top metabolites 50 metabolites are examined and presented in order of their AUROC. Only those correlations that are significant (p-value < 0.05) are presented.

Metabolite	Correlation Coefficient	p-Value
Indole		
Carnitine	0.67	<0.001
Indole-lactate	0.56	<0.001
Saccharopine	0.42	0.007
Stearoyl-carnitine	0.39	0.015
3-(3-hydroxyphenyl)propionate	0.33	0.043
Oxalate	0.33	0.043
Imidazole Propionate		
Galactonate	0.78	<0.001
Gulonate	0.76	<0.001
Palmitoyl-carnitine	0.72	<0.001
Saccharopine	0.7	<0.001
Phosphocholine	0.69	<0.001
Cystathionine	0.62	<0.001
Phenethylamine	0.61	<0.001
Betaine	0.61	<0.001
3-(4-hydroxyphenyl)lactate	0.6	<0.001
N-propionyl-methionine	0.58	<0.001
N-palmitoyl-sphingosine	0.41	0.011
3,5-dihydroxybenzoic	0.4	0.014
3-(3-hydroxyphenyl)propionate	0.39	0.017
Stearoyl-carnitine	0.38	0.018
1-palmitoylglycerol	0.37	0.023
Gamma-glutamyl-histidine	0.36	0.027
Biliverdin	0.34	0.037
Carnitine	0.32	0.048
Adenosine		
Adenine	0.74	<0.001
2′-deoxyadenosine	0.54	<0.001
5-hydroxylysine	0.36	0.0254
Hydroxyproline	0.36	0.0256
5-hydroxylysine	0.36	0.0254
1-(1-enyl-oleoyl)-GPE	0.34	0.0366
Theobromine **		
None		
Hydroxyproline		
2-hydroxy-3-methylvalerate ***	0.61	<0.001
delta-tocopherol	0.41	0.011
2′-deoxyadenosine	0.38	0.017
Adenosine	0.36	0.026
Copro-stanol	0.36	0.026
5alpha-androstan-3beta,17alpha-diol	0.35	0.030
p-cresol	−0.32	0.050
Betaine	−0.33	0.043
Oxalate	−0.35	0.031
N-palmitoyl-sphingosine	−0.37	0.023

Table 3. *Cont.*

Metabolite	Correlation Coefficient	*p*-Value
*2-hydroxy-3-methylvalerate ****		
Gulonate	0.81	<0.001
Imidazole propionate	0.79	<0.001
Galactonate	0.78	<0.001
Phosphocholine	0.75	<0.001
5-hydroxylysine	0.72	<0.001
Hydroxyproline	0.61	<0.001
Betaine	0.6	<0.001
Phenethylamine	0.59	<0.001
1-(1-enyl-oleoyl)-GPE (P-18:1)	0.55	<0.001
Cystathionine	0.53	<0.001
1-palmitoylglycerol (16:0)	0.51	<0.001
Biliverdin	0.51	0.001
Propionyl-glycine (C3)	0.45	0.005
3-(4-hydroxyphenyl)lactate (HPLA)	0.43	0.008
3-(3-hydroxyphenyl)propionate	0.34	0.039
Delta-tocopherol	−0.33	0.042
Copro-stanol	−0.35	0.033

** Theobromine was not found to be significantly correlated with any of the top 50 metabolites.
*** 2-hydroxy-3-methylvalerate is not among the top 50 metabolites as ranked by AUROC but present in both OFM-I/A panels.

The OFM-I/A models were applied to the ASD samples at all distinct time points to assess their accuracy for classifying a sample as belonging to the ASD or TD cohort. The effectiveness of OFM-I/A for classification changed significantly before and after MTT. The type II error rate was initially observed to be 5% for both models, indicating that the ASD and TD distributions are quite distinct, but was observed to rise to 56% eight weeks after MTT was completed (Table 4), thereby indicating that distinguishing between the ASD and TD cohort is not reliably possible after MTT. The PDF curves are shown in Figure 4 to demonstrate the changes in the ASD cohort over time with respect to the values of the FDA score. The distributions indicate that the ASD cohort became more metabolically similar to the TD cohort after treatment, since the curves are shifted towards the TD curve. Notably, the distribution of scores for the ASD cohort become somewhat bimodal at the later time points for both models. The discriminant score for both models decreased substantially as time progressed, indicating that the metabolites of the ASD group were becoming more similar to that of the TD group.

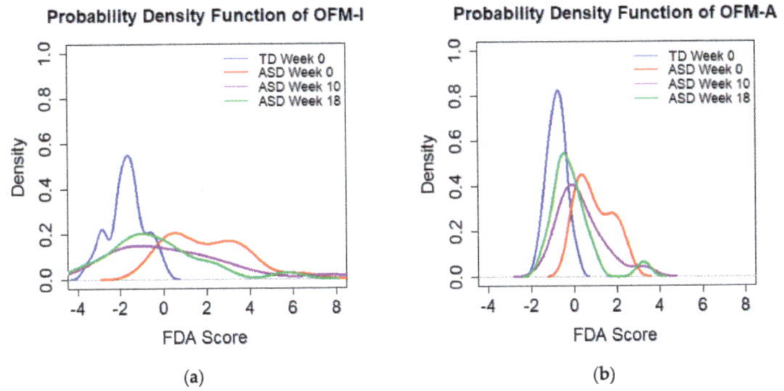

Figure 4. PDF curves for the (**a**) OFM-I and (**b**) OFM-A model when assessing the ASD cohort over the course of the study. The overlap between the TD cohort and the ASD cohorts increases at Week 10 and Week 18, indicating that the metabolite profile of the ASD group after MTT treatment has become more similar to the ones of the TD group.

Table 4. Change in the difference between OFM-I/A metabolites measured in the TD and ASD cohort over the course of the study. The discriminant score was calculated by first taking the absolute value of the difference between measurements at each time point and the median of the TD group, then normalizing the difference by the standard deviation of the TD Week 0 measurements, and then adding the normalized absolute difference for each of the five metabolites. The background color distinguished the individual metabolites from the multivariate models.

	ASD Week 0	ASD Week 3	ASD Week 10	ASD Week 18	TD Week 0
Imidazole Propionate (25th/75th percentile)	0.37 (0.19, 3.38)	0.55 (0.08, 8.57)	0.29 (0.08, 0.80)	0.14 (0.03, 0.46)	0.12 (0.09, 0.29)
Hydroxyproline (25th/75th percentile)	0.96 (0.72, 4.83)	1.06 (0.42, 3.67)	1.27 (0.24, 3.34)	0.80 (0.54, 3.60)	0.60 (0.29, 1.20)
Theobromine (25th/75th percentile)	0.89 (0.47, 2.38)	0.47 (0.47, 1.68)	0.47 (0.16, 0.47)	0.47 (0.43, 0.47)	0.46 (0.34, 0.64)
2-hydroxy-3-methylvalerat (25th/75th percentile)	0.53 (0.43, 0.75)	0.43 (0.18, 0.56)	0.34 (0.06, 0.50)	0.52 (0.21, 0.63)	0.44 (0.21, 0.61)
Indole (25th/75th percentile)	1.13 (0.25, 1.83)	0.66 (0.32, 1.75)	0.85 (0.18, 1.86)	0.86 (0.26, 1.52)	0.39 (0.15, 0.59)
Adenosine (25th/75th percentile)	0.67 (0.36, 0.88)	0.77 (0.50, 1.01)	0.73 (0.47, 0.90)	0.57 (0.26, 0.86)	0.40 (0.18, 0.86)
OFM-I Median discriminant score (25th/75th percentile)	3.90 (2.33, 5.72)	1.90 (0.72, 9.52)	1.84 (0.90, 3.71)	1.73 (0.71, 2.62)	0.46 (0.21, 1.35)
Type II error	5%	53%	50%	56%	-
OFM-A Median discriminant score (25th/75th percentile)	3.51 (2.28, 5.73)	2.87 (1.13, 9.43)	2.18 (1.07, 4.18)	1.36 (0.54, 2.44)	0.62 (0.35, 1.05)
Type II error	5%	53%	39%	56%	-

4. Discussion

Preliminary analysis using univariate methods revealed that none of the individual fecal metabolites achieved a high AUROC value by itself. Interpretations regarding the threshold value needed for an AUROC to be deemed an effective classifier vary by discipline. AUROC values between 0.9–1.0 are desirable for diagnostic tests and are seen to be reflective of excellent classification [35]. However, this value was not chosen here as the AUROC is employed here as a pre-screening tool for reducing the number of metabolites for classification, and not for determining a metabolite that by itself can distinguish between the two groups. The highest AUROC value for an individual metabolite was 0.77, corresponding to carnitine, indicating that the ASD group is somewhat heterogeneous. In contrast, all optimized multivariate models using three or more elements were able to achieve an AUROC greater than 0.9, highlighting that a multivariate analysis can provide better classification than that which can be determined using univariate analysis alone. Nonetheless, 94% of the top 50 univariate metabolites report lower AUROC (Table 1) eight weeks following MTT, which indicates greater similarity between the ASD and TD measurements after treatment.

Analysis of all possible significant metabolites at Week 0 resulted in the OFM-I and OMF-A models, consisting of five metabolites. Four of these five metabolites were identical between the two models and both achieved AUROC values greater than 0.99. Interestingly, the two metabolites that differed between them, Adenosine and Indole, are associated with different metabolic processes and have no significant correlation. Furthermore, cross-validation revealed that using the OFM-I/A models at the Week 0 timepoint resulted in a 0.95 TPR and 0.94 TNR. Subsequently, there was an overall 94.7% accuracy for correctly classifying an individual into the ASD/TD groups after leave-one-out cross-validation.

Many of the metabolites identified as being differentially expressed between the ASD and TD cohorts have also been previously examined for their relationship to ASD. Specifically, among the top five metabolites ranked by their AUROC value, carnitine, indole and sphingosine have all been found to be differentially expressed in some capacity among individuals with ASD [14,17,18,36]. In a meta-analysis, 10–20% of individuals with ASD were found to have disorders with synthesizing carnitine, which was the metabolite that had achieved the largest AUROC value [36]. Plasma carnitine concentration has also previously been shown to be lower among cohorts with ASD [36]. It should be noted that following MTT the AUROC values of carnitine reduced to 0.68, which indicates that the ASD and TD carnitine distributions were less different after MTT (see Table A1). Sphingolipids such as sphingosine have been found to play an active role in the crosstalk between microbiota and intestinal cells [37]. The significant change in concentration for metabolites such as N-palmitoyl-sphingosine (d18:1/16:0) may have been associated with the changed microbiome composition resulting from MTT (Table 1). Approximately 68% of the variance observed in the fecal metabolome can be explained by the gut microbiome [38], which underscores the potential impact FMT can have on reshaping metabolite concentrations.

Among the metabolites which form part of the OFM-I/A models, theobromine exhibited a significant change between its measurements at Week 0 compared to the Week 18 value for the ASD cohort when a sign ranked test was applied at both timepoints (Table 1). Theobromine is not a microbial metabolite, and its source in fecal samples likely stems from dietary intake and from human metabolism of caffeine [38]. Consequently, this may account for the reason why it was not observed to be correlated with any other metabolite and why the median discriminate score often took the value of the detection limit. However, the metabolization of theobromine is primarily via hepatic demethylation and oxidation, which are processes that have at least been hypothesized to be perturbed in ASD [39,40]. The median concentration for this metabolite was also not found to change following the bowel cleanse measurement (see Table A1). We conducted a secondary analysis of a five-metabolite model without theobromine and found that it results in significantly lower sensitivity and specificity, so including theobromine seems to be important for developing a classification model.

Nonetheless, in the case of all metabolites present in the OFM-I/A models, the average difference between the Week 0 TD measurements and ASD group decreased greatly (82–88%) by the end of the study (Table 4). Hydroxyproline, which is another of the OFM metabolites, has been previously determined to be expressed in significantly higher concentration in the plasma of children with ASD, consistent with the higher levels in feces [41] and in the present study. Indole, which was also one of the OFM metabolites, has been found in higher concentration in fecal samples in children with ASD and other neurodevelopmental conditions [17], consistent with the results of this study, and is an important metabolite for tryptophan metabolism [42]. Thus, the shift to a lower discriminant score following the completion of the treatment is consistent with measurements of ASD fecal metabolites becoming more like those of their TD counterparts following MTT.

The OFM-I/A models in their totality demonstrated similar behavior when contrasting measurements taken at Week 0 and Week 18 of the ASD cohort. This study found that some metabolic changes had begun by Week 3 (after vancomycin, bowel cleanse, and approximately five days of FMT). It is also notable that the distributions of FDA scores within both the five-metabolite models at later timepoints (Week 10 and Week 18) are bimodal. This suggests that some individuals may respond differently to MTT than others. This finding was similar to the analysis performed on plasma metabolites where a steep decline in median discriminant score was also observed at Week 3 and Week 10 [29].

The OFM-I/A metabolites demonstrated limited correlation among themselves. This was to be expected as FDA seeks to maximize the amount of discriminating information with a minimal number of utilized metabolites. For this reason, within this subset of fecal metabolites, those with few correlations tended to appear more frequently in the top 1000 models. Specifically, there was a high proportion of top 1000 models featuring theobromine (28.5%), which was ranked as the fourth most common metabolite present in the models. Notably, this metabolite was not significantly correlated with any of the other top 50 metabolites as discussed above. In total, 44 of the 50 metabolites with the highest AUROC were correlated with the OFM metabolite panel, suggesting that there are at least six common types of metabolic abnormalities associated with ASD. Although adenosine and indole were not found to be correlated, they were included in the OFM-A and OFI-I models, respectively, and both metabolites are related to distinct biological pathways, with adenosine being associated with purine metabolism, while indole is associated with tryptophan metabolism. It was observed in one study that metabolites associated with these two pathways were the most different in urine of ASD and TD children [43].

While there are several metabolic pathways that are related to the top 50 metabolites identified, about 45% of the top metabolites were connected to phenylalanine and tyrosine metabolism, fatty acid metabolism or sphingolipid metabolism. Differences in tyrosine metabolites such as decreased concentration of phenylalanine and increased concentration of p-cresol have been previously observed in studies examining the gut metabolite composition in TD and ASD children [14,44]. The role of the microbiota in this pathway is also very significant. Tyrosine metabolism pathway downregulation was observed in an ASD cohort to be associated with an increased prevalence of *Bacteroides vulgatus* while upregulation was associated with *Eggerthella lenta* [44]. Similarly, the relationship between sphingolipid metabolism and microbiome crosstalk has been suggested, and differences in short chain fatty acids of children with ASD and their TD peers have been noted [24,36].

Several metabolites related to mitochondrial metabolism and regulation such as carnitine, betaine, and adenine were also determined to have particularly high AUROC values [35,45–47]. Carnitine serves as the cofactor that transports long-chain fatty acids to the mitochondria matrix, and betaine plays a role in increasing mitochondrial membrane potential [45,47]. There has been considerable investigation into the relationship between ASD and mitochondrial dysfunction. It is estimated that around 4–7% of children with ASD are affected by mitochondrial disease, but it is speculated that up to 80% may have abnormalities in mitochondrial function [48,49].

Prior work has shown similar relationships between ASD fecal metabolite profiles as were observed in this study. GABA, an important neurotransmitter, was one of the metabolites identified as having a lower concentration in the ASD group prior to MTT, which is consistent with prior work [16,17]. Similarly, the fecal concentrations of free carnitine have been previously observed to be higher in children with ASD, which was also observed in this study [14]. The fecal metabolite measurements are consistent with prior work as the average indole measurements for the ASD cohort were more than twice the value of their TD counterparts at Week 0 (see Table A1) [17]. It has also been observed that fecal metabolites associated with glutamate metabolism such as 2-Keto-glutaramic acid and l-Aspartic acid were downregulated in children with ASD [44]. These metabolites were not measured in this study. Nonetheless, one of the metabolites associated with glutamate metabolism, carboxyethyl-GABA, was identified in significantly lower concentration in the ASD + GI cohort at baseline.

While there are indeed some similarities between the analysis of fecal metabolites and prior assessment of plasma samples taken from these participants, there are key distinctions. None of the metabolites identified as being utilized in the optimum multivariate models were previously identified as being significant for classification in the multivariate plasma models. The general performance of the fecal metabolites when subjected to univariate analysis had generally lower AUROC values than plasma metabolites [29]. However, despite having lower AUROC scores, multivariate analysis achieved high accuracy in distinguishing ASD and TD children. That being said, we were able to achieve greater separation using three plasma metabolites than with five fecal metabolites. This may be due to the greater homogeneity in plasma samples vs. stool samples. There have also been far more studies conducted examining plasma metabolite concentrations in individuals with ASD than studies focused on fecal samples [50,51].

Although the models were able to classify between the ASD + GI and TD cohorts with high accuracy, this study also has several limitations. The study focused exclusively on children with ASD with initially moderate to severe GI problems, which were compared to TD children with no GI issues. Therefore, assessments regarding ASD were confounded with GI problems in this analysis. ASD subgroups differentiated by variations in GI abnormalities were ignored in the analysis as subgroups were too small for a robust statistical assessment [52,53]. Furthermore, the study-cohort was not large and the ASD cohort was further split up into two different initial treatments. Future studies with a larger sample size examining cohorts with and without GI symptoms would allow for an assessment on the effectiveness of MTT in ameliorating behavioral symptoms in addition to GI related pathology.

5. Conclusions

This study investigated differences in fecal metabolites between a group of children diagnosed with ASD and GI symptoms and their typically developing peers with no history of GI symptoms. The univariate analysis demonstrated that individual fecal metabolites had limited potential to distinguish between ASD+GI and TD cohorts, unlike the previous study of plasma; this may be due to greater heterogeneity in stool compared to plasma. However, multivariate statistical analysis resulted in five-metabolite models that had high accuracy even after cross-validation. Both the OFM metabolite panels were shown to be capable of achieving 95% specificity and 94% sensitivity.

Following MTT, 14% of the top 50 metabolites that were found to have the greatest difference in concentration between the TD and ASD group shifted such that their distributions were significantly different eight weeks after the treatment ended. Furthermore, 94% of these metabolites reported lower AUROC following treatment, indicating diminished capacity to distinguish between the ASD and TD group. When considering a normalized average of the metabolites in the OFM models, the difference between the ASD and TD groups decreased by 82–88% at 18 weeks. These findings are similar, although less pronounced, as those determined using plasma metabolites, and both suggest that MTT resulted in shifting the metabolic profile of the ASD group towards becoming more similar to the TD group. Future work should be performed to validate the effect of MTT on fecal metabolites using a larger study cohort and a placebo arm.

Author Contributions: J.A., D.-W.K., R.K.-B. and J.H. conceived of the current study and contributed to its design and coordination. R.K.-B. received grant for FMT trial funding, helped design FMT trial, directed microbiome analysis J.A., D.-W.K. and R.K.-B. collected and interpreted the clinical data. F.Q. and K.H. analyzed the data and generated the tables and figures. Statistical results were interpreted by J.A., F.Q. and J.H. All authors have read and agreed to the published version of the manuscript.

Funding: The authors gratefully acknowledge partial financial support from the National Institutes of Health (grant 1R01AI110642).

Acknowledgments: We would like to acknowledge the contributions of Troy Vargason, Uwe Kruger and Kathryn Hollowood Jones for the initial help with the analysis. We would also like to thank Sharon McDonough-Means, Thomas Borody, Alex Khoruts, Michael Sadowsky, Alessio Fasano, Devon Coleman, and Elena Pollard for their help with the treatment portion of the Microbiota Transfer Therapy study.

Conflicts of Interest: The authors have filed an invention disclosure on the results presented here.

Appendix A

Table A1. Univariate assessment of all metabolites with an AUROC greater than 0.60. The AUROC is provided at Week 0 for the TD and ASD cohort as well as average ultrahigh performance liquid chromatography-tandem mass spectroscopy (UHPLC-MS/MS) signal intensity measurements for both cohorts. The *p*-value for the significance between the ASD and TD cohorts at Week 0 and between the ASD cohort at Week 0 and Week 18 are also shown. Finally, the results of leave-n-out (n = 1–3) cross-validation are provided.

Metabolite	Week 0 AUROC	Week 18 AUROC	TD Mean Week 0	ASD Mean Week 0	Week 0 vs. Week 18 ASD *p*-Value	Week 0 ASD vs. TD Un-Adjusted *p*-Value	Leave-1-Out	Leave 2-Out	Leave 3-Out
carnitine	0.77	0.68	9.81×10^6	3.35×10^7	7.64×10^{-1}	4.78×10^{-3}	0.00	0.00	0.00
sphingosine	0.75	0.58	7.18×10^6	2.13×10^7	1.10×10^{-1}	8.15×10^{-3}	0.00	0.00	0.00
2′-deoxyadenosine	0.75	0.59	8.08×10^5	2.32×10^5	1.83×10^{-2}	9.59×10^{-3}	0.00	0.00	0.00
indole	0.74	0.72	4.74×10^5	1.05×10^6	5.80×10^{-1}	1.04×10^{-2}	0.00	0.00	0.00
adenine	0.74	0.81	6.70×10^6	2.91×10^6	5.17×10^{-1}	1.35×10^{-2}	0.00	0.00	0.03
N-stearoyl-sphingosine	0.73	0.61	1.01×10^6	4.05×10^6	1.03×10^{-1}	1.40×10^{-2}	0.00	0.00	0.04
imidazole	0.71	0.64	1.02×10^7	3.95×10^7	1.50×10^{-1}	1.83×10^{-2}	0.00	0.00	0.13
10-nonadecenoate	0.71	0.59	2.42×10^6	5.49×10^6	1.19×10^{-2}	2.18×10^{-2}	0.00	0.01	0.25
p-cresol	0.71	0.53	1.55×10^6	4.00×10^6	6.42×10^{-2}	2.53×10^{-2}	0.00	0.16	0.27
cystathionine	0.71	0.65	6.07×10^4	9.12×10^4	5.98×10^{-1}	2.53×10^{-2}	0.00	0.17	0.25
5alpha-androstan-3beta,17alpha-diol	0.71	0.63	9.86×10^4	6.65×10^4	4.50×10^{-3}	2.55×10^{-2}	0.00	0.31	0.32
3-(3-hydroxyphenyl)propionate	0.71	0.66	2.24×10^7	2.67×10^7	8.62×10^{-1}	2.73×10^{-2}	0.00	0.24	0.30
1-(1-enyl-oleoyl)-GPE	0.71	0.87	3.31×10^5	2.57×10^5	2.47×10^{-1}	2.81×10^{-2}	0.00	0.24	0.29
gamma-glutamyl-histidine	0.71	0.58	1.90×10^5	1.95×10^5	1.83×10^{-1}	2.94×10^{-2}	0.00	0.25	0.38
Deoxy-carnitine	0.71	0.68	2.82×10^8	1.09×10^9	6.46×10^{-1}	2.94×10^{-2}	0.00	0.26	0.42
diaminopimelate	0.70	0.62	8.57×10^5	1.14×10^6	7.16×10^{-1}	3.11×10^{-2}	0.00	0.32	0.40
tyramine	0.70	0.70	2.17×10^7	8.33×10^6	7.86×10^{-1}	3.17×10^{-2}	0.21	0.27	0.36
gulonate	0.70	0.53	2.43×10^5	1.52×10^6	9.12×10^{-2}	3.40×10^{-2}	0.11	0.42	0.46
gamma-tocotrienol	0.70	0.62	5.04×10^6	3.24×10^6	3.51×10^{-1}	3.49×10^{-2}	0.26	0.42	0.46
4-hydroxyphenylacetate	0.70	0.56	9.97×10^5	2.75×10^6	2.75×10^{-1}	3.66×10^{-2}	0.32	0.42	0.44
delta-tocopherol	0.70	0.53	2.50×10^6	1.62×10^5	7.38×10^{-2}	3.85×10^{-2}	0.42	0.49	0.48
phenethylamine	0.69	0.55	4.35×10^5	$9.09 \times 10^{[illegible]}$	6.42×10^{-2}	3.93×10^{-2}	0.39	0.45	0.49
Propionyl-glycine	0.69	0.61	1.56×10^5	$3.92 \times 10^{[illegible]}$	6.09×10^{-1}	3.93×10^{-2}	0.47	0.51	0.53
N-acetyl-sphingosine	0.69	0.63	9.84×10^4	$2.63 \times 10^{[illegible]}$	3.33×10^{-1}	4.22×10^{-2}	0.45	0.51	0.47

Table A1. *Cont.*

Metabolite	Week 0 AUROC	Week 18 AUROC	TD Mean Week 0	ASD Mean Week 0	Week 0 vs. Week 18 ASD p-Value	Week 0 ASD vs. TD Un-Adjusted p-Value	Leave-1-Out	Leave 2-Out	Leave 3-Out
betaine	0.69	0.60	3.39×10^{6}	5.05×10^{6}	5.37×10^{-1}	4.55×10^{-2}	0.63	0.50	0.47
adenosine	0.69	0.65	5.81×10^{5}	3.41×10^{5}	5.58×10^{-1}	4.84×10^{-2}	0.50	0.59	0.60
ornithine	0.68	0.51	2.05×10^{7}	2.74×10^{7}	6.89×10^{-2}	5.19×10^{-2}	0.71	0.61	0.65
N-palmitoyl-sphingosine	0.68	0.54	3.01×10^{6}	1.04×10^{7}	2.57×10^{-2}	5.33×10^{-2}	1.00	1.00	0.67
galactonate	0.68	0.67	4.63×10^{5}	2.05×10^{6}	7.63×10^{-1}	5.37×10^{-2}	0.66	0.62	0.67
N1-Methyl-2-pyridone-5-carboxamide	0.68	0.74	1.63×10^{5}	4.37×10^{5}	7.62×10^{-1}	5.44×10^{-2}	1.00	1.00	0.69
1-palmitoylglycerol	0.68	0.54	1.08×10^{7}	1.55×10^{7}	1.69×10^{-1}	5.72×10^{-2}	1.00	1.00	0.71
phosphocholine	0.67	0.59	3.01×10^{5}	1.25×10^{7}	5.36×10^{-2}	5.93×10^{-2}	0.79	0.72	0.72
theobromine	0.67	0.62	2.60×10^{6}	5.81×10^{6}	1.56×10^{-2}	5.93×10^{-2}	0.76	0.70	0.72
hydroxyproline	0.67	0.60	2.96×10^{6}	9.08×10^{6}	6.92×10^{-1}	6.10×10^{-2}	0.79	0.73	0.74
L-urobilin	0.67	0.56	4.11×10^{7}	3.08×10^{7}	1.55×10^{-2}	6.35×10^{-2}	0.71	0.80	0.73
3,5-dihydroxybenzoic	0.67	0.60	1.61×10^{5}	9.06×10^{4}	3.29×10^{-1}	6.52×10^{-2}	1.00	1.00	0.95
carboxyethyl-GABA	0.67	0.55	1.52×10^{7}	1.01×10^{7}	2.00×10^{-1}	6.52×10^{-2}	1.00	1.00	0.95
oxalate	0.67	0.53	1.03×10^{6}	2.11×10^{6}	7.91×10^{-2}	6.58×10^{-2}	0.74	0.80	0.78
Palmitoyl-carnitine	0.67	0.53	4.93×10^{5}	4.68×10^{6}	5.18×10^{-2}	6.77×10^{-2}	0.79	0.79	0.79
Copro-stanol	0.67	0.60	2.21×10^{6}	1.31×10^{6}	3.17×10^{-1}	6.86×10^{-2}	0.87	0.79	0.79
5-hydroxylysine	0.66	0.57	1.03×10^{6}	2.53×10^{6}	3.35×10^{-1}	6.99×10^{-2}	0.82	0.82	0.80
Saccharopine	0.66	0.53	1.50×10^{6}	4.10×10^{5}	9.49×10^{-2}	7.22×10^{-2}	0.89	0.82	0.79
3-(4-hydroxyphenyl)lactate	0.66	0.58	1.56×10^{6}	1.88×10^{6}	2.37×10^{-2}	7.22×10^{-2}	0.82	0.82	0.81
Stearoyl-carnitine	0.66	0.60	1.65×10^{6}	4.06×10^{6}	1.03×10^{-1}	7.69×10^{-2}	0.92	0.85	0.82
biliverdin	0.66	0.59	1.29×10^{5}	2.88×10^{5}	3.67×10^{-1}	7.69×10^{-2}	0.89	0.85	0.82
carnosine	0.66	0.57	8.48×10^{4}	8.23×10^{4}	3.44×10^{-1}	8.31×10^{-2}	0.87	0.91	0.85
pentadecanoate	0.66	0.64	2.40×10^{8}	1.97×10^{8}	8.62×10^{-1}	8.44×10^{-2}	0.87	0.87	0.87
hexadecanedioate	0.66	0.55	4.54×10^{5}	4.28×10^{5}	1.25×10^{-1}	8.72×10^{-2}	0.89	0.90	0.87
10-hydroxystearate	0.66	0.60	1.16×10^{9}	1.93×10^{9}	8.25×10^{-3}	9.27×10^{-2}	0.95	0.92	0.88
Sphinganine	0.66	0.54	1.67×10^{7}	2.34×10^{7}	3.19×10^{-1}	9.28×10^{-2}	0.89	0.91	0.89
trigonelline	0.66	0.81	3.08×10^{6}	6.92×10^{6}	1.41×10^{-1}	9.28×10^{-2}	0.92	0.92	0.88

Table A1. *Cont.*

Metabolite	Week 0 AUROC	Week 18 AUROC	TD Mean Week 0	ASD Mean Week 0	Week 0 vs. Week 18 ASD p-Value	Week 0 ASD vs. TD Un-Adjusted p-Value	Leave-1-Out	Leave 2-Out	Leave 3-Out
Indole-lactate	0.66	0.64	4.74×10^{5}	1.80×10^{6}	8.80×10^{-3}	9.46×10^{-2}	1.00	1.00	0.87
Dihomo-linoleate	0.65	0.58	1.11×10^{7}	2.92×10^{7}	7.38×10^{-2}	9.76×10^{-2}	1.00	1.00	1.00
Phyto-sphingosine	0.65	0.60	8.22×10^{5}	1.25×10^{6}	5.58×10^{-1}	9.77×10^{-2}	1.00	0.95	0.90
gamma-tocopherol/beta-tocopherol	0.65	0.51	5.43×10^{7}	4.05×10^{7}	1.03×10^{-1}	9.86×10^{-2}	0.92	0.91	0.89
acesulfame	0.65	0.59	3.59×10^{4}	7.24×10^{5}	6.27×10^{-1}	9.86×10^{-2}	0.92	0.92	0.90
N-methyl-pipecolate	0.65	0.63	4.88×10^{6}	9.71×10^{6}	7.16×10^{-1}	9.86×10^{-2}	0.97	0.94	0.88
2-methylserine	0.65	0.66	9.22×10^{5}	7.05×10^{5}	7.16×10^{-1}	9.86×10^{-2}	0.97	0.93	0.90
2-aminobutyrate	0.65	0.61	1.27×10^{7}	2.65×10^{7}	4.02×10^{-1}	1.02×10^{-1}	0.97	0.94	0.92
N-palmitoyl-sphinganine	0.65	0.64	1.99×10^{6}	4.43×10^{6}	1.55×10^{-2}	1.02×10^{-1}	0.95	0.94	0.91
caffeate	0.65	0.60	4.23×10^{5}	4.23×10^{5}	5.19×10^{-1}	1.06×10^{-1}	0.97	0.95	0.94
piperine	0.65	0.59	2.41×10^{7}	1.59×10^{7}	1.96×10^{-2}	1.11×10^{-1}	1.00	0.96	0.93
N-propionyl-methionine	0.65	0.65	1.55×10^{5}	3.58×10^{5}	8.87×10^{-1}	1.11×10^{-1}	1.00	0.96	0.93
alpha-CEHC	0.65	0.50	1.02×10^{5}	5.68×10^{5}	6.53×10^{-2}	1.11×10^{-1}	0.97	0.96	0.93
5-aminovalerate	0.65	0.55	3.29×10^{7}	1.15×10^{8}	4.57×10^{-1}	1.11×10^{-1}	1.00	1.00	0.94
2-aminophenol	0.65	0.56	7.90×10^{5}	6.54×10^{5}	4.02×10^{-1}	1.17×10^{-1}	1.00	1.00	0.93
O-sulfo-L-tyrosine	0.65	0.50	9.04×10^{4}	3.24×10^{5}	1.26×10^{-1}	1.17×10^{-1}	0.97	0.95	0.93
N-acetyl-valine	0.64	0.69	1.99×10^{5}	9.35×10^{5}	9.50×10^{-1}	1.18×10^{-1}	1.00	0.96	0.94
norvaline	0.64	0.52	4.20×10^{6}	1.65×10^{7}	2.05×10^{-1}	1.18×10^{-1}	1.00	0.96	0.94
tryptamine	0.64	0.93	3.40×10^{5}	1.68×10^{6}	1.19×10^{-2}	1.18×10^{-1}	1.00	0.96	0.94
myristate	0.64	0.73	3.65×10^{8}	3.05×10^{8}	3.04×10^{-1}	1.18×10^{-1}	1.00	1.00	0.94
Eicosenoate	0.64	0.59	5.55×10^{7}	1.30×10^{8}	7.91×10^{-2}	1.19×10^{-1}	1.00	1.00	0.95
cholesterol	0.64	0.56	3.70×10^{6}	1.35×10^{7}	3.67×10^{-1}	1.20×10^{-1}	1.00	0.98	0.95
3-ureidopropionate	0.64	0.58	6.14×10^{5}	3.25×10^{5}	6.92×10^{-1}	1.24×10^{-1}	1.00	0.95	0.93
diglycerol	0.64	0.60	3.13×10^{6}	1.50×10^{6}	5.17×10^{-1}	1.25×10^{-1}	1.00	0.97	0.95
N-acetylneuraminate	0.64	0.52	4.66×10^{6}	9.65×10^{6}	1.25×10^{-1}	1.25×10^{-1}	1.00	0.96	0.94
Succinyl-carnitine	0.64	0.65	6.00×10^{5}	3.55×10^{6}	8.87×10^{-1}	1.29×10^{-1}	1.00	0.97	0.97
2′-deoxyinosine	0.64	0.76	4.88×10^{6}	7.84×10^{6}	1.69×10^{-1}	1.30×10^{-1}	1.00	0.99	0.97

Table A1. *Cont.*

Metabolite	Week 0 AUROC	Week 18 AUROC	TD Mean Week 0	ASD Mean Week 0	Week 0 vs. Week 18 ASD *p*-Value	Week 0 ASD vs. TD Un-Adjusted *p*-Value	Leave-1-Out	Leave 2-Out	Leave 3-Out
3-aminoisobutyrate	0.64	0.54	2.82×10^5	3.10×10^6	3.41×10^{-1}	1.32×10^{-1}	1.00	0.99	0.96
D-urobilin	0.64	0.54	7.74×10^5	2.68×10^6	6.42×10^{-2}	1.36×10^{-1}	1.00	0.99	0.97
1-methylnicotinamide	0.64	0.68	1.02×10^5	2.95×10^5	5.58×10^{-1}	1.36×10^{-1}	1.00	0.98	0.97
N-acetyl-alanine	0.64	0.58	3.06×10^6	3.98×10^6	3.84×10^{-1}	1.38×10^{-1}	1.00	1.00	0.98
aspartate	0.64	0.54	1.90×10^8	2.44×10^8	1.03×10^{-1}	1.40×10^{-1}	1.00	0.98	0.96
trans-urocanate	0.64	0.50	4.71×10^7	3.96×10^7	1.17×10^{-1}	1.40×10^{-1}	1.00	0.98	0.97
3-carboxyadipate	0.64	0.66	8.99×10^6	1.47×10^7	5.58×10^{-1}	1.40×10^{-1}	1.00	0.98	0.96
1,7-dimethylurate	0.64	0.60	8.91×10^5	2.31×10^6	2.87×10^{-2}	1.40×10^{-1}	1.00	0.98	0.97
2-piperidinone	0.64	0.64	2.17×10^7	3.82×10^7	9.37×10^{-1}	1.40×10^{-1}	1.00	1.00	0.97
pheophorbide	0.64	0.61	4.12×10^6	4.78×10^5	6.94×10^{-1}	1.41×10^{-1}	1.00	1.00	1.00
acisoga	0.63	0.63	3.52×10^5	6.39×10^5	6.92×10^{-1}	1.41×10^{-1}	1.00	1.00	1.00
sulfate	0.63	0.55	6.68×10^6	1.65×10^7	1.10×10^{-1}	1.41×10^{-1}	1.00	1.00	1.00
1-(1-enyl-palmitoyl)-GPE	0.63	0.79	8.53×10^5	7.57×10^5	5.11×10^{-2}	1.41×10^{-1}	0.97	0.96	0.95
histidine	0.63	0.55	9.65×10^7	1.10×10^8	2.00×10^{-1}	1.43×10^{-1}	1.00	1.00	0.97
Maltotetraose	0.63	0.53	5.10×10^5	6.33×10^5	2.66×10^{-1}	1.48×10^{-1}	1.00	1.00	0.98
maltose	0.63	0.63	7.98×10^6	5.18×10^6	9.62×10^{-1}	1.48×10^{-1}	1.00	1.00	0.98
2-methylcitrate/homocitrate	0.63	0.66	6.24×10^5	9.91×10^5	9.87×10^{-1}	1.48×10^{-1}	1.00	0.98	0.97
trimethylamine	0.63	0.55	3.98×10^5	1.53×10^6	3.35×10^{-1}	1.48×10^{-1}	1.00	0.99	0.97
linoleoyl-linolenoyl-glycerol	0.63	0.53	8.05×10^6	2.50×10^6	1.33×10^{-1}	1.48×10^{-1}	1.00	0.99	0.97
thymidine	0.63	0.66	5.10×10^6	7.32×10^6	9.87×10^{-1}	1.52×10^{-1}	1.00	0.98	0.98
Pyri-doxate	0.63	0.52	1.40×10^7	1.76×10^7	1.69×10^{-1}	1.52×10^{-1}	1.00	0.98	0.98
sarcosine	0.63	0.66	2.59×10^5	6.59×10^5	6.12×10^{-1}	1.56×10^{-1}	0.97	0.95	0.94
2-hydroxy-3-methylvalerate	0.63	0.54	1.27×10^6	1.74×10^6	5.06×10^{-1}	1.56×10^{-1}	1.00	0.99	0.98
gamma-glutamyl-phenylalanine	0.63	0.61	2.27×10^5	2.94×10^5	9.50×10^{-1}	1.56×10^{-1}	1.00	0.99	0.98
Linolenate	0.63	0.59	1.98×10^8	9.80×10^7	9.87×10^{-1}	1.56×10^{-1}	1.00	0.98	0.97
3-hydroxy-3-methylglutarate	0.63	0.59	1.40×10^7	1.99×10^7	5.17×10^{-1}	1.56×10^{-1}	1.00	0.98	0.97
2′-deoxyuridine	0.63	0.69	2.81×10^6	3.79×10^6	6.46×10^{-1}	1.56×10^{-1}	1.00	1.00	0.98

Table A1. *Cont.*

Metabolite	Week 0 AUROC	Week 18 AUROC	TD Mean Week 0	ASD Mean Week 0	Week 0 vs. Week 18 ASD p-Value	Week 0 ASD vs. TD Un-Adjusted p-Value	Leave-1-Out	Leave 2-Out	Leave 3-Out
Quino-linate	0.63	0.52	4.89×10^{4}	$1.[illegible]5 \times 10^{5}$	9.77×10^{-2}	1.57×10^{-1}	1.00	1.00	0.98
I-urobilinogen	0.63	0.60	1.77×10^{6}	1.02×10^{7}	3.91×10^{-2}	1.65×10^{-1}	1.00	1.00	0.98
N-acetyl-cadaverine	0.63	0.61	4.95×10^{7}	1.14×10^{8}	7.64×10^{-1}	1.65×10^{-1}	1.00	1.00	0.99
7-ketolithocholate	0.63	0.51	4.53×10^{6}	1.32×10^{6}	1.92×10^{-1}	1.69×10^{-1}	1.00	1.00	0.98
Carboxy-ibuprofen	0.63	0.53	1.47×10^{6}	1.75×10^{4}	1.48×10^{-1}	1.74×10^{-1}	1.00	0.99	0.98
Phenyl-lactate	0.62	0.57	1.83×10^{6}	1.83×10^{6}	4.13×10^{-2}	1.74×10^{-1}	1.00	0.99	0.98
kynurenate	0.62	0.59	1.30×10^{6}	9.03×10^{5}	9.05×10^{-2}	1.74×10^{-1}	1.00	0.99	0.98
citrate	0.62	0.58	1.29×10^{6}	2.64×10^{6}	5.91×10^{-1}	1.74×10^{-1}	1.00	1.00	0.99
5alpha-androstan-3beta,17beta-diol	0.62	0.53	1.85×10^{5}	7.81×10^{4}	1.06×10^{-1}	1.74×10^{-1}	1.00	1.00	0.99
Octadecane-dioate	0.62	0.66	1.10×10^{6}	8.50×10^{5}	2.67×10^{-2}	1.74×10^{-1}	1.00	0.99	0.98
Oleoyl-carnitine	0.62	0.54	4.89×10^{5}	4.10×10^{6}	1.35×10^{-1}	1.74×10^{-1}	1.00	0.99	0.98
4-androsten-3alpha,17alpha-diol	0.62	0.50	2.30×10^{5}	7.59×10^{4}	2.02×10^{-1}	1.83×10^{-1}	1.00	1.00	0.99
8-hydroxyguanine	0.62	0.55	1.15×10^{5}	1.50×10^{5}	1.58×10^{-1}	1.83×10^{-1}	1.00	1.00	0.98
skatol	0.62	0.50	5.08×10^{5}	3.95×10^{5}	1.71×10^{-1}	1.83×10^{-1}	1.00	1.00	0.99
Ethyl-malonate	0.62	0.66	5.50×10^{6}	6.23×10^{6}	4.20×10^{-1}	1.83×10^{-1}	1.00	1.00	0.99
lactate	0.62	0.52	2.39×10^{6}	3.29×10^{6}	1.41×10^{-1}	1.83×10^{-1}	1.00	1.00	0.99
N6-carboxymethyllysine	0.62	0.60	2.90×10^{6}	$3.6[illegible] \times 10^{6}$	5.37×10^{-1}	1.86×10^{-1}	1.00	1.00	1.00
Nervonate	0.62	0.53	6.63×10^{6}	$1.6[illegible] \times 10^{7}$	3.67×10^{-1}	1.86×10^{-1}	1.00	1.00	1.00
inosine	0.62	0.57	3.45×10^{6}	$6.3[illegible] \times 10^{6}$	7.16×10^{-1}	1.86×10^{-1}	1.00	1.00	0.99
Docosapentaenoate	0.61	0.55	3.98×10^{6}	1.35×10^{7}	7.90×10^{-2}	1.89×10^{-1}	1.00	1.00	0.99
Acetyl-carnitine	0.61	0.54	7.50×10^{5}	$8.0[illegible] \times 10^{6}$	4.77×10^{-1}	1.89×10^{-1}	1.00	1.00	0.98
N-methyl-GABA	0.61	0.59	5.35×10^{6}	$6.3[illegible] \times 10^{6}$	9.35×10^{-1}	1.93×10^{-1}	1.00	1.00	0.99
2-aminoadipate	0.61	0.66	1.11×10^{6}	1.27×10^{6}	7.40×10^{-1}	1.95×10^{-1}	1.00	1.00	0.99
N-methyl-phenylalanine	0.61	0.57	1.65×10^{6}	1.25×10^{6}	7.38×10^{-2}	1.95×10^{-1}	1.00	1.00	0.99
cystine	0.61	0.59	8.29×10^{4}	1.14×10^{5}	9.49×10^{-3}	1.98×10^{-1}	1.00	1.00	1.00
3-hydroxystearate	0.61	0.54	6.21×10^{6}	4.61×10^{6}	7.88×10^{-1}	2.00×10^{-1}	1.00	1.00	0.99
gluconate	0.61	0.51	1.08×10^{6}	3.21×10^{6}	6.90×10^{-1}	2.02×10^{-1}	1.00	1.00	1.00
diacylglycerol	0.61	0.51	6.93×10^{5}	2.55×10^{5}	3.02×10^{-1}	2.03×10^{-1}	1.00	1.00	0.99
dipicolinate	0.61	0.51	4.99×10^{5}	4.94×10^{5}	2.46×10^{-1}	2.03×10^{-1}	1.00	1.00	0.99
quinate	0.61	0.61	9.58×10^{6}	2.75×10^{7}	9.37×10^{-1}	2.03×10^{-1}	1.00	1.00	0.99

Table A1. *Cont.*

Metabolite	Week 0 AUROC	Week 18 AUROC	TD Mean Week 0	ASD Mean Week 0	Week 0 vs. Week 18 ASD *p*-Value	Week 0 ASD vs. TD Un-Adjusted *p*-Value	Leave-1-Out	Leave 2-Out	Leave 3-Out
O-acetyl-homoserine	0.61	0.52	4.56×10^5	3.96×10^5	4.20×10^{-1}	2.14×10^{-1}	1.00	1.00	0.99
glutamate,	0.61	0.51	2.42×10^6	2.03×10^6	2.75×10^{-1}	2.14×10^{-1}	1.00	1.00	0.99
6-hydroxynicotinate	0.61	0.58	1.82×10^6	8.38×10^5	3.67×10^{-1}	2.18×10^{-1}	1.00	1.00	1.00
pyridoxine	0.61	0.61	1.57×10^6	2.91×10^6	5.47×10^{-2}	2.18×10^{-1}	1.00	1.00	1.00
2,4,6-trihydroxybenzoate	0.61	0.55	3.58×10^4	5.36×10^5	6.48×10^{-1}	2.20×10^{-1}	1.00	1.00	1.00
theophylline	0.61	0.57	1.46×10^5	8.09×10^4	6.37×10^{-1}	2.21×10^{-1}	1.00	1.00	1.00
1-methylimidazoleacetate	0.61	0.53	2.51×10^6	2.47×10^6	1.17×10^{-1}	2.21×10^{-1}	1.00	1.00	1.00
1-methylhistamine	0.61	0.55	1.63×10^5	5.62×10^5	4.69×10^{-1}	2.25×10^{-1}	1.00	1.00	0.99
phenylacetate	0.61	0.58	1.69×10^7	2.48×10^7	7.16×10^{-1}	2.25×10^{-1}	1.00	1.00	0.99
4-hydroxyphenylpyruvate	0.61	0.57	5.26×10^5	5.38×10^5	6.69×10^{-1}	2.25×10^{-1}	1.00	1.00	1.00
cysteine	0.61	0.61	3.35×10^6	4.04×10^6	8.62×10^{-1}	2.25×10^{-1}	1.00	1.00	1.00
N-acetylcysteine	0.61	0.51	3.09×10^5	3.95×10^5	2.23×10^{-1}	2.25×10^{-1}	1.00	1.00	0.99
13-methylmyristate	0.61	0.72	3.09×10^5	3.95×10^5	2.89×10^{-1}	2.27×10^{-1}	1.00	1.00	1.00
AMP	0.61	0.52	3.56×10^8	3.17×10^8	2.44×10^{-1}	2.29×10^{-1}	1.00	1.00	1.00
2′-deoxyguanosine	0.61	0.75	1.20×10^5	5.63×10^4	1.79×10^{-1}	2.36×10^{-1}	1.00	1.00	1.00
5-methyluridine	0.61	0.64	2.32×10^6	3.59×10^6	8.62×10^{-1}	2.36×10^{-1}	1.00	1.00	1.00
1,3-dimethylurate	0.61	0.58	7.67×10^5	9.16×10^5	5.20×10^{-2}	2.36×10^{-1}	1.00	1.00	1.00
adrenate	0.60	0.64	3.54×10^4	2.94×10^4	9.61×10^{-1}	2.45×10^{-1}	1.00	1.00	0.99
tryptophan	0.60	0.51	1.44×10^7	1.86×10^7	3.67×10^{-1}	2.47×10^{-1}	1.00	1.00	1.00
dimethylarginine	0.60	0.52	2.18×10^6	6.82×10^5	4.77×10^{-1}	2.47×10^{-1}	1.00	1.00	1.00
4-acetamidobutanoate	0.60	0.50	7.64×10^7	8.86×10^7	3.34×10^{-1}	2.47×10^{-1}	1.00	1.00	1.00
gamma-glutamyl-glutamine	0.60	0.52	3.61×10^6	5.50×10^6	3.51×10^{-1}	2.48×10^{-1}	1.00	1.00	1.00
caproate	0.60	0.72	1.31×10^6	1.72×10^6	1.83×10^{-3}	2.48×10^{-1}	1.00	1.00	1.00
4-methylcatechol	0.60	0.54	1.41×10^6	1.44×10^6	5.61×10^{-1}	2.48×10^{-1}	1.00	1.00	1.00
nicotiana-amine	0.60	0.55	3.44×10^7	3.48×10^7	9.67×10^{-2}	2.54×10^{-1}	1.00	1.00	0.99
1,3-propanediol	0.60	0.56	3.19×10^4	8.27×10^4	5.73×10^{-1}	2.58×10^{-1}	1.00	1.00	1.00
N-acetylserine	0.60	0.59	1.87×10^6	1.07×10^6	6.42×10^{-2}	2.59×10^{-1}	1.00	1.00	1.00
erythronate	0.60	0.64	9.27×10^4	4.29×10^5	4.38×10^{-1}	2.60×10^{-1}	1.00	1.00	1.00
1-palmitoyl-GPE	0.60	0.64	2.07×10^6	3.41×10^6	6.92×10^{-1}	2.60×10^{-1}	1.00	1.00	1.00
4-androsten-3beta,17beta-diol	0.60	0.61	3.81×10^6	5.96×10^6	6.02×10^{-1}	2.60×10^{-1}	1.00	1.00	1.00

References

1. Maenner, M.J.; Shaw, K.A.; Baio, J.; Washington, A.; Patrick, M.; DiRienzo, M.; Christensen, D.L.; Wiggins, L.D.; Pettygrove, S.; Andrews, J.G. Prevalence of Autism Spectrum Disorder Among Children Aged 8 Years—Autism and Developmental Disabilities Monitoring Network—Autism and Developmental Disabilities Monitoring Network, 11 Sites, United States, 2016. *MMWR. Morb. Mortal. Wkly. Rep. Surveill. Summ.* **2020**, *69*, 1–12. [CrossRef] [PubMed]
2. Gaugler, T.L.; Klei, L.; Sanders, S.J.; Bodea, C.A.; Goldberg, A.P.; Lee, A.B.; Mahajan, M.; Manaa, D.; Pawitan, Y.; Reichert, J.; et al. Most genetic risk for autism resides with common variation. *Nat. Genet.* **2014**, *46*, 881–885. [CrossRef] [PubMed]
3. Mandy, W.; Lai, M.-C. Annual Research Review: The role of the environment in the developmental psychopathology of autism spectrum condition. *J. Child Psychol. Psychiatry* **2016**, *57*, 271–292. [CrossRef] [PubMed]
4. Meltzer, A.; Van De Water, J. The Role of the Immune System in Autism Spectrum Disorder. *Neuropsychopharmacology* **2016**, *42*, 284–298. [CrossRef] [PubMed]
5. Hsiao, E.Y. Gastrointestinal Issues in Autism Spectrum Disorder. *Harv. Rev. Psych.* **2014**, *22*, 104–111. [CrossRef] [PubMed]
6. Frye, R.E.; Rose, S.; Slattery, J.; Macfabe, D.F. Gastrointestinal dysfunction in autism spectrum disorder: The role of the mitochondria and the enteric microbiome. *Microb. Ecol. Heal. Dis.* **2015**, *26*, 27458. [CrossRef]
7. Gorkiewicz, G.; Moschen, A.R. Gut microbiome: A new player in gastrointestinal disease. *Virchows Arch.* **2017**, *472*, 159–172. [CrossRef]
8. Hills, J.R.D.; Pontefract, B.A.; Mishcon, H.R.; Black, C.A.; Sutton, S.C.; Theberge, C.R. Gut Microbiome: Profound Implications for Diet and Disease. *Nutrition* **2019**, *11*, 1613. [CrossRef]
9. Abreu, M.T.; Peek, R.M. Gastrointestinal Malignancy and the Microbiome. *Gastroenterol.* **2014**, *146*, 1534–1546.e3. [CrossRef]
10. Hughes, H.K.; Rose, D.; Ashwood, P. The Gut Microbiota and Dysbiosis in Autism Spectrum Disorders. *Curr. Neurol. Neurosci. Rep.* **2018**, *18*, 81. [CrossRef]
11. Vuong, H.E.; Hsiao, E. Emerging Roles for the Gut Microbiome in Autism Spectrum Disorder. *Boil. Psych.* **2016**, *81*, 411–423. [CrossRef] [PubMed]
12. Kang, D.-W.; Park, J.G.; Ilhan, Z.E.; Wallstrom, G.; LaBaer, J.; Adams, J.B.; Krajmalnik-Brown, R. Reduced Incidence of Prevotella and Other Fermenters in Intestinal Microflora of Autistic Children. *PLoS ONE* **2013**, *8*, e68322. [CrossRef] [PubMed]
13. Li, Q.; Han, Y.; Dy, A.B.C.; Hagerman, R.J. The Gut Microbiota and Autism Spectrum Disorders. *Front. Cell. Neurosci.* **2017**, *11*, 11. [CrossRef] [PubMed]
14. Needham, B.D.; Adame, M.D.; Serena, G.; Rose, D.R.; Preston, G.M.; Conrad, M.C.; Campbell, A.S.; Donabedian, D.H.; Fasano, A.; Ashwood, P.; et al. Plasma and Fecal Metabolite Profiles in Autism Spectrum Disorder. In *Plasma and Fecal Metabolite Profiles in Autism Spectrum Disorder. BioRxiv 2020*; Cold Spring Harbor Laboratory: Cold Spring Harbor, NY, USA, 2020.
15. Mohamadkhani, A. Gut Microbiota and Fecal Metabolome Perturbation in Children with Autism Spectrum Disorder. *Midd. East J. Dig. Dis.* **2018**, *10*, 205–212. [CrossRef]
16. Kang, D.-W.; Ilhan, Z.E.; Isern, N.G.; Hoyt, D.W.; Howsmon, D.P.; Shaffer, M.; Lozupone, C.; Hahn, J.; Adams, J.B.; Krajmalnik-Brown, R. Differences in fecal microbial metabolites and microbiota of children with autism spectrum disorders. *Anaerobe* **2018**, *49*, 121–131. [CrossRef]
17. De Angelis, M.; Piccolo, M.; Vannini, L.; Siragusa, S.; De Giacomo, A.; Serrazzanetti, D.I.; Cristofori, F.; Guerzoni, M.E.; Gobbetti, M.; Francavilla, R. Fecal Microbiota and Metabolome of Children with Autism and Pervasive Developmental Disorder Not Otherwise Specified. *PLoS ONE* **2013**, *8*, e76993. [CrossRef]
18. Wang, H.; Liang, S.; Wang, M.; Gao, J.; Sun, C.; Wang, J.; Xia, W.; Wu, S.; Sumner, S.J.; Zhang, F.; et al. Potential serum biomarkers from a metabolomics study of autism. *J. Psych. Neurosci.* **2016**, *41*, 27–37. [CrossRef]
19. Berding, K.; Donovan, S.M. Diet Can Impact Microbiota Composition in Children with Autism Spectrum Disorder. *Front. Neurosci.* **2018**, *12*, 515. [CrossRef]
20. Coretti, L.; Paparo, L.; Riccio, M.P.; Amato, F.; Cuomo, M.; Natale, A.; Borrelli, L.; Corrado, G.; De Caro, C.; Comegna, M.; et al. Gut Microbiota Features in Young Children With Autism Spectrum Disorders. *Front. Microbiol.* **2018**, *9*, 3146. [CrossRef]

21. Adams, J.B.; Johansen, L.J.; Powell, L.D.; Quig, D.W.; Rubin, R.A. Gastrointestinal flora and gastrointestinal status in children with autism—Comparisons to typical children and correlation with autism severity. *BMC Gastroenterol.* **2011**, *11*, 22. [CrossRef]
22. Liu, S.; Li, E.; Sun, Z.; Fu, D.; Duan, G.; Jiang, M.; Yu, Y.; Mei, L.; Yang, P.; Tang, Y.; et al. Altered gut microbiota and short chain fatty acids in Chinese children with autism spectrum disorder. *Sci. Rep.* **2019**, *9*, 287. [CrossRef] [PubMed]
23. Wang, J.; Pan, J.; Chen, H.; Li, Y.; Amakye, W.K.; Liang, J.; Ma, B.; Chu, X.; Mao, L.; Zhang, Z. Fecal Short-Chain Fatty Acids Levels Were Not Associated With Autism Spectrum Disorders in Chinese Children: A Case–Control Study. *Front. Neurosci.* **2019**, *13*, 1216. [CrossRef] [PubMed]
24. Sharon, G.; Cruz, N.J.; Kang, D.-W.; Gandal, M.J.; Wang, B.; Kim, Y.-M.; Zink, E.M.; Casey, C.P.; Taylor, B.C.; Lane, C.J.; et al. Human Gut Microbiota from Autism Spectrum Disorder Promote Behavioral Symptoms in Mice. *Cell* **2019**, *177*, 1600–1618.e17. [CrossRef] [PubMed]
25. Kang, D.-W.; Adams, J.B.; Gregory, A.C.; Borody, T.J.; Chittick, L.; Fasano, A.; Khoruts, A.; Geis, E.; Maldonado, J.; McDonough-Means, S.; et al. Microbiota Transfer Therapy alters gut ecosystem and improves gastrointestinal and autism symptoms: An open-label study. *Microbiome* **2017**, *5*, 10. [CrossRef] [PubMed]
26. Kang, D.-W.; Adams, J.B.; Coleman, D.M.; Pollard, E.L.; Maldonado, J.; McDonough-Means, S.; Caporaso, J.G.; Krajmalnik-Brown, R. Long-term benefit of Microbiota Transfer Therapy on autism symptoms and gut microbiota. *Sci. Rep.* **2019**, *9*, 5821. [CrossRef] [PubMed]
27. Grimaldi, R.; Gibson, G.R.; Vulevic, J.; Giallourou, N.; Castro-Mejía, J.; Hansen, L.H.; Gibson, E.L.; Nielsen, D.S.; Costabile, A. A prebiotic intervention study in children with autism spectrum disorders (ASDs). *Microbiome* **2018**, *6*, 133. [CrossRef]
28. Wang, Y.; Li, N.; Yang, J.-J.; Zhao, D.-M.; Chen, B.; Zhang, G.-Q.; Chen, S.; Cao, R.-F.; Yu, H.; Zhao, C.-Y.; et al. Probiotics and fructo-oligosaccharide intervention modulate the microbiota-gut brain axis to improve autism spectrum reducing also the hyper-serotonergic state and the dopamine metabolism disorder. *Pharmacol. Res.* **2020**, *157*, 104784. [CrossRef]
29. Adams, J.B.; Vargason, T.; Kang, D.-W.; Krajmalnik-Brown, R.; Hahn, J. Multivariate Analysis of Plasma Metabolites in Children with Autism Spectrum Disorder and Gastrointestinal Symptoms Before and After Microbiota Transfer Therapy. *Processes* **2019**, *7*, 806. [CrossRef]
30. Kang, D.; Adams, J.; Vargason, T.; Santiago, M.; Hahn, J.; Krajmalnik-Brown, R. Distinct fecal and plasma metabolites in children with Autism Spectrum Disorders and their modulation after microbiota transfer therapy. *mShere* **2020**, in press.
31. Long, T.; Hicks, M.A.; Yu, H.-C.; Biggs, W.H.; Kirkness, E.F.; Menni, C.; Zierer, J.; Small, K.S.; Mangino, M.; Messier, H.; et al. Whole-genome sequencing identifies common-to-rare variants associated with human blood metabolites. *Nat. Genet.* **2017**, *49*, 568–578. [CrossRef]
32. Fisher, R.A. The use of multiple measurements in taxonomic problems. *Ann. Eugen.* **1936**, *7*, 179–188. [CrossRef]
33. Cawley, G.C.; Talbot, N.L. Efficient leave-one-out cross-validation of kernel fisher discriminant classifiers. *Pattern Recognit.* **2003**, *36*, 2585–2592. [CrossRef]
34. Loftfield, E.; Vogtmann, E.; Sampson, J.N.; Moore, S.C.; Nelson, H.; Knight, R.; Chia, N.; Sinha, R. Comparison of Collection Methods for Fecal Samples for Discovery Metabolomics in Epidemiologic Studies. *Cancer Epidem. Biomark. Prev.* **2016**, *25*, 1483–1490. [CrossRef] [PubMed]
35. Linden, A. Measuring diagnostic and predictive accuracy in disease management: An introduction to receiver operating characteristic (ROC) analysis. *J. Eval. Clin. Pract.* **2006**, *12*, 132–139. [CrossRef] [PubMed]
36. Demarquoy, C.; Demarquoy, J. Autism and carnitine: A possible link. *World J. Boil. Chem.* **2019**, *10*, 7–16. [CrossRef]
37. Bryan, P.-F.; Carvajal, K.; Alejandro, M.-T.E.; Elva, E.-P.S.; Gemma, F.; Luz, C. Sphingolipids as Mediators in the Crosstalk between Microbiota and Intestinal Cells: Implications for Inflammatory Bowel Disease. *Mediat. Inflamm.* **2016**, *2016*, 1–11. [CrossRef]
38. Zierer, J.; Jackson, M.A.; Kastenmüller, G.; Mangino, M.; Long, T.; Telenti, A.; Mohney, R.P.; Small, K.S.; Bell, J.T.; Steves, C.J.; et al. The fecal metabolome as a functional readout of the gut microbiome. *Nat. Genet.* **2018**, *50*, 790–795. [CrossRef]
39. Gu, L.; Gonzalez, F.J.; Kalow, W.; Tang, B.K. Biotransformation of caffeine, paraxanthine, theobromine and theophylline by cDNA-expressed human CYP1A2 and CYP2E1. *Pharmacogenetics* **1992**, *2*, 73–77. [CrossRef]

40. James, S.J.; Cutler, P.; Melnyk, S.; Jernigan, S.; Janak, L.; Gaylor, D.W.; Neubrander, J.A. Metabolic biomarkers of increased oxidative stress and impaired methylation capacity in children with autism. *Am. J. Clin. Nutr.* **2004**, *80*, 1611–1617. [CrossRef]
41. Vargason, T.; Kruger, U.; McGuinness, D.L.; Adams, J.B.; Geis, E.; Gehn, E.; Coleman, D.; Hahn, J. Investigating plasma amino acids for differentiating individuals with autism spectrum disorder and typically developing peers. *Res. Autism Spectr. Disord.* **2018**, *50*, 60–72. [CrossRef]
42. Agus, A.; Planchais, J.; Sokol, H. Gut Microbiota Regulation of Tryptophan Metabolism in Health and Disease. *Cell Host Microbe* **2018**, *23*, 716–724. [CrossRef] [PubMed]
43. Gevi, F.; Zolla, L.; Gabriele, S.; Persico, A.M. Urinary metabolomics of young Italian autistic children supports abnormal tryptophan and purine metabolism. *Mol. Autism* **2016**, *7*, 47. [CrossRef]
44. Wang, M.; Wan, J.; Rong, H.; He, F.; Wang, H.; Zhou, J.; Cai, C.; Wang, Y.; Xu, R.; Yin, Z.; et al. Alterations in Gut Glutamate Metabolism Associated with Changes in Gut Microbiota Composition in Children with Autism Spectrum Disorder. *mSystems* **2019**, *4*, e00321-18. [CrossRef] [PubMed]
45. Lee, I. Betaine is a positive regulator of mitochondrial respiration. *Biochem. Biophys. Res. Commun.* **2015**, *456*, 621–625. [CrossRef] [PubMed]
46. Palmieri, L.; Papaleo, V.; Porcelli, V.; Scarcia, P.; Gaita, L.; Sacco, R.; Hager, J.; Rousseau, F.; Curatolo, P.; Manzi, B.; et al. Altered calcium homeostasis in autism-spectrum disorders: Evidence from biochemical and genetic studies of the mitochondrial aspartate/glutamate carrier AGC1. *Mol. Psychiatry* **2008**, *15*, 38–52. [CrossRef]
47. Frye, R.E.; Melnyk, S.; Macfabe, D.F. Unique acyl-carnitine profiles are potential biomarkers for acquired mitochondrial disease in autism spectrum disorder. *Transl. Psychiatry* **2013**, *3*, e220. [CrossRef]
48. Frye, R.E. Mitochondrial Dysfunction in Autism Spectrum Disorder: Unique Abnormalities and Targeted Treatments. *Semin. Pediatr. Neurol.* **2020**, *35*, 100829. [CrossRef]
49. Frye, R.E.; Rossignol, D.A. Mitochondrial Dysfunction Can Connect the Diverse Medical Symptoms Associated with Autism Spectrum Disorders. *Pediatr. Res.* **2011**, *69*, 41–47. [CrossRef]
50. Orozco, J.S.; Hertz-Picciotto, I.; Abbeduto, L.; Slupsky, C.M. Metabolomics analysis of children with autism, idiopathic-developmental delays, and Down syndrome. *Transl. Psychiatry* **2019**, *9*, 243. [CrossRef]
51. Karu, N.; Deng, L.; Slae, M.; Guo, A.C.; Sajed, T.; Huynh, H.; Wine, E.; Wishart, D.S. A review on human fecal metabolomics: Methods, applications and the human fecal metabolome database. *Anal. Chim. Acta* **2018**, *1030*, 1–24. [CrossRef]
52. Ousley, O.; Cermak, T. Autism Spectrum Disorder: Defining Dimensions and Subgroups. *Curr. Dev. Disord. Rep.* **2013**, *1*, 20–28. [CrossRef] [PubMed]
53. Sacco, R.; Lenti, C.; Saccani, M.; Curatolo, P.; Manzi, B.; Bravaccio, C.; Persico, A.M. Cluster Analysis of Autistic Patients Based on Principal Pathogenetic Components. *Autism Res.* **2012**, *5*, 137–147. [CrossRef] [PubMed]

© 2020 by the authors. Licensee MDPI, Basel, Switzerland. This article is an open access article distributed under the terms and conditions of the Creative Commons Attribution (CC BY) license (http://creativecommons.org/licenses/by/4.0/).

Journal of *Personalized Medicine*

MDPI

Review

Mitochondria May Mediate Prenatal Environmental Influences in Autism Spectrum Disorder

Richard E. Frye [1,*], Janet Cakir [2], Shannon Rose [3], Raymond F. Palmer [4], Christine Austin [5], Paul Curtin [5] and Manish Arora [5]

1 Barrow Neurological Institute at Phoenix Children's Hospital, Phoenix, AZ 85016, USA
2 Department of Applied Ecology, North Carolina State University, Raleigh, NC 27695, USA; Janet_Cakir@nps.gov
3 Department of Pediatrics, Arkansas Children's Research Institute, University of Arkansas for Medical Sciences, Little Rock, AR 72202, USA; SROSE@uams.edu
4 Department of Family and Community Medicine, University of Texas Health Science Center, San Antonio, TX 78229, USA; palmerr@uthscsa.edu
5 Department of Environmental Medicine and Public Health, Icahn School of Medicine at Mount Sinai, New York, NY 10029, USA; christine.autsin@mssm.edu (C.A.); paul.curtin@mssm.edu (P.C.); manish.arora@mssm.edu (M.A.)
* Correspondence: rfrye@phoenixchildrens.com; Tel.: +1-602-933-1100

Abstract: We propose that the mitochondrion, an essential cellular organelle, mediates the long-term prenatal environmental effects of disease in autism spectrum disorder (ASD). Many prenatal environmental factors which increase the risk of developing ASD influence mitochondria physiology, including toxicant exposures, immune activation, and nutritional factors. Unique types of mitochondrial dysfunction have been associated with ASD and recent studies have linked prenatal environmental exposures to long-term changes in mitochondrial physiology in children with ASD. A better understanding of the role of the mitochondria in the etiology of ASD can lead to targeted therapeutics and strategies to potentially prevent the development of ASD.

Keywords: autism spectrum disorder; mitochondria; oxidative stress; prenatal environment; immune dysfunction

Citation: Frye, R.E.; Cakir, J.; Rose, S.; Palmer, R.F.; Austin, C.; Curtin, P.; Arora, M. Mitochondria May Mediate Prenatal Environmental Influences in Autism Spectrum Disorder. *J. Pers. Med.* **2021**, *11*, 218. https://doi.org/10.3390/jpm11030218

Academic Editor: Guido Krenning

Received: 5 February 2021
Accepted: 17 March 2021
Published: 18 March 2021

Publisher's Note: MDPI stays neutral with regard to jurisdictional claims in published maps and institutional affiliations.

Copyright: © 2021 by the authors. Licensee MDPI, Basel, Switzerland. This article is an open access article distributed under the terms and conditions of the Creative Commons Attribution (CC BY) license (https://creativecommons.org/licenses/by/4.0/).

1. Introduction

Autism spectrum disorder (ASD) is a behaviorally defined disorder [1], with the most recent Center for Disease Control and Prevention estimates suggesting that it affects 1 in 54 children in the United States [2]. Recent studies suggest that inherited single-gene and chromosomal defects account for a minority of ASD cases [3], and that ASD most likely arises from a complicated interaction between genetic predisposition and environmental exposures [4,5]. Given the high recurrent risk in siblings, the prenatal maternal environment has undergone careful study with many prenatal risk factors identified [6,7]. Despite the epidemiological connection between many prenatal risk factors and the development of ASD, the biological mechanisms which link prenatal environmental influences and the increased risk of developing ASD are just beginning to be uncovered.

Three physiological abnormalities which have been increasingly recognized to be associated with ASD are immune system dysfunction, mitochondrial dysfunction, and oxidative stress and redox regulation [1]. Previous reviews examining prenatal physiological abnormalities related to ASD have concentrated on prenatal immune stressors as key and consider mitochondrial dysfunction and oxidative stress to have secondary roles of this "Bad Trio" [8]. In contrast, the current review concentrates on the mitochondria as the central player. Of course, the particular component of the "Bad Trio" that is the initiating culprit may be different for different patients and it is possible that multiple stressors on the various portions of the "Bad Trio" simultaneously may also initiate the pathway to disease.

2. The Mitochondria: Dysfunction Can Be Self-Perpetuating

Mitochondria are essential for a wide range of functions in almost every cell in our body (Figure 1). Best known for their role in the production of adenosine triphosphate (ATP) by oxidative phosphorylation, mitochondria are intimately involved in other cellular functions such as redox metabolism, calcium buffering, lipid homeostasis, and steroid synthesis [9–13]. Mitochondria also have a role in important non-energy-producing metabolic pathways, such as the urea cycle, amino acid and porphyrin production, and as a pathway for the activation of apoptosis. Mitochondria also have important roles in cell signaling, most notably being an essential part of the inflammasome, a complex that initiates immune activation, by releasing damage-associated molecular pattern (DAMP) molecules such as cardiolipin, n-formyl peptides, reactive oxygen species (ROS), and mitochondrial DNA (mtDNA) [14]. Lastly, normal mitochondrial function results in the production of ROS, which can cause cellular injury if not controlled.

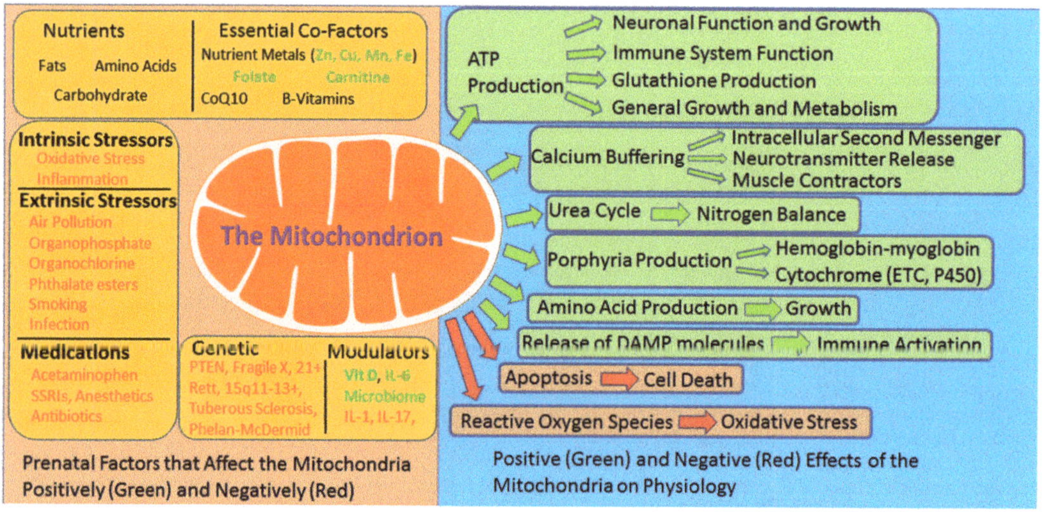

Figure 1. The mitochondria can be negatively affected by many environmental and biological factors associated with autism spectrum disorder (left orange panel) and has many critical roles in cellular physiology (right blue panel). ETC: electron transport chain; DAMP: damage-associated molecular pattern

Since ATP produced by mitochondria is essential for many cellular systems, abnormal mitochondrial function can disproportionally adversely affect cellular physiology. However, there are several pathways in which abnormal mitochondrial function can result in a self-perpetuating destructive cycle causing sustained pathophysiology. Most notably, interactions between mitochondria, redox metabolism, and the immune system can be mutually detrimental; such detrimental interactions have been documented in ASD (Figure 2) [15].

Mitochondria are both a major producer and target of ROS. Dysfunctional mitochondria produce high amounts of ROS which can result in dysfunction of the electron transport chain (ETC) enzymes, particularly complex I and III, as well as aconitase, the first enzyme in the citric acid cycle (CAC). To compound this problem, reduced glutathione (GSH), the main intracellular and mitochondrial antioxidant, requires ATP for its *de novo* production. As such, a decrease in ATP production resulting from reduced mitochondrial function will result in lower GSH production, resulting in poorer control of ROS. In fact, a lower GSH redox ratio has been correlated with lower aconitase activity in post-mortem brain from individuals with ASD [16]. Oxidative damage to cellular lipids, proteins, and nucleic acids [17] has been associated with ASD; this is especially important since mtDNA is vulnerable to oxidative damage, and studies have shown that children with ASD demonstrated mtDNA damage in a pattern consistent with oxidative damage [18].

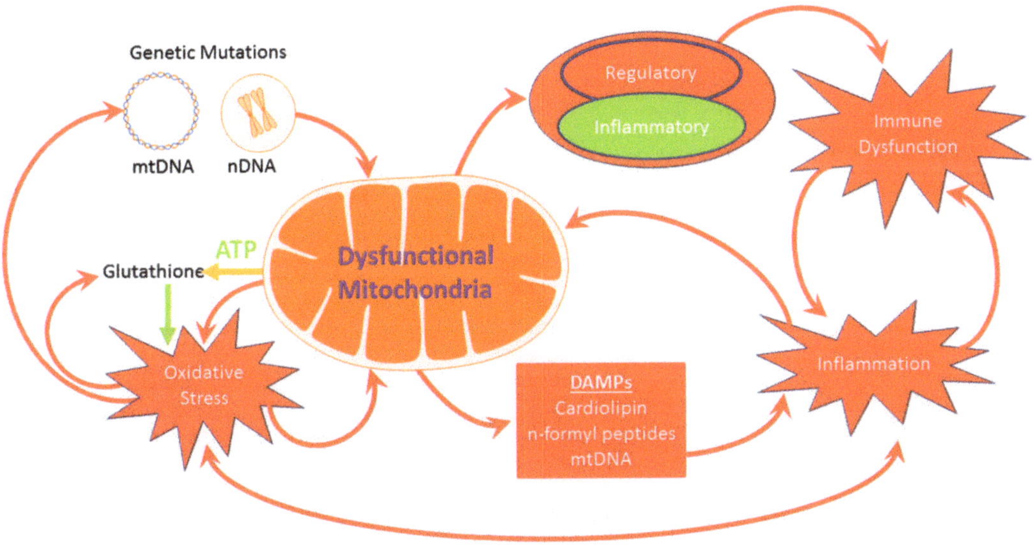

Figure 2. Self-perpetuating destructive cycles which can result in mitochondrial dysfunction.

There are several pathways in which dysfunctional mitochondria can cause a wide variety of abnormalities in immune system function. First, cellular damage due to oxidative stress can activate inflammatory pathways [15,16]. Second, as an essential part of the inflammasome, mitochondria release DAMP molecules such as cardiolipin, n-formyl peptides, ROS, and mtDNA [14]. Third, regulatory immune cells are highly dependent on ATP derived from mitochondrial oxidative phosphorylation, while inflammatory cells are highly glycolytic [19]. Thus, once an immune response has been started, the inflammatory response may be difficult to regulate if mitochondrial dysfunction exists. Fourth, inflammation and immune activation upregulate metabolism and recruit physiological processes, but without mitochondrial support, such resources will not be available. Lastly, the immune system produces ROS as a defense mechanism against potential invaders. Such increases in ROS can result in a further detrimental effect on already dysfunctional mitochondria. In fact, mitochondria appear to have a particularly important role in innate immunity [20], which is an area of immune dysfunction that is implicated in ASD. In addition, an increase in proinflammatory cytokine production has been associated with mitochondrial dysfunction in a subset of children with ASD [21].

3. Prenatal Risk Factors for ASD Modulate Mitochondrial Function

Many prenatal factors associated with an increased risk of ASD are associated with mitochondrial dysfunction; these include nutritional agents, both intrinsic and extrinsic stressors, common medications given during pregnancy, modulators of mitochondrial function, and genetic conditions which might affect the fetus (Figure 1).

Folate is an essential vitamin which is well-known to be important during pregnancy to prevent neural tube defects. Folate is also an essential co-factor for adequate mitochondrial function [22]. Several studies have demonstrated that folate supplementation during pregnancy reduces the risk of ASD. Abnormalities in the folate pathway are associated with ASD, including maternal polymorphisms in the reduced folate carrier [23]. Further, mothers of children with ASD have been shown to have the folate receptor alpha autoantibody [24], an abnormality that prevents folate transport across the placenta, resulting in an ASD phenotype in an animal model [25].

Abnormalities in several nutrient metals have been linked to an increased risk of ASD. Studies have associated an increased risk of ASD with atypical pre- and postnatal Zn and Cu metabolism [26] and found that atypical levels of essential (Zn, Mn) and non-essential (Pb) metals during prenatal development and early life in individuals with ASD are associated with long-term physiological and developmental alternations [27]. Studies have associated low maternal iron (Fe) with increased ASD risk [28]. Prenatal Zn and Cu are essential for the function of the cytoplasmic superoxide dismutase (SOD) which is essential for controlling cellular oxidative stress, while Cu is essential for ETC complex IV function. Mn is essential for mitochondrial SOD function, and Fe is an essential component of cytochromes, which are critical components of the ETC.

Carnitine is an essential nutrient for mitochondrial function and fatty acid metabolism [11,29,30]. Abnormalities in carnitine metabolism have been linked to gestational diabetes [31], a risk factor for ASD [32]. A genetic defect in carnitine synthesis is a risk factor for ASD [33], carnitine metabolism is known to be disrupted in ASD [29,30] and a mouse model of ASD is associated with alternations in carnitine biosynthesis [34]. Due to its importance in energy metabolism in neural stem cells of the developing mammalian brain, carnitine deficiency has been proposed to be a prenatal risk factor for ASD [35].

As noted above, increased oxidative stress as well as inflammation is associated with mitochondrial dysfunction. Abnormalities in maternal trans-sulfuration metabolism and chronic oxidative stress are found in mothers of children with ASD during [36] and following [37] pregnancy and, in general, infection during pregnancy is a risk factor for ASD [38]. In fact, the maternal immune activation (MIA) mouse model of ASD demonstrates long-term mitochondrial dysfunction in brain [39] and leukocytes [40] after birth. Pregnancies resulting in a child with ASD have demonstrated increases in proinflammatory cytokines IL-1α [41] and IL-6 [41] in blood, while maternal elevation in IL-17a has been strongly implicated in the MIA model [42]. In laboratory studies, IL-17 [43,44] induces mitochondrial dysfunction through activation of the mitochondria-induced apoptosis pathway and IL-1 suppresses mitochondrial function [45], while IL-6 promotes mitochondrial biogenesis and fatty acid oxidation [46].

Prenatal exposure to many environmental toxicants is linked to an increased risk of developing ASD, including cigarette smoke, phthalates, air pollution, and pesticides such as organophosphate insecticides (e.g., chlorpyrifos) and organochlorine pesticides (e.g., dicofol and endosulfan) [7]. These toxicants have been associated with mitochondrial dysfunction. Organophosphate induces mitochondrial ultrastructure changes and inhibits ETC and CAC enzyme function, while organochlorine pesticides influence mitochondrial dysfunction indirectly by increasing ROS and reactive nitrogen species by altering antioxidant systems including SOD and GSH [47]. Phthalates, common plasticizers present in everyday products, have also been linked to increased oxygen consumption, mitochondrial mass, and fatty-acid metabolism in neonatal rat cardiomyocytes [48] and detrimental changes in mitochondrial membrane potential in human semen [49]. Mitochondrial-derived peptides in cord blood have been associated with prenatal exposure to non-freeway traffic-related air pollution [50]. Cigarette smoke causes mitochondrial dysfunction in the lung epithelium [51].

Several medications commonly used during pregnancy have been linked to an increased risk of developing ASD including acetaminophen [52] and selective serotonin reuptake inhibitors [53]. Acetaminophen has known toxicity by increasing reactive metabolites leading to suppression of mitochondrial function [54]. Fluoxetine, a commonly used selective serotonin reuptake inhibitor, has been shown to inhibit multiple mitochondrial enzymes in several laboratory studies [55] and may result in long-term changes in energy metabolism with neonatal exposure [56]. Other medications commonly used in pregnancy with less certain association with ASD are associated with mitochondrial dysfunction. For example, commonly used antibiotics, including quinolones, aminoglycosides, and β-lactams, can cause mitochondrial dysfunction [57], and commonly used anesthesia may be particularly detrimental to the developing brain, partially through mitochondrial mechanisms [58].

Interestingly, mitochondrial abnormalities have been documented in genetic syndromes associated with ASD such as PTEN mutations [59] and tuberous sclerosis [60,61], Fragile X [62,63], Rett [64–66], Phelan–McDermid [67], 15q11-13 duplication [68,69], Angelman [70] and Down [71,72] syndromes as well as septo-optic dysplasia [73]. Thus, a fetus with these genetic changes may already have vulnerable mitochondria that might be sensitive to environmental stressors.

Common nutritional deficiencies are prenatal ASD risk factors which have been suggested to modulate mitochondrial function. Decreased vitamin D in the first [74] or second [75] trimester as well as lifetime [76] is associated with more severe ASD [74,75] or increased ASD risk [76]. Vitamin D deficiency is associated with oxidative stress and reduced mitochondrial respiration that is mediated through the vitamin D receptor [77,78].

Several lines of evidence suggest that ASD is associated with disruption of the microbiome in individuals with ASD as well as their mother during pregnancy [79]. Although a recent landmark study provided preliminary evidence that transplanting the microbiome in individuals with ASD can improve gastrointestinal and ASD symptoms [63], studies in pregnant women are more difficult to conduct, leading to animal studies addressing this possibility. Environmentally induced rodent models of ASD, including the MIA [80] and the valproic acid exposure models [81–83], have an altered microbiome. Manipulations which can affect the microbiome have been shown to mitigate the effects of these maternal exposures. Treating pups born from maternal valproic acid exposure demonstrate reduced ASD-like behaviors [84,85] as well as normalization of mitochondrial abnormalities [84], while treatment of pups born from MIA with *Bacteroides fragilis* normalizes gut permeability and microbial composition and reduces ASD-like behaviors [86]. Interestingly, several prenatal environmental exposures linked to ASD, including air pollution [87], glyphosate [88], prenatal antibiotic use [89], maternal stress [90] and organophosphate herbicides [91], have evidence for disrupting the microbiome, suggesting a potential biological pathway for their effects. The microbiome can influence mitochondrial function through several mechanisms, although the most compelling is through the production of short chain fatty acids [92].

4. Unique Abnormalities in Mitochondrial Function Are Prevalent in ASD

The possibility that environmentally induced mitochondrial dysfunction could have a role in ASD is particularly compelling because abnormal mitochondrial function is one of the most prevalent metabolic disorders found in individuals with ASD, with prevalence ranging from 5% for classically defined mitochondrial disease to 8–47% for biomarkers of mitochondrial dysfunction [11,16], to 62–65% for abnormal ETC/CAC enzymology [93,94], and to 80% for abnormal ETC activity in lymphocytes and granulocytes [95,96]. Particularly compelling is that the great majority of the time, genetic defects cannot explain the mitochondrial abnormalities, suggesting that the abnormality could be acquired as a result of an environmental exposure. There is also a tremendous practical appeal in this hypothesis, as environmental determinants may be particularly amenable to modification.

In classic mitochondrial disease, ETC activity is, by definition, depressed. However, what is unique about abnormalities in mitochondrial function in individuals with ASD is that ETC activity is significantly increased in many cases. The first case reported was a boy with ASD who demonstrated a significant increase in ETC complex I activity while his sister, who was diagnosed with a classic mitochondrial disease known as Leigh syndrome, showed depressed ETC activity [97]. Interestingly, both siblings manifested the same mtDNA mutation, but the sister had a greater genetic mutational load (i.e., higher heteroplasmy). Subsequently, a case-series of five patents with ASD with muscle ETC complex IV activity about 200% of normal was reported [98]. The association of elevated ETC complex IV activity with ASD has subsequently been confirmed in fresh frozen superior temporal gyrus [99], buccal swabs enzymology [93] and lymphoblastoid cell lines (LCLs) using high-resolution respirometry [100].

5. The Significance of Mitochondrial Dysfunction in ASD: Sensitivity to Physiological Stress

Since increased ROS is a key mechanism by which environmental stressors, such as toxicants [101–108] and inflammation [1,11], can disrupt mitochondrial function, an assay has been developed which systematically increases ROS *in vitro* [109]. This assay, called the Mitochondrial Oxidative Stress Test (MOST), systematically increases ROS *in vitro* using 2,3–dimethoxy–1,4-napthoquinone (DMNQ), an agent that generates intracellular superoxide and hydrogen peroxide but does not directly deplete thiols [110]. The model was initially developed using LCLs from boys with ASD and age-matched healthy controls (CNT) where DMNQ was shown to increase ROS in CNT and ASD LCLs [110].

In this model, mitochondrial respiratory rates were significantly higher in ASD LCLs as compared to CNT LCLs. Most compelling, indices of mitochondrial health, reserve capacity and maximal respiratory rate, decreased to a greater extent in ASD LCLs when challenged with DMNQ in the MOST assay. Increases in ROS, using the MOST assay, resulted in a depletion of these respiratory parameters at lower DMNQ concentrations in the ASD LCLs, despite these parameters being higher at baseline. This suggests that the ASD LCLs demonstrated a greater vulnerability to ROS.

To determine if these bioenergetics changes were specific to a subset of ASD LCLs, a cluster analysis was used to separated ASD LCLs into those with normal bioenergetics (AD-N) and those with atypical bioenergetics (AD-A) [109]. When the AD-A LCLs were compared to the CNT LCLs, the bioenergetic differences were found to be large. Baseline respiratory rates were ~200% higher in AD-A as compared to the CNT LCLs. Most notably, maximal respiratory capacity and reserve capacity markedly decreased as DMNQ increased, such that reserve capacity was rapidly depleted as DMNQ increased despite being much higher at baseline. This pattern of abnormal respiration in this subset of LCLs has been confirmed over eight studies [61,109,111–116].

Despite these experiments, the question remained whether this pattern of mitochondrial dysfunction was specific to ASD or simply a consequence of higher levels of chronic ongoing intrinsic oxidative stress. Since neurotypical siblings (SIBs) of children with ASD manifest similar chronic ongoing elevation in oxidative stress in their LCLs, mitochondrial function was compared between 10 LCLs from boys with ASD and their 10 male SIBs and 10 age-matched CNT males [117]. Mitochondrial function was similar between SIBs and CNTs, but both were different from ASD. In the ASD LCLs, mitochondrial respiration was elevated at baseline and reserve capacity declined more precipitously with increasing DMNQ, as compared to SIB and CNT LCLs. Most notably, the severity of mitochondrial abnormalities in ASD LCLs was related to the severity of stereotyped behaviors and restricted interests as measured on the gold-standard Autism Diagnostic Observation Schedule evaluation years earlier when the blood samples were original collected. Thus, atypical mitochondrial activity in the ASD LCLs is not simply a product of abnormal redox metabolism but rather associated with atypical mitochondrial function specifically. Furthermore, this atypical mitochondrial function is related to more severe core ASD behaviors, suggesting an association with molecular mechanisms of ASD.

Individuals with ASD demonstrate three developmental trajectories: in the early onset subtype, symptoms are obvious from early in infancy, perhaps at birth; in the plateau subtype, infants develop normally throughout the first year of life but then plateau in the rate of gaining skills, followed by the development of ASD symptoms; lastly is a subset that demonstrates neurodevelopmental regression (NDR). The NDR category is intriguing: children attain all their normal developmental milestones but then lose previously attained skills followed by the development of ASD-like behaviors. Often, NDR is associated with a trigger such as seizure [118] and/or fever [119]. NDR is not uncommon in individuals with mitochondrial disease when an illness occurs [120]. Thus, it is not surprising that a meta-analysis showed that NDR was more common in children with ASD that were also diagnosed with mitochondrial disease [11].

Given that the subset of ASD LCLs with elevated respiratory rates have increased vulnerability to physiological stress, a recent study hypothesized that children with ASD and NDR would demonstrate increase mitochondrial respiratory rates. Mitochondrial function was measured in cryopreserved peripheral blood mononuclear cells (PBMCs) from children with ASD, with and without NDR, as well as CNT using the Seahorse XF96 respirometer [121]. Viability was measured and 600 k viable PBMCs were plated per well. As hypothesized, mitochondrial respiration was elevated in children with ASD and NDR. Specifically, the maximal oxygen consumption rate, maximal respiratory capacity, and reserve capacity were higher in the individuals with ASD and NDR as compared to the other groups. Additionally, comparing ASD twins discordant on NDR demonstrated that the twin with NDR showed a significantly elevated maximal oxygen consumption rate. Thus, the NDR ASD phenotype may be a hallmark of abnormal mitochondrial physiology.

6. Unique ASD Mitochondrial Abnormalities May Be Linked to Both Environmental and Genetic Factors

Interestingly, the unique elevations in mitochondrial respiration reported in human tissue have been associated with both genetic and environmentally induced animal models of ASD. Elevated mitochondrial respiration has been documented in genetic syndromes associated with ASD, including Phelan–McDermid [122], Fragile X [62,63], 22q13 dup [67], and Rett [66] syndromes, the PTEN haploinsufficient mouse model of ASD [59] and the Drosophila model of the ASD associated CYFIP1 mutation [123]. Similar changes have been associated with prenatal environmental exposures, specifically prenatal exposure to inflammation as in the MIA mouse, a model of ASD induced by prenatal immune environmental stress [39], and prenatal exposure to toxins as in the maternal valproic acid exposure mouse model of ASD [84].

Consistent with evidence from these prenatal environmental animal models of ASD, several studies have examined the relationship between alternations in long-term mitochondrial function and prenatal environmental stressors in ASD.

Prenatal exposure to air pollution, as measured by average and maximum $PM_{2.5}$, has been found to be related to mitochondrial respiration in childhood, as measured in PBMCs. The relationship was significantly different for those children with and without a history of NDR. For those with a history of NDR, higher prenatal $PM_{2.5}$ exposure was associated with higher mitochondrial respiration rates, while for those without a history of NDR, higher prenatal $PM_{2.5}$ exposure was related to lower mitochondrial respiration [27]. Additional research has linked prenatal air pollution exposure to mitochondrial-derived peptides in cord blood that are associated with long-term changes in mitochondrial physiology [50].

Both prenatal exposures to nutritional and toxic metal were measured in deciduous teeth using laser ablation inductively coupled plasma mass-spectrometry. Prenatal exposure to Mn and Zn was associated with mitochondrial respiration, but only in children with ASD and NDR [29]. The prenatal Cu to Zn ratio was associated with two independent measures of language development in all children with ASD (both those with and without NDR) [29]. This latter study extends previous findings linking prenatal nutrient metal (Zn, Mn, Cu) exposure and ASD [26,27,124–127].

To determine whether the long-term changes associated with ASD could be induced by exposure to environmental toxicants, one study exposed LCLs to low levels of ROS for a prolonged time (96 h) to simulate chronic ROS exposure which might occur with prolonged exposure to environmental toxicants or other physiological stressors [61]. Prolonged exposure to low levels of ROS induced bioenergetic changes in respiratory parameters involved in ATP production. After prolonged ROS exposure, the LCLs demonstrated increased respiratory rates at baseline, similar to the AD–A LCLs and the ETC activity seen in children with ASD in multiple tissues. These data suggest that a prolonged exposure to a pro-oxidant microenvironment can have chronic effects on the mitochondria.

7. Long-Term Induced Changes in Mitochondrial Function: Adaptive or Maladaptive

Mitochondria undergo long-term adaptive changes in physiology as a result of environmental stressors through a process known as mitoplasticity, which is one compelling mechanism for long-term changes in mitochondrial function associated with prenatal exposures [9]. Several studies may provide insight into the molecular mechanisms associated with long-term changes in mitochondrial function.

Matched typically developing siblings have similar abnormalities in oxidative stress compared to their ASD siblings, but the mitochondria of the ASD siblings appear to have difficulty regulating the mitochondrial ROS (mtROS). mtROS is regulated at the inner mitochondrial membrane through several mechanisms. Uncoupling proteins regulate mtROS by leaking protons across the inner mitochondrial membrane, a process known as proton leak. Studies have demonstrated increased proton leak respiration along with high oxidative stress in both cytoplasm and mitochondria in ASD LCLs [16,128]. Studies have associated ASD with an increase in mechanisms of proton leak. Three previous studies have found an increase in uncoupling protein (UCP2) gene expression [61,116] and protein concentration [109] in LCLs derived from children with ASD, particularly in the LCLs with high respiratory rates (i.e., AD–A LCLs). The adenine nucleotide translocator (ANT) has a significant role in the regulation of inner mitochondrial membrane proton leak. Microdeletion including the SLC25A5 (ANT2) has been associated with non-syndromic intellectual disability with ASD [129]. Heteroplasmic levels of the mtDNA 3243A > G mutation associated with ASD are also associated with significant changes in ANT gene expression [130]. Consistent with this evidence, increased protein leak is also a feature of mitochondrial abnormalities in the Fragile X syndrome mouse, where it is found to directly affect synaptic growth [131]. Thus, dysregulation in inner membrane proton leak seems to be associated with an ASD phenotype.

One of the key processes which maintains optimal mitochondrial function in the face of physiological stress is mitophagy. Several studies have linked ASD to a failure to induce this important process. Mutations in WDFY3 which result in ASD with intellectual disability have been linked to bioenergetic abnormalities in the brain through decreased mitophagy [132], and PARK2, a gene known to be involved in mitophagy, has been identified as a candidate gene for ASD [133]. Examination of the post-mortem temporal cortex has demonstrated ETC activity abnormalities along with alternation in levels of fission (Fis1, Drp1) and fusion (Mfn1, Mfn2 and Opa1) protein essential for regulating mitophagy [134]. Neurons deficient in TSC1/TSC2, a model of tuberous sclerosis, demonstrate impaired mitophagy through a mTORC1 mechanism [60,135]. This is consistent with studies which have demonstrated that ASD LCLs with elevated respiratory rates (i.e., AD–A LCLs) fail to upregulate genes associated with mitophagy through a mTORC1 pathway related mechanism [61]. Recently, ASD-derived fibroblasts were found to have elevated respiratory rates, atypical mitochondrial morphology, and alteration in the mitophagy pathway [136]. Interestingly, a loss of mitophagy can lead to a build-up of cytosolic ROS and mtDNA damage and an increase in proinflammatory cytokines, including IL–1α, IL–1β, IL–18, IFNα, MIF, IL–23, and IL–17 [137].

Alternative to regulatory changes within the body is the possibility that long-term alternation in the microbiome environment (technically outside of the body) could account for long-term changes in mitochondrial function. The connection between the microbiome and mitochondrial dysfunction in ASD is supported by the compelling propionic acid (PPA) rodent model of ASD. Adult rats intraventricularly injected with PPA [138], juvenile rates intraperitoneally injected with PPA [139], and prenatally PPA exposed rodents [140,141] demonstrated ASD-like behaviors. The importance of this model is that fact that enteric microbiome producers of PPA, particularly *Clostridia* sp, are relatively overrepresented in the ASD microbiome [142]. PPA exposure results in several physiological abnormalities, including mitochondrial dysfunction, particularly disruption of the fatty acid metabolism, as manifested by unique elevations in acyl-carnitines, as well as redox abnormalities as manifested by GSH alternations [142]. Parallel to the unique acyl-carnitine elevations in the rodent model, the same pattern was reported in a case series of ASD patients [143] with the parallel mitochondrial and GSH abnormalities later reported in a more detailed study [144]. Further *in vitro* studies with ASD LCLs demonstrated the potential detrimental effects of PPA [114] and the protective effect of another prominent enteric microbiome derived short chain fatty acid butyrate [115]. Thus, long-term changes in the microbiome could also account for long-term changes in mitochondrial function in individuals with ASD.

8. Conclusions

One of the critical knowledge gaps in environmental medicine is how an environmental exposure can result in disease when the symptoms arise years after the exposure. Mitochondrial metabolism is a promising mechanism through which the environment can cause long-term effects. For ASD, we have discussed the many prenatal environmental exposures which are linked to ASD and can cause detrimental changes in mitochondrial function. This is compelling because mitochondrial dysfunction is prevalent in ASD. ASD is also associated with a unique type of mitochondrial dysfunction which may be related to environmental exposures. Studies support the notion that specific prenatal exposures linked to ASD, most notably air pollution and prenatal nutritional metal exposure, is associated with long-term alterations in mitochondrial physiology. A better understanding of these biological processes may lead to prevention and treatment strategies.

Prenatal mitochondrial function is important for brain development, as recent animal studies have shown that mitochondrial dysfunction during gestation alters white matter brain connectivity [145] and non-radial interneuron migration [146]. Mitochondrial function is essential for optimal neuronal function and is essential for transport of essential nutrients into the brain such as folate [30]. Mitochondria are also essential for important core metabolic pathways as well as for optimal function of the immune system, which is now known to have an important role in brain development [30]. Thus, mitochondrial dysfunction during the prenatal period can have a profound effect on long-term development.

In this manuscript, we discuss studies with findings that link prenatal environmental exposures to long-term mitochondrial function and ASD. These studies remain intriguing yet preliminary. These findings need to be confirmed and further studies need to be conducted to expand on these findings. One important caveat is a consideration of the measurement of mitochondrial function, as mitochondrial function can differ from tissue to tissue and various assays reflect different aspects of mitochondrial function. For example, the use of PBMCs to measure mitochondrial function is a relatively newly developed biomarker which will require further validation in the future [147].

The applications of these findings may be far reaching, as interventions to correct metabolic and mitochondrial abnormalities are under development, potentially providing targeted treatments for preventing ASD and other diseases from developing if implemented prenatally.

Author Contributions: All authors have read and agreed to the published version of the manuscript.

Funding: This research received no external funding.

Acknowledgments: This research was supported by the Arkansas Biosciences Institute (Little Rock, AR, USA), The Jonty Foundation (St Paul, MN, USA), The Autism Research Institute (San Diego, CA, USA), the Gupta Family Foundation (Atherton, CA, USA), The Jane Bostford Johnson Foundation (New York, NY, USA) and the Jager Family Foundation (Chicago, IL, USA).

Conflicts of Interest: The authors declare no conflict of interest.

References

1. Rossignol, D.A.; Frye, R.E. A review of research trends in physiological abnormalities in autism spectrum disorders: Immune dysregulation, inflammation, oxidative stress, mitochondrial dysfunction and environmental toxicant exposures. *Mol. Psychiatry* **2012**, *17*, 389–401. [CrossRef] [PubMed]
2. Maenner, M.J.; Shaw, K.A.; Baio, J.; Washington, A.; Patrick, M.; DiRienzo, M.; Christensen, D.L.; Wiggins, L.D.; Pettygrove, S.; Andrews, J.G.; et al. Prevalence of autism spectrum disorder among children aged 8 years—Autism and developmental disabilities monitoring network, 11 sites, United States, 2016. *Morb. Mortal. Wkly. Rep. Surveill. Summ.* **2020**, *69*, 1–12. [CrossRef] [PubMed]
3. Schaefer, G.B.; Mendelsohn, N.J. Professional Practice Guidelines Committee. Clinical genetics evaluation in identifying the etiology of autism spectrum disorders: 2013 guideline revisions. *Genet. Med.* **2013**, *15*, 399–407. [CrossRef] [PubMed]
4. Hallmayer, J.; Cleveland, S.; Torres, A.; Phillips, J.; Cohen, B.; Torigoe, T.; Miller, J.; Fedele, A.; Collins, J.; Smith, K.; et al. Genetic heritability and shared environmental factors among twin pairs with autism. *Arch. Gen. Psychiatry* **2011**, *68*, 1095–1102. [CrossRef]
5. Sandin, S.; Lichtenstein, P.; Kuja-Halkola, R.; Larsson, H.; Hultman, C.M.; Reichenberg, A. The familial risk of autism. *JAMA* **2014**, *311*, 1770–1777. [CrossRef]
6. Hertz-Picciotto, I.; Schmidt, R.J.; Krakowiak, P. Understanding environmental contributions to autism: Causal concepts and the state of science. *Autism Res. Off. J. Int. Soc. Autism Res.* **2018**, *11*, 554–586. [CrossRef]
7. Rossignol, D.A.; Genuis, S.J.; Frye, R.E. Environmental toxicants and autism spectrum disorders: A systematic review. *Transl. Psychiatry* **2014**, *4*, e360. [CrossRef] [PubMed]
8. Panisi, C.; Guerini, F.R.; Abruzzo, P.M.; Balzola, F.; Biava, P.M.; Bolotta, A.; Brunero, M.; Burgio, E.; Chiara, A.; Clerici, M.; et al. Autism spectrum disorder from the womb to adulthood: Suggestions for a paradigm shift. *J. Pers. Med.* **2021**, *11*, 70. [CrossRef]
9. Jose, C.; Melser, S.; Benard, G.; Rossignol, R. Mitoplasticity: Adaptation biology of the mitochondrion to the cellular redox state in physiology and carcinogenesis. *Antioxid. Redox Signal.* **2013**, *18*, 808–849. [CrossRef]
10. Frye, R.E.; Rossignol, D.A. Mitochondrial dysfunction can connect the diverse medical symptoms associated with autism spectrum disorders. *Pediatr. Res.* **2011**, *69*, 41R–47R. [CrossRef]
11. Rossignol, D.A.; Frye, R.E. Mitochondrial dysfunction in autism spectrum disorders: A systematic review and meta-analysis. *Mol. Psychiatry* **2012**, *17*, 290–314. [CrossRef] [PubMed]
12. Frye, R.E.; Rossignol, D. Mitochondrial physiology and autism spectrum disorder. *OA Autism* **2013**, 1. [CrossRef]
13. Wallace, D.C.; Fan, W. Energetics, epigenetics, mitochondrial genetics. *Mitochondrion* **2010**, *10*, 12–31. [CrossRef]
14. Banoth, B.; Cassel, S.L. Mitochondria in innate immune signaling. *Transl. Res.* **2018**, *202*, 52–68. [CrossRef] [PubMed]
15. Rossignol, D.A.; Frye, R.E. Evidence linking oxidative stress, mitochondrial dysfunction, and inflammation in the brain of individuals with autism. *Front. Physiol.* **2014**, *5*, 150. [CrossRef]
16. Rose, S.; Melnyk, S.; Pavliv, O.; Bai, S.; Nick, T.G.; Frye, R.E.; James, S.J. Evidence of oxidative damage and inflammation associated with low glutathione redox status in the autism brain. *Transl. Psychiatry* **2012**, *2*, e134. [CrossRef] [PubMed]
17. Frustaci, A.; Neri, M.; Cesario, A.; Adams, J.B.; Domenici, E.; Dalla Bernardina, B.; Bonassi, S. Oxidative stress-related biomarkers in autism: Systematic review and meta-analyses. *Free Radic. Biol. Med.* **2012**, *52*, 2128–2141. [CrossRef]
18. Napoli, E.; Wong, S.; Giulivi, C. Evidence of reactive oxygen species-mediated damage to mitochondrial DNA in children with typical autism. *Mol. Autism* **2013**, *4*, 2. [CrossRef]
19. O'Neill, L.A.; Kishton, R.J.; Rathmell, J. A guide to immunometabolism for immunologists. *Nat. Rev. Immunol.* **2016**, *16*, 553–565. [CrossRef] [PubMed]
20. West, A.P.; Shadel, G.S.; Ghosh, S. Mitochondria in innate immune responses. *Nat. Rev. Immunol.* **2011**, *11*, 389–402. [CrossRef] [PubMed]
21. Jyonouchi, H.; Geng, L.; Rose, S.; Bennuri, S.C.; Frye, R.E. Variations in mitochondrial respiration differ in IL-1ß/IL-10 ratio based subgroups in autism spectrum disorders. *Front. Psychiatry* **2019**, *10*, 71. [CrossRef] [PubMed]
22. Delhey, L.M.; Nur Kilinc, E.; Yin, L.; Slattery, J.C.; Tippett, M.L.; Rose, S.; Bennuri, S.C.; Kahler, S.G.; Damle, S.; Legido, A.; et al. The effect of mitochondrial supplements on mitochondrial activity in children with autism spectrum disorder. *J. Clin. Med.* **2017**, *6*, 18. [CrossRef] [PubMed]
23. James, S.J.; Melnyk, S.; Jernigan, S.; Pavliv, O.; Trusty, T.; Lehman, S.; Seidel, L.; Gaylor, D.W.; Cleves, M.A. A functional polymorphism in the reduced folate carrier gene and DNA hypomethylation in mothers of children with autism. *Am. J. Med Genet. Part B Neuropsychiatr. Genet. Off. Publ. Int. Soc. Psychiatr. Genet.* **2010**, *153b*, 1209–1220. [CrossRef]
24. Quadros, E.V.; Sequeira, J.M.; Brown, W.T.; Mevs, C.; Marchi, E.; Flory, M.; Jenkins, E.C.; Velinov, M.T.; Cohen, I.L. Folate receptor autoantibodies are prevalent in children diagnosed with autism spectrum disorder, their normal siblings and parents. *Autism Res. Off. J. Int. Soc. Autism Res.* **2018**, *11*, 707–712. [CrossRef]
25. Sequeira, J.M.; Desai, A.; Berrocal-Zaragoza, M.I.; Murphy, M.M.; Fernandez-Ballart, J.D.; Quadros, E.V. Exposure to folate receptor alpha antibodies during gestation and weaning leads to severe behavioral deficits in rats: A pilot study. *PLoS ONE* **2016**, *11*, e0152249. [CrossRef]
26. Curtin, P.; Austin, C.; Curtin, A.; Gennings, C.; Arora, M.; Tammimies, K.; Willfors, C.; Berggren, S.; Siper, P.; Rai, D.; et al. Dynamical features in fetal and postnatal zinc-copper metabolic cycles predict the emergence of autism spectrum disorder. *Sci. Adv.* **2018**, *4*, eaat1293. [CrossRef]

27. Frye, R.E.; Cakir, J.; Rose, S.; Delhey, L.; Bennuri, S.C.; Tippett, M.; Melnyk, S.; James, S.J.; Palmer, R.F.; Austin, C.; et al. Prenatal air pollution influences neurodevelopment and behavior in autism spectrum disorder by modulating mitochondrial physiology. *Mol. Psychiatry* **2020**. [CrossRef]
28. Zhong, C.; Tessing, J.; Lee, B.K.; Lyall, K. Maternal dietary factors and the risk of autism spectrum disorders: A systematic review of existing evidence. *Autism Res. Off. J. Int. Soc. Autism Res.* **2020**. [CrossRef]
29. Frye, R.E. Mitochondrial dysfunction in autism spectrum disorder: Unique abnormalities and targeted treatments. *Semin. Pediatr. Neurol.* **2020**, *35*, 100829. [CrossRef] [PubMed]
30. Rose, S.; Niyazov, D.M.; Rossignol, D.A.; Goldenthal, M.; Kahler, S.G.; Frye, R.E. Clinical and molecular characteristics of mitochondrial dysfunction in autism spectrum disorder. *Mol. Diagn. Ther.* **2018**, *22*, 571–593. [CrossRef]
31. Sun, M.; Zhao, B.; He, S.; Weng, R.; Wang, B.; Ding, Y.; Huang, X.; Luo, Q. The alteration of carnitine metabolism in second trimester in GDM and a nomogram for predicting macrosomia. *J. Diabetes Res.* **2020**, *2020*, 4085757. [CrossRef] [PubMed]
32. Wan, H.; Zhang, C.; Li, H.; Luan, S.; Liu, C. Association of maternal diabetes with autism spectrum disorders in offspring: A systemic review and meta-analysis. *Medicine* **2018**, *97*, e9438. [CrossRef] [PubMed]
33. Celestino-Soper, P.B.; Violante, S.; Crawford, E.L.; Luo, R.; Lionel, A.C.; Delaby, E.; Cai, G.; Sadikovic, B.; Lee, K.; Lo, C.; et al. A common X-linked inborn error of carnitine biosynthesis may be a risk factor for nondysmorphic autism. *Proc. Natl. Acad. Sci. USA* **2012**, *109*, 7974–7981. [CrossRef] [PubMed]
34. Lee, H.; Kim, H.K.; Kwon, J.T.; Park, S.; Park, H.J.; Kim, S.K.; Park, J.K.; Kang, W.S.; Kim, Y.J.; Chung, J.H.; et al. BBOX1 is down-regulated in maternal immune-activated mice and implicated in genetic susceptibility to human schizophrenia. *Psychiatry Res.* **2018**, *259*, 197–202. [CrossRef] [PubMed]
35. Bankaitis, V.A.; Xie, Z. The neural stem cell/carnitine malnutrition hypothesis: New prospects for effective reduction of autism risk? *J. Biol. Chem.* **2019**, *294*, 19424–19435. [CrossRef]
36. Hollowood, K.; Melnyk, S.; Pavliv, O.; Evans, T.; Sides, A.; Schmidt, R.J.; Hertz-Picciotto, I.; Elms, W.; Guerrero, E.; Kruger, U.; et al. Maternal metabolic profile predicts high or low risk of an autism pregnancy outcome. *Res. Autism Spectr. Disord.* **2018**, *56*, 72–82. [CrossRef]
37. James, S.J.; Melnyk, S.; Jernigan, S.; Hubanks, A.; Rose, S.; Gaylor, D.W. Abnormal transmethylation/transsulfuration metabolism and DNA hypomethylation among parents of children with autism. *J. Autism Dev. Disord.* **2008**, *38*, 1966–1975. [CrossRef]
38. Bauman, M.D.; Van de Water, J. Translational opportunities in the prenatal immune environment: Promises and limitations of the maternal immune activation model. *Neurobiol. Dis.* **2020**, *141*, 104864. [CrossRef]
39. Naviaux, R.K.; Zolkipli, Z.; Wang, L.; Nakayama, T.; Naviaux, J.C.; Le, T.P.; Schuchbauer, M.A.; Rogac, M.; Tang, Q.; Dugan, L.L.; et al. Antipurinergic therapy corrects the autism-like features in the poly(IC) mouse model. *PLoS ONE* **2013**, *8*, e57380. [CrossRef]
40. Giulivi, C.; Napoli, E.; Schwartzer, J.; Careaga, M.; Ashwood, P. Gestational exposure to a viral mimetic poly(i:C) results in long-lasting changes in mitochondrial function by leucocytes in the adult offspring. *Mediat. Inflamm.* **2013**, *2013*, 609602. [CrossRef]
41. Jones, K.L.; Croen, L.A.; Yoshida, C.K.; Heuer, L.; Hansen, R.; Zerbo, O.; DeLorenze, G.N.; Kharrazi, M.; Yolken, R.; Ashwood, P.; et al. Autism with intellectual disability is associated with increased levels of maternal cytokines and chemokines during gestation. *Mol. Psychiatry* **2017**, *22*, 273–279. [CrossRef] [PubMed]
42. Wong, H.; Hoeffer, C. Maternal IL-17A in autism. *Exp. Neurol.* **2018**, *299*, 228–240. [CrossRef] [PubMed]
43. Kim, E.K.; Kwon, J.E.; Lee, S.Y.; Lee, E.J.; Kim, D.S.; Moon, S.J.; Lee, J.; Kwok, S.K.; Park, S.H.; Cho, M.L. IL-17-mediated mitochondrial dysfunction impairs apoptosis in rheumatoid arthritis synovial fibroblasts through activation of autophagy. *Cell Death Dis.* **2017**, *8*, e2565. [CrossRef]
44. Kakareko, M.; Jabłońska, E.; Ratajczak-Wrona, W. Role of rhIL-17 in regulating the mitochondrial pathway proteins in peripheral blood neutrophils. *Clin. Lab.* **2015**, *61*, 345–351. [CrossRef]
45. Zhou, H.; Wang, H.; Yu, M.; Schugar, R.C.; Qian, W.; Tang, F.; Liu, W.; Yang, H.; McDowell, R.E.; Zhao, J.; et al. IL-1 induces mitochondrial translocation of IRAK2 to suppress oxidative metabolism in adipocytes. *Nat. Immunol.* **2020**, *21*, 1219–1231. [CrossRef]
46. Xu, Y.; Zhang, Y.; Ye, J. IL-6: A potential role in cardiac metabolic homeostasis. *Int. J. Mol. Sci.* **2018**, *19*, 2474. [CrossRef]
47. Karami-Mohajeri, S.; Abdollahi, M. Toxic influence of organophosphate, carbamate, and organochlorine pesticides on cellular metabolism of lipids, proteins, and carbohydrates: A systematic review. *Hum. Exp. Toxicol.* **2011**, *30*, 1119–1140. [CrossRef]
48. Posnack, N.G.; Swift, L.M.; Kay, M.W.; Lee, N.H.; Sarvazyan, N. Phthalate exposure changes the metabolic profile of cardiac muscle cells. *Environ. Health Perspect.* **2012**, *120*, 1243–1251. [CrossRef] [PubMed]
49. Pant, N.; Shukla, M.; Kumar Patel, D.; Shukla, Y.; Mathur, N.; Kumar Gupta, Y.; Saxena, D.K. Correlation of phthalate exposures with semen quality. *Toxicol. Appl. Pharmacol.* **2008**, *231*, 112–116. [CrossRef]
50. Breton, C.V.; Song, A.Y.; Xiao, J.; Kim, S.J.; Mehta, H.H.; Wan, J.; Yen, K.; Sioutas, C.; Lurmann, F.; Xue, S.; et al. Effects of air pollution on mitochondrial function, mitochondrial DNA methylation, and mitochondrial peptide expression. *Mitochondrion* **2019**, *46*, 22–29. [CrossRef]
51. Aghapour, M.; Remels, A.H.V.; Pouwels, S.D.; Bruder, D.; Hiemstra, P.S.; Cloonan, S.M.; Heijink, I.H. Mitochondria: At the crossroads of regulating lung epithelial cell function in chronic obstructive pulmonary disease. *Am. J. Physiol. Lung Cell. Mol. Physiol.* **2020**, *318*, L149–l164. [CrossRef]

52. Bauer, A.Z.; Kriebel, D.; Herbert, M.R.; Bornehag, C.G.; Swan, S.H. Prenatal paracetamol exposure and child neurodevelopment: A review. *Horm. Behav.* **2018**, *101*, 125–147. [CrossRef]
53. Andalib, S.; Emamhadi, M.R.; Yousefzadeh-Chabok, S.; Shakouri, S.K.; Høilund-Carlsen, P.F.; Vafaee, M.S.; Michel, T.M. Maternal SSRI exposure increases the risk of autistic offspring: A meta-analysis and systematic review. *Eur. Psychiatry J. Assoc. Eur. Psychiatr.* **2017**, *45*, 161–166. [CrossRef]
54. Ramachandran, A.; Jaeschke, H. Acetaminophen hepatotoxicity: A mitochondrial perspective. *Adv. Pharmacol.* **2019**, *85*, 195–219. [CrossRef] [PubMed]
55. De Oliveira, M.R. Fluoxetine and the mitochondria: A review of the toxicological aspects. *Toxicol. Lett.* **2016**, *258*, 185–191. [CrossRef] [PubMed]
56. Da L.D. Barros, M.; Manhães-de-Castro, R.; Alves, D.T.; Quevedo, O.G.; Toscano, A.E.; Bonnin, A.; Galindo, L. Long term effects of neonatal exposure to fluoxetine on energy balance: A systematic review of experimental studies. *Eur. J. Pharmacol.* **2018**, *833*, 298–306. [CrossRef]
57. Kalghatgi, S.; Spina, C.S.; Costello, J.C.; Liesa, M.; Morones-Ramirez, J.R.; Slomovic, S.; Molina, A.; Shirihai, O.S.; Collins, J.J. Bactericidal antibiotics induce mitochondrial dysfunction and oxidative damage in Mammalian cells. *Sci. Transl. Med.* **2013**, *5*, 192ra85. [CrossRef]
58. Bodolea, C. Anaesthesia in early childhood—Is the development of the immature brain in danger? *Rom. J. Anaesth. Intensive Care* **2016**, *23*, 33–40. [CrossRef]
59. Napoli, E.; Ross-Inta, C.; Wong, S.; Hung, C.; Fujisawa, Y.; Sakaguchi, D.; Angelastro, J.; Omanska-Klusek, A.; Schoenfeld, R.; Giulivi, C. Mitochondrial dysfunction in Pten haplo-insufficient mice with social deficits and repetitive behavior: Interplay between Pten and p53. *PLoS ONE* **2012**, *7*, e42504. [CrossRef]
60. Ebrahimi-Fakhari, D.; Saffari, A.; Wahlster, L.; Sahin, M. Using tuberous sclerosis complex to understand the impact of MTORC1 signaling on mitochondrial dynamics and mitophagy in neurons. *Autophagy* **2017**, *13*, 754–756. [CrossRef] [PubMed]
61. Bennuri, S.C.; Rose, S.; Frye, R.E. Mitochondrial dysfunction is inducible in lymphoblastoid cell lines from children with autism and may involve the TORC1 pathway. *Front. Psychiatry Mol. Psychiatry* **2019**, *10*, 269. [CrossRef]
62. D'Antoni, S.; de Bari, L.; Valenti, D.; Borro, M.; Bonaccorso, C.M.; Simmaco, M.; Vacca, R.A.; Catania, M.V. Aberrant mitochondrial bioenergetics in the cerebral cortex of the Fmr1 knockout mouse model of fragile X syndrome. *Biol. Chem.* **2020**, *401*, 497–503. [CrossRef]
63. Griffiths, K.K.; Wang, A.; Wang, L.; Tracey, M.; Kleiner, G.; Quinzii, C.M.; Sun, L.; Yang, G.; Perez-Zoghbi, J.F.; Licznerski, P.; et al. Inefficient thermogenic mitochondrial respiration due to futile proton leak in a mouse model of fragile X syndrome. *FASEB J. Off. Publ. Fed. Am. Soc. Exp. Biol.* **2020**, *34*, 7404–7426. [CrossRef]
64. Grosser, E.; Hirt, U.; Janc, O.A.; Menzfeld, C.; Fischer, M.; Kempkes, B.; Vogelgesang, S.; Manzke, T.U.; Opitz, L.; Salinas-Riester, G.; et al. Oxidative burden and mitochondrial dysfunction in a mouse model of Rett syndrome. *Neurobiol. Dis.* **2012**, *48*, 102–114. [CrossRef]
65. Gibson, J.H.; Slobedman, B.; KN, H.; Williamson, S.L.; Minchenko, D.; El-Osta, A.; Stern, J.L.; Christodoulou, J. Downstream targets of methyl CpG binding protein 2 and their abnormal expression in the frontal cortex of the human Rett syndrome brain. *BMC Neurosci.* **2010**, *11*, 53. [CrossRef]
66. Condie, J.; Goldstein, J.; Wainwright, M.S. Acquired microcephaly, regression of milestones, mitochondrial dysfunction, and episodic rigidity in a 46,XY male with a de novo MECP2 gene mutation. *J. Child Neurol.* **2010**, *25*, 633–636. [CrossRef] [PubMed]
67. Frye, R.E. Mitochondrial disease in 22q13 duplication syndrome. *J. Child Neurol.* **2012**, *27*, 942–949. [CrossRef] [PubMed]
68. Frye, R.E. 15q11.2-13 duplication, mitochondrial dysfunction, and developmental disorders. *J. Child Neurol.* **2009**, *24*, 1316–1320. [CrossRef] [PubMed]
69. Filipek, P.A.; Juranek, J.; Smith, M.; Mays, L.Z.; Ramos, E.R.; Bocian, M.; Masser-Frye, D.; Laulhere, T.M.; Modahl, C.; Spence, M.A.; et al. Mitochondrial dysfunction in autistic patients with 15q inverted duplication. *Ann. Neurol.* **2003**, *53*, 801–804. [CrossRef]
70. Su, H.; Fan, W.; Coskun, P.E.; Vesa, J.; Gold, J.A.; Jiang, Y.H.; Potluri, P.; Procaccio, V.; Acab, A.; Weiss, J.H.; et al. Mitochondrial dysfunction in CA1 hippocampal neurons of the UBE3A deficient mouse model for Angelman syndrome. *Neurosci. Lett.* **2011**, *487*, 129–133. [CrossRef]
71. Pagano, G.; Castello, G. Oxidative stress and mitochondrial dysfunction in Down syndrome. *Adv. Exp. Med. Biol.* **2012**, *724*, 291–299. [CrossRef] [PubMed]
72. Pallardo, F.V.; Lloret, A.; Lebel, M.; d'Ischia, M.; Cogger, V.C.; Le Couteur, D.G.; Gadaleta, M.N.; Castello, G.; Pagano, G. Mitochondrial dysfunction in some oxidative stress-related genetic diseases: Ataxia-telangiectasia, Down syndrome, Fanconi anaemia and Werner syndrome. *Biogerontology* **2010**, *11*, 401–419. [CrossRef]
73. Schuelke, M.; Krude, H.; Finckh, B.; Mayatepek, E.; Janssen, A.; Schmelz, M.; Trefz, F.; Trijbels, F.; Smeitink, J. Septo-optic dysplasia associated with a new mitochondrial cytochrome b mutation. *Ann. Neurol.* **2002**, *51*, 388–392. [CrossRef] [PubMed]
74. Chen, J.; Xin, K.; Wei, J.; Zhang, K.; Xiao, H. Lower maternal serum 25(OH) D in first trimester associated with higher autism risk in Chinese offspring. *J. Psychosom. Res.* **2016**, *89*, 98–101. [CrossRef]
75. Vinkhuyzen, A.A.E.; Eyles, D.W.; Burne, T.H.J.; Blanken, L.M.E.; Kruithof, C.J.; Verhulst, F.; White, T.; Jaddoe, V.W.; Tiemeier, H.; McGrath, J.J. Gestational vitamin D deficiency and autism spectrum disorder. *Bjpsych. Open* **2017**, *3*, 85–90. [CrossRef]

76. Magnusson, C.; Lundberg, M.; Lee, B.K.; Rai, D.; Karlsson, H.; Gardner, R.; Kosidou, K.; Arver, S.; Dalman, C. Maternal vitamin D deficiency and the risk of autism spectrum disorders: Population-based study. *Bjpsych. Open* **2016**, *2*, 170–172. [CrossRef]
77. Dzik, K.P.; Kaczor, J.J. Mechanisms of vitamin D on skeletal muscle function: Oxidative stress, energy metabolism and anabolic state. *Eur. J. Appl. Physiol.* **2019**, *119*, 825–839. [CrossRef]
78. Silvagno, F.; Pescarmona, G. Spotlight on vitamin D receptor, lipid metabolism and mitochondria: Some preliminary emerging issues. *Mol. Cell. Endocrinol.* **2017**, *450*, 24–31. [CrossRef] [PubMed]
79. Slattery, J.; MacFabe, D.F.; Kahler, S.G.; Frye, R.E. Enteric ecosystem disruption in autism spectrum disorder: Can the microbiota and macrobiota be restored? *Curr. Pharm. Des.* **2016**, *22*, 6107–6121. [CrossRef]
80. Lammert, C.R.; Frost, E.L.; Bolte, A.C.; Paysour, M.J.; Shaw, M.E.; Bellinger, C.E.; Weigel, T.K.; Zunder, E.R.; Lukens, J.R. Cutting edge: Critical roles for microbiota-mediated regulation of the immune system in a prenatal immune activation model of autism. *J. Immunol.* **2018**, *201*, 845–850. [CrossRef]
81. Liu, F.; Horton-Sparks, K.; Hull, V.; Li, R.W.; Martínez-Cerdeño, V. The valproic acid rat model of autism presents with gut bacterial dysbiosis similar to that in human autism. *Mol. Autism* **2018**, *9*, 61. [CrossRef] [PubMed]
82. Wang, J.P.; Xu, Y.C.; Hou, J.Q.; Li, J.Y.; Xing, J.; Yang, B.X.; Zhang, Z.H.; Zhang, B.L.; Li, H.H.; Li, P. Effects of dietary fat profile on gut microbiota in valproate animal model of autism. *Front. Med.* **2020**, *7*, 151. [CrossRef]
83. De Theije, C.G.; Wopereis, H.; Ramadan, M.; van Eijndthoven, T.; Lambert, J.; Knol, J.; Garssen, J.; Kraneveld, A.D.; Oozeer, R. Altered gut microbiota and activity in a murine model of autism spectrum disorders. *Brain Behav. Immun.* **2014**, *37*, 197–206. [CrossRef] [PubMed]
84. Ahn, Y.; Narous, M.; Tobias, R.; Rho, J.M.; Mychasiuk, R. The ketogenic diet modifies social and metabolic alterations identified in the prenatal valproic acid model of autism spectrum disorder. *Dev. Neurosci.* **2014**, *36*, 371–380. [CrossRef]
85. Castro, K.; Baronio, D.; Perry, I.S.; Riesgo, R.D.S.; Gottfried, C. The effect of ketogenic diet in an animal model of autism induced by prenatal exposure to valproic acid. *Nutr. Neurosci.* **2017**, *20*, 343–350. [CrossRef] [PubMed]
86. Hsiao, E.Y.; McBride, S.W.; Hsien, S.; Sharon, G.; Hyde, E.R.; McCue, T.; Codelli, J.A.; Chow, J.; Reisman, S.E.; Petrosino, J.F.; et al. Microbiota modulate behavioral and physiological abnormalities associated with neurodevelopmental disorders. *Cell* **2013**, *155*, 1451–1463. [CrossRef]
87. Vallès, Y.; Francino, M.P. Air pollution, early life microbiome, and development. *Curr. Environ. Health Rep.* **2018**, *5*, 512–521. [CrossRef] [PubMed]
88. Pu, Y.; Yang, J.; Chang, L.; Qu, Y.; Wang, S.; Zhang, K.; Xiong, Z.; Zhang, J.; Tan, Y.; Wang, X.; et al. Maternal glyphosate exposure causes autism-like behaviors in offspring through increased expression of soluble epoxide hydrolase. *Proc. Natl. Acad. Sci. USA* **2020**, *117*, 11753–11759. [CrossRef]
89. Hamad, A.F.; Alessi-Severini, S.; Mahmud, S.M.; Brownell, M.; Kuo, I.F. Prenatal antibiotics exposure and the risk of autism spectrum disorders: A population-based cohort study. *PLoS ONE* **2019**, *14*, e0221921. [CrossRef]
90. Beversdorf, D.Q.; Stevens, H.E.; Margolis, K.G.; Van de Water, J. Prenatal stress and maternal immune dysregulation in autism spectrum disorders: Potential points for intervention. *Curr. Pharm. Des.* **2019**, *25*, 4331–4343. [CrossRef]
91. Dong, T.; Guan, Q.; Hu, W.; Zhang, M.; Zhang, Y.; Chen, M.; Wang, X.; Xia, Y. Prenatal exposure to glufosinate ammonium disturbs gut microbiome and induces behavioral abnormalities in mice. *J. Hazard. Mater.* **2020**, *389*, 122152. [CrossRef]
92. Frye, R.E.; Rose, S.; Slattery, J.; MacFabe, D.F. Gastrointestinal dysfunction in autism spectrum disorder: The role of the mitochondria and the enteric microbiome. *Microb. Ecol. Health Dis.* **2015**, *26*, 27458. [CrossRef]
93. Delhey, L.; Kilinc, E.N.; Yin, L.; Slattery, J.; Tippett, M.; Wynne, R.; Rose, S.; Kahler, S.; Damle, S.; Legido, A.; et al. Bioenergetic variation is related to autism symptomatology. *Metab. Brain Dis.* **2017**, *32*, 2021–2031. [CrossRef]
94. Goldenthal, M.J.; Damle, S.; Sheth, S.; Shah, N.; Melvin, J.; Jethva, R.; Hardison, H.; Marks, H.; Legido, A. Mitochondrial enzyme dysfunction in autism spectrum disorders; a novel biomarker revealed from buccal swab analysis. *Biomark. Med.* **2015**, *9*, 957–965. [CrossRef]
95. Giulivi, C.; Zhang, Y.F.; Omanska-Klusek, A.; Ross-Inta, C.; Wong, S.; Hertz-Picciotto, I.; Tassone, F.; Pessah, I.N. Mitochondrial dysfunction in autism. *JAMA* **2010**, *304*, 2389–2396. [CrossRef]
96. Napoli, E.; Wong, S.; Hertz-Picciotto, I.; Giulivi, C. Deficits in bioenergetics and impaired immune response in granulocytes from children with autism. *Pediatrics* **2014**, *133*, e1405–e1410. [CrossRef] [PubMed]
97. Graf, W.D.; Marin-Garcia, J.; Gao, H.G.; Pizzo, S.; Naviaux, R.K.; Markusic, D.; Barshop, B.A.; Courchesne, E.; Haas, R.H. Autism associated with the mitochondrial DNA G8363A transfer RNA(Lys) mutation. *J. Child Neurol.* **2000**, *15*, 357–361. [CrossRef]
98. Frye, R.E.; Naviaux, R.K. Autistic disorder with complex IV overactivity: A new mitochondrial syndrome. *J. Pediatr. Neurol.* **2011**, *9*, 427–434.
99. Palmieri, L.; Papaleo, V.; Porcelli, V.; Scarcia, P.; Gaita, L.; Sacco, R.; Hager, J.; Rousseau, F.; Curatolo, P.; Manzi, B.; et al. Altered calcium homeostasis in autism-spectrum disorders: Evidence from biochemical and genetic studies of the mitochondrial aspartate/glutamate carrier AGC1. *Mol. Psychiatry* **2010**, *15*, 38–52. [CrossRef] [PubMed]
100. Hassan, H.; Gnaiger, E.; Zakaria, F.; Makpol, S.; Karim, N.A. Alterations in mitocohndrial respiratiory capacity and membrane potential: A link between mitochondrial dysregulation and autism. *MitoFit* **2020**, in press.
101. Fowler, B.A.; Woods, J.S. Ultrastructural and biochemical changes in renal mitochondria during chronic oral methyl mercury exposure: The relationship to renal function. *Exp. Mol. Pathol.* **1977**, *27*, 403–412. [CrossRef]

102. Shenker, B.J.; Guo, T.L.; O, I.; Shapiro, I.M. Induction of apoptosis in human T-cells by methyl mercury: Temporal relationship between mitochondrial dysfunction and loss of reductive reserve. *Toxicol. Appl. Pharmacol.* **1999**, *157*, 23–35. [CrossRef] [PubMed]
103. Goyer, R.A. Toxic and essential metal interactions. *Annu. Rev. Nutr.* **1997**, *17*, 37–50. [CrossRef]
104. Pourahmad, J.; Mihajlovic, A.; O'Brien, P.J. Hepatocyte lysis induced by environmental metal toxins may involve apoptotic death signals initiated by mitochondrial injury. *Adv. Exp. Med. Biol.* **2001**, *500*, 249–252. [CrossRef]
105. Hiura, T.S.; Li, N.; Kaplan, R.; Horwitz, M.; Seagrave, J.C.; Nel, A.E. The role of a mitochondrial pathway in the induction of apoptosis by chemicals extracted from diesel exhaust particles. *J. Immunol.* **2000**, *165*, 2703–2711. [CrossRef]
106. Wong, P.W.; Garcia, E.F.; Pessah, I.N. Ortho-substituted PCB95 alters intracellular calcium signaling and causes cellular acidification in PC12 cells by an immunophilin-dependent mechanism. *J. Neurochem.* **2001**, *76*, 450–463. [CrossRef] [PubMed]
107. Sherer, T.B.; Richardson, J.R.; Testa, C.M.; Seo, B.B.; Panov, A.V.; Yagi, T.; Matsuno-Yagi, A.; Miller, G.W.; Greenamyre, J.T. Mechanism of toxicity of pesticides acting at complex I: Relevance to environmental etiologies of Parkinson's disease. *J. Neurochem.* **2007**, *100*, 1469–1479. [CrossRef] [PubMed]
108. Yamano, T.; Morita, S. Effects of pesticides on isolated rat hepatocytes, mitochondria, and microsomes II. *Arch. Environ. Contam. Toxicol.* **1995**, *28*, 1–7. [CrossRef]
109. Rose, S.; Frye, R.E.; Slattery, J.; Wynne, R.; Tippett, M.; Pavliv, O.; Melnyk, S.; James, S.J. Oxidative stress induces mitochondrial dysfunction in a subset of autism lymphoblastoid cell lines in a well-matched case control cohort. *PLoS ONE* **2014**, *9*, e85436. [CrossRef]
110. Hill, B.G.; Higdon, A.N.; Dranka, B.P.; Darley-Usmar, V.M. Regulation of vascular smooth muscle cell bioenergetic function by protein glutathiolation. *Biochim. Biophys. Acta* **2010**, *1797*, 285–295. [CrossRef]
111. Frye, R.E.; Rose, S.; Wynne, R.; Bennuri, S.C.; Blossom, S.; Gilbert, K.M.; Heilbrun, L.; Palmer, R.F. Oxidative stress challenge uncovers trichloroacetaldehyde hydrate-induced mitoplasticity in autistic and control lymphoblastoid cell lines. *Sci. Rep.* **2017**, *7*, 4478. [CrossRef] [PubMed]
112. Rose, S.; Frye, R.E.; Slattery, J.; Wynne, R.; Tippett, M.; Melnyk, S.; James, S.J. Oxidative stress induces mitochondrial dysfunction in a subset of autistic lymphoblastoid cell lines. *Transl. Psychiatry* **2015**, *5*, e526. [CrossRef] [PubMed]
113. Rose, S.; Wynne, R.; Frye, R.E.; Melnyk, S.; James, S.J. Increased susceptibility to ethylmercury-induced mitochondrial dysfunction in a subset of autism lymphoblastoid cell lines. *J. Toxicol.* **2015**, *2015*, 573701. [CrossRef] [PubMed]
114. Frye, R.E.; Rose, S.; Chacko, J.; Wynne, R.; Bennuri, S.C.; Slattery, J.C.; Tippett, M.; Delhey, L.; Melnyk, S.; Kahler, S.G.; et al. Modulation of mitochondrial function by the microbiome metabolite propionic acid in autism and control cell lines. *Transl. Psychiatry* **2016**, *6*, e927. [CrossRef]
115. Rose, S.; Bennuri, S.C.; Davis, J.E.; Wynne, R.; Slattery, J.C.; Tippett, M.; Delhey, L.; Melnyk, S.; Kahler, S.G.; MacFabe, D.F.; et al. Butyrate enhances mitochondrial function during oxidative stress in cell lines from boys with autism. *Transl. Psychiatry* **2018**, *8*, 42. [CrossRef] [PubMed]
116. Rose, S.; Bennuri, S.C.; Wynne, R.; Melnyk, S.; James, S.J.; Frye, R.E. Mitochondrial and redox abnormalities in autism lymphoblastoid cells: A sibling control study. *FASEB J. Off. Publ. Fed. Am. Soc. Exp. Biol.* **2017**, *31*, 904–909. [CrossRef]
117. Melnyk, S.; Fuchs, G.J.; Schulz, E.; Lopez, M.; Kahler, S.G.; Fussell, J.J.; Bellando, J.; Pavliv, O.; Rose, S.; Seidel, L.; et al. Metabolic imbalance associated with methylation dysregulation and oxidative damage in children with autism. *J. Autism Dev. Disord.* **2012**, *42*, 367–377. [CrossRef]
118. Canitano, R.; Zappella, M. Autistic epileptiform regression. *Funct. Neurol.* **2006**, *21*, 97–101.
119. Shoffner, J.; Hyams, L.; Langley, G.N.; Cossette, S.; Mylacraine, L.; Dale, J.; Ollis, L.; Kuoch, S.; Bennett, K.; Aliberti, A.; et al. Fever plus mitochondrial disease could be risk factors for autistic regression. *J. Child Neurol.* **2010**, *25*, 429–434. [CrossRef]
120. Edmonds, J.L.; Kirse, D.J.; Kearns, D.; Deutsch, R.; Spruijt, L.; Naviaux, R.K. The otolaryngological manifestations of mitochondrial disease and the risk of neurodegeneration with infection. *Arch. Otolaryngol. Head Neck Surg.* **2002**, *128*, 355–362. [CrossRef]
121. Singh, K.; Singh, I.N.; Diggins, E.; Connors, S.L.; Karim, M.A.; Lee, D.; Zimmerman, A.W.; Frye, R.E. Developmental regression and mitochondrial function in children with autism. *Ann. Clin. Transl. Neurol.* **2020**, *7*, 683–694. [CrossRef]
122. Frye, R.E.; Cox, D.; Slattery, J.; Tippett, M.; Kahler, S.; Granpeesheh, D.; Damle, S.; Legido, A.; Goldenthal, M.J. Mitochondrial dysfunction may explain symptom variation in Phelan-McDermid syndrome. *Sci. Rep.* **2016**, *6*, 19544. [CrossRef]
123. Kanellopoulos, A.K.; Mariano, V.; Spinazzi, M.; Woo, Y.J.; McLean, C.; Pech, U.; Li, K.W.; Armstrong, J.D.; Giangrande, A.; Callaerts, P.; et al. Aralar sequesters GABA into hyperactive mitochondria, causing social behavior deficits. *Cell* **2020**, *180*, 1178–1197.e20. [CrossRef]
124. Curtin, P.; Curtin, A.; Austin, C.; Gennings, C.; Tammimies, K.; Bolte, S.; Arora, M. Recurrence quantification analysis to characterize cyclical components of environmental elemental exposures during fetal and postnatal development. *PLoS ONE* **2017**, *12*, e0187049. [CrossRef]
125. Arora, M.; Bradman, A.; Austin, C.; Vedar, M.; Holland, N.; Eskenazi, B.; Smith, D.R. Determining fetal manganese exposure from mantle dentine of deciduous teeth. *Environ. Sci. Technol.* **2012**, *46*, 5118–5125. [CrossRef]
126. Arora, M.; Hare, D.; Austin, C.; Smith, D.R.; Doble, P. Spatial distribution of manganese in enamel and coronal dentine of human primary teeth. *Sci. Total Environ.* **2011**, *409*, 1315–1319. [CrossRef]
127. Arora, M.; Reichenberg, A.; Willfors, C.; Austin, C.; Gennings, C.; Berggren, S.; Lichtenstein, P.; Anckarsater, H.; Tammimies, K.; Bolte, S. Fetal and postnatal metal dysregulation in autism. *Nat. Commun.* **2017**, *8*, 15493. [CrossRef] [PubMed]

128. Rose, S.; Melnyk, S.; Trusty, T.A.; Pavliv, O.; Seidel, L.; Li, J.; Nick, T.; James, S.J. Intracellular and extracellular redox status and free radical generation in primary immune cells from children with autism. *Autism Res. Treat.* **2012**, *2012*, 986519. [CrossRef] [PubMed]
129. Vandewalle, J.; Bauters, M.; Van Esch, H.; Belet, S.; Verbeeck, J.; Fieremans, N.; Holvoet, M.; Vento, J.; Spreiz, A.; Kotzot, D.; et al. The mitochondrial solute carrier SLC25A5 at Xq24 is a novel candidate gene for non-syndromic intellectual disability. *Hum. Genet.* **2013**, *132*, 1177–1185. [CrossRef] [PubMed]
130. Picard, M.; Zhang, J.; Hancock, S.; Derbeneva, O.; Golhar, R.; Golik, P.; O'Hearn, S.; Levy, S.; Potluri, P.; Lvova, M.; et al. Progressive increase in mtDNA 3243A>G heteroplasmy causes abrupt transcriptional reprogramming. *Proc. Natl. Acad. Sci. USA* **2014**, *111*, E4033–E4042. [CrossRef] [PubMed]
131. Licznerski, P.; Park, H.A.; Rolyan, H.; Chen, R.; Mnatsakanyan, N.; Miranda, P.; Graham, M.; Wu, J.; Cruz-Reyes, N.; Mehta, N.; et al. ATP Synthase c-subunit leak causes aberrant cellular metabolism in fragile X syndrome. *Cell* **2020**, *182*, 1170–1185.e9. [CrossRef]
132. Napoli, E.; Song, G.; Panoutsopoulos, A.; Riyadh, M.A.; Kaushik, G.; Halmai, J.; Levenson, R.; Zarbalis, K.S.; Giulivi, C. Beyond autophagy: A novel role for autism-linked Wdfy3 in brain mitophagy. *Sci. Rep.* **2018**, *8*, 11348. [CrossRef] [PubMed]
133. Yin, C.-L.; Chen, H.-I.; Li, L.-H.; Chien, Y.-L.; Liao, H.-M.; Chou, M.C.; Chou, W.-J.; Tsai, W.-C.; Chiu, Y.-N.; Wu, Y.-Y.; et al. Genome-wide analysis of copy number variations identifies PARK2 as a candidate gene for autism spectrum disorder. *Mol. Autism* **2016**, *7*, 23. [CrossRef] [PubMed]
134. Tang, G.; Gutierrez Rios, P.; Kuo, S.-H.; Akman, H.O.; Rosoklija, G.; Tanji, K.; Dwork, A.; Schon, E.A.; Dimauro, S.; Goldman, J.; et al. Mitochondrial abnormalities in temporal lobe of autistic brain. *Neurobiol. Dis.* **2013**, *54*, 349–361. [CrossRef]
135. Ebrahimi-Fakhari, D.; Saffari, A.; Wahlster, L.; Di Nardo, A.; Turner, D.; Lewis, T.L., Jr.; Conrad, C.; Rothberg, J.M.; Lipton, J.O.; Kölker, S.; et al. Impaired mitochondrial dynamics and mitophagy in neuronal models of tuberous sclerosis complex. *Cell Rep.* **2016**, *17*, 1053–1070. [CrossRef]
136. Pecorelli, A.; Ferrara, F.; Messano, N.; Cordone, V.; Schiavone, M.L.; Cervellati, F.; Woodby, B.; Cervellati, C.; Hayek, J.; Valacchi, G. Alterations of mitochondrial bioenergetics, dynamics, and morphology support the theory of oxidative damage involvement in autism spectrum disorder. *FASEB J. Off. Publ. Fed. Am. Soc. Exp. Biol.* **2020**, *34*, 6521–6538. [CrossRef] [PubMed]
137. Harris, J.; Deen, N.; Zamani, S.; Hasnat, M.A. Mitophagy and the release of inflammatory cytokines. *Mitochondrion* **2018**, *41*, 2–8. [CrossRef]
138. Meeking, M.M.; MacFabe, D.F.; Mepham, J.R.; Foley, K.A.; Tichenoff, L.J.; Boon, F.H.; Kavaliers, M.; Ossenkopp, K.P. Propionic acid induced behavioural effects of relevance to autism spectrum disorder evaluated in the hole board test with rats. *Prog. Neuro Psychopharmacol. Biol. Psychiatry* **2020**, *97*, 109794. [CrossRef] [PubMed]
139. Shams, S.; Foley, K.A.; Kavaliers, M.; MacFabe, D.F.; Ossenkopp, K.P. Systemic treatment with the enteric bacterial metabolic product propionic acid results in reduction of social behavior in juvenile rats: Contribution to a rodent model of autism spectrum disorder. *Dev. Psychobiol.* **2019**, *61*, 688–699. [CrossRef]
140. Foley, K.A.; MacFabe, D.F.; Kavaliers, M.; Ossenkopp, K.P. Sexually dimorphic effects of prenatal exposure to lipopolysaccharide, and prenatal and postnatal exposure to propionic acid, on acoustic startle response and prepulse inhibition in adolescent rats: Relevance to autism spectrum disorders. *Behav. Brain Res.* **2015**, *278*, 244–256. [CrossRef]
141. Foley, K.A.; MacFabe, D.F.; Vaz, A.; Ossenkopp, K.P.; Kavaliers, M. Sexually dimorphic effects of prenatal exposure to propionic acid and lipopolysaccharide on social behavior in neonatal, adolescent, and adult rats: Implications for autism spectrum disorders. *Int. J. Dev. Neurosci. Off. J. Int. Soc. Dev. Neurosci.* **2014**, *39*, 68–78. [CrossRef] [PubMed]
142. Macfabe, D. Autism: Metabolism, mitochondria, and the microbiome. *Glob. Adv. Health Med.* **2013**, *2*, 52–66. [CrossRef] [PubMed]
143. Frye, R.E. Biomarkers of abnormal energy metabolism in children with autism spectrum disorder. *N. Am. J. Med. Sci.* **2012**, *5*, 141–147. [CrossRef]
144. Frye, R.E.; Melnyk, S.; Macfabe, D.F. Unique acyl-carnitine profiles are potential biomarkers for acquired mitochondrial disease in autism spectrum disorder. *Transl. Psychiatry* **2013**, *3*, e220. [CrossRef] [PubMed]
145. Fernandez, A.; Meechan, D.W.; Karpinski, B.A.; Paronett, E.M.; Bryan, C.A.; Rutz, H.L.; Radin, E.A.; Lubin, N.; Bonner, E.R.; Popratiloff, A.; et al. Mitochondrial dysfunction leads to cortical under-connectivity and cognitive impairment. *Neuron* **2019**, *102*, 1127–1142.e3. [CrossRef]
146. Lin-Hendel, E.G.; McManus, M.J.; Wallace, D.C.; Anderson, S.A.; Golden, J.A. Differential mitochondrial requirements for radially and non-radially migrating cortical neurons: Implications for mitochondrial disorders. *Cell Rep.* **2016**, *15*, 229–237. [CrossRef]
147. Chacko, B.K.; Kramer, P.A.; Ravi, S.; Benavides, G.A.; Mitchell, T.; Dranka, B.P.; Ferrick, D.; Singal, A.K.; Ballinger, S.W.; Bailey, S.M.; et al. The Bioenergetic Health Index: A new concept in mitochondrial translational research. *Clin. Sci.* **2014**, *127*, 367–373. [CrossRef]

Journal of *Personalized Medicine*

MDPI

Article

Mitochondrial Fatty Acid β-Oxidation and Resveratrol Effect in Fibroblasts from Patients with Autism Spectrum Disorder

Rita Barone [1,2,*,†], Jean Bastin [3,†], Fatima Djouadi [3], Indrapal Singh [4,5], Mohammad Azharul Karim [4,5], Amrit Ammanamanchi [4,5], Patrick John McCarty [4,5], Leanna Delhey [6], Rose Shannon [6], Antonino Casabona [7], Renata Rizzo [1] and Richard Eugene Frye [4,5,*]

1 Department of Clinical and Experimental Medicine, Child Neuropsychiatry Section, University of Catania, 95124 Catania, Italy; rerizzo@unict.it
2 CNR-Institute for Polymers, Composites and Biomaterials IPCB, 95124 Catania, Italy
3 Centre de Recherche des Cordeliers, INSERM U1138, Sorbonne Université, Université de Paris, 75006 Paris, France; jean.bastin@inserm.fr (J.B.); fatima.djouadi@inserm.fr (F.D.)
4 Barrow Neurological Institute at Phoenix Children's Hospital, Phoenix, AZ 85016, USA; isingh@arizona.edu (I.S.); karim2@arizona.edu (M.A.K.); aammanamanchi@arizona.edu (A.A.); pmccarty@phoenixchildrens.com (P.J.M.)
5 Department of Child Health, University of Arizona College of Medicine—Phoenix, Phoenix, AZ 85004, USA
6 Arkansas Children's Research Institute, Little Rock, AR 72758, USA; LMDelhey@uams.edu (L.D.); SROSE@uams.edu (R.S.)
7 Department of Biomedical and Biotechnological Sciences, Physiology Section, University of Catania, 95124 Catania, Italy; casabona@unict.it
* Correspondence: rbarone@unict.it (R.B.); rfrye@phoenixchildrens.com (R.E.F.)
† R.B. and J.B. contributed equally.

Citation: Barone, R.; Bastin, J.; Djouadi, F.; Singh, I.; Karim, M.A.; Ammanamanchi, A.; McCarty, P.J.; Delhey, L.; Shannon, R.; Casabona, A.; et al. Mitochondrial Fatty Acid β-Oxidation and Resveratrol Effect in Fibroblasts from Patients with Autism Spectrum Disorder. *J. Pers. Med.* **2021**, *11*, 510. https://doi.org/10.3390/jpm11060510

Academic Editor: Farah R. Zahir

Received: 3 May 2021
Accepted: 31 May 2021
Published: 4 June 2021

Publisher's Note: MDPI stays neutral with regard to jurisdictional claims in published maps and institutional affiliations.

Copyright: © 2021 by the authors. Licensee MDPI, Basel, Switzerland. This article is an open access article distributed under the terms and conditions of the Creative Commons Attribution (CC BY) license (https://creativecommons.org/licenses/by/4.0/).

Abstract: Patients with autism spectrum disorder (ASD) may have an increase in blood acyl-carnitine (AC) concentrations indicating a mitochondrial fatty acid β-oxidation (mtFAO) impairment. However, there are no data on systematic mtFAO analyses in ASD. We analyzed tritiated palmitate oxidation rates in fibroblasts from patients with ASD before and after resveratrol (RSV) treatment, according to methods used for the diagnosis of congenital defects in mtFAO. ASD participants ($N = 10$, 60%; male; mean age (SD) 7.4 (3.2) years) were divided in two age-equivalent groups based on the presence ($N = 5$) or absence ($N = 5$) of elevated blood AC levels. In addition, electron transport chain (ETC) activity in fibroblasts and muscle biopsies and clinical characteristics were compared between the ASD groups. Baseline fibroblast mtFAO was not significantly different in patients in comparison with control values. However, ASD patients with elevated AC exhibited significantly decreased mtFAO rates, muscle ETC complex II activity, and fibroblast ETC Complex II/III activity ($p < 0.05$), compared with patients without an AC signature. RSV significantly increased the mtFAO activity in all study groups ($p = 0.001$). The highest mtFAO changes in response to RSV were observed in fibroblasts from patients with more severe symptoms on the Social Responsiveness Scale total ($p = 0.001$) and Awareness, Cognition, Communication and Motivation subscales (all $p < 0.01$). These findings suggested recognition of an ASD patient subset characterized by an impaired mtFAO flux associated with abnormal blood AC. The study elucidated that RSV significantly increased fibroblast mtFAO irrespective of plasma AC status, and the highest changes to RSV effects on mtFAO were observed in the more severely affected patients.

Keywords: autism spectrum disorder; energy metabolism; fatty acid oxidation; acyl-carnitines; resveratrol

1. Introduction

Autism spectrum disorder (ASD) is a neurodevelopmental condition characterized by early social communication deficits and repetitive motor behavior, sensory abnormalities, and restricted interests, with a global prevalence of about 1% [1] and, according to the most recent estimates, of about 2% in the United States (US) [2]. ASD biology is particularly complex, including individual genetic contributions interacting with multiple environmental factors. Genetic risk points to a complex inheritance, with additive contributions from common variants or through rare variants with larger effect sizes [3]. The vast majority of ASD is idiopathic, with a specific cause identified in only 4–20% of patients, including a genetic etiology. Association of ASD behavioral phenotypes to specific genetic subtypes is envisaged; however, patients with molecularly defined ASD are not easily clinically identified because clinical and neurobehavioral correlates of a given genetic contribution vary widely [3,4].

Immune dysregulation/inflammation, oxidative stress, and mitochondrial dysfunction are all key pathologic underpinning of ASD [5,6]. Complex biological changes play a role in ASD clinical heterogeneity, hindering the discovery of universal biomarkers for diagnosis and treatments. Currently, ASD diagnosis is based on measurements of behavioral symptoms according to the Diagnostic Statistical Manual of Mental Disorders Version 5 (DSM-5) diagnostic criteria [7]. Recent data point to identifying patient subsets to better define the contribution of certain biological changes in individual patients. In this context, considerable evidence highlights energy metabolism abnormalities in ASD, pointing to acquired mitochondrial dysfunction in a proportion of patients [8,9]. Impaired mitochondrial metabolism may influence neuronal development and synaptic plasticity, which play a major role in neurodevelopment and contribute to ASD. Low free carnitine [10] and abnormal levels of blood acyl-carnitines (AC) were repeatedly found in ASD clinical studies [11,12]. We recently tested the metabolic profile in dried blood spots to support early recognition of young children at risk for ASD diagnosis. We found a significant increase in blood short-chain and long-chain AC and, to a lesser extent, medium-chain AC. Using machine learning analyses, we found a high classification performance of this AC signature to support diagnosis at younger ages (<5 years) [13]. Interestingly, a similar pattern of increased AC had been detected in patients with ASD from the US [12] and in rodent models, where ASD-like behavior was induced by propionic acid [14]. Recently, a global metabolome analysis of plasma and feces found differential levels of AC among the most discriminant metabolites in ASD compared with typically developing (TD) populations. Furthermore, blood C2–C14 AC levels were positively correlated with a more severe impairment of social behavior, supporting a key role for mitochondrial dysfunction in ASD pathophysiology [15].

The mitochondrial fatty acid β-oxidation (mtFAO) is a major energy-producing metabolic pathway, which uses fatty acids to produce adenosine triphosphate (ATP). First, the import of long-chain fatty-acids (LCFA) into mitochondria requires the activity of a multi-enzymatic carnitine-dependent shuttle, with formation of AC intermediates. Within mitochondria, AC are converted back to acyl-CoA, and the various β-oxidation enzymes isoforms progressively shorten the acyl-CoA to produce acetyl-CoA, NADH, and $FADH_2$ via the Lynen helix [16]. Re-oxidation of produced NADH and $FADH_2$ by the mitochondrial respiratory chain ultimately results in the production of large amounts of ATP. In addition, very recent data unveiled the involvement of mtFAO in instructing non-energy-related functions, such as chromatin modification or neural stem cell activity [17,18].

Thus, AC enables the transport of fatty acids across mitochondrial membranes, and these conjugated fatty acids typically accumulate when β-oxidation is disturbed. This led to widespread clinical applications in the screening for inborn mtFAO disorders in newborns, implemented in many countries, which is based on the detection of specific accumulating AC in the blood of newborns [19]. In line with this, it can be hypothesized that the increase in plasma AC levels in patients with ASD points to an impairment of mtFAO. To date, the implication of mtFAO in the pathophysiology of ASD is largely unknown, but there are consistent findings documenting AC accumulation, and thereby possible mtFAO impairments, as biomarkers and therapeutic targets in a subset of patients with ASD. In the present study, we therefore analyzed the mtFAO flux and respiratory chain activities on primary cultured fibroblasts from ASD patients with elevated plasma AC (w-AC) or without elevated plasma AC (w/o-AC).

Resveratrol (RSV) (3,5,4-trihydroxy-trans-stilbene) is a natural polyphenol produced in plants and enriched in grapes and red fruits. Pre-clinical studies showed that RSV ameliorated social behavior and sensory alterations in the rat model of ASD induced by valproic acid [20,21]. At the molecular level, RSV decreased neuroimmune dysregulation through the inhibition of neuronal toll-like receptors and COX-2 signaling [22] and by downregulation of the chemokine receptor in the BTBR T^+ $Itpr3^{tf}/J$ mice model [23]. Interestingly, RSV was also shown to stimulate mtFAO in control human fibroblasts and could restore normal mtFAO rates in fibroblasts from patients with mild forms of inborn mtFAO deficiencies [24]. This further supports a putative therapeutic effect of RSV in patients with ASD [25] and led us to test whether RSV might induce up-regulation of mtFAO in fibroblasts from ASD patients.

Altogether, the present study had several objectives. At first, we aimed to determine if fibroblasts from ASD patients exhibited mitochondrial mtFAO and respiratory chain deficiencies, compared with fibroblasts from control individuals. In parallel, we sought to determine whether cellular mtFAO rates correlated with the AC status of the ASD patients. Then, we tested the effects of RSV on fibroblasts mtFAO rates in patients with ASD and we evaluated whether the mtFAO response upon RSV treatment was depended on clinical characteristics.

2. Materials and Methods

2.1. Participants

Protocols used in this study were registered in clinicaltrials.gov as NCT02000284 and NCT02003170 and approved by the Institutional Review Board at the University of Arkansas for Medical Sciences (Little Rock, AR, USA). Parents of participants provided written informed consent. All participants were recruited from the Arkansas Children's Hospital Autism Multispecialty clinic directed by Dr Richard E. Frye (senior author). The ASD diagnosis was documented by at least one of the following: (i) a gold-standard diagnostic instrument, such as the Autism Diagnostic Observation Schedule and/or Autism Diagnostic Interview-Revised (ADI-R); (ii) the state of Arkansas diagnostic standard, defined as agreement of a physician, psychologist, and speech therapist who specializes in ASD; and/or (iii) Diagnostic Statistical Manual of Mental Disorders diagnosis by a physician along with standardized validated questionnaires including the Social Responsiveness Scale (SRS), the Social Communication Questionnaire and the Autism Symptoms Questionnaire, all of which have excellent correspondence to the gold-standard instruments, along with diagnosis confirmation by the referral investigator (senior author). In our recent clinical trial [26], we found that methods (ii) and (iii) were consistent with the ADI-R diagnostic criteria for ASD.

In general, fibroblast samples were obtained for clinical use and then transferred to the research laboratory. For individuals that underwent sedated procedures, most commonly muscle biopsy, the samples were obtained under sedation by the surgeon. For individuals that did not undergo other procedures, Dr Richard E. Frye (senior author) personally obtained the sample by a punch biopsy with local anesthesia.

Overall, fibroblast samples were available from 10 children diagnosed with ASD for this study, 6 males and 4 females aged 7.4 ± 3.2 years (mean $\pm$ SD) (range: 3–13). Seven patients (70%) were diagnosed with regressive ASD. Five control fibroblasts from children of similar age who did not manifest any known medical disease or genetic abnormalities were obtained from Coriell Institute for Medical Research (Camden, NJ, USA).

2.2. Neurodevelopmental and Behavioral Measurements

Neurodevelopment assessment was accomplished by the Vineland Adaptive Behavior Scale (VABS) 2nd edition. The VABS is a valid tool based on structured interview with a caretaker allowing to measure age-appropriate abilities in everyday skills including social and motor skills, communication, and daily living. The VABS provides standard scores (m = 100, SD = 15) and higher scores indicate better functioning. The Aberrant Behavior Checklist (ABC), a 58-item parent-reported questionnaire, was used to measure behavioral symptoms across 5 subscales (social withdrawal, hyperactivity, stereotypy, inappropriate speech, and irritability) (0–30 raw scores, higher is worse). Multiple ASD clinical trials have used it and it has both convergent and divergent validity [26]. ASD symptoms severity was assessed by the SRS, a 65-item questionnaire completed by a parent or close family member that measures the severity of social skill deficits across five domains (awareness, cognition, communication, motivation and restricted interests, and repetitive behavior) (clinical cut-off $\geq$ 60).

2.3. Cell Culture and Metabolic Evaluation

Fibroblasts were derived from skin biopsies obtained with written informed consent from the parents. Control and patient fibroblasts were cultured at 37 °C, 5% CO_2 in RPMI with Glutamax™ (Carlsbad, CA, USA) supplemented with 10% (*v*/*v*) fetal bovine serum and 0.2% (*v*/*v*) primocin (InvivoGen, San Diego, CA, USA). For treatment, the media were removed and vehicle (0.04% DMSO) or RSV (75 µM *trans*-RSV, Cayman Chemical, Bertin technologies, Montigny-le-Bretonneux, France), were added to a fresh medium for the last 48 h of culture before mtFAO measurement, as previously described [27]. The mtFAO flux was measured in cultured fibroblasts from w-AC (N = 5) and w/o-AC (N = 5) patients, and in control fibroblasts (N = 5) obtained from healthy subjects with equivalent age and gender distribution. Metabolic evaluation was blinded to patient group, specifically fibroblast assignments were retained confidential and were unveiled at the end of the mtFAO assay for statistical analysis. The FAO flux was determined by quantifying the production of ^3H_2O from (9,10-^{3}H) palmitate, as described previously [27]. The FAO assay was run in triplicate and was repeated twice for each cell line. The FAO assay on resveratrol-treated fibroblasts was performed once. Results (mean ± SD) were expressed in nmol of tritiated-palmitate oxidized per hour per milligram of protein. The electron transport chain (ETC) activity was tested in frozen muscle biopsies and/or cultured fibroblast cultures as previously reported (Baylor Medical Genetics Laboratory, Houston TX, USA) [28]. Values corrected and uncorrected for citrate synthase (CS) activity were considered.

2.4. Statistical Analyses

Data were presented as means and standard deviations (SDs) for continuous variables. Statistical analyses on FAO rates were conducted in the three groups of fibroblasts (w-AC, w/o-AC, and controls). The data were preliminarily subjected to the Shapiro–Wilk test to verify the presence of a normal distribution of the sample, and to the Levene's test to verify the homogeneity of the variances between the groups. Two-way analysis of variance (ANOVA) with repeated measures was used to verify whether FAO was influenced by the group itself (inter-group effect) and presence/absence of RSV (intra-group effect). We used the ANOVA to compare the three groups and all combinations of paired groups. Possible differences between paired groups in the ANOVA analyses were then evaluated by *t*-test with the Bonferroni correction. Student's *t*-test was used to compare the mean values of ETC activity and the clinical scores between the ASD study groups. Correlations among study variables were analyzed by the Pearson correlation analysis. Differences with $p < 0.05$ were considered significant. We assumed that the data were normally distributed based on previous studies which have examined these measures in larger sample sizes as well as by examination of our current dataset. Thus, parameter statistical analyses—especially the technique used here within which are robust to small differences in parameter distribution—were considered appropriate for analysis.

Additionally, to interpret differences between groups, especially in the context of small sample sizes where biological variability can prevent differences from being statistically significant, we compared differences between groups with the minimally clinical important difference (MCID), a value which indicates whether the difference could be considered clinically significant. These values for the VABS, SRS, and ABC are provided in previous clinical studies [26]. Data were analyzed using the SPSS Statistics software, version 23 (SPSS, Inc., Chicago, IL, USA, IBM, Somers, NY, USA).

3. Results

3.1. Blood AC Levels in Patients with ASD

Participants were divided in two groups: w-AC (n:5; age 7.2 ± 3.7) or w/o-AC (n:5; age 7.6 ± 3.1). Mean age was not significantly different in the two study groups ($p = 0.429$). Patients with high plasma AC levels had consistent AC elevation defined as at least three AC significantly elevated ($p < 0.05$) in repeated analyses [12] (Figure 1).

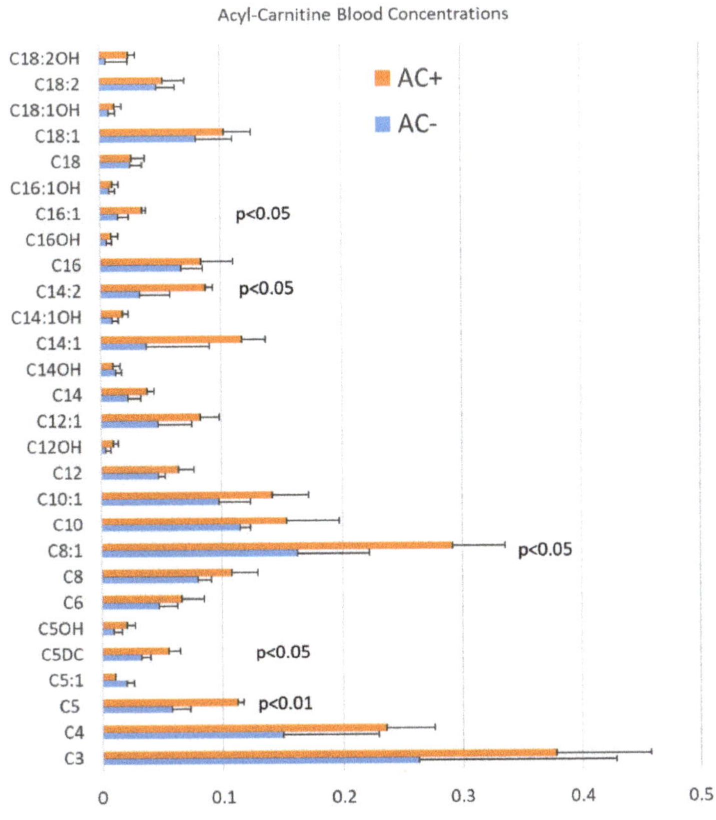

Figure 1. Average blood acyl-carnitine (AC) levels in studied patients with autism spectrum disorder (ASD) with (AC+, orange bars) and without (AC−, blue bars) elevations in acyl-carnitines. Short-chain (C5, C5DC), medium-chain (C8:1), and long-chain (C14:2, C16:1) acyl-carnitines (AC) were significantly elevated in a subset of studied patients with ASD. Patients with high plasma AC levels had consistent AC elevation defined as at least three AC clinically significantly elevated (outside the normal reference range) in repeated analyses.

3.2. mtFAO Activity in Fibroblast Cultures from Patients with ASD

There was no overall significant difference in FAO rates between controls and the ASD fibroblasts (Figure 2; $F_{1,8} = 1.107$; $p = 0.368$) indicating that under basal conditions, FAO was not significantly impaired in ASD children's fibroblasts, regardless of the AC status. However, significant differences were found between the two ASD patient groups ($F_{1,8} = 5.374$; $p = 0.049$). Pairwise t-test revealed that the effect found between the ASD groups in the ANOVA was driven by differences between the two groups of children with ASD, before RSV supplementation. In fact, under basal conditions, the w-AC patients' fibroblasts exhibited significantly decreased FAO values (5.20 ± 0.42) compared with those measured in the w/o-AC group (5.9 ± 0.53) (p = 0.044). Basal FAO rates (5.85 ± 1.12) appeared higher in the control compared with the w-AC patients, but no significant differences were found in paired comparisons, likely because of higher variability of FAO rates in controls. Overall, although not significantly impaired compared with controls, baseline FAO values were significantly lower in patients w-AC elevations compared with patients with normal AC blood levels (Figure 2).

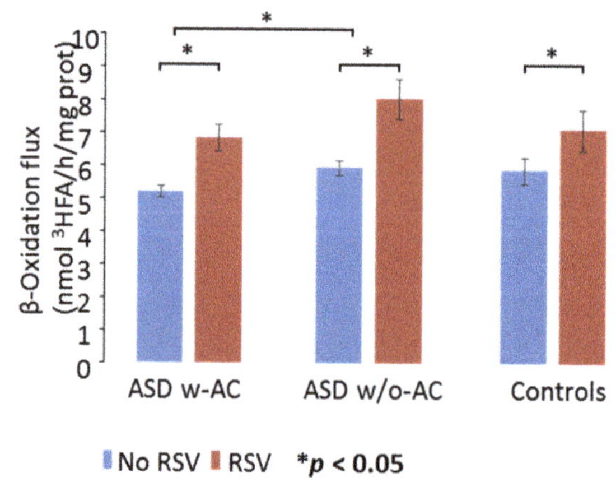

Figure 2. Mitochondrial fatty acid oxidation (FAO) rates (blue bars) and effects of resveratrol (RSV) (red bars) in fibroblasts of ASD patients and healthy control individuals. Figure shows participants with autism spectrum disorder (ASD) that also have acyl-carnitine (AC) elevations (ASD w-AC) and participants with ASD without AC elevations (ASD w/o-AC) as well as control participants. Under basal conditions, the β-oxidation flux (nmol ^{3}HFA/h/mg protein) measured in fibroblasts of patients with ASD w-AC were significantly decreased compared with the ASD w/o-AC. RSV significantly increased mtFAO values in all the study groups. The results are means (±SD) of three different experiments. * $p < 0.05$.

3.3. Electron Transport Chain Complex Activity

Measurements of activities of the ETC complexes were performed on frozen muscle biopsies (N = 8) and cultured fibroblasts (N = 10). Percentages of normal ETC function, uncorrected or corrected for citrate synthase, were compared between the w-AC and w/o-AC groups (Figure 3).

The graph values represent percentages of normal ETC function, uncorrected (Figure 3A,C) or corrected for citrate synthase (Figure 3B,D). Activities of the complex II in the muscle (M; Figure 3B) and the complex II/III in fibroblasts (FB; Figure 3D) were significantly reduced in the patients with ASD with plasma AC elevations as compared with patients with ASD without plasma AC elevations ($p < 0.05$).

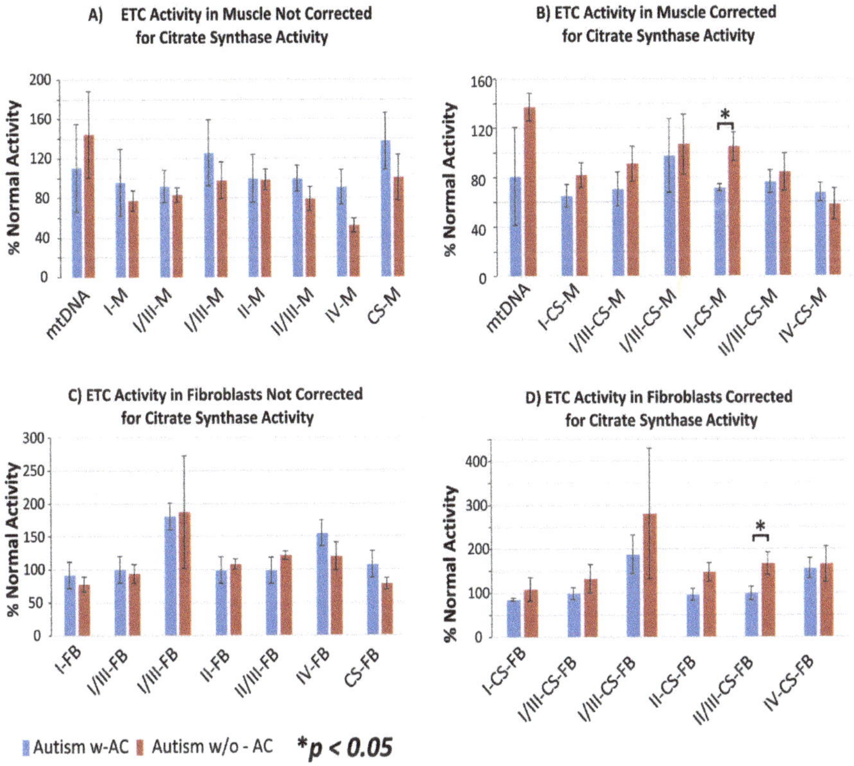

Figure 3. Electron transport chain (ETC) activity in muscle (M; Panels (**A**,**B**)) and fibroblast (FB) culture (Panels (**C**,**D**)) without (Panels (**A**,**C**)) and with (Panels (**B**,**D**)) correction for citrate synthase (CS) activity, in patients with autism spectrum disorder (ASD) that also have acyl-carnitine (AC) elevations (ASD w-AC, blue bars) and participants with ASD without AC elevations (ASD w/o-AC, red bars). Mitochondrial DNA copy number (mtDNA) is also provided in the graphs for muscle samples.

3.4. Clinical Characteristics

Standardized clinical assessment in participants with ASD is reported in Table S1. On average, VABS indicated mildly impaired functioning in all three domains [daily living SS (70.1 ± 16.3), communication SS (73.1 ±16.3); and socialization SS (70.5 ± 16)] in all participants with ASD. The levels of functional disability for ASD symptoms, communication, and socialization measured by the VABS subscales were lower in the participants without AC elevations as compared with those with AC elevations, and these differences exceeded the MCID, suggesting that they were clinically observable. However, these differences were not statistically significant, probably because of the small sample size. On average, patients had disruptive behavioral symptoms, such as irritability and hyperactivity, at least of moderate severity (defined as scores greater than or equal to 13 on the ABC). Patients in the w-AC group had higher scores on the ABC social withdrawal, inappropriate speech, and stereotypy subscales compared with the w/o-AC group, and these differences exceeded the MCID, suggesting that they were clinically observable. Patients in the w/o-AC group had higher scores on the ABC hyperactivity and irritability, and they exceeded the MCID. However, all these differences were not statistically significant, probably because of the small sample size.

All participants with ASD had social impairment severity in the clinical range (T-scores > 60 on SRS total), with no significant differences between the study groups. However, those with ASD with AC elevations demonstrated less impaired social awareness and cognition but greater repetitive behaviors (mannerism) on the SRS as compared with those with ASD but without AC elevation, and these differences exceeded the MCID.

Then we evaluated whether fibroblast mtFAO at baseline and upon RSV treatment was depended on clinical characteristics (Table S2). We found that patients who had the highest mtFAO activity in response to RSV were the most impaired on the SRS–total (r = 0.65; p = 0.044), SRS–awareness (r = 0.72; p = 0.019), and SRS–cognition (r = 0.76; p = 0.011). Moreover, the highest changes to RSV with respect to baseline were observed in patients most impaired on the SRS–total (r = 0.87; p = 0.001; Figure 4A) as well as on SRS subscales including awareness (r = 0.89; p < 0.001; Figure 4B), cognition (r = 0.88; p < 0.001; Figure 4C), communication (r = 0.78; p = 0.008; Figure 4D), and motivation (r = 0.77; p = 0.009; Figure 4E).

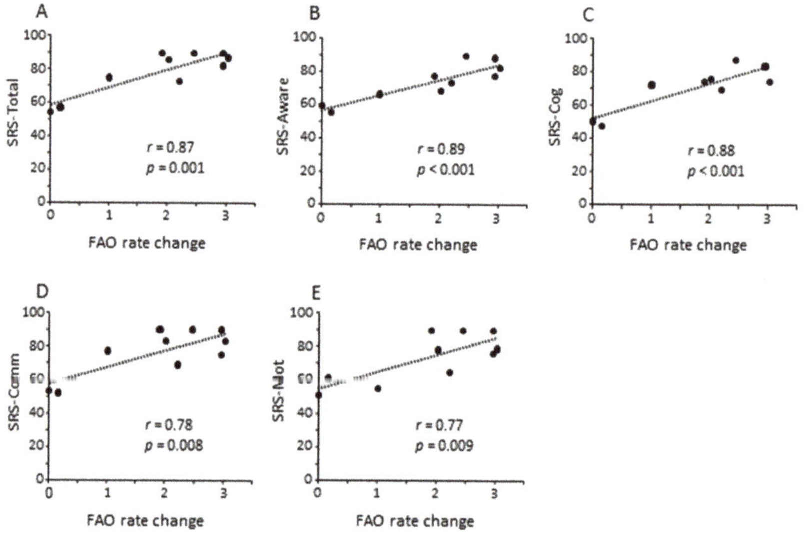

Figure 4. Correlation analyses among clinical characteristics of patients with ASD as measured by the Social Responsiveness Scale (SRS) and resveratrol (RSV) effect on fatty acid oxidation (FAO) in fibroblasts. Highest changes of mtFAO in response to RSV were significantly associated with clinical impairment (higher scores) on the SRS–total (**A**) as well as on SRS awareness (**B**), cognition (**C**), communication (**D**), and motivation (**E**) subscales.

4. Discussion

In the present study, we systematically applied palmitate oxidation rate measurements in fibroblasts to investigate ex vivo mtFAO levels in a series of patients with ASD. We found that under basal conditions, mtFAO in fibroblasts was not significantly different in children with ASD compared with healthy controls. However, the mtFAO flux was significantly decreased in patients with elevated blood AC compared with patients with normal blood AC. Significant differences in basal mtFAO rate between ASD groups may be consistent with recurrent findings of elevated blood AC in subgroups of children with ASD [12,13].

As mentioned above, screening of inborn mtFAO deficiencies in newborns is based on acyl-carnitines analysis in dried blood spots, which needs to be followed by confirmatory testing to define the ultimate diagnosis [19]. Importantly, patients diagnosed in this way at birth are mostly asymptomatic, and the AC pattern is not predictive of symptomatology [29]. In many cases, the symptom-free period will last for years, and the disease manifestations will only develop in the adolescence or adulthood, generally triggered by exercise, cold, fever, or other metabolic stress situations. This is true in particular for the

VLCAD deficiency, one of the most common inborn mtFAO disorders. In the mild—most frequent—form of this disorder, the typical C (14:1) AC accumulation detected at birth can be associated with near-normal FAO flux values in the patients' fibroblasts and with the absence of clinical manifestations [30–32]. In adult patients with the muscular form of carnitine-palmitoyl transferase II (CPT-II) deficiency, high plasma levels of long-chain AC can be measured in the absence of disease symptoms, and mtFAO values in patient fibroblasts may also appear marginally modified [33]. In sum, evidence from genetic mtFAO defects suggests that an inefficient mtFAO flux with accumulation of AC biomarkers may arise without obvious symptoms affecting mtFAO-dependent organs and even in the presence of a relatively high residual mtFAO activity. The occurrence of developmental delay, autistic-like behavior, or ASD in genetic defects of mtFAO, particularly VLCAD [34] and LCHAD [35], suggests that impaired mtFAO may contribute to dysfunctional energy metabolism in subsets of patients with ASD. Furthermore, interestingly, post-hoc analysis of newborn screening data in a large (>9000 individuals) cohort showed that high levels of ACs could be associated with an increased risk of ASD [36]. Specific abnormalities in AC also characterize an animal model of ASD in which propionic acid, a microbiome-produced short chain fatty acid, results in ASD-like behavior, mitochondrial dysfunction, and neuroinflammation [37].

In addition to reduced mtFAO oxidation rate, patients with ASD and plasma AC elevations had significantly lower ETC complex II and complex II/III activities in muscle and fibroblasts, respectively, when compared with patients with normal AC blood levels. This is consistent with a previous study that demonstrated a partial deficit in complexes I/III and I/III RS functions in muscle of patients with ASD and elevated blood AC [12]. As a whole, the current findings support recognition of an ASD patient subset characterized by impaired mtFAO efficiency associated with abnormal blood AC underlying decreased energy production in different cell types.

It is noteworthy that our finding of a >200% increase in the ETC complex I/III activity in patients with ASD is consistent with recent findings illustrating that an elevation of the respiratory chain activity may be abnormal and associated with ASD. An increase in the baseline respiratory chain activity in lymphoblastoid cell lines from subsets of patients with ASD is associated with increased vulnerability to environmental toxicants and to physiological stress [38,39]. It was shown that patients with ASD and mitochondrial dysfunction have higher rates of neurodevelopmental regression with loss of acquired abilities following fever or infections [40] as not uncommonly seen in patients with ETC mitochondrial disorders [41]. Such abnormalities are consistent with acquired mitochondrial dysfunction in ASD patients with neurodevelopmental regression [42] and with studies which demonstrated that mitochondrial dysfunction in ASD can be associated with environmental factors, such as fever [40], immune activation and oxidative stress [43], microbiome metabolites [37], air pollution [44], and prenatal nutritional deficiencies [45]. Some other symptoms of mitochondrial disease, including hypotonia and motor delay, seizures, and gastrointestinal disturbances are frequently encountered in ASD as well [5].

Previous research established that ex vivo measurements of palmitate oxidation rate provide a sensitive approach to test the efficiency of compounds potentially capable to stimulate mtFAO, such as fibrates and RSV [24,27,46]. Pre-clinical studies using different ASD models showed the effects of RSV on several pathways involved in ASD, such as decreasing microglia-induced neuroinflammation and oxidative stress, by reducing oxygen and nitrogen reactive species and neurotransmitter imbalance [22,47]. More recently, RSV was found capable of ameliorating social behavioral deficits in the oxytocin receptor gene knockout by up-regulation of the silent information regulator 1 (Sirt1) gene and early growth response factor 3 (Egr3) gene expressions in the amygdala of Oxtr-KO mice [48]. In 2020, a double-blind, placebo-controlled clinical trial investigated the effects of RSV as an adjunctive treatment in decreasing disruptive behavioral symptoms measured by SRS in patients with ASD. RSV add-on therapy to Risperidone did not yield any significant improvement on the irritability subscale compared with placebo but led to significant improvement on the hyperactivity/non-compliance subscale after a 10-week period [49]. No severe adverse effects were observed and no significant difference in the frequency of adverse effects was documented between RSV-treated versus placebo group, thus supporting further clinical studies using RSV monotherapy in patients with ASD.

For the first time, the current study explored the effects of RSV on mtFAO in fibroblasts from patients with ASD. It showed that RSV significantly increased mtFAO activity in fibroblasts from patients with ASD as well as in controls. RSV effects on FAO are mediated by peroxisome proliferator activated receptor gamma co-activator-1-alpha (PGC-1α). PGC-1α serves as a co-activator of various transcription factors [PPARs, NRF 1 and 2 (nuclear respiratory factors), hepatic nuclear factor 4], thus regulating the expression of several enzymes involved in the mtFAO pathway, mitochondrial biogenesis, oxidative phosphorylation, and energy production [24]. Importantly, we showed an association between RSV effects on mtFAO activity in fibroblasts from children with ASD and pertinent clinical characteristics. We found that the highest changes to RSV with respect to baseline were observed in patients with more severe ASD symptoms on the SRS scale, such as impaired awareness, cognition, social communication, and motivation.

The main limitations of the present study include the small size of the samples used for ex vivo analyses of mtFAO. This suggests that the study is underpowered, so non-significant differences cannot be claimed to signify that no difference exists. Clearly, further studies with larger sample sizes will be needed to follow up this work. Secondly, it should be noted that results from pre-clinical studies such as the present one may partially apply to the in vivo condition and will ultimately require to be tested in clinical trials. As ASD is heterogeneous in nature, there is a need to characterize patients also considering what possible differences in metabolic profiling might lead to different clinical responses to the same therapies. Taken into account that ASD is unequivocally associated with mtFAO impairment in patient subsets, the effects of RSV in ameliorating mtFAO in patient cells may be relevant for understanding the therapeutic response.

5. Conclusions

In conclusion, we found a significant difference in fibroblasts basal mtFAO rates between ASD groups that differ by the presence or absence of elevated blood acyl-carnitines. The study showed for the first time that the mtFAO activity in fibroblasts of ASD children increased significantly after RSV and that the highest changes to RSV effects on mtFAO occurred in the most severely affected patients. In the light of the present findings, future clinical trials might well consider whether possible RSV effects in ameliorating behavioral symptoms are associated with baseline symptoms severity in patients with ASD. Moreover, further studies should take into account how and to what extent different metabolic profiles may influence response to therapies in patients with ASD.

Supplementary Materials: The following are available online at https://www.mdpi.com/article/10.3390/jpm11060510/s1, Table S1: Standardized clinical assessment scores in participants with ASD. Table S2: Correlation analysis (*r*) among clinical severity and mitochondrial fatty acid oxidation (mtFAO) activity in fibroblasts from patients with ASD under basal conditions and after resveratrol (RSV+) treatment.

Author Contributions: Conceptualization, R.B., J.B. and R.E.F.; Data curation, R.B., J.B., F.D., R.S. and R.E.F.; Formal analysis, J.B., F.D., R.S. and A.C.; Investigation, J.B., F.D., I.S., M.A.K., A.A., P.J.M. and L.D.; Methodology, R.B., J.B., A.C. and R.E.F.; Project administration, R.S. and R.E.F.; Writing—original draft, R.B., J.B. and R.E.F.; Writing—review & editing, R.B., J.B., R.R. and R.E.F.; Funding Acquisition: R.R., R.E.F. All authors have read and agreed to the published version of the manuscript.

Funding: This research was funded, in part, by the N of 1 Foundation (Dallas, TX, USA), the Phoenix Children's Hospital Foundation (Phoenix, AZ, USA), the Arkansas Biosciences Institute (Little Rock, AR, USA), The Jonty Foundation (St Paul, MN, USA), the Gupta Family Foundation (Atherton, CA, USA), and the Jager Family Foundation (Chicago, IL, USA)to R.E.F. and by Piano di Ricerca di Ateneo 2020-22 linea 2 grant from the University of Catania (Catania, Italy) to R.B. and R.R.

Institutional Review Board Statement: The study was conducted according to the guidelines of the Declaration of Helsinki. Protocols used in this study were registered in clinicaltrials.gov as NCT02000284 and NCT02003170 and approved by the Institutional Review Board at the University of Arkansas for Medical Sciences (Little Rock, AR, USA).

Informed Consent Statement: Informed consent was obtained from all subjects involved in the study.

Data Availability Statement: All data presented in the study are included in the article. Further inquiries can be directed to the corresponding authors.

Acknowledgments: The authors would like to thank John Slattery for his help with coordination participants, Sirish C. Bennuri for help coordinating samples, Stephen Kahler for his help with patient recruitment, and the families who have volunteered to be involved in the research despite their demanding lives.

Conflicts of Interest: The authors declare no conflict of interest.

References

1. Lord, C.; Brugha, T.S.; Charman, T.; Cusack, J.; Dumas, G.; Frazier, T.; Jones, E.J.H.; Jones, R.M.; Pickles, A.; State, M.W.; et al. Autism spectrum disorder. *Nat. Rev. Dis. Prim.* **2020**, *6*, 5. [CrossRef]
2. Maenner, M.J.; Shaw, K.A.; Baio, J.; Washington, A.; Patrick, M.; DiRienzo, M.; Christensen, D.L.; Wiggins, L.D.; Pettygrove, S.; Andrews, J.G.; et al. Prevalence of Autism Spectrum Disorder Among Children Aged 8 Years—Autism and Developmental Disabilities Monitoring Network, 11 Sites, United States, 2016. *MMWR Surveill. Summ.* **2020**, *69*, 1–12. [CrossRef]
3. Havdahl, A.; Niarchou, M.; Starnawska, A.; Uddin, M.; van der Merwe, C.; Warrier, V. Genetic contributions to autism spectrum disorder. *Psychol. Med.* **2021**, *26*, 1–14.
4. Barone, R.; Gulisano, M.; Amore, R.; Domini, C.; Milana, M.C.; Giglio, S.; Madia, F.; Mattina, T.; Casabona, A.; Fichera, M.; et al. Clinical correlates in children with autism spectrum disorder and CNVs: Systematic investigation in a clinical setting. *Int. J. Dev. Neurosci.* **2020**, *80*, 276–286. [CrossRef]
5. A Rossignol, D.; E Frye, R. Mitochondrial dysfunction in autism spectrum disorders: A systematic review and meta-analysis. *Mol. Psychiatry* **2011**, *17*, 290–314.
6. Masi, A.; Quintana, D.S.; Glozier, N.; Lloyd, A.R.; Hickie, I.B.; Guastella, A.J. Cytokine aberrations in autism spectrum disorder: A systematic review and meta-analysis. *Mol. Psychiatry* **2014**, *20*, 440–446. [CrossRef] [PubMed]
7. American Psychiatric Association. *Diagnostic and Statistical Manual of Mental Disorders (DSM–5)*; American Psychiatric Association: Washington, DC, USA, 2013.
8. Rose, S.; Niyazov, D.M.; Rossignol, D.A.; Goldenthal, M.; Kahler, S.G.; Frye, R.E. Clinical and Molecular Characteristics of Mitochon-drial Dysfunction in Autism Spectrum Disorder. *Mol. Diagn. Ther.* **2018**, *22*, 571–593. [CrossRef] [PubMed]
9. Frye, R.E. Mitochondrial Dysfunction in Autism Spectrum Disorder: Unique Abnormalities and Targeted Treatments. *Semin. Pediatr. Neurol.* **2020**, *35*, 100829. [CrossRef]
10. Filipek, P.A.; Juranek, J.; Nguyen, M.T.; Cummings, C.; Gargus, J.J. Relative carnitine deficiency in autism. *J. Autism Dev. Disord.* **2004**, *34*, 615–623. [CrossRef]
11. Clark-Taylor, T.; Clark-Taylor, B.E. Is autism a disorder of fatty acid metabolism? Possible dysfunction of mitochondrial be-ta-oxidation by long chain acyl-CoA dehydrogenase. *Med. Hypotheses* **2004**, *62*, 970–975. [CrossRef]
12. E Frye, R.; Melnyk, S.; MacFabe, D.F. Unique acyl-carnitine profiles are potential biomarkers for acquired mitochondrial disease in autism spectrum disorder. *Transl. Psychiatry* **2013**, *3*, e220. [CrossRef]
13. Barone, R.; Alaimo, S.; Messina, M.; Pulvirenti, A.; Bastin, J.; Ferro, A.; Frye, R.E.; Rizzo, R.; MIMIC-Autism Group. A Subset of Patients with Autism Spectrum Disorders Show a Distinctive Metabolic Profile by Dried Blood Spot Analyses. *Front. Psychiatry* **2018**, *9*, 636. [CrossRef] [PubMed]
14. Thomas, R.H.; Foley, K.A.; Mepham, J.R.; Tichenoff, L.J.; Possmayer, F.; MacFabe, D.F. Altered brain phospholipid and acylcarnitine profiles in propionic acid infused rodents: Further development of a potential model of autism spectrum disorders. *J. Neuro-Chem.* **2010**, *113*, 515–529. [CrossRef]
15. Needham, B.D.; Adame, M.D.; Serena, G.; Rose, D.R.; Preston, G.M.; Conrad, M.C.; Campbell, A.S.; Donabedian, D.H.; Fasano, A.; Ashwood, P.; et al. Plasma and Fecal Metabolite Profiles in Autism Spectrum Disorder. *Biol. Psychiatry* **2021**, *89*, 451–462. [CrossRef] [PubMed]
16. Houten, S.M.; Wanders, R.J.A. A general introduction to the biochemistry of mitochondrial fatty acid β-oxidation. *J. Inherit. Metab. Dis.* **2010**, *33*, 469–477. [CrossRef]
17. Menzies, K.J.; Zhang, H.; Katsyuba, E.; Auwerx, J. Protein acetylation in metabolism—Metabolites and cofactors. *Nat. Rev. Endocrinol.* **2015**, *12*, 43–60. [CrossRef] [PubMed]
18. Knobloch, M.; Pilz, G.-A.; Ghesquière, B.; Kovacs, W.J.; Wegleiter, T.; Moore, D.L.; Hruzova, M.; Zamboni, N.; Carmeliet, P.; Jessberger, S. A Fatty Acid Oxidation-Dependent Metabolic Shift Regulates Adult Neural Stem Cell Activity. *Cell Rep.* **2017**, *20*, 2144–2155. [CrossRef]

19. Wanders, R.J.A.; Visser, G.; Ferdinandusse, S.; Vaz, F.M.; Houtkooper, R.H. Mitochondrial Fatty Acid Oxidation Disorders: Labora-tory Diagnosis, Pathogenesis, and the Complicated Route to Treatment. *J. Lipid Atheroscler.* **2020**, *9*, 313–333. [CrossRef]
20. Bambini-Junior, V.; Zanatta, G.; Nunes, G.D.F.; de Melo, G.M.; Michels, M.S.; Fontes-Dutra, M.; Freire, V.N.; Riesgo, R.; Gottfried, C. Resveratrol prevents social deficits in animal model of autism induced by valproic acid. *Neurosci. Lett.* **2014**, *583*, 176–181. [CrossRef] [PubMed]
21. Fontes-Dutra, M.; Santos-Terra, J.; Deckmann, I.; Schwingel, G.B.; Nunes, G.D.-F.; Hirsch, M.M.; Bauer-Negrini, G.; Riesgo, R.S.; Bambini-Júnior, V.; Hedin-Pereira, C.; et al. Resveratrol Prevents Cellular and Behavioral Sensory Alterations in the Animal Model of Autism Induced by Valproic Acid. *Front. Synaptic Neurosci.* **2018**, *10*, 9. [CrossRef]
22. Ahmad, S.F.; Ansari, M.A.; Nadeem, A.; Alzahrani, M.Z.; Bakheet, S.A.; Attia, S.M. Resveratrol Improves Neuroimmune Dysregula-tion Through the Inhibition of Neuronal Toll-Like Receptors and COX-2 Signaling in BTBR T+ Itpr3tf/J Mice. *Neuromol. Med.* **2018**, *20*, 133–146. [CrossRef]
23. Bakheet, S.A.; Alzahrani, M.Z.; Nadeem, A.; Ansari, M.A.; Zoheir, K.M.A.; Attia, S.M.; Al-Ayadhi, L.Y.; Ahmad, S.F. Resveratrol treat-ment attenuates chemokine receptor expression in the BTBR T+tf/J mouse model of autism. *Mol. Cell Neurosci.* **2016**, *77*, 1–10. [CrossRef]
24. Djouadi, F.; Bastin, J. Mitochondrial Genetic Disorders: Cell Signaling and Pharmacological Therapies. *Cells* **2019**, *8*, 289. [CrossRef]
25. Barone, R.; Rizzo, R.; Tabbì, G.; Malaguarnera, M.; Frye, R.E.; Bastin, J. Nuclear Peroxisome Proliferator-Activated Receptors (PPARs) as Therapeutic Targets of Resveratrol for Autism Spectrum Disorder. *Int. J. Mol. Sci.* **2019**, *20*, 1878. [CrossRef] [PubMed]
26. Frye, R.E.; Slattery, J.; Delhey, L.; Furgerson, B.; Strickland, T.; Tippett, M.; Sailey, A.; Wynne, R.; Rose, S.; Melnyk, S.; et al. Folinic acid improves verbal communication in children with autism and language impairment: A randomized double-blind placebo-controlled trial. *Mol. Psychiatry* **2018**, *23*, 247–256. [CrossRef]
27. Aires, V.; Delmas, D.; Le Bachelier, C.; Latruffe, N.; Schlemmer, D.; Benoist, J.F.; Djouadi, F.; Bastin, J. Stilbenes and resveratrol metab-olites improve mitochondrial fatty acid oxidation defects in human fibroblasts. *Orphanet. J. Rare Dis.* **2014**, *9*, 79. [CrossRef] [PubMed]
28. Kirby, D.M.; Thorburn, D.R.; Turnbull, D.M.; Taylor, R.W. Biochemical assays of respiratory chain complex activity. *Methods Cell Biol.* **2007**, *80*, 93–119.
29. Bastin, J. Regulation of mitochondrial fatty acid ß-oxidation in human:what can we learn from inborn fatty acid ß-oxidation deficiencies? *Biochimie* **2014**, *96*, 113–120. [CrossRef]
30. Gobin-Limballe, S.; Djouadi, F.; Aubey, F.; Olpin, S.; Andresen, B.S.; Yamaguchi, S.; Mandel, H.; Fukao, T.; Ruiter, J.P.N.; Wanders, R.J.A.; et al. Genetic basis for correction of very-long-chain acyl-coenzyme A dehydrogenase deficiency by bezafi-brate in patient fibroblasts: Toward a genotype-based therapy. *Am. J. Hum. Genet.* **2007**, *81*, 1133–1143. [CrossRef] [PubMed]
31. Hesse, J.; Braun, C.; Behringer, S.; Matysiak, U.; Spiekerkoetter, U.; Tucci, S. The diagnostic challenge in very-long chain acyl-CoA dehydrogenase deficiency (VLCADD). *J. Inherit. Metab. Dis.* **2018**, *41*, 1169–1178. [CrossRef]
32. Bleeker, J.C.; Kok, I.L.; Ferdinandusse, S.; van der Pol, L.W.; Cuppen, I.; Bosch, A.M.; Langeveld, M.; Derks, T.G.J.; Williams, M.; de Vries, M.; et al. Impact of newborn screening for very-long-chain acyl-CoA dehydrogenase deficiency on genetic, enzymatic, and clinical outcomes. *J. Inherit. Metab. Dis.* **2019**, *42*, 414–423. [CrossRef]
33. Bonnefont, J.P.; Bastin, J.; Laforêt, P.; Aubey, F.; Mogenet, A.; Romano, S.; Ricquier, D.; Gobin-Limballe, S.; Vassault, A.; Behin, A.; et al. Long-term follow-up of bezafibrate treatment in patients with the myopathic form of carnitine palmito-yltransferase 2 deficiency. *Clin. Pharmacol. Ther.* **2010**, *88*, 101–108. [CrossRef]
34. Brown, A.; Crowe, L.; Andresen, B.S.; Anderson, V.; Boneh, A. Neurodevelopmental profiles of children with very long chain acyl-CoA dehydrogenase deficiency diagnosed by newborn screening. *Mol. Genet. Metab.* **2014**, *113*, 278–282. [CrossRef]
35. Strandqvist, A.; Haglind, C.B.; Zetterström, R.H.; Nemeth, A.; von Döbeln, U.; Stenlid, M.H.; Nordenström, A. Neuropsychological Development in Patients with Long-Chain 3-Hydroxyacyl-CoA Dehydrogenase (LCHAD) Deficiency. *JIMD Rep.* **2016**, *28*, 75–84. [PubMed]
36. Canfield, M.A.; Langlois, P.H.; Rutenberg, G.W.; Mandell, D.J.; Hua, F.; Reilly, B.; Ruktanonchai, D.J.; Jackson, J.F.; Hunt, P.; Freedenberg, D.; et al. The association between newborn screening analytes and childhood autism in a Texas Medicaid popula-tion, 2010–2012. *Am. J. Med. Genet. B Neuropsychiatr. Genet.* **2019**, *180*, 291–304. [CrossRef] [PubMed]
37. Frye, R.E.; Rose, S.; Slattery, J.; MacFabe, D.F. Gastrointestinal dysfunction in autism spectrum disorder: The role of the mitochon-dria and the enteric microbiome. *Microb. Ecol. Health Dis.* **2015**, *26*, 27458. [CrossRef]
38. Rose, S.; Wynne, R.; Frye, R.E.; Melnyk, S.; James, S.J. Increased susceptibility to ethylmercury-induced mitochondrial dysfunction in a subset of autism lymphoblastoid cell lines. *J. Toxicol.* **2015**, *2015*, 573701. [CrossRef]
39. Rose, S.; Bennuri, S.; Wynne, R.; Melnyk, S.; James, S.J.; Frye, R.E. Mitochondrial and redox abnormalities in autism lymphoblas-toid cells: A sibling control study. *FASEB J.* **2016**, *31*, 904–909. [CrossRef]
40. Shoffner, J.; Hyams, L.; Langley, G.N.; Cossette, S.; Mylacraine, L.; Dale, J.; Ollis, L.; Kuoch, S.; Bennett, K.; Aliberti, A.; et al. Fever plus mitochondrial disease could be risk factors for autistic regression. *J. Child Neurol.* **2009**, *25*, 429–434. [CrossRef]
41. Edmonds, J.L.; Kirse, D.J.; Kearns, D.; Deutsch, R.; Spruijt, L.; Naviaux, R.K. The otolaryngological manifestations of mitochondrial disease and the risk of neurodegeneration with infection. *Arch. Otolaryngol. Head Neck Surg.* **2002**, *128*, 355–362. [CrossRef]
42. Singh, K.; Singh, I.N.; Diggins, E.; Connors, S.L.; Karim, M.A.; Lee, D.; Zimmerman, A.W.; Frye, R.E. Developmental regression and mi-tochondrial function in children with autism. *Ann. Clin. Transl. Neurol.* **2020**, *7*, 683–694. [CrossRef]

43. Rossignol, D.A.; Frye, R.E. Evidence linking oxidative stress, mitochondrial dysfunction, and inflammation in the brain of indi-viduals with autism. *Front Physiol.* **2014**, *5*, 150. [CrossRef]
44. Frye, R.E.; Cakir, J.; Rose, S.; Delhey, L.; Bennuri, S.C.; Tippett, M.; Melnyk, S.; James, S.J.; Palmer, R.F.; Austin, C.; et al. Prenatal air pollution influences neurodevelopment and behavior in autism spectrum disorder by modulating mitochondrial physiology. *Mol. Psychiatry* **2020**, 1–17. [CrossRef] [PubMed]
45. Frye, R.E.; Cakir, J.; Rose, S.; Delhey, L.; Bennuri, S.C.; Tippett, M.; Palmer, R.F.; Austin, C.; Curtin, P.; Arora, M. Early life metal exposure dysregulates cellular bioenergetics in children with regressive autism spectrum disorder. *Transl. Psychiatry* **2020**, *10*, 223. [CrossRef]
46. Bastin, J.; Lopes-Costa, A.; Djouadi, F. Exposure to resveratrol triggers pharmacological correction of fatty acid utilization in human fatty acid oxidation-deficient fibroblasts. *Hum. Mol. Genet.* **2011**, *20*, 2048–2057. [CrossRef] [PubMed]
47. Malaguarnera, M.; Khan, H.; Cauli, O. Resveratrol in Autism Spectrum Disorders: Behavioral and Molecular Effects. *Antioxidants* **2020**, *9*, 188. [CrossRef]
48. Hidema, S.; Kikuchi, S.; Takata, R.; Yanai, T.; Shimomura, K.; Horie, K.; Nishimori, K. Single administration of resveratrol improves social behavior in adult mouse models of autism spectrum disorder. *Biosci. Biotechnol. Biochem.* **2020**, *84*, 2207–2214. [CrossRef]
49. Hendouei, F.; Sanjari Moghaddam, H.; Mohammadi, M.R.; Taslimi, N.; Rezaei, F.; Akhondzadeh, S. Resveratrol as adjunctive ther-apy in treatment of irritability in children with autism: A double-blind and placebo-controlled randomized trial. *J. Clin. Pharm. Ther.* **2020**, *45*, 324–334. [CrossRef]

Journal of *Personalized Medicine*

MDPI

Review

Folate Receptor Alpha Autoantibodies in Autism Spectrum Disorders: Diagnosis, Treatment and Prevention

Natasha Bobrowski-Khoury [1], Vincent T. Ramaekers [2], Jeffrey M. Sequeira [3] and Edward V. Quadros [3,*]

1 School of Graduate Studies, SUNY Downstate Medical Center, Brooklyn, NY 11203, USA; natasha.bobrowski-khoury@downstate.edu
2 The Autism Center, University of Liège, 4000 Liège, Belgium; vramaekers@skynet.be
3 Department of Medicine, SUNY Downstate Medical Center, Brooklyn, NY 11203, USA; jeffrey.sequeira@downstate.edu
* Correspondence: edward.quadros@downstate.edu

Abstract: Folate deficiency and folate receptor autoimmune disorder are major contributors to infertility, pregnancy related complications and abnormal fetal development including structural and functional abnormalities of the brain. Food fortification and prenatal folic acid supplementation has reduced the incidence of neural tube defect (NTD) pregnancies but is unlikely to prevent pregnancy-related complications in the presence of folate receptor autoantibodies (FRAb). In pregnancy, these autoantibodies can block folate transport to the fetus and in young children, folate transport to the brain. These antibodies are prevalent in neural tube defect pregnancies and in developmental disorders such as cerebral folate deficiency (CFD) syndrome and autism spectrum disorder (ASD). In the latter conditions, folinic acid treatment has shown clinical improvement in some of the core ASD deficits. Early testing for folate receptor autoantibodies and intervention is likely to result in a positive outcome. This review discusses the first identification of FRAb in women with a history of neural tube defect pregnancy and FRAb's association with sub-fertility and preterm birth. Autoantibodies against folate receptor alpha (FRα) are present in about 70% of the children with a diagnosis of ASD, and a significant number of these children respond to oral folinic acid with overall improvements in speech, language and social interaction. The diagnosis of folate receptor autoimmune disorder by measuring autoantibodies against FRα in the serum provides a marker with the potential for treatment and perhaps preventing the pathologic consequences of folate receptor autoimmune disorder.

Keywords: autism spectrum disorders; folate receptor alpha; folates; pregnancy; brain development; fetal development

Citation: Bobrowski-Khoury, N.; Ramaekers, V.T.; Sequeira, J.M.; Quadros, E.V. Folate Receptor Alpha Autoantibodies in Autism Spectrum Disorders: Diagnosis, Treatment and Prevention. *J. Pers. Med.* **2021**, *11*, 710. https://doi.org/10.3390/jpm11080710

Academic Editors: Richard E. Frye, Richard Boles, Shannon Rose and Daniel Rossignol

Received: 27 June 2021
Accepted: 21 July 2021
Published: 24 July 2021

Publisher's Note: MDPI stays neutral with regard to jurisdictional claims in published maps and institutional affiliations.

Copyright: © 2021 by the authors. Licensee MDPI, Basel, Switzerland. This article is an open access article distributed under the terms and conditions of the Creative Commons Attribution (CC BY) license (https://creativecommons.org/licenses/by/4.0/).

1. Background

Folate, an umbrella term used for metabolically active forms of folic acid (B9), is an essential B-complex vitamin necessary for basic cellular metabolism including, but not limited to, essential cellular DNA synthesis, repair and methylation including regulation of synthesis and metabolism of monoamine neurotransmitters. As a nutrient found in green leafy vegetables, legumes and fruits, it is readily absorbed by the upper small intestine after breakdown from polyglutamates to monoglutamates. Folate in its active forms facilitates one-carbon transfer reactions and contributes to the synthesis of purines, pyrimidines and amino acids [1]. One of its most characterized roles is facilitating single carbon transfer to homocysteine to form methionine. This reaction is critical for maintaining intracellular S-adenosyl methionine, an essential compound for methylation reactions. Folate also has a co-dependent relationship with vitamin B_{12} in that both vitamins must be present in adequate amounts for conversion to the physiologic forms that participate in metabolic reactions. If folate and B_{12} are not adequate, cellular metabolism and replication is interrupted [2,3]. This is most critical during fetal and neonatal development because inadequate folate during this period can result in interruptions in brain development leading to structural abnormalities that produce functional deficits of the CFD syndrome. Low cerebro-spinal fluid (CSF) folate is a characteristic feature of CFD syndrome, as first described by Ramaekers and Blau [4]. On rare occasions, CFD can also result from mutations in the FRα gene [5–7], but the most common cause of low CSF folate in CFD is the presence of anti-folate receptor antibodies (FRAb) that can block folate transport across the choroid plexus [8,9]. A recent report has identified mutations in the *CIC* transcription factor gene in children diagnosed with CFD syndrome. Mutations in the *CIC* gene decrease the expression of FRα to reduce folate transport across the choroid plexus [10]. No abnormalities of the FRα gene are found in ASD, but a majority of these children are positive for FRAb and have low CSF folate [11,12]. This is *a priori* proof that FRα is the primary transporter of folate into the brain under physiologic folate status.

2. Folate Requirements during Pregnancy

Since the discovery of its role in megaloblastic anemia and spina bifida, folate supplementation during pregnancy and fortification of food products have become two of the most globally accepted methods of treating and preventing folate deficiency. The basic folate requirement increases 75 to 100% (approximately 300–400 μg per day) in pregnancy because folate has a critical role in the growth and development of the embryo/fetus, especially during early stages of development [13]. It is, therefore, common practice to recommend that women supplement their diet with folate before conception and throughout pregnancy. The prevention of folate deficiency during pregnancy is achieved by consumption of at least 0.4 mg/day of folic acid during the first trimester of pregnancy [14,15]. In light of the recently discovered FRAb that can block folate transport, women positive for these antibodies may need additional supplementation with folinic acid to provide adequate folate to the developing fetus [16,17].

3. Folate and Fetal Brain Development

The importance of folate during embryonic and fetal brain development has been demonstrated in genetic animal models and dietary manipulations of folate deficiency [18,19]. If either folate transport or folate concentration in circulation is adversely manipulated, embryonic and fetal development is significantly altered. Mouse knockout models of genes such as FOLR1 that encode for folate receptor alpha (FRα) produce lethality in litters along with orbito-facial abnormalities, congenital heart defects and/or neural tube defects [20]. In FOLR1 knockout mouse, these lethalities can be prevented with adequate folinic acid (N5-formyltetrahydrofolate, a reduced form of folate) supplementation. These dramatic results occur because folate transport is lacking in the KO mouse during the early stages of neurulation and in regions where abnormalities arise [21]. In rodent models, folate deficiency causes a decrease in progenitor cells and an increase in apoptosis, and this could lead to infertility or resorption of embryos or fetal malformations [22]. Behavioral deficits are seen in rat pups born to folate-deficient mothers [23] and on methyl donor deficient diet during pregnancy [24]. In a rat model of exposure to rat folate receptor antibodies during pregnancy, resorption of embryos and malformations of the cranio-facial region and the brain were reported [25]. When the antibodies were administered at lower doses, embryos were carried to term with normal appearing pups born. However, these pups showed severe behavioral deficits [23,26]. The behavioral phenotype can be rescued by treatment with folinic acid and dexamethasone prior to antibody exposure [27]. These studies provide strong evidence in support of the pathologic consequences of exposure to FRα antibodies and the protective role of folinic acid.

4. Folate and Neonatal Brain Development

After birth, it is crucial for the offspring to have an adequate amount of folate in their diet. Instead of rapid cell division as embryogenesis calls for, postnatal development requires folate for neural progenitor differentiation as well as proliferation [28]. It has yet to be fully elucidated what the detailed mechanisms of folate action are, but the folate deficiency produced in animal models during early postnatal development illustrates the importance of folate in preventing developmental and cognitive deficits [23,27]. Researchers have also reported changes in neuronal excitability and maintenance that arise with a decrease in brain folate in a rat model [29]. Others have reported an increase in p53 and signs of homocysteine accumulation in the neurons and astrocytes [30]. There was a long-term effect on locomotor function and cognition in these animals. Therefore, folate is necessary for maintenance of neuronal function, as well. Based on this, further investigations into the mechanisms of folate metabolism in neurons and support cells of the brain are necessary. Thus far, folate has been linked to neuronal repair and differentiation after injury, myelin formation and maintenance and neuronal plasticity [30–32]. Figure 1 provides a summary of the effects of folate deficiency on fetal and post-natal brain development and the consequent sequelae that contribute to neurologic deficits.

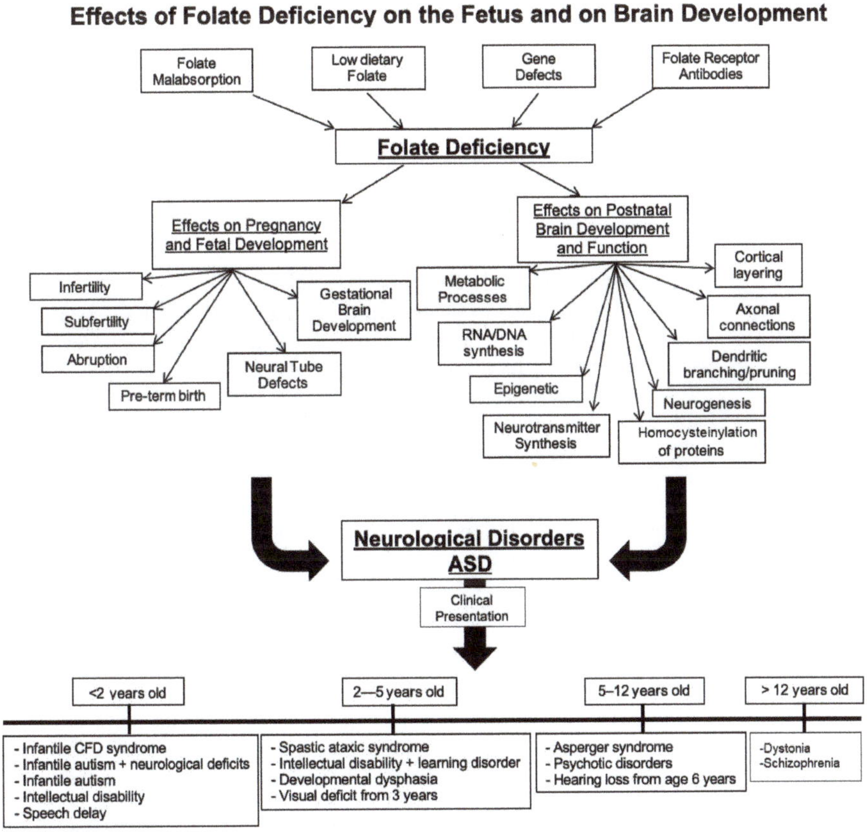

Figure 1. Effects of folate deficiency on the fetus and on brain development. Multiple causes lead to systemic as well as fetal folate deficiency. Folate receptor autoantibodies can block folate transport to the fetus and to the fetal as well as neonatal brain. In addition to folate deficiency, immune-mediated inflammation can contribute to the pathology. This has multipronged effects on brain development and function.

5. Folate Receptors: Expression and Function

In humans, there are four genes that code for folate receptors (see Table 1). The most characterized of these receptors is folate receptor alpha (FRα). As extracellular receptors, FRα, FRβ, FRγ and FRδ function as transporters of folate across different target tissues [33,34]. FRα can also act as a transcription factor [33]. Other transporters of folate include the reduced folate carrier (RFC), which requires high local concentrations (micromolar) of biologically active reduced forms of folates, and the proton-coupled folate transporter (PCFT), which can only transport folates and folic acid under acidic conditions and is the primary transporter involved in folate absorption in the gut [35].

Table 1. Summary of folate transporters.

Protein	Gene	Chromosome	GPI Anchor?	Localization	Cofactors?	Refs.
FRα	FOLR1	11q13.3	Yes	Liver, kidney, uterus, placenta, choroid plexus, retinal pigment epithelium	LRP2	[33,35–38]
FRβ	FOLR2	11q13.4	Yes	Placenta, spleen, bone marrow, thymus, macrophages	NA	[33,35–39]
FRγ	FOLR3	11q13.4	NA	Secretory granules of neutrophil granulocytes	NA	[33,35–39]
FRδ	FOLR4	11q14	Yes	Oocytes	NA	[33,35–39]
RFC	SLC19A1	21q22.3	No	Liver, kidney, placenta, choroid plexus, intestinal tract	Vitamin D, thiamine pyrophosphate	[34,40]
PCFT	SLC46A1	17q11.2	No	Liver, kidney, choroid plexus, placenta, intestinal epithelium, human tumors	Proton gradient	[34,40]

6. FRα Role in Maternofetal Transport of Folate

The high demand for folate during pregnancy requires homeostatic mechanisms to ensure that sufficient folate is provided to the fetus throughout development. As the most characterized receptor in the folate transporter family of proteins, the accepted mechanism of FRα-mediated transport is translocation/endocytosis of the holo receptor subsequent to folate binding [35]. FRα is expressed on all epithelial cells including the choroid plexus. It is highly expressed in the reproductive tissues including the placenta and the fetus. To determine the mechanism of folate transport in the placenta during pregnancy, Yasuda et al. [41] manipulated osmolarity, concentrations of phosphatidylinositol-specific phospholipase C inhibition and concentrations of ^{3}H-folic acid *in vitro* culture of human placental brush border membrane vesicles and determined that FRα, RFC and PCFT could transport various forms of folate, but that approximately 60% of folate was binding to FRα. They also noted that the folate requirements of Wistar rats increased across gestation, and expression of the mRNA of the transporters increased as well.

7. FRα Role in Folate Transport to the Brain

FRα is accepted as the main transporter of folate into the brain. However, there have been limitations to studying how FRα transports folate across the blood–brain barrier. A potential mechanism of folate transport across the choroid plexus and into the brain has been described by Grapp et al. [42]. In their experiments using immortalized Z310n rat choroid plexus cells in culture and a mouse model, they determined that transport of folate required shuttling of folates via exosomes from the basolateral side of the choroid plexus to the brain parenchyma of the apical side. Alternative transporters such as RFC and PCFT may only play a role when there is a disruption of FRα expression and transport, and adequate folate concentration is made available locally at the receptor [43]. The shuttling across the epithelial lining of the choroid plexus is a mechanism presumed to be conserved in all tissues that express FRα [44].

8. Folate Receptor Autoantibodies: Their Role in Disrupting Folate Transport

In some conditions, there is disruption in folate utilization that is not related to a dietary deficiency but is most likely due to a disturbance in the folate's transport due to genetic or metabolic abnormalities. An emerging culprit of folate transport disruption is folate receptor autoimmune disorder, where autoantibodies against the FRα can interfere with folate transport to the fetus; it has been associated with subfertility, difficulty in conceiving, miscarriage and neural tube defects in the fetus [16,17,45,46].

In infants and young children, these antibodies can block folate transport to the brain. Approximately 70% of the children diagnosed with cerebral folate deficiency syndrome or autism spectrum disorder have low CSF folate and respond to folinic acid treatment [47,48]. The majority of the autoantibodies are of the IgG class and, therefore, can readily cross the placenta and affect the fetus. Two distinct types of antibodies have been identified. One binds to FRα at the active site where folate binds and, as a consequence, blocks folate binding (blocking Ab). Another type of antibody binds to an antigenic site not involved in folate binding (binding Ab) but can trigger an immune reaction and inflammation and render the receptor nonfunctional. In most cases, one or both types of antibodies are present [49,50]. Thus, functional blocking of folate transport and inflammation are an integral part of the pathology [44].

9. Pathologic Consequences of Folate Receptor Antibodies

The presence of folate receptor autoantibodies can disrupt the transport of folate, and the consequences of decreased folate uptake by cells can impact development of the fetus, especially the central nervous system. There is also a correlation of folate receptor antibodies with neural tube defect pregnancy [16]. In less severe cases, a subset of children born with exposure to maternal FRα autoantibodies *in utero* develop low-functioning autism with or without neurological deficits after birth. Recent studies show significant association of folate receptor autoantibodies with autism spectrum disorder in children [11,51,52].

10. Diagnosis of Folate Receptor Autoimmune Disorder

Early indications of cerebral folate deficiency that are potentially due to maternal folate deficiency or folate receptor autoantibodies can be deduced by measuring serum folate and homocysteine and folate receptor autoantibodies in the mother during pregnancy. Other than dietary folate deficiency, folate receptor autoantibodies in the pregnant mother can contribute to fetal folate deficiency. In the latter case, blocking of folate transport across the placenta and antibody-mediated inflammation could contribute to the pathology, as shown in the rat model of exposure to rat folate receptor antibodies during pregnancy [26,27]. In infants, the presence of folate receptor autoantibodies in the blood could provide a mechanism by which folate transport to the brain via the choroid plexus could be blocked, thus leading to cerebral folate deficiency [51,52]. Therefore, determining the presence of folate receptor autoantibodies in the blood of pregnant mothers and children becomes a necessary test to prove or rule out folate receptor autoimmune disorder.

Methodology for determination of the antibody titer in serum is well-established. Two distinct types of IgG and/or IgM antibodies have been described [50]. These antibodies can be blocking and/or binding antibodies. Both types of antibodies are capable of triggering an immune reaction due to antigen/antibody interaction, leading to local inflammation, and this could interfere with folate transport via the FR protein. Both types of assays can be performed in a laboratory setting as described below.

11. Assay for Blocking Antibodies

Blocking autoantibodies to FRα are determined using a functional binding radio assay. Patient's serum (200 μL) is acidified with 300 μL 0.1 M glycine/HCl pH 2.5/0.5% Triton X-100/10 mM EDTA and added to 12.5 mg charcoal pellets in a separate tube (250 μL of 5% charcoal/1% dextran in 0.1 M Na PO4 pH 7.4/0.5% Triton X-100/10 mM

EDTA, spun down and supernatant-aspirated) to remove any endogenous folate, and the pH of the supernatant fluid is neutralized with 40 μL of 1 M dibasic NaPO4 prior to using it in the assay. This assay is performed by adding purified apo human FRα protein (40 ng) to the processed serum and incubating overnight at 4 °C. The next day, ^{3}H-folic acid (700 pg) (Moravek) is added and incubated for 20 min at room temperature. Unbound ^{3}H folic acid is removed with dextran-coated charcoal (200 μL) and the ^{3}H folate bound to FRα determined by counting the sample in a liquid scintillation counter. The reduction in binding of ^{3}H-folic acid to the apo human FRα when compared to the negative control serum sample provides a measure of the blocking autoantibody present in the sample [50]. Blocking antibody can be IgG or IgM; the values are expressed as pico moles of ^{3}HPGA blocked per ml serum, and the titer can range from >0.2 to 0.5 (low titer), >0.5 to 1.0 (medium titer) or >1.0 (high titer).

12. Assay for Binding Antibody

Binding of the IgG autoantibody to folate receptor alpha (FRα) is determined by an ELISA-based method. FRα (1 μg in 100 μL) purified from human milk is added to each well of an ELISA plate to covalently bind the protein to maleic anhydride-coated wells (Thermo Fisher, Waltham, MA, USA). Following blocking of additional sites by treatment with normal goat serum (200 μL) overnight to prevent non-specific binding to the wells, serum samples (4 and 8 μL) (negative control, positive control and patient samples) are added to wells along with 100 μL fresh goat serum and incubated at 4 °C overnight to facilitate binding of autoantibodies to the FRα in the wells. Following washing of the wells to remove unbound proteins, the specific IgG autoantibody bound in each well is detected by incubating with a peroxidase-conjugated, anti-human IgG secondary antibody (1:6000 dilution) (Vector Labs) for 1 h at room temperature. After washing to remove the unbound secondary antibody, the bound peroxidase-conjugated secondary antibody is determined by incubation with ultra TMB (Thermo Fisher) for 10 min. The resultant blue colored reaction is converted to yellow with 100 μL of 1.0 M HCl, and then absorbance is read at 450 nm in an ELISA plate reader. In a second set of wells, known amounts of human IgG captured in protein A-coated plates are used to construct a standard curve [50]. Values are expressed as pico moles of IgG antibody per ml serum and can range from >0.1 to 0.5 (low titer); >0.5 to 2.0 (medium titer) and >2.0 (high titer).

Among other criteria, specific diagnosis of folate receptor autoimmune disorder is confirmed using the above tests. After correcting for background, for the blocking antibody, values of 0.2 pmoles or greater are considered positive and for the binding antibody, 0.1 pmoles or greater are considered positive. Because folate receptor alpha is a peripheral membrane protein, the antibody titer measured in the serum should be considered as excess antibody appearing in the circulation after saturating the membrane-bound antigen. Fluctuations in antibody titer have been reported in the same individual over time and can range from low to medium titer or to undetectable levels. While the reason for these changes in antibody titer are not identified, it is likely that changes in FR antigen on cells, exposure to milk FR antigen in the gut and the specific B-cell population may be contributory factors.

13. Treatment of FRα Autoimmune Disorder in ASD

Among the developmental disorders, ASD is most prevalent and has continued to increase over the past decade. Based on available publications, the WHO reports the worldwide prevalence at 1 in 162 births [53]. In the USA and Canada, the prevalence is reported at 1 in 50, and this rate is predicted to increase over the next few years [54]. While the clinical phenotype of ASD may result from multiple genetic, epigenetic and environmental factors, nutrient deficiencies such as folate can play a significant role. Folate receptor antibodies and cerebral folate deficiency are prevalent in ASD. Treatment of FRα autoimmunity in ASD is based on our previous findings in infantile-onset CFD syndrome and low-functioning autism associated with neurological deficits [11]. In these children, a repeat CSF analysis after three to six months of treatment with folinic acid showed normalization of 5-methyl-tetrahydrofolate levels [11,51]. Supplementation with high-dose dl-folinic acid (Leucovorin) (0.5–2 mg/kg body weight or 0.25–1.0 mg levofolinate) given in 1 or 2 divided daily doses increases 5-methyltetrahydrofolate concentration by more than 100-fold compared to physiological folate concentrations in plasma. Despite the autoantibody-induced blocking of the FRα-pathway to transport folate across the choroid plexus, the significant increase of 5-methyltetrahydrofolate and folinic acid in plasma will enable reduced folate carrier-1 (RFC-1), a high capacity/low affinity transmembrane folate transporter at the blood–brain barrier, to transport sufficient 5-methyltetrahydrofolate and folinic acid to the brain. In this context, it appears important to verify a normal vitamin D status because RFC-1 gene transcription depends on vitamin D availability within microvasculature cells at the blood–brain barrier [40].

Another important therapeutic intervention represents a diet strictly free of animal-derived milk or milk products, which can be replaced by other vegetal milk products (for example soya-, almond- and rice-based and coconut milk). Although many previous studies on a casein/gluten-free diet have been conducted, there has been no final evidence yet to consider these dietary treatments as beneficial in the management of ASD. Many studies have been conducted for a maximum of only 3 months, although some studies on a small number of patients were conducted over 1 to 2 years and indicated that part of the core symptoms of autism had improved [55–58]. The conclusion was that a casein/gluten-free diet should be tried for at least 6 months to see a positive response in a subset of the ASD population. One suggested hypothesis was that opioid peptides derived from milk casein contributed to the pathogenesis of autism [59]. Because bovine milk contains a soluble form of the FRα protein with 91% homology with human FRα, we examined the binding properties of human FRα autoantibodies with different FRα antigens isolated from human placenta; human milk; and bovine, goat and camel milk. The highest cross-reactivity of the autoantibody was found for soluble FRα protein from bovine and camel milk (Figure 2). To determine if FRα in the milk consumed contributed to the autoimmune disorder, we studied the effects of a milk-free diet in children positive for the FRα antibody. Patients with infantile CFD syndrome associated with FRα antibodies were randomized to receive either a cow's milk-free diet or a normal, milk-containing diet. Among children on a normal diet, FRα antibodies increased from baseline toward higher titers during 6–12 months of evaluation. However, the children receiving a milk-free diet showed a significant drop in FRα antibody titers after 3–6 months that rose again after re-introduction of bovine milk. These studies confirmed down-regulation of the FRα antibodies following a strict animal milk-free diet [55]. In this group of patients with infantile CFD syndrome, a number also suffered from low-functioning autism with neurological deficits and showed a clinical response after a milk-free diet. These findings suggest that in predisposed individuals, the soluble FRα antigen derived from bovine and other animal-derived milk products acts as the antigen that triggers a gut immune response with the formation of specific B-cell clones that produce autoantibodies that enter the circulation, cross-reacts with the human FRα anchored to the choroid plexus and blocks folate transport from the circulation into the CSF [44,60]. Thyroid dysfunction is common in children with ASD. Even though FRα expression in the thyroid gland is decreased in older children and adults, it is highly expressed in the fetal and neonatal thyroid, and FRα antibodies can affect development of the thyroid gland [61]. A preferred strategy for individuals with autism spectrum disorder is to take a serum sample for determination of FRα autoantibodies after exposure to milk products for about 2–3 weeks. After this diagnostic blood test, autistic children can be placed on an animal milk-free diet. As soon as the FRα autoantibodies test positive, a milk-free dietary intervention can be continued along with high oral doses of folinic acid. Other treatment strategies to reduce FRα autoantibodies may be immunosuppression using steroids or intravenously administered immunoglobulins, but these therapeutic options should be reserved for emergency situations such as refractory epileptic seizures or dramatic movement disorders such as dystonia, choreoathetosis or ballism.

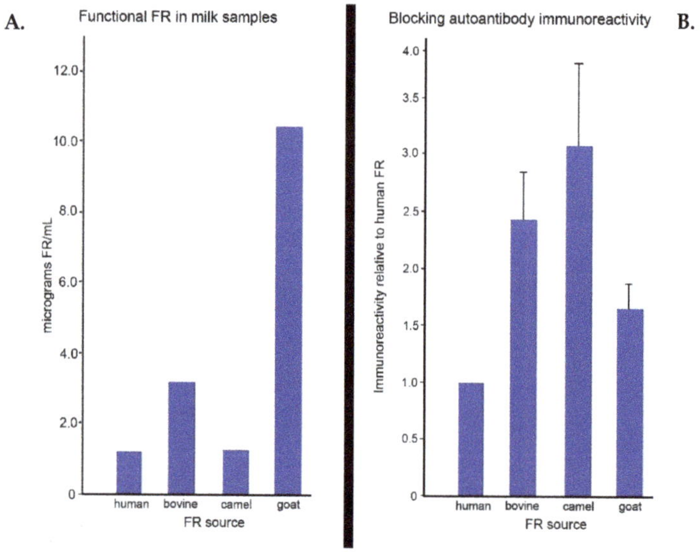

Figure 2. (**A**) Folate receptor concentrations in milk. (**B**) Immune cross-reactivity of blocking autoantibodies against various FR antigens. The blocking assay was performed by testing a known amount of blocking activity in serum samples from 8 different patients with molar equivalent amounts of FR antigens from milk. Blocking activity was determined as pico moles of ^{3}HPGA blocked and was compared to blocking in human milk antigen.

Treatment with high-dose folinic acid in a subgroup of ASD children positive for FRα autoimmunity, i.e., low-functioning autism with neurological deficits, showed clinical improvement of core autistic symptoms and normalization of previously lowered CSF 5-methyltetrahydrofolate [51]. A double-blind, placebo-controlled study conducted among children with ASD without additional neurologic deficits showed significant improvements in verbal scores in subjects positive for FRAb following treatment with folinic acid [48]. A recent, self-controlled clinical trial was conducted among children with low-functioning autism without additional neurological complications. In these, a high, 76% prevalence of FRα antibodies was found. These children also had multiple nutrient deficiencies attributed to selective eating habits and malnutrition. Combined correction of deficient nutrients and high dose folinic acid administration resulted in an overall significant recovery from severe autism to mild–moderate autism (Figure 3A). Comparison of the Childhood Autism Rating Scale (CARS) after 2 years of treatment (folinic acid supplementation and correction of abnormal nutrient values) with the CARS at baseline showed better outcomes for children having negative or low FRα antibody titers of the blocking type, up to 0.44 pmol FRα blocked/mL serum, versus the group whose FRα antibody titers were above 0.44. The baseline CARS score increased as a function of the age at which treatment was initiated. The outcome became poorer for the older subgroup of treated autistic children (Figure 3B). This outcome may be further compounded by the presence of maternal and paternal autoantibodies and embryonic exposure to these. Preliminary data suggested that in the event of maternal or parental FRα autoantibodies, the child´s outcome after treatment was also less favorable (Figure 3C).

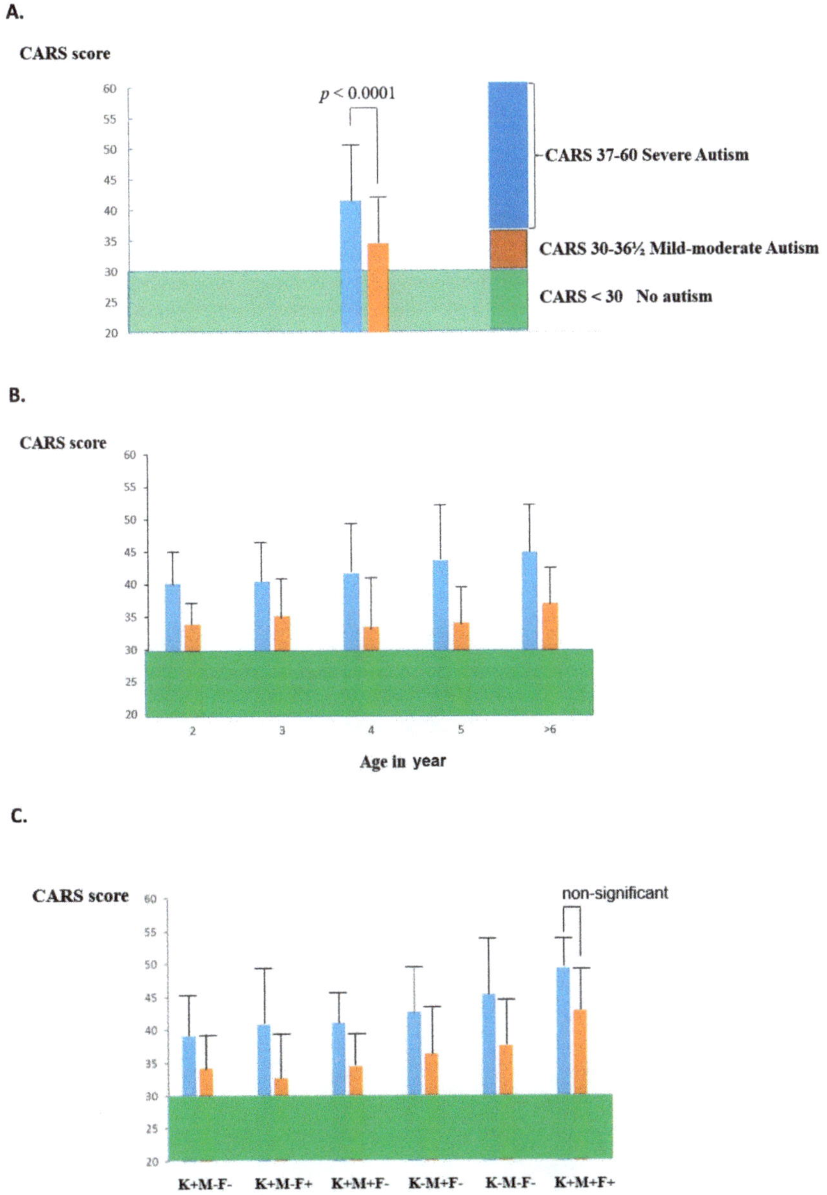

Figure 3. (**A**). Compared to untreated autistic patients (n = 84) whose CARS remained unchanged, a group treated with folinic acid and with their nutritional deficits corrected showed a decrease in baseline CARS score from severe (n = 82; CARS mean ± SD: 41.34 ± 6.47) to moderate or mild autism (mean ± SD: 34.35 ± 6.25; paired t-test $p < 0.0001$). (**B**). As a function of age, the baseline CARS (blue bars) increased slowly with advancing age, while the CARS after a 2-year treatment period (orange bars) diminished significantly for all age subgroups. The increase of baseline CARS with advancing age will adversely influence the final outcome for older age groups, particularly above 6 years. (**C**). This graph represents the outcome of treatment as a function of the particular FRα antibody profile in the child (K), mother (M) and father (F). The presence of maternal FRα antibodies or presence of antibodies in both parents will negatively affect the treatment outcome (adapted from [51]).

Compared to infantile-onset CFD syndrome where FRα antibody testing remained negative in the parents, testing of the parents of children with autism revealed a prevalence of 34% in mothers and 29% in fathers versus 3% in healthy controls [51]. Another study also confirmed an equal prevalence of FRα autoimmunity in children with autism (76%) and even higher autoantibody prevalence in their unaffected siblings (75%), fathers (69%) and mothers (59%) [62]. The appearance of these antibodies may have a familial heritable origin, but the risk of developing ASD is likely influenced by other unknown factors because some siblings positive for these antibodies have been asymptomatic. Two of the suspected determinant factors for the development of autism are the appearance of antibodies at a critical stage of neurodevelopmental processes during the first 18 months of life and fetal exposure to maternal antibodies.

The outcome after folinic acid treatment of autism associated with FRα autoimmunity appears to be influenced by several factors such as the level of FRα antibody titer and age at which treatment was initiated as well as the FRα antibody profile amongst parents. In our studies on the treatment outcome after folinic acid therapy for two years we only included the group of children with infantile-onset autism in whom genetic abnormalities had been excluded because genetic defects might constitute a bias to statistical assessment regarding the influence of FRα autoimmunity (Figure 4).

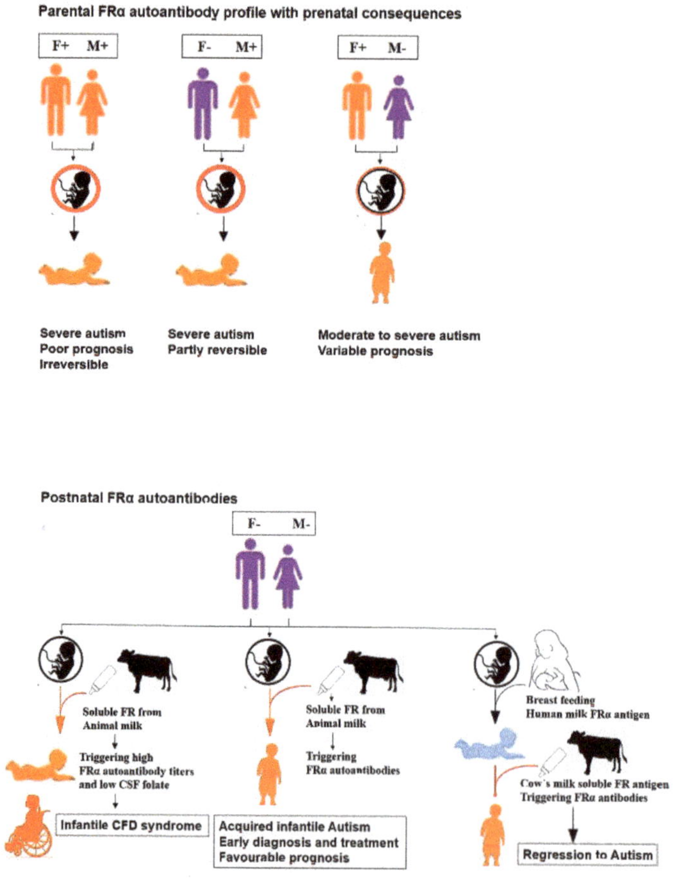

Figure 4. The significance of parental antibody status on developmental outcomes in offspring (top panel) and postnatal antibody development in offspring (bottom panel).

14. Treatment of FR Autoimmune Disorder in Pregnancy

FRα autoimmunity has been associated with a high risk of neural tube defects (NTD) and other congenital malformations in offspring [16,17]. This has been confirmed by other independent studies [63,64]. Even though the incidence of NTD is high in the Irish population, evaluation of FRα autoantibodies in this population has failed to show a statistically significant correlation with NTD pregnancies [65]. However, the study showed a higher prevalence (35–40%) of FR antibodies in the mothers and both male and female controls. Because FRα antibodies were not assessed in the fathers of the children with NTD and only in unrelated males of the control group, the contribution of the possibility of both parents being positive for FRα antibodies to the NTD outcome cannot be ruled out. Parental studies in ASD have shown both maternal and paternal influences on the incidence and severity of ASD outcome [51]. The folic acid fortification of foods has reduced the prevalence of NTD by 30–50 percent. However, for women having a normal folate status but testing positive for FRα autoantibodies, we suspect that even the addition of a daily dose of 400–800 μg or 1000 μg for twin pregnancies may not prevent NTD or congenital malformations due to the persistence of embryonic and fetal folate deficiency in the presence of FRα antibodies.

One case report described a woman who, upon follow-up after three pregnancies, was found to have high titers of serum FRα autoantibodies of the blocking and binding types. She had previously had two miscarriages and a third pregnancy with monozygotic twins, during which she took 1 mg folic acid per day. However, one twin was reduced at 12 weeks because of an encephalocele, and the pregnancy was terminated because the other twin had hypoplastic left-heart syndrome and choroid plexus cysts. At this time, extensive genetic testing did not reveal any abnormalities. After finding FRα autoantibodies, treatment with a milk-free diet was able to reduce FRα antibody titers, but a fourth pregnancy by IVF also resulted in a miscarriage after 5 months. It was only after continuation of the milk-free diet combined with 4 mg folic acid, 2.5 mg leucovorin and 5 mg prednisone that FRα antibody titers fell to undetectable levels, and a fifth pregnancy was carried to term and resulted in the birth of a healthy baby boy [17]. FRα autoantibodies are significantly associated with subfertility and preterm birth [45,46], and preterm babies have a higher prevalence of ASD [66]. Therefore, testing for FRα antibodies in women of child-bearing age may help in preventing some of these disorders by early intervention.

15. Prevention of ASD and Related Complications Due to FR Antibodies

Prevention of ASD has not been reported yet. However, it seems extremely important to diagnose ASD at the earliest age possible in order to be able to perform further evaluation including testing for serum FRα autoantibodies. We believe that as soon as ASD is strongly suspected and FRα antibodies identified as early as possible prior to the age of three years, the outcome following prompt treatment with high-dose folinic acid in combination with an animal milk-free diet will have a favorable outcome if maternal FRα antibodies or the presence of antibodies in both parents were negative [51].

Currently, FRα antibody testing is only performed after ASD is suspected or has been diagnosed. However, this procedure postpones treatment and causes a significant delay, affecting prognosis unfavorably. Therefore, the early screening of autism at 18 or 24 months using the Modified Checklist for Autism in Toddlers (M-CHAT test) or other instruments can be used by health workers, although there is lack of optimal sensitivity and specificity for ASD when using these tests at an early age.

Another option would be to perform the screening test for FRα antibodies at an early age between 12 and 18 months, particularly among those children suspected to manifest one or more autistic signs or symptoms. The children testing positive for FRα antibodies could be placed on an animal milk-free diet and receive folinic acid supplementation with a mandatory follow-up of these children.

16. Clinical Significance of the Findings

Since the discovery of folic acid more than a century ago, the hematologic consequences of its deficiency and its role in DNA synthesis and treatment of megaloblastic anemia has been well defined. Emerging research aims to define its role in methylation reactions, epigenetic regulation of gene expression, reproductive function, pregnancy and fetal development. It is becoming evidently clear that folate plays a major role not only in fetal brain development but also in post-natal development and refinement of functional integration of the mature brain. Clinical improvement seen in response to folinic acid treatment in ASD, schizophrenia, depression and dementia attests to the role of folate in metabolic regulation of brain function, potentially by regulating the expression and processing of neurotransmitters. While conventional thinking would associate disruption of folate metabolism with nutritional folate deficiency and gene defects of folate pathways, the identification of folate receptor autoantibodies contributing to fetal and cerebral folate deficiency has thrown a monkey wrench into our current thinking regarding folate transport into the brain and its role in regulating brain function. Therefore, clinical recognition of cerebral folate deficiency is critical to our understanding of neuro–developmental as well as neuro–psychiatric disorders.

To prevent fetal folate deficiency, specific guidelines for treatment of future parents testing positive for FRα antibodies should consider the time frame and dose for folinic acid supplementation prior to conception and for mothers, the folinic acid dose to be used during pregnancy. It will be extremely important to assess optimal dosage in order to provide sufficient folate supplementation but avoid excess dosing, especially since data are lacking on the safety profile of high-dose folinic acid administered throughout pregnancy. Based on the safety profile of high-dose folinic acid used in the treatment of CFD and ASD, one may speculate that a daily dose of 5–10 mg may be in the safe range. The future availability of levofolinate could reduce this dose by half. For favorable outcomes in CFD and ASD, early testing for FRAb and treatment with folinic acid could potentially prevent the development of neurologic deficits.

17. Concluding Remarks

Decades of research into neural tube defect pregnancies have only managed to reduce their incidence through folic acid supplementation, but not prevent them altogether. ASD incidence, on the other hand, has continued to rise with no definitive contributing cause identified. Both public and private funding agencies have poured a major share of available funds toward identifying gene defects and genomic polymorphisms to no avail. An enormous sum of money has been expended in developing gene deletion mouse and rat models to identify the autism gene(s). It is now clear that ASD is not a congenital genetic disorder and does not follow Mendelian inheritance. Therefore, the answer to the pathogenesis of ASD must lie in epigenetic and environmental factors that broadly affect gene expression. Folate plays a pivotal role in DNA/RNA synthesis, methylation and epigenetic control of gene expression, and therefore, decreased folate availability during critical stages of development, albeit by the presence of FRAb-blocking folate transport as well as triggering inflammation, may play a significant role in the pathology of ASD.

Author Contributions: All authors contributed equally to the conceptualization, writing and finalization of the manuscript. All authors have read and agreed to the published version of the manuscript.

Funding: Ongoing research in the Quadros Laboratory is supported by a grant from the Brain Foundation and by the Vembu Srinivasan family fund. N.B.-K. is supported by a graduate student fellowship from the NY City-funded Institute for Basic Science Research, Staten Island, NY, USA.

Institutional Review Board Statement: Not Applicable.

Informed Consent Statement: Informed consent was obtained from all subjects reported in this study.

Data Availability Statement: Not Applicable.

Conflicts of Interest: Two of the authors (J.M.S. and E.V.Q.) are inventors on a US patent for the detection of FRalpha autoantibodies issued to the Research Foundation of SUNY.

References

1. Rucker, R.B.; Zempleni, J.; Suttie, J.W.; McCormick, D.B. *Handbook of Vitamins*, 4th ed.; Taylor & Francis: Boca Raton, FL, USA, 2007. Available online: https://books.google.com/books?id=AasGngEACAAJ (accessed on 4 November 2019).
2. Mikkelsen, K.; Apostolopoulos, V. Vitamin B12, Folic Acid, and the Immune System. In *Nutrition and Immunity*; Mahmoudi, M., Rezaei, N., Eds.; Springer: Cham, Switzerland, 2019. [CrossRef]
3. Scott, J.M. Folate and vitamin B12. *Proc. Nutr. Soc.* **1999**, *58*, 441–448. [CrossRef]
4. Ramaekers, V.T.; Blau, N. Cerebral folate deficiency. *Dev. Med. Child. Neurol.* **2004**, *46*, 843–851. [CrossRef]
5. Cario, H.; Bode, H.; Debatin, K.M.; Opladen, T.; Schwarz, K. Congenital null mutations of the FOLR1 gene: A progressive neurologic disease and its treatment. *Neurology* **2009**, *73*, 2127–2129. [CrossRef]
6. Pérez-Dueñas, B.; Toma, C.; Ormazábal, A.; Muchart, J.; Sanmartí, F.; Bombau, G.; Serrano, M.; García-Cazorla, A.; Cormand, B.; Artuch, R. Progressive ataxia and myoclonic epilepsy in a patient with a homozygous mutation in the FOLR1 gene. *J. Inherit. Metab. Dis.* **2010**, *33*, 795–802. [CrossRef]
7. Delmelle, F.; Thöny, B.; Clapuyt, P.; Blau, N.; Nassogne, M.C. Neurological improvement following intravenous high-dose folinic acid for cerebral folate transporter deficiency caused by FOLR-1 mutation. *Eur. J. Paediatr. Neurol.* **2016**, *20*, 709–713. [CrossRef]
8. Ramaekers, V.T.; Rothenberg, S.P.; Sequeira, J.M.; Opladen, T.; Blau, N.; Quadros, E.V.; Selhub, J. Autoantibodies to folate receptors in the cerebral folate deficiency syndrome. *N. Engl. J. Med.* **2005**, *352*, 1985–1991. [CrossRef]
9. Ramaekers, V.T.; Segers, K.; Sequeira, J.M.; Koenig, M.; Van Maldergem, L.; Bours, V.; Kornak, U.; Quadros, E.V. Genetic assessment and folate receptor autoantibodies in infantile-onset cerebral folate deficiency (CFD) syndrome. *Mol. Genet. Metab.* **2018**, *124*, 87–93. [CrossRef] [PubMed]
10. Cao, X.; Wolf, A.; Kim, S.E.; Cabrera, R.M.; Wlodarczyk, B.J.; Zhu, H.; Parker, M.; Lin, Y.; Steele, J.W.; Han, X.; et al. CIC de novo loss of function variants contribute to cerebral folate deficiency by downregulating FOLR1 expression. *J. Med. Genet.* **2020**, 1–11. [CrossRef]
11. Ramaekers, V.T.; Blau, N.; Sequeira, J.M.; Nassogne, M.C.; Quadros, E.V. Folate receptor autoimmunity and cerebral folate deficiency in low-functioning autism with neurological deficits. *Neuropediatrics* **2007**, *38*, 276–281. [CrossRef] [PubMed]
12. Ramaekers, V.T.; Sequeira, J.M.; Thöny, B.; Quadros, E.V. Oxidative Stress, Folate Receptor Autoimmunity, and CSF Findings in Severe Infantile Autism. *Autism Res. Treat.* **2020**, *2020*, 9095284. [CrossRef] [PubMed]
13. Fekete, K.; Berti, C.; Trovato, M.; Lohner, S.; Dullmeijer, C.; Souverein, O.W.; Cetin, I.; Decsi, T. Effect of folate intake on health outcomes in pregnancy: A systematic review and meta-analysis on birth weight, placental weight and length of gestation. *Nutr. J.* **2012**, *11*, 1–8. [CrossRef] [PubMed]
14. Greenberg, J.A.; Bell, S.J.; Guan, Y.; Yu, Y. Folic acid supplementation and pregnancy—More than just neural tube defect prevention. *Rev. Obs. Gynecol.* **2011**, *4*, 52–59.
15. Bailey, L.B.; Stover, P.J.; McNulty, H.; Fenech, M.F.; Gregory, J.F., 3rd; Mills, J.L.; Pfeiffer, C.M.; Fazili, Z.; Zhang, M.; Ueland, P.M.; et al. Biomarkers of nutrition for development-Folate Review. *J. Nutr.* **2015**, *145*, 1636S–1680S. [CrossRef]
16. Rothenberg, S.P.; da Costa, M.P.; Sequeira, J.M.; Cracco, J.; Roberts, J.L.; Weedon, J.; Quadros, E.V. Autoantibodies against folate receptors in women with a pregnancy complicated by a neural-tube defect. *N. Engl. J. Med.* **2004**, *350*, 134–142. [CrossRef]
17. Shapira, I.; Sequeira, J.M.; Quadros, E.V. Folate receptor autoantibodies in pregnancy related complications. *Birth Defects Res. Part A Clin. Mol. Teratol.* **2015**, *103*, 1028–1030. [CrossRef]
18. Peng, L.; Dreumont, N.; Coelho, D.; Guéant, J.L.; Arnold, C. Genetic animal models to decipher the pathogenic effects of vitamin B12 and folate deficiency. *Biochimie* **2016**, *126*, 43–51. [CrossRef] [PubMed]
19. Kappen, C. Folate supplementation in three genetic models: Implications for understanding folate-dependent developmental pathways. *Am. J. Med. Genet. Part C Semin Med. Genet.* **2005**, *135C*, 24–30. [CrossRef]
20. Piedrahita, J.A.; Oetama, B.; Bennett, G.D.; van Waes, J.; Kamen, B.A.; Richardson, J.; Lacey, S.W.; Anderson, R.G.; Finnell, R.H. Mice lacking the folic acid-binding protein Folbp1 are defective in early embryonic development. *Nat. Genet.* **1999**, *23*, 228–232. [CrossRef] [PubMed]
21. Tang, L.S.; Santillano, D.R.; Wlodarczyk, B.J.; Miranda, R.C.; Finnell, R.H. Role of Folbp1 in the regional regulation of apoptosis and cell proliferation in the developing neural tube and craniofacies. *Am. J. Med. Genet. Part C Semin. Med. Genet.* **2005**, *135C*, 48–58. [CrossRef]
22. Craciunescu, C.N.; Brown, E.C.; Mar, M.H.; Albright, C.D.; Nadeau, M.R.; Zeisel, S.H. Folic acid deficiency during late gestation decreases progenitor cell proliferation and increases apoptosis in fetal mouse brain. *J Nutr.* **2004**, *134*, 162–166. [CrossRef] [PubMed]
23. Berrocal-Zaragoza, M.I.; Sequeira, J.M.; Murphy, M.M.; Fernandez-Ballart, J.D.; Abdel Baki, S.G.; Bergold, P.J.; Quadros, E.V. Folate deficiency in rat pups during weaning causes learning and memory deficits. *Br. J. Nutr.* **2014**, *112*, 1323–1332. [CrossRef]
24. Blaise, S.A.; Nédélec, E.; Schroeder, H.; Alberto, J.M.; Bossenmeyer-Pourié, C.; Guéant, J.L.; Daval, J.L. Gestational vitamin B deficiency leads to homocysteine-associated brain apoptosis and alters neurobehavioral development in rats. *Am. J. Pathol.* **2007**, *170*, 667–679. [CrossRef] [PubMed]

25. da Costa, M.; Sequeira, J.M.; Rothenberg, S.P.; Weedon, J. Antibodies to Folate Receptors Impair Embryogenesis and Fetal Development in the Rat. *Birth Defects Res. Part A Clin. Mol. Teratol.* **2003**, *67*, 837–847. [CrossRef]
26. Sequeira, J.M.; Desai, A.; Berrocal-Zaragoza, M.I.; Murphy, M.M.; Fernandez-Ballart, J.D.; Quadros, E.V. Exposure to folate receptor alpha antibodies during gestation and weaning leads to severe behavioral deficits in rats: A pilot study. *PLoS ONE* **2016**, *11*, e0152249. [CrossRef]
27. Desai, A.; Sequeira, J.M.; Quadros, E.V. Prevention of behavioral deficits in rats exposed to folate receptor antibodies: Implication in autism. *Mol. Psychiatry* **2017**, *22*, 1291–1297. [CrossRef]
28. Balashova, O.A.; Visina, O.; Borodinsky, L.N. Folate action in nervous system development and disease. *Dev. Neurobiol.* **2018**, *78*, 391–402. [CrossRef]
29. Mann, A.; Portnoy, E.; Han, H.; Inbar, D.; Blatch, D.; Shmuel, M.; Ben-Hur, T.; Eyal, S.; Ekstein, D. Folate homeostasis in epileptic rats. *Epilepsy Res.* **2018**, *142*, 64–72. [CrossRef]
30. Kruman, I.I.; Mouton, P.R.; Emokpae, R., Jr.; Cutler, R.G.; Mattson, M.P. Folate deficiency inhibits proliferation of adult hippocampal progenitors. *NeuroReport.* **2005**, *16*, 1055–1059. [CrossRef] [PubMed]
31. Weng, Q.; Wang, J.; Wang, J.; Tan, B.; Wang, J.; Wang, H.; Zheng, T.; Lu, Q.R.; Yang, B.; He, Q. Folate Metabolism Regulates Oligodendrocyte Survival and Differentiation by Modulating AMPKα Activity. *Sci. Rep.* **2017**, *7*, 1705. [CrossRef] [PubMed]
32. Kim, G.B.; Chen, Y.; Kang, W.; Guo, J.; Payne, R.; Li, H.; Wei, Q.; Baker, J.; Dong, C.; Zhang, S.; et al. The critical chemical and mechanical regulation of folic acid on neural engineering. *Biomaterials.* **2018**, *178*, 504–516. [CrossRef]
33. Mayanil, C.S.; Siddiqui, M.R.; Tomita, T. Novel functions of folate receptor alpha in CNS development and diseases. *Neurosci. Discov.* **2014**, *2*, 5. [CrossRef]
34. Hou, Z.; Matherly, L.H. Biology of the major facilitative folate transporters SLC19A1 and SLC46A1. *Curr. Top. Membr.* **2014**, *73*, 175–204. [CrossRef]
35. Antony, A.C. Folate receptors. *Annu. Rev. Nutr.* **1996**, *16*, 501–521. [CrossRef] [PubMed]
36. Machacek, C.; Supper, V.; Leksa, V.; Mitulovic, G.; Spittler, A.; Drbal, K.; Suchanek, M.; Ohradanova-Repic, A.; Stockinger, H. Folate Receptor β Regulates Integrin CD11b/CD18 Adhesion of a Macrophage Subset to Collagen. *J. Immunol.* **2016**, *197*, 2229–2238. [CrossRef]
37. Kelemen, L.E. The role of folate receptor alpha in cancer development, progression and treatment: Cause, consequence or innocent bystander? *Int. J. Cancer* **2006**, *119*, 243–250. [CrossRef] [PubMed]
38. Spiegelstein, O.; Eudy, J.D.; Finnell, R.H. Identification of two putative novel folate receptor genes in humans and mouse. *Gene* **2000**, *258*, 117–125. [CrossRef]
39. Holm, J.; Hansen, S.I. Characterization of soluble folate receptors (folate binding proteins) in humans. Biological roles and clinical potentials in infection and malignancy. *Biochim. Biophys. Acta Proteins Proteom.* **2020**, *1868*, 140466. [CrossRef] [PubMed]
40. Alam, C.; Hoque, M.T.; Finnell, R.H.; Goldman, I.D.; Bendayan, R. Regulation of Reduced Folate Carrier (RFC) by Vitamin D Receptor at the Blood-Brain Barrier. *Mol. Pharm.* **2017**, *14*, 3848–3858. [CrossRef]
41. Yasuda, S.; Hasui, S.; Yamamoto, C.; Yoshioka, C.; Kobayashi, M.; Itagaki, S.; Hirano, T.; Iseki, K. Placental folate transport during pregnancy. *Biosci. Biotechnol. Biochem.* **2008**, *72*, 2277–2284. [CrossRef] [PubMed]
42. Grapp, M.; Wrede, A.; Schweizer, M.; Hüwel, S.; Galla, H.J.; Snaidero, N.; Simons, M.; Bückers, J.; Low, P.S.; Urlaub, H.; et al. Choroid plexus transcytosis and exosome shuttling deliver folate into brain parenchyma. *Nat. Commun.* **2013**, *4*, 2123. [CrossRef]
43. Alam, C.; Kondo, M.; O'Connor, D.L.; Bendayan, R. Clinical Implications of Folate Transport in the Central Nervous System. *Trends Pharmacol. Sci.* **2020**, *41*, 349–361. [CrossRef] [PubMed]
44. Desai, A.; Sequeira, J.M.; and Quadros, E.V. The metabolic basis for developmental disorders due to defective folate transport. *Biochimie* **2016**, *126*, 31–42. [CrossRef] [PubMed]
45. Berrocal-Zaragoza, M.I.; Fernandez-Ballart, J.D.; Murphy, M.M.; Cavallé-Busquets, P.; Sequeira, J.M.; Quadros, E.V. Association between blocking folate receptor autoantibodies and subfertility. *Fertil. Steril.* **2009**, *91* (Suppl. 4), 1518–1521. [CrossRef] [PubMed]
46. Vo, H.D.; Sequeira, J.M.; Quadros, E.V.; Schwarz, S.M.; Perenyi, A.R. The role of folate receptor autoantibodies in preterm birth. *Nutrition* **2015**, *31*, 1224–1227. [CrossRef]
47. Ramaekers, V.; Sequeira, J.M.; Quadros, E.V. Clinical recognition and aspects of the cerebral folate deficiency syndromes. *Clin. Chem. Lab. Med.* **2013**, *51*, 497–511. [CrossRef] [PubMed]
48. Frye, R.E.; Slattery, J.; Delhey, L.; Furgerson, B.; Strickland, T.; Tippett, M.; Sailey, A.; Wynne, R.; Rose, S.; Melnyk, S.; et al. Folinic acid improves verbal communication in children with autism and language impairment: A randomized double-blind placebo-controlled trial. *Mol. Psychiatry* **2018**, *23*, 247–256. [CrossRef]
49. Frye, R.E.; Delhey, L.; Slattery, J.; Tippett, M.; Wynne, R.; Rose, S.; Kahler, S.G.; Bennuri, S.C.; Stepan, M.; Sequeira, J.M.; et al. Blocking and binding folate receptor alpha autoantibodies identify novel autism spectrum disorder subgroups. *Front. Neurosci.* **2016**, *10*, 80. [CrossRef]
50. Sequeira, J.M.; Ramaekers, V.T.; Quadros, E.V. The diagnostic utility of folate receptor autoantibodies in blood. *Clin. Chem. Lab. Med.* **2013**, *51*, 545–554. [CrossRef]
51. Ramaekers, V.T.; Sequeira, J.M.; DiDuca, M.; Vrancken, G.; Thomas, A.; Philippe, C.; Peters, M.; Jadot, A.; Quadros, E.V. Improving Outcome in Infantile Autism with Folate Receptor Autoimmunity and Nutritional Derangements: A Self-Controlled Trial. *Autism Res. Treat.* **2019**, *2019*, 7486431. [CrossRef] [PubMed]

52. Zhou, J.; Liu, A.; He, F.; Jin, Y.; Zhou, S.; Xu, R.; Guo, H.; Zhou, W.; Wei, Q.; Wang, M. High prevalence of serum folate receptor autoantibodies in children with autism spectrum disorders. *Biomarkers* **2018**, *23*, 622–624. [CrossRef] [PubMed]
53. Elsabbagh, M.; Divan, G.; Koh, Y.J.; Shin Kim, Y.; Kauchali, S.; Marcin, C.; Montiel-Nava, C.; Patel, P.; Paula, C.S.; Wang, C.; et al. Global Prevalence of Autism and Other Pervasive Developmental Disorders. *Autism Res.* **2012**, *5*, 160–179. [CrossRef]
54. Chiarotti, F.; Venerosi, A. Epidemiology of Autism Spectrum Disorders: A Review of Worldwide Prevalence Estimates Since 2014. *Brain Sci.* **2020**, *10*, 274. [CrossRef] [PubMed]
55. Ramaekers, V.T.; Sequeira, J.M.; Blau, N.; Quadros, E.V. A milk-free diet downregulates folate receptor autoimmunity in cerebral folate deficiency syndrome. *Dev. Med. Child. Neurol.* **2008**, *50*, 346–352. [CrossRef] [PubMed]
56. Whiteley, P.; Shattock, P.; Knivsberg, A.M.; Seim, A.; Reichelt, K.L.; Todd, L.; Carr, K.; Hooper, M. Gluten- and casein-free dietary intervention for autism spectrum conditions. *Front. Hum. Neurosci.* **2013**, *6*, 344. [CrossRef] [PubMed]
57. Whiteley, P.; Haracopos, D.; Knivsberg, A.M.; Reichelt, K.L.; Parlar, S.; Jacobsen, J.; Seim, A.; Pedersen, L.; Schondel, M.; Shattock, P. The ScanBrit randomised, controlled, single-blind study of a gluten- and casein-free dietary intervention for children with autism spectrum disorders. *Nutr. Neurosci.* **2010**, *13*, 87–100. [CrossRef] [PubMed]
58. Knivsberg, A.M.; Reichelt, K.L.; Høien, T.; Nødland, M. A randomised, controlled study of dietary intervention in autistic syndromes. *Nutr. Neurosci.* **2002**, *5*, 251–261. [CrossRef]
59. Jarmołowska, B.; Bukało, M.; Fiedorowicz, E.; Cieślińska, A.; Kordulewska, N.K.; Moszyńska, M.; Świątecki, A.; Kostyra, E. Role of Milk-Derived Opioid Peptides and Proline Dipeptidyl Peptidase-4 in Autism Spectrum Disorders. *Nutrients* **2019**, *11*, 87. [CrossRef]
60. Schwartz, R.S. Autoimmune folate deficiency and the rise and fall of "horror autotoxicus". *N. Engl. J. Med.* **2005**, *352*, 1948–1950. [CrossRef] [PubMed]
61. Frye, R.E.; Wynne, R.; Rose, S.; Slattery, J.; Delhey, L.; Tippett, M.; Kahler, S.G.; Bennuri, S.C.; Melnyk, S.; Sequeira, J.M.; et al. Thyroid dysfunction in children with autism spectrum disorder is associated with folate receptor α autoimmune disorder. *J. Neuroendocrinol.* **2017**, *29*. [CrossRef] [PubMed]
62. Quadros, E.V.; Sequeira, J.M.; Brown, W.T.; Mevs, C.; Marchi, E.; Flory, M.; Jenkins, E.C.; Velinov, M.T.; Cohen, I.L. Folate receptor autoantibodies are prevalent in childrendiagnosed with autism spectrum disorder, their normal siblings and parents. *Autism Res.* **2018**, *11*, 707–712. [CrossRef]
63. Cabrera, R.M.; Shaw, G.M.; Ballard, J.L.; Carmichael, S.L.; Yang, W.; Lammer, E.J.; Finnell, R.H. Autoantibodies to folate receptor during pregnancy and neural tube defect risk. *J. Reprod. Immunol.* **2008**, *79*, 85–92. [CrossRef] [PubMed]
64. Boyles, A.L.; Ballard, J.L.; Gorman, E.B.; McConnaughey, D.R.; Cabrera, R.M.; Wilcox, A.J.; Lie, R.T.; Finnell, R.H. Association between inhibited binding of folic acid to folate receptor alpha in maternal serum and folate-related birth defects in Norway. *Hum. Reprod.* **2011**, *26*, 2232–2238. [CrossRef]
65. Molloy, A.M.; Quadros, E.V.; Sequeira, J.M.; Troendle, J.F.; Scott, J.M.; Kirke, P.N.; Mills, J.L. Lack of association between folate-receptor autoantibodies and neural-tube defects. *N. Engl. J. Med.* **2009**, *361*, 152–160. [CrossRef] [PubMed]
66. Harel-Gadassi, A.; Friedlander, E.; Yaari, M.; Bar-Oz, B.; Eventov-Friedman, S.; Mankuta, D.; Yirmiya, N. Risk for ASD in Preterm Infants: A Three-Year Follow-Up Study. *Autism Res. Treat.* **2018**, *2018*, 8316212. [CrossRef] [PubMed]

Journal of
*Personalized
Medicine*

MDPI

Review

Cerebral Folate Deficiency, Folate Receptor Alpha Autoantibodies and Leucovorin (Folinic Acid) Treatment in Autism Spectrum Disorders: A Systematic Review and Meta-Analysis

Daniel A. Rossignol [1,*] and Richard E. Frye [2,3]

1 Rossignol Medical Center, 24541 Pacific Park Drive, Suite 210, Aliso Viejo, CA 92656, USA
2 Barrow Neurological Institute at Phoenix Children's Hospital, Phoenix, AZ 85016, USA; rfrye@phoenixchildrens.com
3 Department of Child Health, University of Arizona College of Medicine, Phoenix, AZ 85004, USA
* Correspondence: rossignolmd@gmail.com

Abstract: The cerebral folate receptor alpha (FRα) transports 5-methyltetrahydrofolate (5-MTHF) into the brain; low 5-MTHF in the brain causes cerebral folate deficiency (CFD). CFD has been associated with autism spectrum disorders (ASD) and is treated with *d,l*-leucovorin (folinic acid). One cause of CFD is an autoantibody that interferes with the function of the FRα. FRα autoantibodies (FRAAs) have been reported in ASD. A systematic review was performed to identify studies reporting FRAAs in association with ASD, or the use of *d,l*-leucovorin in the treatment of ASD. A meta-analysis examined the prevalence of FRAAs in ASD. The pooled prevalence of ASD in individuals with CFD was 44%, while the pooled prevalence of CFD in ASD was 38% (with a significant variation across studies due to heterogeneity). The etiology of CFD in ASD was attributed to FRAAs in 83% of the cases (with consistency across studies) and mitochondrial dysfunction in 43%. A significant inverse correlation was found between higher FRAA serum titers and lower 5-MTHF CSF concentrations in two studies. The prevalence of FRAA in ASD was 71% without significant variation across studies. Children with ASD were 19.03-fold more likely to be positive for a FRAA compared to typically developing children without an ASD sibling. For individuals with ASD and CFD, meta-analysis also found improvements with *d,l*-leucovorin in overall ASD symptoms (67%), irritability (58%), ataxia (88%), pyramidal signs (76%), movement disorders (47%), and epilepsy (75%). Twenty-one studies (including four placebo-controlled and three prospective, controlled) treated individuals with ASD using *d,l*-leucovorin. *d,l*-Leucovorin was found to significantly improve communication with medium-to-large effect sizes and have a positive effect on core ASD symptoms and associated behaviors (attention and stereotypy) in individual studies with large effect sizes. Significant adverse effects across studies were generally mild but the most common were aggression (9.5%), excitement or agitation (11.7%), headache (4.9%), insomnia (8.5%), and increased tantrums (6.2%). Taken together, *d,l*-leucovorin is associated with improvements in core and associated symptoms of ASD and appears safe and generally well-tolerated, with the strongest evidence coming from the blinded, placebo-controlled studies. Further studies would be helpful to confirm and expand on these findings.

Keywords: autism spectrum disorder; cerebral folate deficiency; folate receptor alpha autoantibodies; folinic acid; leucovorin

Citation: Rossignol, D.A.; Frye, R.E. Cerebral Folate Deficiency, Folate Receptor Alpha Autoantibodies and Leucovorin (Folinic Acid) Treatment in Autism Spectrum Disorders: A Systematic Review and Meta-Analysis. *J. Pers. Med.* **2021**, *11*, 1141. https://doi.org/10.3390/jpm11111141

Academic Editor: Guido Krenning

Received: 10 October 2021
Accepted: 1 November 2021
Published: 3 November 2021
Corrected: 29 April 2022

Publisher's Note: MDPI stays neutral with regard to jurisdictional claims in published maps and institutional affiliations.

Copyright: © 2021 by the authors. Licensee MDPI, Basel, Switzerland. This article is an open access article distributed under the terms and conditions of the Creative Commons Attribution (CC BY) license (https://creativecommons.org/licenses/by/4.0/).

1. Introduction

Autism spectrum disorder (ASD) is a behaviorally defined disorder that affects approximately 2% of children in the United States [1]. A number of medical comorbidities have been reported in individuals with ASD, with some studies reporting an average of 4–5 comorbidities [2], including allergic rhinitis [3], irritable bowel syndrome [3], attention deficit hyperactivity disorder [4], ophthalmological conditions [4], sleep problems [5], immune problems [5], mitochondrial dysfunction [6], gastrointestinal abnormalities [7] and epilepsy [8]. Recently, cerebral folate deficiency (CFD) has been reported in a number of studies in individuals with ASD and its treatment, *d,l*-leucovorin calcium (also known as folinic acid) has undergone investigation as a treatment for ASD [9].

The importance of folate for the development of the central nervous system (CNS) was first discovered in animal models of dietary folate deficiency where findings such as hydrocephalus [10], decreased myelin cerebroside [11] and impaired synthesis of neuronal RNA [12] were reported. In humans, studies of serum folate deficiency reported neurological findings including ataxia, nystagmus, areflexia, and confusion [13] as well as organic brain syndrome and damage to the pyramidal tracts [14]. In 1974, low levels of cerebrospinal fluid (CSF) folate were reported in patients with epilepsy that improved with tetrahydrofolate but not folic acid [15]. A study in 1976 reported 2 children with low CSF folate who developed intracranial calcifications [16]. In 1979, cerebral atrophy was reported in a 48-year-old woman with low serum and CSF folate [17]. In 1983, a case of a 23 year old woman with Kearns-Sayre syndrome and CNS deterioration was found to have decreased serum and CSF folate while taking phenytoin and improved with folic acid treatment [18].

In 2002, Ramaekers reported a novel neurometabolic syndrome in five children with low CSF 5-MTHF [19] who manifested severe neurodevelopmental symptoms including irritability, seizures, lower extremity pyramidal signs, spastic paraplegia, psychomotor retardation, dyskinesias, cerebellar ataxia, acquired microcephaly and developmental regression which occurred as young as 4 months of age. Unlike previous studies of folate deficiency associated with CNS abnormalities, this new neurometabolic disorder demonstrated below normal concentration of 5-methyltetrahydrofolate (5-MTHF), one of the active metabolites of folate, in the CSF, but normal systemic folate levels. This condition improved with folinic acid (*d,l*-leucovorin) treatment. In these patients, no genetic abnormalities were identified. Ramaekers et al., later described this condition as "idiopathic CFD" [20].

CFD occurs due to the impaired transport of folates across the blood-brain barrier. CFD is usually caused by dysfunction of the folate receptor-alpha (FRα) [21]. FRα is a receptor which has a high affinity for 5-MTHF and is found on the basolateral endothelial surface of the choroid plexus. FRα transports folates across the blood-brain barrier through adenosine triphosphate (ATP) dependent receptor-mediated endocytosis. Dysfunction of the FRα can occur through several mechanisms. In only rare cases, genetic mutations in the gene encoding for FRα (FOLR1) is a cause of CFD [22,23]. Two other mechanisms are more prevalent in causing FRα dysfunction. First, in the seminal paper describing CFD, two autoantibodies to the FRα (blocking and binding autoantibodies) were described that interfere with the function of the FRα [21]. Second, mitochondrial disease is associated with CFD since folate transportation through the FRα is dependent on ATP [24–27].

Another folate transporter, the reduced folate carrier (RFC/SLC19A1), lies on both the basolateral and apical surface of the choroid plexus and has a lower affinity for folates. *d,l*-leucovorin is a reduced (active) form of folate which can enter the CNS through the RFC and has been reported to normalize 5-MTHF levels in the CSF in individuals with CFD [21]. In some cases, clinical response to *d,l*-leucovorin is dramatic, especially if this treatment is started early in life [19,28] but sometimes improvements can be marked even in adults [29]. *d,l*-leucovorin consists of two diastereomers designated as *d*-leucovorin and *l*-leucovorin. *l*-Leucovorin (5-formyl-(6S)-tetrahydrofolate) is the biologically active isomer. It is rapidly metabolized (via 5,10-methenyltetrahydrofolate then 5,10-methylenetetrahydrofolate) to 5-methyl-(6S)-tetrahydrofolate (L-methyl-folate or 5-MTHF), which, in turn, can be metabolized via other pathways back to tetrahydrofolate and 5,10-methenyltetrahydrofolate. 5,10-methylenetetrahydrofolate is converted to 5-MTHF by an irreversible enzyme-catalyzed reduction using the cofactors $FADH_2$ and NADPH. The major mechanism of transportation of folates into the brain occurs through the FRα. FRα binds to folate at lower serum concentrations than the RFC; the latter functions at relatively high concentrations of serum folate and is the predominant method of folate transport in the intestine. Genetic defects in RFC can lead to a rare disorder in intestine folate absorption and genetic abnormalities in FRα may lead to neural tube defects [19].

d,l-leucovorin was first approved in the United States in the 1950s and has been used continuously since then to reduce toxicities associated with folate pathway antagonists such as methotrexate (which is typically used in the treatment of osteosarcoma, other cancers and autoimmune diseases). By replenishing intracellular pools of reduced folates, *d,l*-leucovorin can counteract the toxic effects of folate pathway antagonists such as methotrexate which act by inhibiting dihydrofolate reductase (DHFR). The *d*-isomer of leucovorin is not metabolically active and is not metabolized *in vivo* to any significant degree; therefore, only the *l*-isomer can contribute to the direct replenishment of the pools of active folate cofactors. One of the main advantages reported for *d,l*-leucovorin over folic acid (pteroylmonoglutamic acid) is that folic acid is oxidized and must be reduced by DHFR to a biologically active folate in order to become active. High doses of folic acid may also block the FRα which can potentially exacerbate CFD [30]. Many individuals, including those with ASD, have polymorphisms in the DHFR gene which makes the function of this enzyme less efficient [31]. Currently, the most prescribed form of leucovorin in the United States is *d,l*-leucovorin calcium. *d,l*-Leucovorin is only form of folate that has been used to treat CFD except for one case report using 5-MTHF [32].

Since its original description, the phenotype of CFD has expanded. A number of studies have reported ASD in a subset of children with CFD [20,21,33–36]. This is not particularly surprising as two mechanisms for FRα dysfunction, FRα autoantibodies (FRAAs) and mitochondrial dysfunction, are common in ASD. Indeed, studies have reported a high prevalence of FRAAs in individuals with ASD ranging from 58% to 76% [37–45]. Mitochondrial dysfunction is a common medical comorbidity in ASD, with studies reporting 30–50% of individuals with ASD possessing biomarkers of mitochondrial dysfunction [6,46] and up to 80% having abnormal electron transport chain (ETC) activity in immune cells [47,48]. Treatment in some children with CFD and ASD with oral *d,l*-leucovorin has led to clinical improvements ranging from partial improvements in communication, social interaction, attention and stereotypies [21,33,35,36] to complete recovery of both neurological and ASD symptoms [21,34] in up to 21% of treated patients [44]. Of note, *d,l*-leucovorin has been reported to improve symptoms in Down syndrome [49], Rett syndrome [50–52] and schizophrenia [53].

This paper systematically reviews the studies examining an association between CFD and ASD, then examines the prevalence of the major cause of CFD, namely FRAAs, in ASD, typically developing (TD) siblings of individuals with ASD and their parents and TD non-related controls, followed by reviewing the evidence for treatment with *d,l*-leucovorin, the primary treatment for CFD, in individuals with ASD and any associated adverse effects (AEs).

2. Materials and Methods

2.1. Search Process

A prospective protocol for this review was developed a priori and the search terms and selection criteria were chosen to capture all pertinent publications. The search included individuals with autistic disorder, Asperger syndrome, pervasive developmental disorder-not otherwise specified (PDD-NOS) and ASD. A computer-aided search of PUBMED, Google Scholar, CINAHL, EmBase, Scopus, and ERIC databases from inception through September 2021 was conducted to identify pertinent publications using the search terms "autism", "autistic", "Asperger", "pervasive", "ASD", and "PDD" in all combinations with "folinic acid", "leucovorin", "folate", "folic", "methyl-folate", "5MTHF", "levofolinic", "folinate", and "formyltetrahydrofolate." The references cited in identified publications were also searched to locate additional studies.

2.2. Study Selection and Assessment

This systematic review and meta-analysis followed PRISMA guidelines [33], the PRISMA Checklist is found in Supplementary Table S1 and the PRISMA Flowchart for *d,l*-leucovorin treatment in ASD is displayed as Figure 1. Studies were included in this systematic review if they: (a) involved individuals with ASD, and (b) either reported on the use of leucovorin in at least one individual with ASD and/or described FRAAs in at least one individual with ASD. Articles that did not present new or unique data (such as review articles or letters to the editor), and animal studies were excluded. Studies on Rett syndrome and Childhood Disintegrative Disorder were also excluded. One reviewer (DR) screened titles and abstracts of all potentially relevant studies for identification purposes. Both reviewers then examined each identified study in-depth and assessed factors such as the risk of bias. As per standardized guidelines [54], selection, performance detection, attrition, and reporting biases were considered.

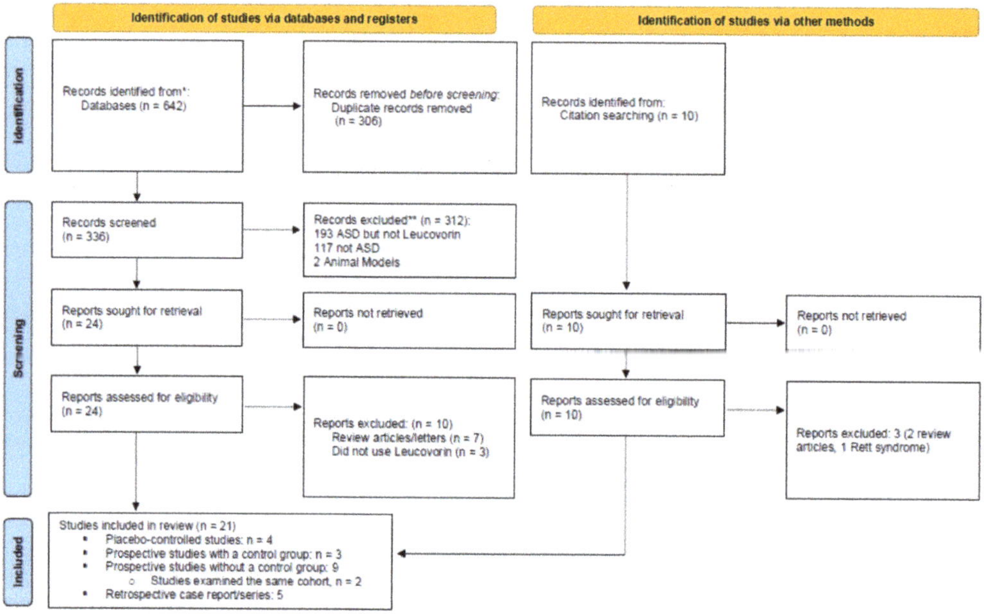

Figure 1. PRISMA 2020 flow diagram for this systematic review.

As a result of the in-depth review, several studies were excluded from further consideration. One study [55] reported on a child with "autistic personal characteristics" who had CFD, but it was unclear whether this child was diagnosed with ASD. Two studies reported treatment of children with ASD using **folic acid** [56,57]. Finally, one study [43] used an unvalidated, non-clinical FRAA assay in which the functional significance of the autoantibody is unknown.

2.3. Meta-Analysis

MetaXL Version 5.2 (EpiGear International Pty Ltd., Sunrise Beach, QLD, Australia) was used with Microsoft Excel Version 16.0.12827.20200 (Redmond, WA, USA) to perform the meta-analysis. Random-effects models, which assume variability in effects from both sampling error and study level differences [58,59], were used to calculate pooled prevalence and odds ratios. The Luis Furuya-Kanamori (LFK) Index derived from Doi plots was reviewed for significant asymmetries ($>\pm 2$) in the prevalence distribution when there were three or more studies [60,61]. Cochran's Q was calculated to determine heterogeneity of effects across studies and, when significant, the I^2 statistic (Heterogeneity Index) was calculated to determine the percentage of variation across studies that is due to heterogeneity rather than chance [62,63]. Funnel plots were also reviewed.

Mean FRAA titers were pooled across studies using standard methodology [64]. To compare FRAA titers across groups, pooled Cohen's d' (a measure of effect size) was calculated from the standardized mean difference of outcome measures using the inverse variance heterogeneity model, since it has been shown to resolve issues with underestimation of the statistical error and spuriously overconfident estimates with the random effects model when analyzing continuous outcome measures [65].

The outcome measures used across treatment studies were different in most cases, making a formal meta-analysis of any particular outcome not possible. Thus, the effect size, as measured by Cohen's d', was calculated where possible so the strengths of effects could be compared across studies. For controlled studies, the effect size represented the difference between the treatment and the control groups, whereas for uncontrolled studies the effect size was calculated only for the treatment group. Only a subset of studies contained the information needed to calculate the effect size. For example, for the calculation of effect size, the change in the outcome needed to be reported across the treatment period; reported mean values of the outcome before and after treatment were insufficient to calculate an effect size. Effect sizes were considered small if Cohen's d' was 0.2; medium for Cohen's d' was 0.5; and large if Cohen's d' was 0.8 [66].

3. Results

This section will first discuss folate pathway abnormalities related to ASD, followed by treatment of folate pathway abnormalities.

3.1. *Central Folate Pathway Abnormalities and the Folate Receptor Alpha Autoantibody*

3.1.1. ASD Prevalence in CFD

Five case-series [20,21,33,35,67] described 79 children with CFD in which ASD was assessed (Supplementary Table S2) resulting in a prevalence of 44% (21%, 70%) of ASD in CFD (Table 1). Removing the one study with a very high prevalence rate because of asymmetry [33] lowered the pooled prevalence rate to 32% (19%, 45%).

3.1.2. Cerebral Folate Deficiency in Autism Spectrum Disorder

Two case-series [34,68], two case-reports [36,69] and four prospective cohort-studies [37,45,70,71] described 172 individuals with idiopathic ASD who had CSF measurements (See Supplementary Table S3). The pooled prevalence of CFD in ASD was 38% (11%, 71%) with a significant variation across studies due to heterogeneity driven by three studies with very high prevalence rates [34,36,68] and four studies with very low prevalence rates [37,45,70,71]. Two studies with high prevalence rates reported severe patients; one study was an older case series specifically examining low-functioning ASD with neurological deficits [34]; and one was a case report of a child with mental retardation and seizures [36]. Two case series examined patients with mitochondrial disorders with very different prevalence; the series which reported a new type of non-traditional mitochondrial disorder reported a high prevalence (100%) of CFD [68], while the series which reported classical mitochondrial disorders reported a low (5%) prevalence of CFD [71]. The overall pooled prevalence was 43% (0%, 100%) with significant heterogeneity. One study found no correlation between CSF levels of 5-MTHF and measures of autism symptomatology as measured by the Autism Diagnostic Observation Schedule (ADOS) calibrated severity score, adaptive behavior as measured by the Vineland Adaptive Behavior Scale (VABS), and cognitive functioning as measured by the Mullen Scales of Early Learning [70].

Table 1. Meta-analysis results for the prevalence of cerebral folate deficiency and folate receptor alpha autoantibodies. Pooled prevalence with 95% confidence interval, Cochran's Q (Q), Heterogeneity Index (I^2), Luis Furuya-Kanamori (LFK) Index and number of studies involved (N). Statistics are estimated by a random-effects model. * $p < 0.05$; ** $p < 0.01$; ^{T} Significant Asymmetry.

	Prevalence (95% CI)	Q	I^2	LFK	N
Cerebral Folate Deficiency					
Prevalence of ASD in CFD	44% (21%, 70%)	16.14 **	75%	2.57 ^{T}	5
Prevalence of CFD in ASD	38% (11%, 71%)	85.50 **	92%	4.20 ^{T}	8
Etiology of CFD in ASD:					
• Either FRα autoantibody	83% (69%, 94%)	5.19			5
• Mitochondrial Dysfunction	43% (0%, 100%)	9.15 **	89%		2
• Genetic abnormalities	14% (0%, 39%)	12.4 *	60%	4.63 ^{T}	6
Prevalence of FRα Autoantibody					
Autism Spectrum Disorder (ASD)					
• Blocking FRα autoantibody	46% (27%, 64%)	52.34 **	92%	0.42	5
• Binding FRα autoantibody	49% (43%, 55%)	2.34			4
• Either FRα autoantibody	71% (64%, 77%)	10.07			5
Parents of ASD children					
• Blocking FRα autoantibody	30% (19%, 44%)	9.39 *	79%	−0.78	3
• Binding FRα autoantibody	23% (0%, 61%)	13.45 **	93%		2
• Either FRα autoantibody	45% (27%, 60%)	89.90 **	89%	0.05	4
Typically Developing Siblings of ASD					
• Blocking FRα autoantibody	38% (19%, 58%)	1.39			2
• Binding FRα autoantibody	40% (9%, 77%)	2.93			2
• Either FRα autoantibody	61% (28%, 97%)	3.86			2
Typically Developing Non-sibling					
• Blocking FRα autoantibody	4% (1%, 10%)	0.00			2
• Binding FRα autoantibody	10% (10%, 48%)	16.33 **	94%		2
• Either FRα autoantibody	15% (0%, 46%)	9.60 **	90%		2
Developmentally Delayed without ASD					
• Blocking FRα autoantibody	5% (0%, 14%)				1

3.1.3. Prevalence of Autoantibodies to the Folate Receptor Alpha in ASD

Nine studies examined the prevalence of FRAAs in ASD [37–42,44,45,72]. Two sets of studies [37,39] and [40,41,72] reported on the same cohort of patients. Additionally, one study reported the prevalence in two subsets of patients; those treated with *d,l*-leucovorin (n = 82) and those untreated (n = 84) [44]. This resulted in six unique studies that examined the prevalence of FRAAs in children with ASD (See Supplementary Table S4).

The correlation between FRAAs and patient characteristics have been outlined in several studies. Two studies [35,37] reported a significant inverse correlation between higher blocking FRAA serum titers and lower 5-MTHF CSF concentrations. One study found that blocking FRAA decreased with age [37] with another study reporting increased blocking FRAA over a 2-year period with continued use of cow's milk [35]. One study suggested that children with ASD were significantly different in physiological and developmental characteristics depending on whether they had the blocking or binding FRAA; the binding FRAA was associated with higher serum B12 concentration, while the blocking FRAA was associated with better redox metabolism, inflammation markers, communication on the VABS, stereotyped behavior on the Aberrant Behavioral Checklist (ABC) and mannerisms on the Social Responsiveness Scale (SRS) [40]. In another study, FRAA positive children were more likely to have a medical diagnosis of hypothyroidism [37]. Two studies found a positive correlation between the blocking FRAA titers and thyroid stimulating hormone (TSH) concentrations [39,41]. One study examined this relationship in detail, finding that thyroid hormone was rarely outside the normal range, suggesting that the relationship between TSH and thyroid hormone levels were altered in some children with ASD. Interestingly, this study also found that FRAAs bind to prenatal thyroid tissue in early gestation (prior to 18 weeks) suggesting that FRAAs during gestation could affect the programing of the hypothalamic-pituitary-axis regulation of thyroid hormone [37].

Five studies [37,38,40,42,45] from three sets of investigators found a blocking FRAA prevalence of 46% (27%, 64%) in ASD with a significant heterogeneity but no asymmetry, indicating variation in the underlying ASD samples across studies. Four studies [37,40,42,45] from two sets of investigators found a binding FRAA prevalence of 49% (43%, 55%) without significant variation across studies. Five studies [37,40,42,44,45] from three sets of investigators found an overall FRAA prevalence of 71% (64%, 77%) without significant variation across studies. From the three studies reporting both FRAA titers [37,40,42] and one study only measuring blocking FRAAs [38] in ASD, pooled mean blocking FRAA titers was 0.85 pmol of IgG antibody per ml of serum (95% CI: 0.59, 1.11) and binding FRAA was 0.42 pmol of IgG antibody per ml of serum (95% CI: 0.35, 0.49).

One study that looked at the blocking FRAA over a five-week period found that in four patients with predominately negative titers, if tested over several weeks, they may have low positive (~0.3–0.4 pmol of IgG antibody per ml of serum) at some point, while others with the most high titers can have low or negative titers at some time points [45].

Four studies [37,38,42,44] from three sets of investigators examined blocking and binding FRAA prevalence in parents and TD siblings of children with ASD. Prevalence of the blocking, binding and either FRAA was 30% (19%, 44%), 23% (0%, 61%) and 45% (27%, 60%) in parents of children with ASD, respectively. All studies demonstrated significant heterogeneity without asymmetry suggesting variation in the underlying ASD samples across studies. Interestingly, TD siblings of children with ASD appear to have a similar prevalence as the children with ASD themselves with a pooled prevalence of 38% (19%, 58%), 40% (9%, 77%) and 61% (28%, 97%) for blocking, binding and either FRAA, respectively, without significant variation across studies.

The prevalence of FRAAs in TD children without ASD siblings was assessed in two studies [42,45] with a pooled prevalence of 4% (1%, 10%), 10% (10%, 48%) and 15% (0%, 46%) for blocking, binding and either FRAA, respectively; this is much lower than the FRAA prevalence in children with ASD or their siblings. However, there was significant variability in the binding FRAA across these two studies, demonstrating the need for larger cohorts of non-sibling control samples.

One study [38] examined the prevalence of the blocking FRAA in developmentally delayed children without ASD and found a pooled prevalence of 5% (0%, 14%); this is much lower than the FRAAs prevalence in children with ASD or their TD siblings.

3.1.4. Comparison of Prevalence of Autoantibodies to the Folate Receptor Alpha in ASD to Other Groups

A meta-analysis was used to calculate the odds ratio of having FRAAs in children with ASD compared to various groups. Five studies [37,38,42,44,45] reported FRAAs in both children with ASD and their parents. The odds of being positive for the blocking or either FRAA, but not binding alone, was significantly increased in children with ASD as compared to their parents (Table 2). The odds of being positive for the FRAA was not different between children with ASD and their TD siblings. However, children with ASD demonstrated a significantly increased odds of being positive for the blocking, binding and either FRAA as compared to TD children without an ASD sibling, and as compared to developmentally delayed children without ASD for the blocking FRAA.

Table 2. Meta-analysis of Odds Ratios with 95% confidence interval for differences between the prevalence of Folate Receptor Alpha Autoantibodies in children with ASD to Various Comparison Groups. Odd ratios that are significant are bolded and italicized. Also listed are Cochran's Q (Q), Heterogeneity Index (I2), Luis Furuya-Kanamori (LFK) Index and number of studies involved (N). Statistics are estimated by a random-effects model. $^{\Gamma}$ $p < 0.05$, ** $p \leq 0.001$.

Comparison Group	Odds Ratio (95% CI)	Q	I^2	LFK	N
Parents of ASD children					
• Blocking FRα autoantibody	**2.10 (1.05, 4.21)** $^{\Gamma}$	6.37			3
• Binding FRα autoantibody	3.62 (0.70, 18.84)	4.40			2
• Either FRα autoantibody	**3.56 (1.62, 7.79) ****	8.60 $^{\Gamma}$	65%	−0.77	4
Typically Developing Siblings of ASD					
• Blocking FRα autoantibody	2.00 (0.26, 15.21)	3.31			2
• Binding FRα autoantibody	1.32 (0.44, 3.99)	1.41			2
• Either FRα autoantibody	2.12 (0.40, 11.30)	3.12			2
Typically Developing Non-sibling					
• Blocking FRα autoantibody	***26.84 (7.84, 91.86) *****	1.02			2
• Binding FRα autoantibody	***7.90 (0.70, 89.13) *****	2.81			2
• Either FRα autoantibody	***19.03 (2.36, 153.58) *****	3.58			2
Developmentally Delayed without ASD					
• Blocking FRα autoantibody	***25.38 (3.29, 196.02) *****				1

Two studies [37,42] compared the serum concentrations of FRAAs in children with ASD compared to parents and/or TD siblings while one study compared FRAA in children with ASD to TD children without ASD siblings [42]. Meta-analysis found that the mean blocking FRAA titer in ASD was significantly higher than parents (d' = 0.26 (0.116, 0.36), $p < 0.0001$) and siblings (d' = 0.29 (0.15, 0.43), $p < 0.0001$) with small-to-medium effect sizes and significantly higher than controls with a very large effect size (d' = 2.93 (1.85, 4.01), $p < 0.0001$). However, the mean binding FRAA titer in ASD was significantly higher than in parents (d' = 0.14 (0.06, 0.22), $p < 0.001$) but not siblings (d' = 0.06 (−0.04, 0.17), p = n.s.) with small effect sizes and significantly higher than controls but with a small effect size (d' = 0.16 (0.07, 0.25), $p < 0.001$).

Finally, in one study that measured blocking FRAAs in children with CFD with and without ASD there was no significant difference between groups (Mean (SD) 1.17 (0.84) pmol/mL and 1.78 (1.99) pmol/mL, respectively, t(23) = 0.91, $p = 0.37$) [35].

3.2. *Treatment of ASD with d,l-Leucovorin*

As seen in Figure 1, 20 studies were identified which studied *d,l*-leucovorin treatment in individuals with ASD including four placebo-controlled studies [72–75], three prospective, controlled studies [37,44,76], nine prospective studies without a control group [20,21,33–35,77–80] (two studies examined the same cohort of patients [78,79]), and four case reports/series [36,67–69].

A review of these studies on treatment of children with ASD with *d,l*-leucovorin appears to fall into three categories. Firstly, children with ASD and concomitant CFD were studied. Secondly, *d,l*-leucovorin was studied in isolation for treating idiopathic ASD. Thirdly, some studies used *d,l*-leucovorin in combination with other nutritional supplements to treat ASD symptoms. Each of these approaches to using *d,l*-leucovorin is outlined in separate sections below.

3.2.1. Treatment with *d,l*-Leucovorin in ASD and Comorbid CFD

Nine unique case-series/reports describe children with ASD and comorbid CFD treated with *d,l*-leucovorin (See Supplementary Tables S2 and S3) [20,21,33–36,67–69]. Two studies, one [36] case report and one case series [33], reported on the same child. A meta-analysis was conducted to determine the prevalence of improvement in symptoms as a result of *d,l*-leucovorin treatment in children with CFD with and without ASD (See Table 3; Supplementary Table S5). Six studies [21,33–35,67,69] reported a response rate of 67% for improvement in ASD symptoms with *d,l*-leucovorin treatment. Response to *d,l*-leucovorin in irritability was studied in children with ASD in three studies [21,34,35] and in children without ASD in three studies [21,33,35]. For those with ASD, irritability improved in 58% while in those without ASD irritability improved in 47% with a wide variation among studies, because one study demonstrated a high response rate of 88% [21] while the other two studies demonstrated much lower response rates of 22% [35] and 0% [33].

Table 3. Meta-analysis results for the prevalence response to *d,l*-leucovorin treatment in children with CFD with and without autism spectrum disorder (ASD). Pooled prevalence with 95% confidence interval, Cochran's Q (Q), Heterogeneity Index (I2), Luis Furuya-Kanamori (LFK) Index and number of studies involved (N). Statistics are estimated by a random-effects model. * $p < 0.01$; [T] Significant Asymmetry.

	Prevalence (95% CI)	Q	I^2	LFK	N
Children with ASD					
• Autism	67% (43%, 87%)	9.23			6
• Irritability	58% (40%, 76%)	2.24			3
• Ataxia	88% (75%, 97%)	3.16			5
• Pyramidal Signs	76% (19%, 100%)	13.83 *	75%	−2.27 [T]	4
• Movement Disorder	47% (20%, 75%)	3.85			4
• Epilepsy	75% (54%, 91%)	4.48			5
Children without ASD					
• Irritability	47% (0%, 100%)	12.11 *	84%	−5.54 [T]	2
• Ataxia	72% (24%, 100%)	5.82			2
• Pyramidal Signs	33% (0%, 100%)	13.41	92%		2
• Movement Disorder	18% (1%, 46%)	2.07			3
• Epilepsy	54% (0%, 100%)	12.90 *	77%	−2.31 [T]	4

Five studies examined ataxia in ASD [21,33–35,67] while two studies examined ataxia in children without ASD [21,35] with both groups of children demonstrating a high rate of response of ataxia to *d,l*-leucovorin treatment (88% and 72%, respectively). Pyramidal signs were reported in four studies for those with ASD [21,34,35,67] and in two studies for those without ASD [21,35]. Response was relatively high for those with ASD (76%) while relatively low for those without ASD (33%), although there was wide variation in response rates across studies in both groups.

The response of dyskinesias and other movement disorders to *d,l*-leucovorin treatment was examined in ASD in four studies [21,33–35] and in children without ASD in three studies [21,33,35]. Movement disorders improved with *d,l*-leucovorin in 47% of those with ASD while the response rate was much lower for those without ASD (18%).

Six studies examined epilepsy response for those with ASD [21,33–35,67,69] while four studies examined response to epilepsy for those without ASD [21,33,35,67]. Epilepsy improved in 75% of children with ASD, but the response rate was somewhat lower (54%) and much more variable for those without ASD since there was a large variation across studies, perhaps driven by the overall small number of cases.

Treatment with *d,l*-leucovorin was reported to improve CSF 5-MTHF concentrations in several studies. One year of 0.5–1 mg/kg/day *d,l*-leucovorin treatment normalized 5-MTHF CSF concentrations in 90% of children in one case-series [20]; 0.5–1 mg/kg/day *d,l*-leucovorin improved CSF 5-MTHF concentrations in seven children in another study [35]; *d,l*-leucovorin 1–3 mg/kg/day over a 12-month period led to improvements in CSF 5-MTHF concentrations in 21 patients in a third study [34]; *d,l*-leucovorin, 0.5–9.0 mg/kg/day orally, followed by *d,l*-leucovorin, 6 mg/kg Q6 h for 1d IV monthly for 6 months normalized CSF 5-MTHF in a fourth study [69]. Additional treatments which resulted in clinical improvements included the removal of cow's milk in one study [35]. One study reported a trend towards more robust improvements in younger children as compared to older children [34].

3.2.2. Treatment with *d,l*-Leucovorin in General ASD: Leucovorin Only

Supplementary Table S6 lists the five studies [37,72,74,80,81] performed by three different sets of investigators which have examined the use of *d,l*-leucovorin in children with idiopathic ASD without additional treatments in order to determine if *d,l*-leucovorin administered by itself is a useful treatment for ASD. Table 4 outlines the effect sizes of some of the key outcome measures used in these studies.

Table 4. Outcome measures represented in effect size in key studies which have used *d,l*-leucovorin. Cohen's d' was calculated for studies which provided enough information to make such calculations. For controlled studies, the effect size represented the difference between the treatment and the control group, whereas for uncontrolled studies, the effect size was calculated only for the treatment. Effect sizes were considered small if Cohen's d' was 0.2; medium for Cohen's d' of 0.5, and large if Cohen's d' was 0.8. Effects in bold are statistically significant.

Core ASD Symptoms	Communication	Behaviors	Other Symptoms
	_d,l_-leucovorin Only Studies		
Frye et al., 2013 [37] (Non-Treated Wait List Controlled)			
Stereotypy d' = 1.02	**Verbal Comm d' = 0.91** **Expressive Lang d' = 0.81** **Receptive Lang d' = 0.76**	**Attention d' = 1.01** Hyperactivity d' = 0.25	
Frye et al., 2018 [72] (Double Blind Placebo Controlled)			
ABC Social Withdrawal d' = 0.27 **ABC Stereotypy d' = 0.60**	**Verbal Comm (All) d' = 0.70** **Verbal Comm (FRAA+) d' = 0.91**	**Hyperactivity d' = 0.05**	
Renard et al., 2020 [74] (Single Blind Placebo Controlled)			
ADOS total score d' = 1.16 **Social interaction d' = 1.11** **SRS Total d' = 0.03**	**Communication d' = 0.66**		
	_d,l_-leucovorin Combined with Other Supplements		
Adams et al., 2011 [73] (Double Blind Placebo Controlled; PGI-R Outcome)			
Play d' = 0.23 Sociability d' = 0.15	Expressive Language d' = 0.37 **Receptive Language d' = 0.44**	**Hyperactivity d' = 0.60** **Tantrums d' = 0.53**	Cognition d' = 0.34 Gastrointestinal d' = 0.30 Sleep d' = 0.18
Adams et al., 2018 [76] (Prospective Non-Treatment Controlled; PGI-2 Outcome)			
Play d' = 1.50 **Sociability d' = 1.44** **Eye Contact d' = 1.41** **Perseveration d' = 1.33** **Sound Sensitivity d' = 1.14**	**Expressive Language d' = 1.60** **Receptive Language d' = 1.99**	**Attention d' = 1.19** **Hyperactivity d' = 1.46** **Tantrums d' = 1.00** **Aggression d' = 0.96** Self-Injury d' = 0.69	**Cognition d' = 1.49** **Gastrointestinal d' = 2.09** **Sleep d' = 0.92** **Mood d' = 1.58** **Anxiety d' = 0.95**
Ramaekers et al., 2019 [44] (Baseline Controlled)			
CARS d' = 1.01–1.32			
Frye et al., 2013 [79] (Baseline Controlled)			
Interpersonal d' = 0.43 **Play d' = 0.59** **Coping d' = 0.66**	**Expressive Language d' = 0.59** **Receptive Language d' = 0.97** **Written Language d' = 0.56**		**Personal d' = 0.65** **Domestic d' = 0.37** **Community d' = 0.52**

In a medium-sized (n = 44) open-label, prospective, controlled study which used a wait-list control group that did not receive any new interventions, children with ASD who were known to be positive for a FRAA were treated with 2 mg/kg/day (max 50 mg per day) of *d,l*-leucovorin over a mean period of 4 months [37]. Using the Parent Rated Autism Symptomatic Change Scale, significant improvements were reported in verbal communication, expressive and receptive language, attention and stereotypy with mostly large effect sizes (See Table 4). Interestingly, improvement in verbal communication and expression language demonstrated greater improvement as age increased in children who were negative for the binding FRAA but demonstrated lesser improvement as age increased for children who were positive for the binding FRAA.

One study reported nonsignificant improvements with *d,l*-leucovorin in 12 patients with ASD using 2 mg/kg/day (max 50 mg/day) of *d,l*-leucovorin over 12 weeks. Nonsignificant improvements were observed on the ABC (2.4-point improvement) and SRS (7.8-point improvement) while a 0.8-point nonsignificant worsening on the PedsQL was also observed. Urinary metabolites showed changes during the study including a 24.8-fold increase in 5MTHF concentrations; a 10.1-fold increase in 1-stearoyl-2-arachidonoyl-GPC; a 9.3-fold increase in 1-stearoyl-2-oleoylGPC; a 9.2-fold increase in alpha-tocopherol; and a 7.8-fold increase in 1-stearoyl-2linoleoyl-GPC (7.8); however, the authors noted that the study lacked to power to determine if changes in urinary metabolites predicted treatment response [80].

Two placebo-controlled studies of *d,l*-leucovorin used *d,l*-leucovorin in children with idiopathic ASD without additional treatments. In a medium-sized (n = 48) double-blind, placebo controlled (DBPC) study of 48 children with ASD without known CFD, 23 children received *d,l*-leucovorin calcium (2 mg/kg/day; maximum 50 mg/day) and 25 received a placebo [72]. Significant improvements were seen in the primary outcome measure of verbal communication with an overall medium-to-large effect size and a larger effect size for those positive for at least one FRAA (Table 4). The primary outcome measure exceeded the minimal clinically important difference defined as a change of five standardized points on the language assessments over 3 months. Improvements were also observed in the secondary outcome measures of the VABS daily living skills, ABC irritability, social withdrawal, stereotypy, hyperactivity and inappropriate speech; and in the Autism Symptom Questionnaire (ASQ) stereotypic behavior and total score. ABC social withdrawal, stereotypy, and inappropriate speech and ASQ stereotypic behavior and total score exceeded the predefined minimal clinically important difference. The number needed to treat (NNT) for improvements in verbal communication was 2.4 in all treated children, and 1.8 in children who were positive for at least one FRAA [72].

The second placebo-controlled study was a smaller (n = 19) single-blind, placebo-controlled study of 19 children with ASD; 9 children received *d,l*-leucovorin (5 mg twice daily; 0.29–0.63 mg/kg/day) for 12 weeks and 10 children received a placebo [74]. Significant improvements were found in ADOS total score and social interaction subscale with large to very large effect sizes and in the communication subscale with a medium effect size (See Table 4). These changes were significant in the treated group but not in the placebo-control group. The SRS, completed by the parents, showed nonsignificant improvement with a very small effect size.

In a retrospective national survey of 1286 participants with ASD or their parents/caregivers, a number of nutritional supplements were rated for changes in behaviors and AEs. Higher dose folinic acid (more than 5 mg/day orally) improved cognition in 33%, attention in 29%, and language/communication in 24%. A moderate dose of folinic acid (below 5 mg/day orally) improved language/communication (20%). The overall adverse effect rating was minimal [81].

These series of studies provide evidence that *d,l*-leucovorin is helpful for a wide variety of core and associated ASD symptoms. The three sets of investigators used very different doses of *d,l*-leucovorin. Three studies [37,72,80] used a relatively high dose (2 mg/kg/day; maximum 50 mg/day) while one study [74] used a much lower dose

(5 mg twice daily; 0.29–0.63 mg/kg/day) but both dosing parameters were associated with significant clinical improvements.

3.2.3. Treatment with *d,l*-Leucovorin in General ASD: Combined with Other Supplements

Six studies (spanning seven reports) from four sets of investigators used *d,l*-leucovorin in combination with nutritional supplements or other medications to treat ASD (Supplementary Table S7). The most recent study added *d,l*-leucovorin or placebo to risperidone in a DBPC study [75]. One set of investigators examined a multivitamin-mineral complex (MVMC) in two controlled studies [73,76] (one study was controlled with a placebo group and one utilized untreated children as controls), while another set of investigators examined *d,l*-leucovorin along with other indicated treatments using a prospective clinical protocol with a control group of ASD children receiving only standard behavioral and educational therapy without medical interventions [44]. Finally, one set of investigators examined *d,l*-leucovorin along with other treatments in an open-label fashion without comparison groups [77–79]. All of these studies were performed on children with ASD without known CFD.

In a medium-size (n = 55) DBPC study, children received either *d,l*-leucovorin (2 mg/kg/day up to 50 mg daily) or placebo in two divided daily doses along with risperidone for 10 weeks [75]. Risperidone was started at 0.5 mg and increased by 0.5 mg weekly up to 1 mg for children <20 kg and 2 mg for children ≥20 kg. The ABC inappropriate speech was the primary outcome measure with the remainder of the ABC subscales as the secondary outcome measures. All ABC subscales improved more in the leucovorin group as compared to the placebo group with statistical significance in all subscales except for social withdrawal. The authors used two different measures of effect size Cohen d′ and η^2 which provided different estimates of the effect sizes with η^2 showing medium effect sizes and Cohen d′ demonstrating extremely large effect sizes. Due to this discrepancy, these results are not listed in Table 4 because of their ambiguity.

In a large (n = 141) DBPC study, children with ASD were treated with either a MVMC which contained 550 µg of *d,l*-leucovorin (n = 72) or a placebo (n = 69) for 3 months. The Parental Global Impressions-Revised (PGI-R) demonstrated improvements in communication and behavior (See Table 4). In addition to the *d,l*-leucovorin, the active treatment contained vitamins A, C, D3, E, K, B1-B6, B12, folic acid, biotin, choline, inositol, mixed carotenoids, mixed tocopherols, CoEnzyme Q10, N-acetylcysteine, calcium, chromium, copper, iodine, iron, lithium, magnesium, manganese, molybdenum, phosphorus, potassium, selenium, sulfur and zinc [73].

In another medium-sized (n = 67) prospective, open-label, controlled study of 67 individuals with ASD, a MVMC containing 600 µg folate mixture (*d,l*-leucovorin, folic acid and 5-MTHF combined) per day was given to 37 individuals with ASD for 12 months, while 30 individuals were untreated [76]. Improvements were found in several of the Parental Global Impressions-2 (PGI-2) measures (Table 4) as well as in the Childhood Autism Rating Scale 2 (CARS2) score, Short Sensory Profile, SRS, ABC, Autism Treatment Evaluation Checklist (ATEC) and VABS. Besides the folate mixture, the treatment contained vitamins A, C, D3, E, K, B1-B6, B12, biotin, choline, inositol, mixed tocopherols, CoEnzyme Q10, N-acetylcysteine, Acetyl-L-Carnitine, calcium, chromium, vanadium, boron, lithium, magnesium, manganese, molybdenum, potassium, selenium, sulfur and zinc.

In a large (n = 166) prospective, case-control, open-label study, 82 children with ASD (ages 1–15.9 years) were treated with *d,l*-leucovorin 0.5–2 mg/kg/day (maximum 50 mg/day) for 2 years and were compared to 84 untreated children with ASD (ages 1–16.8 years) who were matched for age, gender, CARS score and FRα autoantibody status [44]. The untreated control group of 84 ASD children received only standard behavioral and educational therapy without additional medical interventions. Blood tests were performed to identify nutritional deficiencies and abnormal oxidative stress biomarkers which were treated with other vitamins and minerals (such as vitamins A, C, D, E, zinc, selenium, manganese, and CoEnzyme Q10, when indicated by testing) in the treated children. *d,l*-

Leucovorin was given to the children who had positive FRAAs (62 of 82 children with ASD had FRAAs, 75.6%). The other 20 children without positive FRAAs did not receive *d,l*-leucovorin. This study reported improvements in mean CARS scores from severe ASD (mean (SD): 41.34 (6.47)) to mild or moderate ASD (mean (SD): 34.35 (6.25)) in all age cohorts of the treated group (See Table 4). In the untreated group of 84 children, there was no significant change in the mean CARS score over the study period. The authors reported "complete recovery" in 17 of 82 children (21%).

Two of the open-label, prospective studies from one set of investigators examined the use of *d,l*-leucovorin in a cohort of individuals with ASD without a control group. In the first study which included eight children with ASD, 800 μg of *d,l*-leucovorin and 1000 mg of betaine was given twice a day for 4 months; significant improvements ($p \leq 0.05$) were found in the concentrations of methionine, S-adenosylmethionine (SAM), homocysteine, cystathionine, cysteine, total glutathione (tGSH) concentrations, SAM:S-adenosylhomocysteine (SAH) and tGSH:GSSG; clinical improvements in speech and cognition were noted by the attending physician but were not formally quantified [77]. James et al., 2009 [78] studied 40 children with ASD and administered 400 μg of *d,l*-leucovorin twice a day and 75 μg/kg methyl-cobalamin injected subcutaneously twice a week. This treatment led to significant increases in cysteine, cysteinyl-glycine, and glutathione concentrations (all $p < 0.001$); significant improvements were observed in all subscales of the VABS [79].

3.3. Adverse Effects Reported with d,l-Leucovorin Treatment in ASD

Overall, the placebo-controlled studies support the minimal AEs associated with leucovorin treatment. No significant difference in AE frequency as compared to placebo was reported in the single-blind, placebo-controlled study [74], in two DBPC studies [72,75], or in the last DPBC study for patients who followed the protocol [73].

To investigate the consistency of reported AEs, a meta-analysis was performed on reported AEs for patients on leucovorin treatment, separately for studies examining only leucovorin and for those studies which combined leucovorin with other supplements or treatments (Table 5). For studies which only treated with leucovorin, consistently reported AEs included excitement or agitation (11.7%), aggression (9.5%), insomnia (8.5%), increased tantrums (6.2%), headache (4.9%) and gastroesophageal reflux (2.8%). For studies which used leucovorin in combination with other agents, AEs that were consistently reported included worsening behavior (8.5%) and aggression (1.3%).Interestingly, Frye et al., 2020 [9] examined the reported targeted AE of agitation and excitability every 3 weeks during their previous 12-week study of 2018 [72]. This AE was reported at almost the exact same frequency in the treatment and placebo group until the 9th week of treatment when it precipitously dropped in frequency in the treatment, but not the placebo, group, demonstrating the improvement of this reported AE with longer exposure to the medication.

Table 5. Meta-analysis of Adverse Effects Associated with Leucovorin in Children with ASD. Bold and italics indicate significant effects across studies.

Leucovorin Alone		Leucovorin Combination	
Adverse Effect	**Incidence (95% CI)**	**Adverse Effect**	**Incidence (95% CI)**
Abdominal Pain	1.7% (0.0%, 4.8%)	Abdominal Pain	2.1% (0.0%, 7.2%)
Aggression	***9.5% (4.2%, 16.3%)***	***Aggression***	***1.3% (0.1%, 3.6%)***
Blood in Stool	1.7% (0.0%, 4.8%)	Attention Problems	0.9% (0.0%, 2.9%)
Confusion	1.8% (0.0%, 5.0%)	Constipation/Diarrhea	7.4% (0.0%, 21.5%)
Constipation	2.6% (0.0%, 7.4%)	Dizziness	2.1% (0.0%, 7.2%)
Decreased Appetite	2.6% (0.0%, 7.4%)	Headaches	0.9% (0.0%, 2.5%)
Depression	230% (0.0%, 6.9%)	Hyperactivity	2.5% (0.0%, 8.8%)
Diarrhea	2.3% (0.0%, 7.0%)	Impulsivity	1.0% (0.0%, 2.7%)
Dry Mouth, Excessive Thirst	5.0% (0.0%, 13.6%)	Increased Appetite	3.2% (0.0%, 12.1%)
Emotional Lability	2.0% (0.0%, 7.4%)	Irritability	1.0% (0.0%, 2.7%)

Table 5. *Cont.*

Leucovorin Alone		Leucovorin Combination	
Adverse Effect	**Incidence (95% CI)**	**Adverse Effect**	**Incidence (95% CI)**
Excitement or Agitation	***11.7% (1.1%, 28.8%)***	Nausea/Vomiting	0.9% (0.0%, 2.9%)
Gastroesophageal Reflux	***2.8% (0.2%, 7.5%)***	Rash	0.9% (0.0%, 2.5%)
Headache	***4.9% (1.3%, 10.5%)***	Reduced Sleep	1.9% (0.0%, 6.3%)
Insomnia	***8.5% (0.2%, 23.8%)***	Sedation	1.7% (0.0%, 5.6%)
Increased Motor Activity	7.4% (0.0%, 21.8%)	***Worsening Behavior***	***8.5% (3.9%, 14.6%)***
Increased Tantrums	***6.2% (1.5%, 13.3%)***		
Involuntary Movements	2.6% (0.0%, 7.4%)		
Restlessness	3.4% (0.0%, 10.6%)		
Stiffness	1.7% (0.0%, 5.0%)		
Viral Infection	10.3% (0.0%, 33.8%)		
Weight Gain	2.6% (0.0%, 7.4%)		

4. Discussion

This systemic review found CFD is associated with ASD. One cause of CFD is FRAAs which are a common finding in children with ASD. *d,l*-Leucovorin is a proven treatment for CFD that has been studied in ASD and can normalize 5-MTHF concentrations in the CSF.

The meta-analysis found a pooled prevalence of ASD in CFD of 44%. The pooled prevalence of CFD in ASD was 38% with the etiology attributed to FRAAs in 83% of the cases. The pooled prevalence of blocking, binding and either FRAA in idiopathic ASD was 46%, 49% and 71%, respectively. Children with ASD were more likely than their parents to have blocking or at least one FRAA but were not more likely than typically developing (TD) siblings to have FRAAs. For those with ASD, blocking FRAA titers were significantly higher than their parents or TD siblings, while binding FRAA titers were significantly higher than parents but not TD siblings. Children with ASD were more likely to have positive FRAAs as compared to non-related TD children or children with developmental delay without ASD. Children with ASD demonstrated significantly higher blocking and binding FRAA titers than normal controls with the effect size for blocking FRAAs being very large. FRAAs, particularly blocking FRAAs, are highly prevalent in children with ASD, and may serve as a biomarker for treatment.

This systemic review identified 20 studies which described treating individuals with ASD using *d,l*-leucovorin with a dose typically ranging from 0.5 to 2.5 mg/kg/day. For children with ASD and CFD, *d,l*-leucovorin was particularly effective (>75% response rate) for treating ataxia, pyramidal signs and epilepsy, although it also improved ASD symptoms, irritability and movement disorders in eight case-series. In three controlled studies, *d,l*-leucovorin alone was found to consistently improve communication with medium-to-large effect sizes, but also was shown to have a positive effect on core ASD symptoms and associated behaviors (attention and stereotypy) in individual studies with large effect sizes. In five controlled and uncontrolled studies, *d,l*-leucovorin in combination with vitamin and/or mineral supplements was found to significantly improve core ASD symptoms, communication, behavior and associated symptoms with medium-to-large effect sizes. This systemic review found *d,l*-leucovorin is associated with improvements in core and associated symptoms of ASD with the strongest evidence coming from the blinded, placebo-controlled studies. Most studies reported mild to no AEs, and AEs in the placebo-controlled studies were similar in treated and untreated individuals.

4.1. Dosing of d,l-Leucovorin in ASD

Most studies used 0.5 to 2.5 mg/kg/day of oral *d,l*-leucovorin but one study reported using up to 9 mg/kg/day in a child with ASD and then added 24 mg/kg/day IV (divided into 4 doses) for one day every month for 6 months with a decrease in severity and seizures along with improved eye contact [69]. Therefore, higher doses of *d,l*-leucovorin appear necessary in order to achieve a higher brain folate level and clinical improvements.

4.2. Time Period Needed for Maximal d,l-Leucovorin Treatment Effects

One case report of a child with CFD and mitochondrial disease (this child did not have ASD) reported improvements with *d,l*-leucovorin over a 3 year period [26]. Other studies in ASD reported significant improvements over periods of 1 year [34] to 2 years [35,44]. However, other much shorter studies also demonstrated significant improvement in ASD symptoms [37,72,74]. Therefore, although some individuals might show a relatively quick response to *d,l*-leucovorin, it may take 1–2 years to observe maximal clinical improvements.

4.3. The Effect of d,l-Leucovorin on the Core Symptoms of ASD

Some of the improvements with *d,l*-leucovorin in the reviewed studies were in core ASD symptoms (communication and repetitive and stereotyped behavior). To date, there are no FDA approved medications available to treat the core symptoms of ASD and the only two currently approved medications for ASD (aripiprazole and risperidone) are only approved for treating irritability associated with ASD, which is not considered a core symptom of ASD. In addition, aripiprazole and risperidone have been shown in repeated studies to potentially cause long-term metabolic and neurological adverse effects [82]. Therefore, *d,l*-leucovorin is especially promising since many of the reviewed studies found improvements in core ASD symptomology. *d,l*-Leucovorin also has a much better safety profile and less AEs compared to aripiprazole and risperidone.

4.4. Seizures and Treatment with d,l-Leucovorin

Six studies reported reductions in seizures in children with ASD and CFD using *d,l*-leucovorin [20,33,34,67,69] even in patients with difficult-to-control seizures [20,33]. One child had a breakthrough seizure with discontinuation of *d,l*-leucovorin for 2 weeks [67]. It is possible that epilepsy in these children could be caused by CFD or FRAAs [83]. This is potentially an important finding as many treatments for epilepsy in children treat the seizure condition but not the potential underlying cause or contributing factor. Of note, an animal model reported that certain antiepileptic medications might disrupt folate transportation into the CNS [84]. More studies would be helpful in determining if CFD or FRAAs are an underlying cause of seizures in children with ASD and if treatment with *d,l*-leucovorin is a useful medication for mitigating seizures in these children.

4.5. Treatment of d,l-Leucovorin in Patients with Mitochondrial Dysfunction and ASD

Mitochondrial dysfunction is a common comorbidity in ASD, with studies reporting 30–50% of individuals with ASD possessing biomarkers of mitochondrial dysfunction [6,46] and up to 80% having abnormal electron transport chain activity in immune cells [47,48]. Several studies have linked CFD to mitochondrial disease in individuals without ASD [24–27] and mitochondrial dysfunction in children with ASD [68]. In children with ASD and CFD, meta-analysis revealed a prevalence of mitochondrial dysfunction of 43% as a potential etiology of CFD. Thus, even in the absence of FRAAs, mitochondrial disease and dysfunction should also be considered as a potential cause of CFD in individuals with ASD.

Treatment of mitochondrial dysfunction with mitochondrial-related cofactors and vitamins, including carnitine [85,86], ubiquinol [87] and a "mitochondrial cocktail" containing carnitine, CoEnzyme Q10 and Alpha-Lipoic Acid [88] has been reported to improve some symptoms of ASD. Folate has also been reported to increase ETC Complex I activity in children with ASD and mitochondrial disease and positively modulate the coupling of ETC Complex I and IV and ETC Complex I and Citrate Synthase [89]. *d,l*-Leucovorin rapidly accumulates in mitochondria [90] and is the preferred form of folate in treating mitochondrial dysfunction [91]. *d,l*-Leucovorin has been reported to improve mitochondrial related symptoms and laboratory findings in some patients with mitochondrial disease in doses ranging from 1–8 mg/kg/day [24,26,27,92] including in one child with ASD [68]. Since mitochondrial dysfunction is relatively common in individuals with ASD [6,46–48,93] and *d,l*-leucovorin appears to help patients with mitochondrial dysfunction [24,26,27,92], one mechanism by which *d,l*-leucovorin might help improve ASD symptoms is by improvements in mitochondrial function.

4.6. Safety of d,l-Leucovorin in ASD

d,l-Leucovorin was first approved in the United States in the 1950s and has been used continuously since then to reduce toxicities associated with folate pathway antagonists. Therefore, it has a strong and long track record of safety. Most of the reviewed studies reported mild to no AEs with *d,l*-leucovorin. Some studies reported mild behavioral problems, diarrhea/constipation, and aggressive behaviors. In the placebo-controlled studies, AEs were similar in treated and untreated individuals. Two studies used *d,l*-leucovorin for up to 2 years [35,44] without significant AEs. Two other studies used *d,l*-leucovorin for one year without significant AEs [20,34]. Therefore, the use of *d,l*-leucovorin appears to be safe for at least 2 years of use in most individuals with ASD.

4.7. Screening for FRα Autoantibodies in ASD

The meta-analysis reported a pooled prevalence of a positive FRAA in children with ASD and concomitant CFD [21,34,35,68] of 83% (69%, 94%) with consistency across studies. Two studies [35,37] reported a significant correlation between higher blocking FRAA concentration and lower CSF levels of 5-MTHF. One study reported that children with ASD who had higher titers of FRAAs had less robust improvements [44]. Only two studies reported one child each with a mutation in the FOLR1 gene which could account for CFD [67,69]. These findings suggest that FRAAs are the major cause of CFD in children with ASD. One set of authors suggested screening young children and infants who have developmental delay and ASD features for FRAAs and starting treatment as soon as possible with *d,l*-leucovorin, especially since younger children generally show more robust improvements [34]. Some patients have intermittently positive FRAA levels and may need to be tested several times if they are negative [45]. Another approach which has been suggested by some authors is an empiric trial of *d,l*-leucovorin in children with ASD without performing a lumbar puncture to confirm CFD, especially given the excellent safety profile of *d,l*-leucovorin [94]. Additionally, one study reported improvements with *d,l*-leucovorin in children with ASD who did not have known CFD and did not possess positive FRAAs [72], further suggesting that empiric treatment in individuals with ASD with *d,l*-leucovorin is a reasonable approach.

Evidence has linked the FRAAs with 5-MTHF concentrations in the CSF in ASD and demonstrated that they can predict response to *d,l*-leucovorin treatment, suggesting that FRAAs are involved in the disruption of folate metabolism in patients with ASD. Additionally, animal models have validated their pathophysiological mechanism [95,96]. However, the meta-analysis suggested a high rate of FRAAs not only in children with ASD but also in their parents and TD siblings, but not in unrelated TD controls or children with developmental delay without ASD. This suggests that FRAA may be one of several mechanisms involved in the disruption of folate metabolism that can contribute to CNS folate disruption. Other factors may be involved. For example, if a child with ASD has FRAAs and other medical comorbidities such as mitochondrial dysfunction, this might explain why a sibling (without these medical comorbidities) can have a positive FRAA but not develop ASD. Polymorphisms in folate genes are also overrepresented in children with ASD and their mothers, suggesting that FRAAs are not alone is disrupting folate metabolism. It is possible that combinations of several mechanisms involved in disrupting folate metabolism many be needed to lead to enough disruption in neurodevelopment to lead to ASD. Timing may also be an important factor as FRAAs and CFD have been related to other psychiatric disorders when they occur outside of childhood such as in schizophrenia [53] and depression [97]. Of note, none of the reviewed studies examined a potential correlation between ASD severity and FRAA concentrations. In the future, studies that examine this would be useful.

4.8. Adjunctive Treatments Studied for FRAA Positive Patients

Cow's milk appears to regulate FRAA titers; 6 months of a milk-free diet resulted in a significant decrease in FRAA titers with re-exposure to cow's milk increasing this titer, with the titer often rising above the original titer level before initially discontinuing cow's milk [35]. Concomitant with the decrease in the FRAA titers, patients with CFD who went on a cow's milk free diet demonstrated improvements in ataxia, improved seizure control, and improved ASD symptoms. This is believed to occur because milk contains the FRα protein which may react immunologically in the gut or cause an increase in cross-reactive FRAAs in the blood. Several types of diets (such as a casein-free diet) which have been reported to show some effectiveness in ASD are milk-free diets [98,99] although this has not been found in some studies [100]. Thus, it is possible that dietary treatments not uncommonly used to treat children with ASD may have a therapeutic effect by lowering the concentration of FRAAs in the blood. Unfortunately, large studies have not examined the potential benefit of adding a milk-free diet to *d,l*-leucovorin treatment but it is probably prudent to recommend a milk-free diet when FRAAs are present. Interestingly, in the group of patients with CFD who continued to drink bovine milk, the FRAA concentrations continued to rise over a two-year period [35]. In this study, the use of goat milk caused less elevation in the FRAA concentration and thus might be a better alternative to bovine milk [35]. It is important to recognize that this effect may not generalize to other forms of dairy that do not have intact milk proteins. Indeed, dairy is an important source of calcium, which is a critical nutrient in childhood for bone health.

4.9. Treatments That Support Folate Transport into the Brain

Presumably, when the FRα is partially blocked, the RFC may be the main alternative transportation mechanism of folates into the brain. In a human cerebral microvascular endothelial cell model, 1,25-dihydroxyvitamin D_3 was shown to up-regulation RFC mRNA and protein expression through activation of the vitamin D receptor [101]. In the same cell model, nuclear respiratory factor 1 and peroxisome proliferator-activated receptor-γ coactivator-1α signaling were found to modulate RFC expression and transport activity with this pathway upregulated by treatment with pyrroloquinoline quinone (PQQ) resulting in increased RFC expression and folate transport activity [102]. Furthermore, 1,25-dihydroxyvitamin D_3 was found to rescue CFD in a knockout FOLR1 mouse model [103].

Interestingly, meta-analysis has shown that vitamin D3 800IU to 2,000IU supplementation improves core ASD symptoms as measured by the Social Responsiveness Scale or CARS in three studies in children with ASD who were not vitamin D deficient [104] and PQQ has been shown to improve social behavior in the bilateral whisker trimming for 10 days after birth in a mouse model which is characterized by its abnormal social behavior [105]. Thus, although no studies have been conducted in ASD or CFD to determine whether these supplements may improve function in children with ASD who have FRAAs or CFD, such supplements may have some utility in these children. Future studies will need to address this possibility.

4.10. Adjunctive Treatments to Support Folate Metabolism

Folate is essential for several important biochemical pathways, particularly the function of methylation metabolism and the production of purines and pyrimidines. Several studies used *d,l*-leucovorin in combination with other cofactors which could support its metabolism, including methyl-cobalamin, betaine (trimethyl-glycine) and other important cofactors. Many cofactors are essential for optimal functioning of enzymes in the folate cycle; for example, methionine synthase requires cobalamin, and methylenetetrahydrofolate reductase (MTHFR) requires nicotinamide adenine dinucleotide (NAD) which can be derived from niacin. Other factors like betaine support methylation metabolism. No study has compared the specific cofactors that could best be used in conjunction with *d,l*-leucovorin, but it is likely that other cofactors may be useful to optimize folate metabolism. One intriguing possibility is that, along with a CNS folate deficiency, individuals with ASD may also have a CNS cobalamin deficiency [106], so the addition of cobalamin could be critical in some children with ASD.

4.11. Therapeutic Effect of d,l-Leucovorin on Neurotransmitters

Most important for neurological outcomes for those with a CNS folate deficiency is the connection between folate and the production of neurotransmitters. Being the precursor to purines, folate is essential to produce guanosine-5′-triphosphate which is the precursor of tetrahydrobiopterin (BH_4) [107]. BH_4 is an important cofactor for the production of the monoamine neurotransmitters serotonin, dopamine, norepinephrine and epinephrine which are essential for behavioral regulation, mood, social function and cognition. Interestingly, like folate, a central deficiency of BH_4 is associated with ASD [108]; children with ASD respond to BH_4 supplementation [109]; and there is evidence that BH_4 may be transported into the brain through the FRα [110]. The connection between folate and BH_4 can explain how *d,l*-leucovorin can normalize CSF concentrations of serotonin and dopamine in CFD patients [28].

4.12. Implications of FRAAs during Pregnancy

Rodent models report that exposure of dams to FRAA's during gestation can lead to stereotypies and anxiety in offspring [95]. Further studies showed that *d,l*-leucovorin and/or dexamethasone treatment of dams exposed to FRAAs prevented cognitive, communication and learning problems in the offspring [96]. Human studies have reported an association between FRAAs and subfertility [111], neural tube defects [112], and preterm births [113]. One study found that FRAAs bind to prenatal thyroid tissue, potentially affecting its development and potentially altering hypothalamic-pituitary-axis regulation of thyroid hormones in the offspring [37]. In one case report, a pregnant women with a history of multiple complications in previous pregnancies and who was positive for FRAAs was able to conceive and have a normal pregnancy and delivery with the use of *d,l*-leucovorin, a milk free diet, and a low dose of prednisone given during pregnancy [114].

4.13. Limitation of Published Studies

Many of the reviewed studies had important limitations. First, there is only one medium-sized [72] and one small-sized [74] blinded, placebo controlled, single center studies that examined treatment only with *d,l*-leucovorin. Thus, clearly larger, multisite trials, which are ongoing [9], are necessary to confirm previous findings. Since many of the studies used *d,l*-leucovorin in combination with other treatments [73,76–79], other treatments may have added to the effects of *d,l*-leucovorin. In addition, studies examining CFD are rather small and do not always use standardized outcome measures [20,21,33–36,67,68].

Interestingly, in the blinded controlled studies, standardized measures of language and social functioning which were obtained by objective and blinded examiners tended to have large effect sizes, whereas parent rated measures tended to have very modest effect sizes. This reflects one of the difficulties in research in ASD where the placebo effect can be large, especially as rated by parents [115]. Such large placebo effects have washed out the effect of the treatment in many studies, resulting in many failed clinical trials. Thus, one of the strengths in the currently conducted blinded trials is the use of standard objective measures of function in blinded observers in addition to parent reported measures. This is especially important when studying more mildly affected children with ASD as the placebo effect appears to be inversely proportional to the severity of the ASD symptoms, so studies with less severe children would be expected to have a larger placebo effect [116]. This effect can explain the larger effect size in parent reported outcomes in the studies which used a non-treatment comparison group [37,76] when compared to the trials which were placebo controlled [72–74].

5. Conclusions

This systematic review and meta-analysis found *d,l*-leucovorin is associated with improvements in core and associated symptoms of ASD with the strongest evidence coming from the blinded, placebo-controlled studies. FRAAs, particularly blocking FRAAs, are highly prevalent in children with ASD, and may serve as a biomarker for treatment. The high prevalence of FRAAs in families with children with ASD suggests unknown heritability mechanisms that involve additional genetic or environmental factors which contribute to the expression of ASD in those with FRAAs. *d,l*-Leucovorin is an evidence-based treatment for ASD which has significant promise and appears safe and well-tolerated. Further studies would be helpful to confirm and expand on these findings.

Supplementary Materials: The following are available online at https://www.mdpi.com/article/10.3390/jpm11111141/s1, Table S1: PRISMA Checklist, Table S2: Studies on Children with CFD where ASD was found to be a characteristic, Table S3: Studies on Children with ASD where CSF was measured for possible CFD, Table S4: Studies of FRα autoantibodies in ASD, by year published, Table S5: Response to *d,l*-leucovorin in children with CFD with and without ASD (Total cases with symptoms/total Responses), Table S6: Studies examining only *d,l*-leucovorin in ASD, by year published, Table S7: Studies examining *d,l*-leucovorin along with other supplements or treatments in ASD, by year published.

Author Contributions: Conceptualization, methodology, formal analysis, writing—original draft preparation, review and editing, were performed by both D.A.R. and R.E.F. All authors have read and agreed to the published version of the manuscript.

Funding: The review did not receive any financial or grant support from any sources.

Institutional Review Board Statement: Not applicable. This review is not human research.

Informed Consent Statement: Not applicable. This review is not human research.

Data Availability Statement: All data are presented within the article.

Conflicts of Interest: Frye is funded by the National Institutes of Child Health and Human Development Grant R01HD088528, Department of Defense Grant AR180134 and Autism Speaks Grant 11407 to study the therapeutic effects of leucovorin in autism spectrum disorder. Frye is an uncompensated scientific advisory board member to Iliad Neurosciences Inc. (Plymouth Meeting, PA, USA) which is the commercial laboratory which performs the folate receptor alpha autoantibody tests.

References

1. Maenner, M.J.; Shaw, K.A.; Baio, J.; Washington, A.; Patrick, M.; DiRienzo, M.; Christensen, D.L.; Wiggins, L.D.; Pettygrove, S.; Andrews, J.G.; et al. Prevalence of Autism Spectrum Disorder Among Children Aged 8 Years—Autism and Developmental Disabilities Monitoring Network, 11 Sites, United States, 2016. *MMWR Surveill. Summ.* **2020**, *69*, 1–12. [CrossRef]
2. Soke, G.N.; Maenner, M.J.; Christensen, D.; Kurzius-Spencer, M.; Schieve, L.A. Prevalence of Co-occurring Medical and Behavioral Conditions/Symptoms Among 4- and 8-Year-Old Children with Autism Spectrum Disorder in Selected Areas of the United States in 2010. *J. Autism Dev. Disord.* **2018**, *48*, 2663–2676. [CrossRef] [PubMed]
3. Brondino, N.; Fusar-Poli, L.; Miceli, E.; di Stefano, M.; Damiani, S.; Rocchetti, M.; Politi, P. Prevalence of Medical Comorbidities in Adults with Autism Spectrum Disorder. *J. Gen. Intern. Med.* **2019**, *34*, 1992–1994. [CrossRef]
4. Dizitzer, Y.; Meiri, G.; Flusser, H.; Michaelovski, A.; Dinstein, I.; Menashe, I. Comorbidity and health services' usage in children with autism spectrum disorder: A nested case-control study. *Epidemiology Psychiatr. Sci.* **2020**, *29*, e95. [CrossRef]
5. Vargason, T.; Frye, R.E.; McGuinness, D.L.; Hahn, J. Clustering of co-occurring conditions in autism spectrum disorder during early childhood: A retrospective analysis of medical claims data. *Autism Res.* **2019**, *12*, 1272–1285. [CrossRef] [PubMed]
6. Rossignol, D.; Frye, R. Mitochondrial dysfunction in autism spectrum disorders: A systematic review and meta-analysis. *Mol. Psychiatry* **2011**, *17*, 290–314. [CrossRef]
7. Holingue, C.; Newill, C.; Lee, L.-C.; Pasricha, P.J.; Fallin, M.D. Gastrointestinal symptoms in autism spectrum disorder: A review of the literature on ascertainment and prevalence. *Autism Res.* **2018**, *11*, 24–36. [CrossRef]
8. Anukirthiga, B.; Mishra, D.; Pandey, S.; Juneja, M.; Sharma, N. Prevalence of Epilepsy and Inter-Ictal Epileptiform Discharges in Children with Autism and Attention-Deficit Hyperactivity Disorder. *Indian J. Pediatr.* **2019**, *86*, 897–902. [CrossRef]
9. Frye, R.E.; Rossignol, D.A.; Scahill, L.; McDougle, C.J.; Huberman, H.; Quadros, E.V. Treatment of Folate Metabolism Abnormalities in Autism Spectrum Disorder. *Semin. Pediatr. Neurol.* **2020**, *35*, 100835. [CrossRef]

10. Overholser, M.D.; Whitley, J.R.; O'Dell, B.L.; Hogan, A.G. The ventricular system in hydrocephalic rat brains produced by a deficiency of vitamin B12 or of folic acid in the maternal diet. *Anat. Rec. Adv. Integr. Anat. Evol. Biol.* **1954**, *120*, 917–933. [CrossRef] [PubMed]
11. Chida, N.; Hirono, H.; Arakawa, T. Effects of Dietary Folate Deficiency on Fatty Acid Composition of Myelin Cerebroside in Growth Rats. *Tohoku J. Exp. Med.* **1972**, *108*, 219–224. [CrossRef]
12. Haltia, M. The effect of folate deficiency on neuronal RNA content. A quantitative cytochemical study. *Br. J. Exp. Pathol.* **1970**, *51*, 191–196. [PubMed]
13. Dow, W. Electroencephalogram in anticonvulsant-induced folate deficiency. *BMJ* **1971**, *2*, 207. [CrossRef] [PubMed]
14. Reynolds, E.H.; Rothfeld, P.; Pincus, J.H. Neurological Disease associated with Folate Deficiency. *BMJ* **1973**, *2*, 398–400. [CrossRef]
15. Cerebrospinal Folate Levels in Epileptics and Their Response to Folate Therapy. *Nutr. Rev.* **1974**, *32*, 70–72. [CrossRef]
16. Garwicz, S.; Mortensson, W. Intracranial calcification mimicking the Sturge-Weber syndrome A consequence of cerebral folic acid deficiency? *Pediatr. Radiol.* **1976**, *5*, 5–9. [CrossRef]
17. Botez, M.; Peyronnard, J.-M.; Bérubé, L.; Labrecque, R. Relapsing Neuropathy, Cerebral Atrophy and Folate Deficiency. A Close Association. *Ster. Funct. Neurosurg.* **1979**, *42*, 171–183. [CrossRef]
18. Allen, R.J.; DiMauro, S.; Coulter, D.L.; Papadimitriou, A.; Rothenberg, S.P. Kearns-sayre syndrome with reduced plasma and cerebrospinal fluid folate. *Ann. Neurol.* **1983**, *13*, 679–682. [CrossRef]
19. Ramaekers, V.T.; Häusler, M.; Opladen, T.; Heimann, G.; Blau, N. Psychomotor Retardation, Spastic Paraplegia, Cerebellar Ataxia and Dyskinesia Associated with Low 5-Methyltetrahydrofolate in Cerebrospinal Fluid: A Novel Neurometabolic Condition Responding to Folinic Acid Substitution. *Neuropediatrics* **2002**, *33*, 301–308. [CrossRef]
20. Ramaekers, V.T.; Blau, N. Cerebral folate deficiency. *Dev. Med. Child Neurol.* **2004**, *46*, 843–851. [CrossRef]
21. Ramaekers, V.T.; Rothenberg, S.P.; Sequeira, J.M.; Opladen, T.; Blau, N.; Quadros, E.V.; Selhub, J. Autoantibodies to Folate Receptors in the Cerebral Folate Deficiency Syndrome. *N. Engl. J. Med.* **2005**, *352*, 1985–1991. [CrossRef] [PubMed]
22. Grapp, M.; Just, I.A.; Linnankivi, T.; Wolf, P.; Lücke, T.; Häusler, M.; Gärtner, J.; Steinfeld, R. Molecular characterization of folate receptor 1 mutations delineates cerebral folate transport deficiency. *Brain* **2012**, *135*, 2022–2031. [CrossRef]
23. Zhang, C.; Deng, X.; Wen, Y.; He, F.; Yin, F.; Peng, J. First case report of cerebral folate deficiency caused by a novel mutation of FOLR1 gene in a Chinese patient. *BMC Med. Genet.* **2020**, *21*, 1–5. [CrossRef] [PubMed]
24. Pineda, M.; Ormazabal, A.; López-Gallardo, E.; Nascimento, A.; Solano, A.; Herrero, M.D.; Vilaseca, M.A.; Briones, P.; Ibáñez, L.; Montoya, J.; et al. Cerebral folate deficiency and leukoencephalopathy caused by a mitochondrial DNA deletion. *Ann. Neurol.* **2006**, *59*, 394–398. [CrossRef]
25. Garcia-Cazorla, A.; Quadros, E.V.; Nascimento, A.; Garcia-Silva, M.T.; Briones, P.; Montoya, J.; Ormazabal, A.; Artuch, R.; Sequeira, J.M.; Blau, N.; et al. Mitochondrial Diseases Associated with Cerebral Folate Deficiency. *Neurology* **2008**, *70*, 1360–1362. [CrossRef] [PubMed]
26. Ramaekers, V.T.; Weis, J.; Sequeira, J.M.; Quadros, E.V.; Blau, N. Mitochondrial Complex I Encephalomyopathy and Cerebral 5-Methyltetrahydrofolate Deficiency. *Neuropediatrics* **2007**, *38*, 184–187. [CrossRef] [PubMed]
27. Hasselmann, O.; Blau, N.; Ramaekers, V.T.; Quadros, E.V.; Sequeira, J.; Weissert, M. Cerebral folate deficiency and CNS inflammatory markers in Alpers disease. *Mol. Genet. Metab.* **2010**, *99*, 58–61. [CrossRef]
28. Hansen, F.J.; Blau, N. Cerebral folate deficiency: Life-changing supplementation with folinic acid. *Mol. Genet. Metab.* **2005**, *84*, 371–373. [CrossRef] [PubMed]
29. Karin, I.; Borggraefe, I.; Catarino, C.B.; Kuhm, C.; Hoertnagel, K.; Biskup, S.; Opladen, T.; Blau, N.; Heinen, F.; Klopstock, T. Folinic acid therapy in cerebral folate deficiency: Marked improvement in an adult patient. *J. Neurol.* **2017**, *264*, 578–582. [CrossRef]
30. Antony, A.C. The biological chemistry of folate receptors. *Blood* **1992**, *79*, 2807–2820. [CrossRef]
31. Adams, M.; Lucock, M.; Stuart, J.; Fardell, S.; Baker, K.; Ng, X. Preliminary evidence for involvement of the folate gene polymorphism 19bp deletion-DHFR in occurrence of autism. *Neurosci. Lett.* **2007**, *422*, 24–29. [CrossRef]
32. Knowles, L.; Morris, A.A.; Walter, J.H. Treatment with Mefolinate (5-Methyltetrahydrofolate), but Not Folic Acid or Folinic Acid, Leads to Measurable 5-Methyltetrahydrofolate in Cerebrospinal Fluid in Methylenetetrahydrofolate Reductase Deficiency. *JIMD Rep.* **2016**, *29*, 103–107. [PubMed]
33. Moretti, P.; Peters, S.U.; Del Gaudio, D.; Sahoo, T.; Hyland, K.; Bottiglieri, T.; Hopkin, R.; Peach, E.; Min, S.H.; Goldman, D.; et al. Brief Report: Autistic Symptoms, Developmental Regression, Mental Retardation, Epilepsy, and Dyskinesias in CNS Folate Deficiency. *J. Autism Dev. Disord.* **2008**, *38*, 1170–1177. [CrossRef]
34. Ramaekers, V.T.; Blau, N.; Sequeira, J.M.; Nassogne, M.-C.; Quadros, E.V. Folate Receptor Autoimmunity and Cerebral Folate Deficiency in Low-Functioning Autism with Neurological Deficits. *Neuropediatrics* **2007**, *38*, 276–281. [CrossRef]
35. Ramaekers, V.T.; Sequeira, J.M.; Blau, N.; Quadros, E.V. A Milk-Free Diet Downregulates Folate Receptor Autoimmunity in Cerebral Folate Deficiency Syndrome. *Dev. Med. Child. Neurol.* **2008**, *50*, 346–352. [CrossRef] [PubMed]
36. Moretti, P.; Sahoo, T.; Hyland, K.; Bottiglieri, T.; Peters, S.; Del Gaudio, D.; Roa, B.; Curry, S.; Zhu, H.; Finnell, R.; et al. Cerebral folate deficiency with developmental delay, autism, and response to folinic acid. *Neurology* **2005**, *64*, 1088–1090. [CrossRef]
37. Frye, R.; Sequeira, J.M.; Quadros, E.V.; James, S.J.; Rossignol, D. Cerebral folate receptor autoantibodies in autism spectrum disorder. *Mol. Psychiatry* **2012**, *18*, 369–381. [CrossRef]
38. Ramaekers, V.T.; Quadros, E.V.; Sequeira, J.M. Role of folate receptor autoantibodies in infantile autism. *Mol. Psychiatry* **2012**, *18*, 270–271. [CrossRef]

39. Frye, R.; Sequeira, J.; Quadros, E.; Rossignol, D. Folate Receptor Alpha Autoantibodies Modulate Thyroid Function in Autism Spectrum Disorder. *North Am. J. Med. Sci.* **2014**, *7*, 53–56. [CrossRef]
40. Frye, R.E.; Delhey, L.; Slattery, J.; Tippett, M.; Wynne, R.; Rose, S.; Kahler, S.G.; Bennuri, S.C.; Melnyk, S.; Sequeira, J.M.; et al. Blocking and Binding Folate Receptor Alpha Autoantibodies Identify Novel Autism Spectrum Disorder Subgroups. *Front. Neurosci.* **2016**, *10*, 80. [CrossRef] [PubMed]
41. Frye, R.E.; Wynne, R.; Rose, S.; Slattery, J.; Delhey, L.; Tippett, M.; Kahler, S.G.; Bennuri, S.C.; Melnyk, S.; Sequeira, J.M.; et al. Thyroid Dysfunction in Children with Autism Spectrum Disorder Is Associated with Folate Receptor Alpha Autoimmune Disorder. *J. Neuroendocrinol.* **2017**, *29*, 3. [CrossRef]
42. Quadros, E.V.; Sequeira, J.M.; Brown, W.T.; Mevs, C.; Marchi, E.; Flory, M.; Jenkins, E.C.; Velinov, M.T.; Cohen, I.L. Folate receptor autoantibodies are prevalent in children diagnosed with autism spectrum disorder, their normal siblings and parents. *Autism Res.* **2018**, *11*, 707–712. [CrossRef]
43. Zhou, J.; Liu, A.; He, F.; Jin, Y.; Zhou, S.; Xu, R.; Guo, H.; Zhou, W.; Wei, Q.; Wang, M. High prevalence of serum folate receptor autoantibodies in children with autism spectrum disorders. *Biomarkers* **2018**, *23*, 622–624. [CrossRef] [PubMed]
44. Ramaekers, V.T.; Sequeira, J.M.; Di Duca, M.; Vrancken, G.; Thomas, A.; Philippe, C.; Peters, M.; Jadot, A.; Quadros, E.V. Improving Outcome in Infantile Autism with Folate Receptor Autoimmunity and Nutritional Derangements: A Self-Controlled Trial. *Autism Res. Treat.* **2019**, *2019*, 1–12. [CrossRef]
45. Ramaekers, V.T.; Sequeira, J.M.; Thöny, B.; Quadros, E.V. Oxidative Stress, Folate Receptor Autoimmunity, and CSF Findings in Severe Infantile Autism. *Autism Res. Treat.* **2020**, *2020*, 1–14. [CrossRef]
46. Frye, R.E. Biomarkers of Abnormal Energy Metabolism in Children with Autism Spectrum Disorder. *Am. Chin. J. Med. Sci.* **2012**, *5*, 141. [CrossRef]
47. Giulivi, C.; Zhang, Y.-F.; Omanska-Klusek, A.; Ross-Inta, C.; Wong, S.; Hertz-Picciotto, I.; Tassone, F.; Pessah, I.N. Mitochondrial Dysfunction in Autism. *JAMA* **2010**, *304*, 2389–2396. [CrossRef] [PubMed]
48. Napoli, E.; Wong, S.; Hertz-Picciotto, I.; Giulivi, C. Deficits in Bioenergetics and Impaired Immune Response in Granulocytes from Children with Autism. *Pediatrics* **2014**, *133*, e1405–e1410. [CrossRef]
49. Blehaut, H.; Mircher, C.; Ravel, A.; Conte, M.; de Portzamparc, V.; Poret, G.; de Kermadec, F.H.; Rethore, M.O.; Sturtz, F.G. Effect of Leucovorin (Folinic Acid) on the Developmental Quotient of Children with Down's Syndrome (Trisomy 21) and Influence of Thyroid Status. *PLoS ONE* **2010**, *5*, e8394. [CrossRef]
50. Hagebeuk, E.E.O.; Koelman, J.H.T.M.; Duran, M.; Abeling, N.G.; Vyth, A.; Poll-The, B.-T. Clinical and Electroencephalographic Effects of Folinic Acid Treatment in Rett Syndrome Patients. *J. Child Neurol.* **2011**, *26*, 718–723. [CrossRef] [PubMed]
51. Ramaekers, V.; Hansen, S.; Holm, J.; Opladen, T.; Senderek, J.; Hausler, M.; Heimann, G.; Fowler, B.; Maiwald, R.; Blau, N. Reduced folate transport to the CNS in female Rett patients. *Neurology* **2003**, *61*, 506–515. [CrossRef] [PubMed]
52. Ormazábal, A.; Artuch, R.; Vilaseca, M.A.; Aracil, A.; Pineda, M. Cerebrospinal Fluid Concentrations of Folate, Biogenic Amines and Pterins in Rett Syndrome: Treatment with Folinic Acid. *Neuropediatrics* **2005**, *36*, 380–385. [CrossRef]
53. Ramaekers, V.; Thöny, B.; Sequeira, J.; Ansseau, M.; Philippe, P.; Boemer, F.; Bours, V.; Quadros, E. Folinic acid treatment for schizophrenia associated with folate receptor autoantibodies. *Mol. Genet. Metab.* **2014**, *113*, 307–314. [CrossRef]
54. Higgins, J.P.; Altman, D.G. Assessing Risk of Bias in Included Studies. In *Cochrane Handbook for Systematic Reviews of Interventions*; Higgins, J.P.T., Green, S., Eds.; The Cochrane Collaboration: London, UK, 2011.
55. Kakkassery, V.; Koschmieder, A.; Walther, F.; Lehbrink, R.; Bertsche, A.; Wortmann, S.B.; Buchmann, J.; Jager, M.; Friedburg, C.; Lorenz, B.; et al. Chorioretinal Atrophy in Pediatric Cerebral Folate Deficiency—A Preventable Disease? *Ophthalmologe* **2021**, *118*, 383–390. [CrossRef]
56. Gillberg, C.; Wahlström, J.; Johansson, R.; Törnblom, M.; Albertsson-Wikland, K. Folic acid as an adjunct in the treatment of children with the autism fragile-x syndrome (afrax). *Dev. Med. Child Neurol.* **1986**, *28*, 624–627. [CrossRef]
57. Sun, C.; Zou, M.; Zhao, D.; Xia, W.; Wu, L. Efficacy of Folic Acid Supplementation in Autistic Children Participating in Structured Teaching: An Open-Label Trial. *Nutrients* **2016**, *8*, 337. [CrossRef] [PubMed]
58. Lipsey, M.W.; Wilson, D.B. The Way in Which Intervention Studies Have "Personality" and why it is Important to Meta-Analysis. *Eval. Health Prof.* **2001**, *24*, 236–254. [CrossRef] [PubMed]
59. Senn, S. Trying to be precise about vagueness. *Stat. Med.* **2007**, *26*, 1417–1430. [CrossRef]
60. Barendregt, J.J.; Doi, S.A.; Lee, Y.Y.; Norman, R.E.; Vos, T. Meta-Analysis of Prevalence. *J. Epidemiol. Community Health* **2013**, *67*, 974–978. [CrossRef]
61. Furuya-Kanamori, L.; Barendregt, J.J.; Doi, S.A. A new improved graphical and quantitative method for detecting bias in meta-analysis. *Int. J. Evid.-Based Health* **2018**, *16*, 195–203. [CrossRef]
62. Higgins, J.P.T.; Thompson, S.G. Quantifying heterogeneity in a meta-analysis. *Stat. Med.* **2002**, *21*, 1539–1558. [CrossRef] [PubMed]
63. Higgins, J.P.T.; Thompson, S.G.; Deeks, J.; Altman, D.G. Measuring inconsistency in meta-analyses. *BMJ* **2003**, *327*, 557–560. [CrossRef]
64. Altman, D.G.; Machin, D.; Bryant, T.N.; Gardner, M.J. *Statistics with Confidence*, 2nd ed.; BMJ Books: Hoboken, NJ, USA, 2000.
65. Doi, S.A.; Barendregt, J.J.; Khan, S.; Thalib, L.; Williams, G. Advances in the meta-analysis of heterogeneous clinical trials I: The inverse variance heterogeneity model. *Contemp. Clin. Trials* **2015**, *45*, 130–138. [CrossRef]
66. Cohen, J. *Statistical Power Analysis for the Behavioral Sciences*, 2nd ed.; Lawrence Erlbaum Associates: New York, NY, USA, 2013.

67. Al-Baradie, R.S.; Chaudhary, M.W. Diagnosis and Management of Cerebral Folate Deficiency. A Form of Folinic Acid-Responsive Seizures. *Neurosciences* **2014**, *19*, 312–316.
68. Frye, R.E.; Naviaux, R.K. Autistic disorder with complex IV overactivity: A new mitochondrial syndrome. *J. Pediatr. Neurol.* **2011**, *9*, 427–434.
69. Kanmaz, S.; Simsek, E.; Yilmaz, S.; Durmaz, A.; Serin, H.M.; Gokben, S. Cerebral folate transporter deficiency: A potentially treatable neurometabolic disorder. *Acta Neurol.* **2021**, 1–7. [CrossRef]
70. Shoffner, J.B.; Trommer, A.; Thurm, C.; Farmer, W.A.; Langley, L., III; Soskey, A.N.; Rodriguez, P.; D'Souza, S.J.; Spence, K.; Hyland, S.; et al. Csf Concentrations of 5-Methyltetrahydrofolate in a Cohort of Young Children with Autism. *Neurology* **2016**, *86*, 2258–2263. [CrossRef] [PubMed]
71. Shoffner, J.; Hyams, L.; Langley, G.N.; Cossette, S.; Mylacraine, L.; Dale, J.; Ollis, L.; Kuoch, S.; Bennett, K.; Aliberti, A.; et al. Fever Plus Mitochondrial Disease Could Be Risk Factors for Autistic Regression. *J. Child Neurol.* **2009**, *25*, 429–434. [CrossRef]
72. Frye, R.; Slattery, J.; Delhey, L.; Furgerson, B.; Strickland, T.; Tippett, M.; Sailey, A.; Wynne, R.; Rose, S.; Melnyk, S.; et al. Folinic acid improves verbal communication in children with autism and language impairment: A randomized double-blind placebo-controlled trial. *Mol. Psychiatry* **2018**, *23*, 247–256. [CrossRef]
73. Adams, J.B.; Audhya, T.; McDonough-Means, S.; Rubin, R.; Quig, D.; Geis, E.; Gehn, E.; Loresto, M.; Mitchell, J.; Atwood, S.; et al. Effect of a vitamin/mineral supplement on children and adults with autism. *BMC Pediatr.* **2011**, *11*, 111. [CrossRef]
74. Renard, E.; Leheup, B.; Guéant-Rodriguez, R.-M.; Oussalah, A.; Quadros, E.V.; Guéant, J.-L. Folinic acid improves the score of Autism in the EFFET placebo-controlled randomized trial. *Biochimie* **2020**, *173*, 57–61. [CrossRef]
75. Batebi, N.; Moghaddam, H.S.; Hasanzadeh, A.; Fakour, Y.; Mohammadi, M.R.; Akhondzadeh, S. Folinic Acid as Adjunctive Therapy in Treatment of Inappropriate Speech in Children with Autism: A Double-Blind and Placebo-Controlled Randomized Trial. *Child Psychiatry Hum. Dev.* **2021**, *52*, 928–938. [CrossRef]
76. Adams, J.B.; Audhya, T.; Geis, E.; Gehn, E.; Fimbres, V.; Pollard, E.L.; Mitchell, J.; Ingram, J.; Hellmers, R.; Laake, D.; et al. Comprehensive Nutritional and Dietary Intervention for Autism Spectrum Disorder—A Randomized, Controlled 12-Month Trial. *Nutrients* **2018**, *10*, 369. [CrossRef] [PubMed]
77. James, S.J.; Cutler, P.; Melnyk, S.; Jernigan, S.; Janak, L.; Gaylor, D.W.; Neubrander, J. Metabolic biomarkers of increased oxidative stress and impaired methylation capacity in children with autism. *Am. J. Clin. Nutr.* **2004**, *80*, 1611–1617. [CrossRef] [PubMed]
78. James, S.J.; Melnyk, S.; Fuchs, G.; Reid, T.; Jernigan, S.; Pavliv, O.; Hubanks, A.; Gaylor, D.W. Efficacy of methylcobalamin and folinic acid treatment on glutathione redox status in children with autism. *Am. J. Clin. Nutr.* **2008**, *89*, 425–430. [CrossRef] [PubMed]
79. Frye, R.E.; Melnyk, S.; Fuchs, G.; Reid, T.; Jernigan, S.; Pavliv, O.; Hubanks, A.; Gaylor, D.W.; Walters, L.; James, S.J. Effectiveness of Methylcobalamin and Folinic Acid Treatment on Adaptive Behavior in Children with Autistic Disorder Is Related to Glutathione Redox Status. *Autism Res. Treat.* **2013**, *2013*, 1–9. [CrossRef]
80. Bent, S.; Chen, Y.; McDonald, M.G.; Widjaja, F.; Wahlberg, J.; Hendren, R.L. An Examination of Changes in Urinary Metabolites and Behaviors with the Use of Leucovorin Calcium in Children with Autism Spectrum Disorder (ASD). *Adv. Neurodev. Disord.* **2020**, *4*, 241–246. [CrossRef]
81. Adams, J.B.; Bhargava, A.; Coleman, D.M.; Frye, R.E.; Rossignol, D.A. Ratings of the Effectiveness of Nutraceuticals for Autism Spectrum Disorders: Results of a National Survey. *J. Pers. Med.* **2021**, *11*, 878. [CrossRef]
82. Alfageh, B.H.; Wang, Z.; Mongkhon, P.; Besag, F.M.C.; Alhawassi, T.M.; Brauer, R.; Wong, I.C.K. Safety and Tolerability of Antipsychotic Medication in Individuals with Autism Spectrum Disorder: A Systematic Review and Meta-Analysis. *Pediatr. Drugs* **2019**, *21*, 153–167. [CrossRef]
83. Frye, R.E.; Casanova, M.F.; Fatemi, S.H.; Folsom, T.D.; Reutiman, T.J.; Brown, G.L.; Edelson, S.M.; Slattery, J.C.; Adams, J.B. Neuropathological Mechanisms of Seizures in Autism Spectrum Disorder. *Front. Neurosci.* **2016**, *10*, 192. [CrossRef] [PubMed]
84. Opladen, T.; Blau, N.; Ramaekers, V.T. Effect of antiepileptic drugs and reactive oxygen species on folate receptor 1 (FOLR1)-dependent 5-methyltetrahydrofolate transport. *Mol. Genet. Metab.* **2010**, *101*, 48–54. [CrossRef]
85. Fahmy, S.F.; El-Hamamsy, M.H.; Zaki, O.K.; Badary, O.A. l-Carnitine supplementation improves the behavioral symptoms in autistic children. *Res. Autism Spectr. Disord.* **2013**, *7*, 159–166. [CrossRef]
86. Geier, D.A.; Kern, J.K.; Davis, G.; King, P.G.; Adams, J.B.; Young, J.L.; Geier, M.R. A prospective double-blind, randomized clinical trial of levocarnitine to treat autism spectrum disorders. *Med. Sci. Monit.* **2011**, *17*, PI15–PI23. [CrossRef] [PubMed]
87. Gvozdjáková, A.; Kucharská, J.; Ostatníková, D.; Babinská, K.; Nakladal, D.; Crane, F.L. Ubiquinol Improves Symptoms in Children with Autism. *Oxidative Med. Cell. Longev.* **2014**, *2014*, 1–6. [CrossRef]
88. Legido, A.; Goldenthal, M.; Garvin, B.; Damle, S.; Corrigan, K.; Connell, J.; Thao, D.; Valencia, I.; Melvin, J.; Khurana, D.; et al. Effect of a Combination of Carnitine, Coenzyme Q10 and Alpha-Lipoic Acid (Mitococktail) on Mitochondrial Function and Neurobehavioral Performance in Children with Autism Spectrum Disorder (P3.313). *Neurology* **2018**, *90*, 15.
89. Delhey, L.M.; Kilinc, E.N.; Yin, L.; Slattery, J.C.; Tippett, M.L.; Rose, S.; Bennuri, S.C.; Kahler, S.G.; Damle, S.; Legido, A.; et al. The Effect of Mitochondrial Supplements on Mitochondrial Activity in Children with Autism Spectrum Disorder. *J. Clin. Med.* **2017**, *6*, 18. [CrossRef] [PubMed]
90. Horne, D.W.; Holloway, R.S.; Said, H.M. Uptake of 5-Formyltetrahydrofolate in Isolated Rat Liver Mitochondria Is Carrier-Mediated. *J. Nutr.* **1992**, *122*, 2204–2209. [CrossRef] [PubMed]

91. Ormazabal, A.; Casado, M.; Molero-Luis, M.; Montoya, J.; Rahman, S.; Aylett, S.-B.; Hargreaves, I.; Heales, S.; Artuch, R. Can folic acid have a role in mitochondrial disorders? *Drug Discov. Today* **2015**, *20*, 1349–1354. [CrossRef]
92. Quijada-Fraile, P.; O'Callaghan, M.; Martin-Hernandez, E.; Montero, R.; García-Cazorla, A.; de Aragón, A.M.; Muchart, J.; Malaga, I.; Pardo, R.; García-Gonzalez, P.; et al. Follow-up of folinic acid supplementation for patients with cerebral folate deficiency and Kearns-Sayre syndrome. *Orphanet J. Rare Dis.* **2014**, *9*, 217. [CrossRef]
93. Palmieri, L.; Papaleo, V.; Porcelli, V.; Scarcia, P.; Gaita, L.; Sacco, R.; Hager, J.; Rousseau, F.; Curatolo, P.; Manzi, B.; et al. Altered calcium homeostasis in autism-spectrum disorders: Evidence from biochemical and genetic studies of the mitochondrial aspartate/glutamate carrier AGC1. *Mol. Psychiatry* **2010**, *15*, 38–52. [CrossRef]
94. Geller, B. Does Folinic Acid Improve Language in Children with Autism? *NEJM J. Watch Psychiatry* **2016**. [CrossRef]
95. Sequeira, J.M.; Desai, A.; Berrocal-Zaragoza, M.I.; Murphy, M.M.; Fernández-Ballart, J.D.; Quadros, E.V. Exposure to Folate Receptor Alpha Antibodies during Gestation and Weaning Leads to Severe Behavioral Deficits in Rats: A Pilot Study. *PLoS ONE* **2016**, *11*, e0152249. [CrossRef] [PubMed]
96. Desai, A.; Sequeira, J.M.; Quadros, E.V. Prevention of behavioral deficits in rats exposed to folate receptor antibodies: Implication in autism. *Mol. Psychiatry* **2016**, *22*, 1291–1297. [CrossRef] [PubMed]
97. Pan, L.A.; Martin, P.; Zimmer, T.; Segreti, A.M.; Kassiff, S.; McKain, B.W.; Baca, C.A.; Rengasamy, M.; Hyland, K.; Walano, N.; et al. Neurometabolic Disorders: Potentially Treatable Abnormalities in Patients with Treatment-Refractory Depression and Suicidal Behavior. *Am. J. Psychiatry* **2017**, *174*, 42–50. [CrossRef] [PubMed]
98. Whiteley, P.; Haracopos, D.; Knivsberg, A.-M.; Reichelt, K.L.; Parlar, S.; Jacobsen, J.; Seim, A.; Pedersen, L.; Schondel, M.; Shattock, P. The ScanBrit randomised, controlled, single-blind study of a gluten- and casein-free dietary intervention for children with autism spectrum disorders. *Nutr. Neurosci.* **2010**, *13*, 87–100. [CrossRef]
99. Pennesi, C.M.; Klein, L.C. Effectiveness of the gluten-free, casein-free diet for children diagnosed with autism spectrum disorder: Based on parental report. *Nutr. Neurosci.* **2012**, *15*, 85–91. [CrossRef] [PubMed]
100. Keller, A.; Rimestad, M.L.; Rohde, J.F.; Petersen, B.H.; Korfitsen, C.B.; Tarp, S.; Lauritsen, M.B.; Händel, M.N. The Effect of a Combined Gluten- and Casein-Free Diet on Children and Adolescents with Autism Spectrum Disorders: A Systematic Review and Meta-Analysis. *Nutrients* **2021**, *13*, 470. [CrossRef]
101. Alam, C.; Hoque, T.; Finnell, R.; Goldman, I.D.; Bendayan, R. Regulation of Reduced Folate Carrier (RFC) by Vitamin D Receptor at the Blood-Brain Barrier. *Mol. Pharm.* **2017**, *14*, 3848–3858. [CrossRef]
102. Alam, C.; Hoque, T.; Sangha, V.; Bendayan, R. Nuclear respiratory factor 1 (NRF-1) upregulates the expression and function of reduced folate carrier (RFC) at the blood-brain barrier. *FASEB J.* **2020**, *34*, 10516–10530. [CrossRef] [PubMed]
103. Alam, C.; Aufreiter, S.; Georgiou, C.J.; Hoque, T.; Finnell, R.H.; O'Connor, D.; Goldman, I.D.; Bendayan, R. Upregulation of reduced folate carrier by vitamin D enhances brain folate uptake in mice lacking folate receptor alpha. *Proc. Natl. Acad. Sci. USA* **2019**, *116*, 17531–17540. [CrossRef]
104. Song, L.; Luo, X.; Jiang, Q.; Chen, Z.; Zhou, L.; Wang, D.; Chen, A. Vitamin D Supplementation is Beneficial for Children with Autism Spectrum Disorder: A Meta-analysis. *Clin. Psychopharmacol. Neurosci.* **2020**, *18*, 203–213. [CrossRef] [PubMed]
105. Soumiya, H.; Araiso, H.; Furukawa, S.; Fukumitsu, H. Pyrroloquinoline quinone improves abnormal functional development of whisker-mediated tactile perception and social behaviors caused by neonatal whisker trimming. *Neurosci. Lett.* **2019**, *705*, 67–73. [CrossRef] [PubMed]
106. Zhang, Y.; Hodgson, N.W.; Trivedi, M.S.; Abdolmaleky, H.M.; Fournier, M.; Cuenod, M.; Do, K.Q.; Deth, R.C. Decreased Brain Levels of Vitamin B12 in Aging, Autism and Schizophrenia. *PLoS ONE* **2016**, *11*, e0146797. [CrossRef] [PubMed]
107. Frye, R.E.; Huffman, L.C.; Elliott, G.R. Tetrahydrobiopterin as a novel therapeutic intervention for autism. *Neurotherapeutics* **2010**, *7*, 241–249. [CrossRef] [PubMed]
108. Frye, R.E. Central tetrahydrobiopterin concentration in neurodevelopmental disorders. *Front. Neurosci.* **2010**, *4*, 52. [CrossRef]
109. Frye, R.; De La Torre, R.; Taylor, H.B.; Slattery, J.; Melnyk, S.; Chowdhury, N.; James, S.J. Metabolic effects of sapropterin treatment in autism spectrum disorder: A preliminary study. *Transl. Psychiatry* **2013**, *3*, e237. [CrossRef] [PubMed]
110. Frye, R.E. Tetrahydrobiopterin May Be Transported into the Central Nervous System by the Folate Receptor α. *North Am. J. Med. Sci.* **2013**, *3*, 117.
111. Berrocal-Zaragoza, M.I.; Fernandez-Ballart, J.D.; Murphy, M.M.; Cavallé-Busquets, P.; Sequeira, J.M.; Quadros, E.V. Association between blocking folate receptor autoantibodies and subfertility. *Fertil. Steril.* **2009**, *91*, 1518–1521. [CrossRef]
112. Rothenberg, S.P.; Da Costa, M.P.; Sequeira, J.M.; Cracco, J.; Roberts, J.L.; Weedon, J.; Quadros, E.V. Autoantibodies against Folate Receptors in Women with a Pregnancy Complicated by a Neural-Tube Defect. *N. Engl. J. Med.* **2004**, *350*, 134–142. [CrossRef]
113. Vo, H.D.; Sequeira, J.M.; Quadros, E.V.; Schwarz, S.M.; Perenyi, A.R. The role of folate receptor autoantibodies in preterm birth. *Nutrition* **2015**, *31*, 1224–1227. [CrossRef]
114. Shapira, I.; Sequeira, J.M.; Quadros, E.V. Folate receptor autoantibodies in pregnancy related complications. *Birth Defects Res. Part A Clin. Mol. Teratol.* **2015**, *103*, 1028–1030. [CrossRef] [PubMed]
115. Jones, R.M.; Carberry, C.; Hamo, A.; Lord, C. Placebo-like response in absence of treatment in children with Autism. *Autism Res.* **2017**, *10*, 1567–1572. [CrossRef] [PubMed]
116. King, B.H.K.; Dukes, C.L.; Donnelly, L.; Sikich, J.T.; McCracken, L.; Scahill, E.; Hollander, J.D.; Bregman, E.; Anagnostou, F.; Robinson, L.S.; et al. Baseline Factors Predicting Placebo Response to Treatment in Children and Adolescents with Autism Spectrum Disorders: A Multisite Randomized Clinical Trial. *JAMA Pediatr.* **2013**, *167*, 1045–1052. [CrossRef] [PubMed]

Journal of *Personalized Medicine*

MDPI

Review

The Effectiveness of Cobalamin (B12) Treatment for Autism Spectrum Disorder: A Systematic Review and Meta-Analysis

Daniel A. Rossignol [1,]* and Richard E. Frye [2]

1 Rossignol Medical Center, 24541 Pacific Park Drive, Suite 210, Aliso Viejo, CA 92656, USA
2 Barrow Neurological Institute at Phoenix Children's Hospital, 1919 E Thomas Rd, Phoenix, AZ 85016, USA; rfrye@phoenixchildrens.com
* Correspondence: rossignolmd@gmail.com

Abstract: Autism spectrum disorder (ASD) is a common neurodevelopmental disorder affecting 2% of children in the United States. Biochemical abnormalities associated with ASD include impaired methylation and sulphation capacities along with low glutathione (GSH) redox capacity. Potential treatments for these abnormalities include cobalamin (B12). This systematic review collates the studies using B12 as a treatment in ASD. A total of 17 studies were identified; 4 were double-blind, placebo-controlled studies (2 examined B12 injections alone and 2 used B12 in an oral multivitamin); 1 was a prospective controlled study; 6 were prospective, uncontrolled studies, and 6 were retrospective (case series and reports). Most studies (83%) used oral or injected methylcobalamin (mB12), while the remaining studies did not specify the type of B12 used. Studies using subcutaneous mB12 injections (including 2 placebo-controlled studies) used a 64.5–75 μg/kg/dose. One study reported anemia in 2 ASD children with injected cyanocobalamin that resolved with switching to injected mB12. Two studies reported improvements in markers of mitochondrial metabolism. A meta-analysis of methylation metabolites demonstrated decreased S-adenosylhomocysteine (SAH), and increased methionine, S-adenosylmethionine (SAM), SAM/SAH ratio, and homocysteine (with small effect sizes) with mB12. Meta-analysis of the transsulfuration and redox metabolism metabolites demonstrated significant improvements with mB12 in oxidized glutathione (GSSG), cysteine, total glutathione (GSH), and total GSH/GSSG redox ratio with medium to large effect sizes. Improvements in methylation capacity and GSH redox ratio were significantly associated with clinical improvements (with a mean moderate effect size of 0.59) in core and associated ASD symptoms, including expressive communication, personal and domestic daily living skills, and interpersonal, play-leisure, and coping social skills, suggesting these biomarkers may predict response to B12. Other clinical improvements observed with B12 included sleep, gastrointestinal symptoms, hyperactivity, tantrums, nonverbal intellectual quotient, vision, eye contact, echolalia, stereotypy, anemia, and nocturnal enuresis. Adverse events identified by meta-analysis included hyperactivity (11.9%), irritability (3.4%), trouble sleeping (7.6%), aggression (1.8%), and worsening behaviors (7.7%) but were generally few, mild, not serious, and not significantly different compared to placebo. In one study, 78% of parents desired to continue mB12 injections after the study conclusion. Preliminary clinical evidence suggests that B12, particularly subcutaneously injected mB12, improves metabolic abnormalities in ASD along with clinical symptoms. Further large multicenter placebo-controlled studies are needed to confirm these data. B12 is a promising treatment for ASD.

Keywords: autism spectrum disorder; cobalamin; glutathione; methylation; methylcobalamin; redox metabolism

Citation: Rossignol, D.A.; Frye, R.E. The Effectiveness of Cobalamin (B12) Treatment for Autism Spectrum Disorder: A Systematic Review and Meta-Analysis. *J. Pers. Med.* **2021**, *11*, 784. https://doi.org/10.3390/jpm11080784

Academic Editor: Farah R. Zahir

Received: 12 July 2021
Accepted: 8 August 2021
Published: 11 August 2021

Publisher's Note: MDPI stays neutral with regard to jurisdictional claims in published maps and institutional affiliations.

Copyright: © 2021 by the authors. Licensee MDPI, Basel, Switzerland. This article is an open access article distributed under the terms and conditions of the Creative Commons Attribution (CC BY) license (https://creativecommons.org/licenses/by/4.0/).

1. Introduction

Autism spectrum disorder (ASD) is a common neurodevelopmental disorder affecting 2% of children in the United States [1]. ASD is defined behaviorally by reduced social communication and the existence of restrictive and repetitive behaviors and interests. Although

ASD is currently classified as a psychiatric disorder, a number of medical comorbidities and biochemical abnormalities are associated with ASD and may contribute to symptoms. These include immune disorders [2], mitochondrial dysfunction [3,4], oxidative stress [5], seizures [6], gastrointestinal problems [7], and impaired methylation capacity [8].

The methylation cycle recycles homocysteine to methionine, the precursor of S-adenosylmethionine (SAM), which is the major methyl donor for many chemical processes in the body including DNA methylation. Importantly, the methylation cycle is intricately connected to redox metabolism through the contribution of homocysteine (Figure 1). Homocysteine is metabolized to cystathionine and then to cysteine, which is the rate-limiting precursor of glutathione (GSH), the major antioxidant in the body.

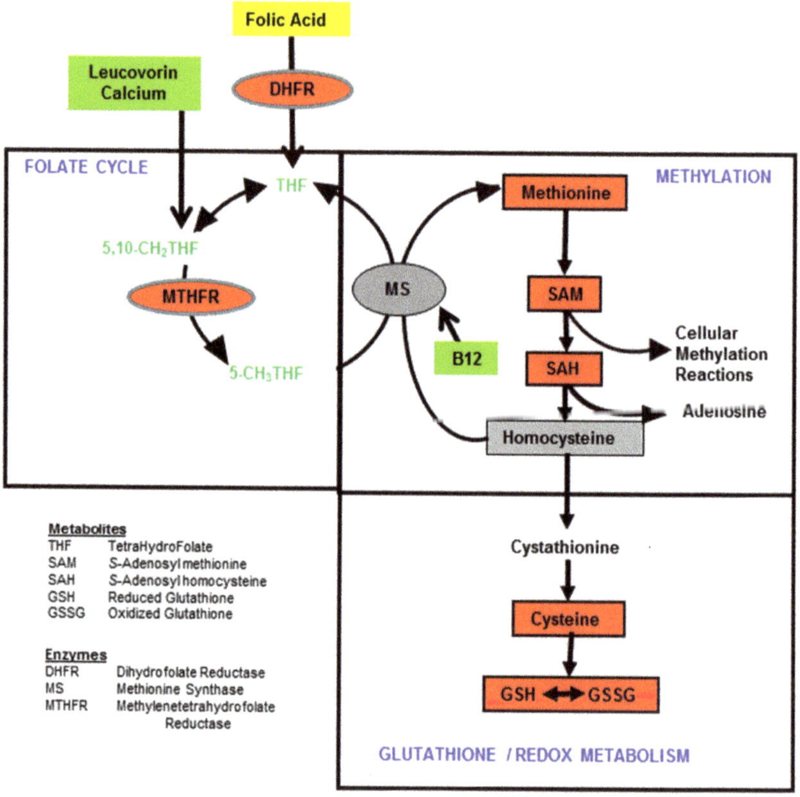

Figure 1. The connected folate, methylation, and redox cycles. Ovals represent enzymes and boxes represent metabolites. Red indicates metabolites and enzymes repeatedly noted to be consistently abnormal in ASD. Green highlights treatments that improve the metabolism of these cycles. Folic acid is shown in yellow as it is a suboptimal treatment because it is oxidized and has to be converted to active forms of folate.

The first study to formally evaluate methylation and redox capacity in ASD reported significantly lower plasma levels of methionine, SAM, homocysteine, cystathionine, cysteine, and total GSH, and significantly higher concentrations of S-adenosylhomocysteine (SAH), adenosine, and oxidized GSH (GSSG) in 20 children with ASD compared to 33 controls. The lower SAM/SAH ratio is indicative of impaired methylation capacity and a lower GSH with elevated GSSG represents impaired redox capacity [8]. These initial findings have been confirmed in several other prospective, controlled studies in blood [9–12] and brain samples [13–15], and a meta-analysis has confirmed the consistency of these findings across multiple studies and multiple laboratories [5]. A meta-analysis of 22 studies confirmed a consistent finding of impaired DNA methylation in ASD [16] and impaired DNA methylation has been associated with mitochondrial dysfunction in ASD [17]. These biochemical abnormalities have even been proposed to be diagnostic of ASD as they could predict the presence of ASD with a 98% correct classification rate using Fisher discriminant analysis [18].

Impairments in the methylation cycle commonly lead to an accumulation in homocysteine, a finding which was reported in a number of studies in ASD [19–21], including a meta-analysis of 31 studies [22]. However, some studies also report lower homocysteine levels in some children with ASD [8,9]. This may be related to the fact that homocysteine is the precursor to two pathways. First, methionine synthase (MS), a B12 and folate-dependent enzyme, converts homocysteine to methionine; one study reported lower MS mRNA in the brains of individuals with ASD (especially in younger children) compared to controls [23]. Lower MS mRNA would presumably result in lower production of the MS enzyme, which would slow the conversion of homocysteine to methionine and result in a build-up of homocysteine. However, homocysteine is also the precursor to cysteine, which is the rate-limiting substrate for the production of GSH. ASD is associated with lowered concentrations of GSH in blood [8,9,24], mitochondria [25], lymphoblasts [25], and brain tissue [15,26], and a recent meta-analysis found consistent depletion of GSH in ASD across 14 studies [5]. Since GSH is produced from homocysteine (and cysteine), GSH depletion may lead to the depletion of homocysteine by consuming it as a precursor. Impaired methylation can also weaken sulphation pathways; lower blood and higher urinary sulfate concentrations have been reported in ASD as early as 1997 [27–29].

Treatments that have been shown to improve methylation and GSH production in ASD include methylcobalamin (mB12), betaine (anhydrous trimethylglycine), and leucovorin (folinic acid) [8,11]. Cobalamin (B12) exists in several forms: cyanocobalamin (cB12, a synthetic form of B12 not found in a natural form; available by injection or orally) and three naturally occurring forms: mB12, hydroxycobalamin (hB12), and adenosylcobalamin (aB12); the latter three natural forms have better bioavailability compared to cB12 and are available in an injectable form or orally [30]. B12 is important for brain development, and B12 deficiency has been associated with regression in social interaction in one child [31] and in another who developed Childhood Disintegration Disorder [32].

Although a number of studies have used B12 as a treatment in children with ASD, these studies have not been systematically reviewed to date. This systematic review identifies and collates the studies using B12 as a treatment in individuals with ASD. When possible, this review lists out the type(s) of B12 used along with dosing, route of administration, types of studies, clinical outcomes, and adverse events (AEs). Meta-analysis was used to examine biochemical changes in methylation and redox metabolism as well as AEs.

2. Materials and Methods

2.1. Search Process

A prospective protocol for this systematic review was developed a priori, and the search terms and selection criteria were chosen in an attempt to capture all pertinent publications. A computer-aided search of PUBMED, Google Scholar, EmBase, Scopus, and ERIC databases from inception through June 2021 was conducted to identify pertinent publications using the search terms 'autism', 'autistic', 'Asperger', 'ASD', 'pervasive', and 'pervasive developmental disorder' in all combinations with the terms "MB12", "Methylcobalamin", "Cobalamin", "B12", "Cyanocobalamin", "Hydroxycobalamin", "Adenosylcobalamin", and "Vitamin B12." References cited in identified publications were also searched to locate additional studies.

2.2. Study Selection and Assessment

This systematic review and meta-analysis followed PRISMA guidelines [33]. The PRISMA Checklist is found in Supplementary Table S1, and the PRISMA Flowchart is displayed as Figure 2. One reviewer screened titles and abstracts of all potentially relevant publications. Studies were initially included if they (1) involved individuals with ASD; and (2) reported on the use of B12 as a treatment in ASD. Articles were excluded if they: (1) did not involve humans (for example, cellular or animal models); and or (2) did not present new or unique data (such as review articles or letters to the editor). After screening all records, 17 publications met inclusion criteria (see Figure 2); two reviewers then independently reviewed these articles for inclusion and assessed factors such as the risk of bias. As per standardized guidelines [34], selection, performance detection, attrition, and reporting biases were considered. Two DBPC studies that used only injected mB12 were identified, but since only one of these studies provided detailed descriptive statistics of the clinical outcome measures [35], a meta-analysis could not be conducted on clinical outcome measures.

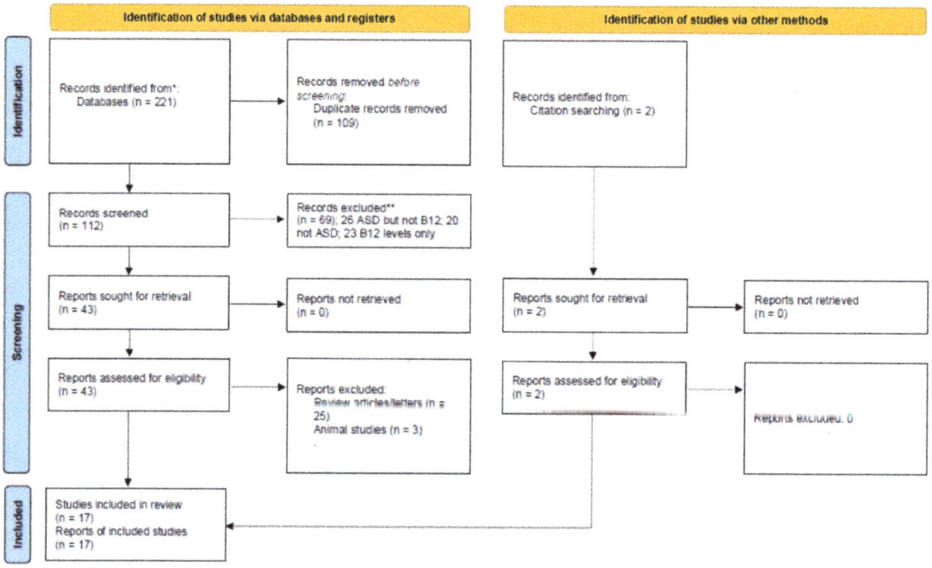

Figure 2. PRISMA 2020 flow diagram for this systematic review.

2.3. Meta-Analysis

MetaXL Version 5.2 (EpiGear International Pty Ltd., Sunrise Beach, Queensland, Australia) was used with Microsoft Excel Version 16.0.12827.20200 (Redmond, WA, USA) to perform the meta-analysis. The data from this meta-analysis is available upon request to the authors. Random-effects models, which assume variability in effects from both sampling error and study level differences [36,37], were used to calculate incidence across studies (AEs Meta-analysis) while pooled Cohen's d' (a measure of effect size) was calculated from the standardized mean difference of outcome measures using the inverse variance heterogeneity model since it has been shown to resolve issues with underestimation of the statistical error and spuriously overconfident estimates with the random effects model when analyzing continuous outcome measures (Biochemistry Meta-analysis) [38]. Effect sizes were considered small if Cohen's d' was 0.2; medium if Cohen's d' was 0.5; and large if Cohen's d' was 0.8 or higher [39]. Cochran's Q was calculated to determine heterogeneity of effects across studies, and when significant, the I^2 statistic (Heterogeneity Index) was calculated to determine the percentage of variation across studies that was due to heterogeneity rather than chance [40,41], and the Luis Furuya-Kanamori (LFK) Index derived from Doi plots was reviewed for significant asymmetries ($>\pm2$) [42,43].

3. Results

This section will discuss the type(s), routes, and dosing parameters of B12 used along with the type of study and phenotypes of patients (Section 3.1), biochemical changes (Section 3.2), clinical outcome measures (Section 3.3), and AEs (Section 3.4) associated with B12 treatment studies. In the clinical outcomes section, the outcomes are presented and organized by study type.

3.1. B12 Administration: Type of B12, Route, Dosing, and Type of Study

3.1.1. Type of B12

Five studies did not specify the type of B12 used [32,44–47]. Two studies used oral cB12 [48,49]. One study used a 50/50 oral mixture of mB12 and cB12 [50]. One study initially used cB12 injections and switched to mB12 injections due to worsening anemia from cB12 in 2 children and also used oral hB12 in one child [51]. The remaining 8 studies used mB12 [8,11,35,52–56]. Thus, of the 12 studies specifying the type of B12 used, 10 (83%) used mB12 by itself or in combination with cB12.

3.1.2. Route Parameters of B12

Two studies did not specify the route of B12 administration [45,52]. Six studies used subcutaneously (SC) injected mB12 [8,11,35,53,55,56] and 4 studies used intramuscularly injected B12 [32,46,47,51]. Five studies used oral B12 [44,48–50,54]. One study used both injected cB12 and oral hB12 [51]. Thus, of the 15 studies specifying the route of administration, 10 (67%) used an injected form.

3.1.3. Dosing of B12

Six studies (including two DBPC studies) used subcutaneous mB12 injections at a dose ranging from 64.5 to 75 µg/kg/dose [8,11,35,53,55,56]. One study used a lower dose of 25–30 µg/kg/dose (up to 1500 µg), but the route of administration was not specified [52]. One study used oral mB12 at a dose of 500 µg per day [54] while 2 studies used oral cB12 in doses of 500–1600 µg per day along with a multivitamin/mineral supplement (MVI) [48,49]. Another study used a 50/50 mixture of mB12 and cB12 500 µg per day combined in an MVI [50]. One study used oral B12 1.2 µg per day but did not specify the type of B12 given [44]. One study used 1000 µg of B12 (type not specified) intramuscularly for 5 days and then weekly for 8 weeks [32]. One study used mB12 intramuscularly at 1 mg once per week in 2 children and 10 mg of oral hB12 in another child [51]. Finally, 3 studies did not list the dose of B12 given [45–47].

3.1.4. Types of B12 Studied

Of the 17 treatments studies, 2 were DBPC studies using mB12 injections alone [35,55], 2 were DBPC studies using oral cB12 in a MVI preparation [48,49], 1 was a prospective, controlled study [50], 6 were prospective, uncontrolled studies [8,11,44,45,52,53], and 6 were retrospective case series/reports [32,46,47,51,54,56]. Two studies reported on the same cohort of patients [11,53].

3.1.5. Phenotypes of Patients in B12 Studies

Table 1 lists the phenotypes for the 17 studies. Six studies used DSM-4 criteria to diagnose ASD [8,11,44,52,55,56]. Six studies used autism diagnostic observation schedule (ADOS) and/or autism diagnostic interview (ADI) to confirm the diagnosis [35,45,50,51,54,55]. Five studies did not specify criteria for autism [32,46–49]. Two studies only enrolled patients with abnormal biochemical findings (such as methylation abnormalities or oxidative stress) [11,53].

Table 1. Phenotypes of autism in the 17 reviewed studies, by year published.

Study	Phenotype
Adams and Holloway, 2004 [48]	20 children with autism (age 3–8 yo); diagnosis of an autism spectrum disorder (autism, pervasive developmental disorder/not otherwise specified [PDD/NOS], or Asperger's syndrome) by a psychiatrist or developmental pediatrician (criteria not specified); no changes in any treatments during the preceding two months; no previous multivitamin/mineral supplement use (except a standard children's multivitamin/mineral)
James, et al., 2004 [8]	20 children with autism (mean age 6.4 yo, all white, 14 boys, 6 girls); 19 with regressive autism, 1 with infantile autism. Autism was based on the criteria for autistic disorder (DSM-4) by a developmental pediatrician; most had speech and socialization impairments and gastrointestinal problems
Nakano, et al., 2005 [52]	13 patients (2–18 yo, 11 male, 2 female) with autism, diagnosed by DSM-4 criteria by a pediatric neurologist; 4 with epilepsy and 1 with periventricular leukomalacia
James, et al., 2009 [11]	40 children with autism (2–7 yo, 33 boys, 7 girls) diagnosed by DSM-4 criteria and a CARS score >30; exclusion criteria included Asperger's disorder, PDD-NOS, genetic disorders, seizures; severe gastrointestinal problems, recent infection, and use of high-dose vitamin or mineral supplements; all children had reduced methylation capacity (SAM:SAH) or reduced GSH redox ratio (GSH:GSSG) as an inclusion criterion
Bertoglio, et al., 2010 [55]	30 children with autism (3–8 yo, 28 boys, 2 girls) diagnosed by DSM-4 criteria and ADOS/ADI. No current use of mB12; nonverbal IQ of 49 or higher confirmed by a psychologist (Wechsler Preschool and Primary Scale of Intelligence, Mullen Scales of Early Learning, or the Wechsler Intelligence Scale for Children)
Geier and Geier, 2010 [56]	24 children with autism (mean age 9.3 yo, 23 white, 3 minorities, 21 boys, 3 girls) diagnosed by DSM-4 criteria
Pineles, et al., 2010 [46]	3 children with autism (6 yo boy, 13 yo boy, 7 yo boy) and vision loss/optic neuropathy (diagnostic criteria not specified)
Adams, et al., 2011 [49]	141 individuals with autism (3–60 yo, 125 boys, 16 girls); diagnosis of autism, PDD/NOS, or Asperger's syndrome by psychiatrist or similar professional (criteria not specified); No vitamin/mineral supplement in the preceding 2 months
Kaluzna-Czaplinska, et al., 2011 [44]	30 children with autism (4–11 yo, 27 boys, 3 girls); autism diagnosed by DSM-4 criteria; all children on a sugar-free diet
Duvall, et al., 2013 [47]	9 yo child with ASD (criteria not specified)
Frye, et al., 2013 [53]	Same cohort as James et al., 2009 [11]
Malhotra, et al., 2013 [32]	14 yo boy with CDD (vegetarian)
Corejova, et al., 2015 [54]	18 yo adult male with autism diagnosed by ADI and CARS-2 by psychologist
Hendren, et al., 2016 [35]	57 children with autism (3–7 yo, 45 boys, 12 girls) with diagnosis confirmed by ADI and ADOS (the latter if needed) performed by a psychiatrist; IQ > 50 (Stanford–Binet 5th edition verbal subtest); excluded children with bleeding disorder, seizures, cancer, or genetic abnormalities, perinatal brain injury, current use of B12, or "other serious medical illness"
Delhey, et al., 2017 [45]	127 children with autism (ages 3–14 yo), diagnosis confirmed with ADOS and/or ADI, the state of Arkansas diagnostic standard, and/or DSM-4; prematurity was an exclusion criterion; 38 had mitochondrial function measured
Nashabat, et al., 2017 [51]	3 children with autism (3–2 yo, all boys); one diagnosed by GARS and PSL4; other 2 diagnosed by ADOS
Adams, et al., 2018 [50]	37 individuals (3–58 yo, 30 male, 7 female) with autism (29), PDD-NOS (3) or Asperger's disorder (3); diagnosis confirmed by ADOS or CARS-2 by a psychiatrist, psychologist, or developmental pediatrician; no current use of nutritional supplements; patients with metabolic or genetic disorders not excluded; 13 had developmental regression, 15 with early-onset autism and 8 with developmental plateau; 9 with asthma; 13 with food allergies; 19 with other allergies

Autism Diagnostic Interview (ADI); Autism Diagnostic Observation Schedule (ADOS); Childhood Autism Rating Scale (CARS); childhood disintegrative disorder (CDD); Diagnostic and Statistical Manual of Mental Disorders, fourth edition (DSM-4); Gilliam Autism Scale (GARS); glutathione (GSH); Preschool Language scale, Fourth Edition (PSL4); oxidized glutathione (GSSG); Pervasive Developmental Disorder, Not Otherwise Specified (PDD-NOS); S-adenosylhomocysteine (SAH); S-adenosylmethionine (SAM); years old (yo).

3.2. Biochemical Changes with B12 Treatment

3.2.1. Review of Studies

Eleven studies examined biochemical changes with B12 treatment and are outlined in Table 2. A 12-week randomized DBPC crossover study of 30 children with ASD (ages 3–8 yo) used mB12 64.5 µg/kg subcutaneous injections every 3 days for 6 weeks or a placebo. GSH and GSH/GSSG were measured before and after treatment. No significant changes in GSH related metabolites were observed comparing the treatment group to the placebo group. However, significant improvements in GSH and the GSH redox ratio were found in a subgroup of 9 children who were considered "responders" based on significant improvements on the CGI and 2 other behavioral outcomes, suggesting these may be biomarkers for identifying children who respond to mB12 treatment [55]. In another randomized DBPC study, 57 children with ASD received 75 µg/kg mB12 subcutaneous injections every 3 days for 8 weeks or placebo injections, and clinical improvements were positively associated with increased plasma methionine, decreased SAH, and improved methylation capacity as measured by the SAM/SAH ratio [35].

Table 2. Biochemical outcomes for treatment studies of cobalamin injections for autism spectrum disorder. Clinical global impression scale (CGI); subcutaneous (SC); years old (yo).

Study	Participants	Treatment	Outcomes
	Subcutaneous Methylcobalamin Injections		
Bertoglio et al., 2010 [55] DBPC Crossover	30	64.5 µg/kg SC every 3 days	Significant improvements in GSH and the GSH redox ratio in a subgroup of 9 children who were considered "responders"
Hendren et al., 2016 [35] DBPC Parallel	57	75 µg/kg SC every 3 days	Clinical improvements were positively associated with increased plasma methionine, decreased SAH, and improved methylation compacity as measured by the SAM/SAH ratio
James et al., 2004 [8] Prospective Uncontrolled	8	75 µg/kg 2x/wk for 1 month with folinic acid and betaine	Decreased adenosine and GSSG; increased methionine, cysteine, tGSH, SAM/SAH, and tGSH/GSSG
James et al., 2009 [11] Prospective Uncontrolled	40	75 µg/kg 2x/wk for 3 months with folinic acid	Increased cysteine, cysteinylglycine, and GSH;decreased GSSG
Frye et al., 2013 [53] Prospective Uncontrolled			Clinical improvements associated with biochemical improvements in GSH redox status
Geier and Geier 2010 [56] Retrospective, controlled	24	75 µg/kg SC every 1–3 days	Urinary and plasma cobalt levels higher in mB12 group
	Intramuscular Methylcobalamin Injections		
Nashabat et al., 2017 [51] Retrospective Uncontrolled		cB12 switched to mB12; one child received hB12	Improvement in anemia and metabolic acidosis when cB12 was changed to mB12; homocysteine normalized with 10 mg of hB12 orally in one child

Table 2. *Cont.*

Subcutaneous Methylcobalamin Injections			
Oral Cobalamin with Other Vitamins			
Adams et al., 2011 [49] DBPC Parallel	141	500mcg Daily Orally	Improvements in total sulfate, SAM, reduced GSH, GSSG:GSH, nitrotyrosine, ATP, NADH, and NADPH
Kaluzna-Czaolinska et al., 2011, [44] Prospective Uncontrolled	30	B12 1200 mcg per day with vitamin B6 200 mg and folic acid 400 μg	Reduction in urinary homocysteine
Cobalamin with Route of Administration Not Specified			
Delhey et al., 2017 [45] Prospective Uncontrolled	127	Any B12 taken in 38% of Patients along with other supplements	Improved coupling of Complex I and Citrate Synthase mitochondrial enzymes
Nakano et al., 2005 [52] Prospective Uncontrolled	13	mB12 25–30 μg/kg/day (up to 1500 μg) for 6–25 months	Increased B12 blood concentrations

In a prospective study of 8 children with ASD, 75 μg/kg mB12 SC two times per week for one month was given along with folinic acid (800 μg twice a day orally) and betaine (1000 mg twice a day orally). This treatment led to significant decreases in adenosine and GSSG as well as significantly increased levels of methionine, cysteine, GSH, SAM/SAH, and GSH/GSSG [8].

In a study of 40 children with ASD, 75 μg/kg mB12 SC 2 times per week for 3 months given with folinic acid (400 μg twice per day) led to increased cysteine, cysteinylglycine, and GSH, and decreased GSSG [11]. Improvements in GSH redox status were associated with improvements in expressive communication, personal and domestic daily living skills, and interpersonal, play-leisure, and coping social skills [53].

In a case series of 3 patients with ASD with transcobalamin deficiency/transcobalamin II (TCN2) mutations (one patient had metabolic acidosis and pancytopenia), cB12 intramuscular injections (1 mg once or twice weekly) were started along with carnitine. However, both patients developed acute anemia on cB12 injections, which improved when switching to mB12 intramuscular injections 1 mg weekly; in the third child, homocysteine levels normalized with 10 mg per day of hB12 orally once per day [51].

In a randomized DBPC study of 141 children and adults with ASD, a MVI containing 500 mcg of oral cB12 led to significant improvements compared to placebo in total sulfate, SAM, reduced glutathione, GSSG:GSH, nitrotyrosine, adenosine triphosphate (ATP), NADH, and NADPH [49].

In a study of 13 patients with ASD, mB12 25–30 μg/kg/day (up to 1500 μg/day; route of administration not specified) was given for 6–25 months. Five patients had normal B12 serum levels and after the study, 4 cases had above normal serum B12 without any apparent AEs [52].

In another study of 30 children with ASD, oral B12 (type not specified) 1.2 μg per day given with vitamin B6 200 mg and folic acid 400 μg led to a significant reduction in urinary homocysteine [44]. In a prospective, uncontrolled study of 127 children with ASD, B12 treatment (type and route of administration not specified) was administered to 38% of the ASD group along with mitochondrial supplements. Analysis showed that B12 treatment improved complex I activity compared to not supplementing with B12. In addition, B12 treatment was associated with the better coupling of Complex I and Citrate Synthase mitochondrial enzymes [45].

Finally, one retrospective study examined 24 children with ASD (mean age 9.3 ± 3.5 years) who received SC mB12 injections (75 μg/kg, given every 1–3 days) and compared urinary and plasma cobalt levels to 48 children (mean age 8.9 ± 3.7 years) who did not receive mB12 injections. The mean plasma cobalt concentration in the mB12 group was 0.82 ± 0.19 μg/L compared to 0.12 ± 0.10 in the untreated group ($p < 0.001$). The investigators noted that the study was limited as it could not determine what form of cobalt was present (free or bound in mB12), how the cobalt was distributed in the body, and what the tissue levels would be. This study did not report clinical outcomes [56].

3.2.2. Meta-Analysis of Biochemical Changes Related to Methylcobalamin

Only three studies [8,11,35] provided enough detailed information about biochemical metabolites before and after treatment to be included in a meta-analysis. All studies used subcutaneously injected mB12. One study [35] was a DBPC study that used mB12 alone, and two studies [8,11] were uncontrolled prospective studies, which used mB12 with additional treatments. Of these latter two studies, one study [8] obtained biochemical measurements three months after starting daily 800 µg of leucovorin (folinic acid) and 1000 mg of betaine and then three months after adding mB12. In the meta-analysis, the biochemical measurements directly before and after adding mB12 were used rather than using the baseline measures obtained before any treatments were added. For the second study [11], mB12 was provided along with daily 800 µg of leucovorin (folinic acid). Common metabolites across all three studies were analyzed, and the results are outlined in Table 3. Even though these 3 studies used different dosing parameters and two used mB12 with folinic and one without, both mB12 and folinic have been shown to lead to biochemical changes in methylation metabolites and work in a synergistic fashion. Therefore, combining these studies to examine biochemical changes was felt to be advantageous.

Table 3. Meta-analysis of biochemical changes with subcutaneously injected methylcobalamin in children with ASD. Oxidized glutathione (GSSG); S-adenosylhomocysteine (SAH); S-adenosylmethionine (SAM); methylation capacity (SAM/SAH); total GSH (tGSH); total glutathione redox ratio (tGSH/GSSG) * $p < 0.05$, ** $p < 0.01$, *** $p < 0.0001$.

Metabolite	Weighted Mean Difference	Cohen's d' (95% CI)	Cochran's Q	I^2	LFK Index
	Methylation Metabolites				
Methionine (µmol/L)	0.95	0.25 (−0.10, 0.59)	0.12		
SAM (nmol/L)	1.80	0.12 (−0.23, 0.47)	2.12		
SAH (nmol/L)	−0.78	−0.19 (−2.14, 0.58)	0.53		
SAM/SAH Ratio	0.22	0.28 (−0.07, 0.62)	0.66		
Homocysteine (µmol/L)	0.01	0.10 (−0.25, 0.45)	6.94 *	71%	1.03
	Transsulfuration/Redox Metabolites				
Cysteine (µmol/L)	13.30	0.70 (0.34, 1.07) ***	15.13 **	87%	0.72
Total GSH (µmol/L)	0.36	0.43 (0.08. 0.79) *	8.73 **	77%	−0.16
GSSG (nmol/L)	−0.004	−0.68 (0.32, 1.04) ***	7.13 *	72%	0.61
Total GSH/GSSG Ratio	7.43	0.84 (0.47. 1.21) ***	18.37 ***	89%	0.88

Meta-analysis of the methylation metabolites demonstrated small effect sizes that were in the direction expected for improvement of methylation metabolism for the majority of the metabolites. Specifically, the weighted mean differences suggested an increase in Methionine, SAM, and SAM/SAH ratio, and a decrease in SAH. None of the effects were overall statistically significant, and the Cochran's Q statistic suggested that the variation was not due to heterogeneity across studies but rather due to random chance. However, for homocysteine, although the overall effect was not significant, the variation in the measurement was found to be largely due to variation across studies with a slight asymmetry in the Doi plots. This was due to one study [35] demonstrating a decrease in homocysteine with treatment and two studies [8,11] demonstrating an increase in homocysteine with treatment.

Meta-analysis of the redox metabolism metabolites demonstrated statistically significant medium to large effect sizes that were in the direction expected for an improvement in redox metabolism for all of the metabolites examined. Specifically, the weighted mean differences demonstrated an increase in cysteine, total GSH, and total GSH/GSSG redox ratio, and a decrease in GSSG. The I^2 statistic suggested that the variation was due to heterogeneity across studies, specifically one study [35] demonstrating more marginal effects as compared to the other two studies [8,11]. However, Doi plots did not demonstrate any significant asymmetries.

3.3. Clinical Outcomes with B12 Treatment

Twelve studies examined clinical outcomes and are outlined in Table 4. Improvements reported in these studies included sleep, hyperactivity, gastrointestinal problems, tantrums, nonverbal IQ, expressive, written and receptive communication skills, daily living skills, social skills domains, vision, eye contact, echolalia, stereotypy, anemia, and nocturnal enuresis.

Table 4. Studies of cobalamin injections for autism spectrum disorder with clinical outcomes. Childhood autism rating scale (CARS); clinical global impression scale (CGI); subcutaneous (SC); years old (yo).

Study	Participants	Treatment	Outcomes	Adverse Effects
Subcutaneous Methylcobalamin Injections: Prospective Double-Blind Placebo Controlled Studies				
Bertoglio et al., 2010 [55] Crossover	30	64.5 μg/kg SC every 3 days	No change in overall behavior	Hyperactivity; mouthing objects
Hendren et al., 2016 [35] Parallel	57	75 μg/kg SC every 3 days	Significant improvement in CGI	No significant difference between groups
Subcutaneous Methylcobalamin Injections: Prospective Uncontrolled Study				
Frye et al., 2013 [53]	40	75 μg/kg 2x/wk for 3 months with folinic acid	Overall improvement in development. Clinical improvement associated with biochemical improvements	Hyperactivity (10%), reduced sleep (6%), impulsiveness (3%)
Intramuscular Cobalamin Injections with Type of B12 not specified: Retrospective Case Series/Reports				
Pineles et al., 2010 [46]	3	B12 IM	Improvement in vision	None reported
Duvall et al., 2013 [47]	1	B12 IM with oral MVI	Improvements in pulmonary hypertension and musculoskeletal problems	None reported
Malhotra et al., 2013 [32]	1	B12 IM with oral MVI	Improvements in eye contact, licking fingers, hyperactivity, pacing, echolalia, and repetitive behaviors and in CARS score	None reported
Oral Multivitamin, which Included Cobalamin: Prospective Double-Blind Placebo-Controlled Studies				
Adams and Holloway 2004 [48] Parallel	30	1200–1600 mcg Daily Orally	Improved gastrointestinal problems and sleep	No adverse events in those adhering to the protocol
Adams et al., 2011 [49] Parallel	141	500 mcg Daily Orally	Improved hyperactivity, tantrums and receptive language	Mild behavioral problems, diarrhea, constipation
Oral Multivitamin, which Included Cobalamin: Prospective Controlled Study				
Adams et al., 2018 [50]	37	500 mcg Daily Orally	Improved non-verbal IQ, daily living skills and social skills	Worsened behaviors, gastrointestinal disturbance, facial rash, aggression, stereotypy

Table 4. *Cont.*

Study	Participants	Treatment	Outcomes	Adverse Effects
Oral Methylcobalamin: Retrospective Case Report				
Corejova et al., 2015 [54]	1	mB12 500 μg orally per day	Nocturnal enuresis resolved; reappeared when treatment was stopped	Increased stereotypy and hyperactivity
Oral Hydroxycobalamin: Retrospective Case Report				
Nashabat, et al., 2017 [51]	3	hB12 10 mg orally pr day	Improved developmental milestones	None
Methylcobalamin with Route of Administration Not Specified: Prospective Uncontrolled Study				
Nakano et al., 2005 [52]	13	25–30 μg/kg/day (up to 1500 μg) mB12 for 6–25 months	Improvements in IQ, developmental quotient and CARS score	No significant events

3.3.1. Double Blind Placebo-Controlled Studies

Four DBPC studies examined B12 use in ASD, with two of the studies administering it alone as an injection in the form of mB12 and two studies using cB12 in an orally administered MVI.

In a 12-week randomized DBPC crossover study, 30 children with ASD (ages 3–8 yo) received mB12 64.5 μg/kg SC injections every 3 days for 6 weeks or placebo injections for 6 weeks; a 6-month extension study was also performed. No significant changes in clinical outcomes were observed comparing the treatment group to the placebo group. A total of 22 children entered the 6-month open-label extension portion of the study, but no clinical outcomes were reported for this time period in the publication. A subgroup of 9 children were considered "responders" based on significant improvements on the CGI and 2 other behavioral outcomes. The authors commented that the crossover design without a washout period between the two treatments might have made it more difficult to see a significant difference between groups [55]. In another randomized DBPC study by some of the same investigators, 57 children with ASD received 75 μg/kg mB12 subcutaneous injections every 3 days for 8 weeks or placebo injections. A significant improvement in CGI-I as rated by clinicians was observed with mB12 treatment, but no significant improvements in the treatment group were observed in the parent-rated aberrant behavior checklist (ABC) or social responsiveness scale (SRS). Notably, this study did not include the crossover design, which was felt to be a weakness in design from the first study [35].

In a randomized DBPC 3-month study of 20 children with ASD (ages 3–8 yo), a MVI, which also contained 1200–1600 mcg of oral cB12, led to significant improvements in sleep and gastrointestinal problems compared to placebo [48]. In another randomized DBPC study of 141 individuals with ASD, a MVI containing 500 mcg of oral cB12 led to significant improvements in several behavioral scales compared to placebo, including hyperactivity, tantrums, and receptive language [49].

3.3.2. Prospective, Controlled Study

In a prospective, controlled, single-blind (clinical evaluators blinded) 12-month study, 37 individuals with ASD were treated with an oral MVI containing 500 mcg of B12 (50% as mB12 and 50% as cB12) along with other nutritional and dietary interventions and were compared to 30 control ASD individuals who were not treated. Significant improvements were observed in nonverbal IQ, communication, daily living skills, and social skills domains in the treated ASD group compared to controls [50].

3.3.3. Prospective, Uncontrolled Studies

There were six prospective, uncontrolled studies of B12 in ASD [8,11,44,45,52,53], but no clinical outcomes were reported in four of these studies [8,11,44,45].

In a study of 13 patients with ASD, mB12 25–30 μg/kg/day (up to 1500 μg/day, route of administration unknown) given for 6–25 months led to significant improvements in IQ, developmental quotient, and Childhood Autism Rating Scale (CARS) score; improvements were similar in older children as in younger children, and in children with lower IQ compared to those with higher IQ [52].

In a study of 40 children with ASD, 75 μg/kg mB12 SC 2 times per week for 3 months given with folinic acid (400 μg twice per day) led to significant improvements on all subscales of the Vineland Adaptive Behavior Scale (VABS), including significant improvements in receptive, expressive, and written communication skills, personal, domestic, and community daily living skills, and interpersonal, play-leisure, and coping social skills. The average effect size of improvement was 0.59 (a moderate effect size), and the average improvement in skills development was 7.7 months [53]. This improvement over a 3-month period was consistent with the notion that the children started "catching up" in development.

3.3.4. Retrospective Studies

Five retrospective studies examined B12 treatment in ASD [32,46,47,51,54]. The first three studies used intramuscular B12 (type not specified) to treat a B12 deficiency. Improvements in vision were found in a case series of 3 children with ASD and optic nerve atrophy [46]. In a 9-year-old child with ASD, pulmonary hypertension and nutritional deficiencies (including B12 deficiency), B12 along with other nutritional supplements led to improvements in pulmonary hypertension and musculoskeletal problems [47]. Improvements in eye contact, licking fingers, hyperactivity, pacing, echolalia, repetitive behaviors, and in the CARS score were observed in a 14-year-old vegetarian boy with Childhood Disintegrative Disorder (CDD) with daily injections of 1000 μg B12 for 5 days and then weekly for 8 weeks along with oral antioxidants and vitamins [32]. In another study, daily oral mB12 500 μg resolved nocturnal enuresis a 18-year-old child with ASD, with the enuresis reoccurring when mB12 was stopped [54]. Finally, in one child, "developmental milestones improved" with 10 mg per day of hB12 orally once per day [51].

3.4. *Adverse Effects of B12*

Here the potential AEs (see Table 4) of injected and oral forms of B12 are discussed separately, followed by the studies in which the route of administration is unknown.

Both DBPC studies [35,55] that used mB12 injections reported AEs. No serious AEs were reported in either study. Hyperactivity and increased mouthing of items were reported as AEs in one study [55], but the study did not indicate whether these AEs were significantly different between the treatment and placebo groups or what percentage of children had one of these side effects. The other DBPC study [35] reported 21 adverse events in the mB12 group compared to 24 in the placebo group (no significant difference). Adverse events in the mB12 group included a cold (11%), fever (7%), flu (4%), growing pains (4%), increased hyperactivity (7%), increased irritability (4%), lack of focus (4%), mouthing (19%), nosebleed (7%), rash (4%), stomach flu (4%), and trouble sleeping (4%); these were not significantly different compared to the placebo group. Two prospective, uncontrolled studies used mB12 injections [8,53], with one reporting AEs [53]. Adverse events in this study included hyperactivity (10%, improved when the folinic acid dose was lowered), sleep disruption (3%), difficulty falling asleep (3%), increased impulsiveness (3%), and irritability (3%). After study completion, 31/40 (78%) of parents indicated a desire to continue treatment (8 parents (20%) did not respond to this question) [11,53]. Of the five case reports using injected B12, only two reported AEs. Two patients who received cB12 injection developed acute anemia, which resolved by changing the cB12 form to mB12 injections [51]. In a child receiving oral mB12, increased motor stereotypy and hyperactivity were noted within 100 days of starting treatment [54]. Finally, one retrospective study reported higher plasma and urinary cobalt levels in patients who received SC mB12 compared to controls, but no apparent adverse events from this finding were observed [56].

Of the two DBPC studies that used B12 incorporated into an oral MVI [48,49], one reported no side effects in patients who followed the correct dosing parameters, but nausea and vomiting in 2 children (18%) in the treatment group when the MVI was taken on an empty stomach (against study protocol) [48]. The other study reported aggression (4%), night terrors (2%), trouble focusing (2%), moodiness (2%), nausea (2%), diarrhea (2%), mild behavioral problems (11% compared to 7% in the placebo group, p = ns), and diarrhea/constipation (11% compared to 7% in the placebo group, p = ns) with 2 participants withdrawing due to aggression and one withdrawing because of nausea and diarrhea [49]. In a prospective controlled single-blind study using an oral MVI, which included a 50/50 mixture of cB12 and mB12, AEs included moderate worsening of behaviors in 2 children (6%) found to have low levels of nutrients, particularly extremely low levels of cobalamin [50].

Three retrospective case series using intramuscular cobalamin with the type of B12 not specified did not report if any side effects occurred [32,46,47]. Two studies did not report the route of administration. One prospective uncontrolled study using mB12 (route not specified) reported there were no significant adverse events [52]. Another study did not examine AEs specifically [45].

Meta-analysis of Adverse Effects Related to Cobalamin

To better understand the AEs associated with cobalamin treatment, a meta-analysis was performed on the reported AEs across studies for studies using injected and oral B12 separately (see Table 5). Case reports were excluded from this analysis due to the potential bias of reporting in such studies, and only studies that included quantitative measures of the AEs in the samples studied were included. For injected B12, only two studies [11,35] met this criterion, with both studies using subcutaneously injected mB12. For oral B12, three studies [48–50] met this criterion, all using an MVI including B12 in various forms.

Table 5. Meta-analysis of adverse effects associated with cobalamin in children with ASD. Multivitamin (MVI) * $p < 0.05$. Adverse effects that were statistically significant are in bold and italic.

Injected mB12		MVI Including B12	
Adverse Effect	**Incidence (95% CI)**	**Adverse Effect**	**Incidence (95% CI)**
Cold Symptoms	4.5% (0.0%, 20.1%)	***Aggression***	***1.8% (0.1%, 5.2%) ****
Fever	3.3% (0.0%, 13.7%)	Attention Problems	1.5% (0.0%, 4.1%)
Flu Symptoms	2.0% (0.0%, 7.4%)	Constipation/Diarrhea	4.1% (0.0%, 14.0%)
Growing Pains	2.0% (0.0%, 7.4%)	Moodiness	1.5% (0.0%, 4.1%)
Increased Hyperactivity	***11.9% (5.2%, 20.8%) ****	Nausea/Vomiting	3.5% (0.0%, 11.0%)
Increased Irritability	***3.4% (0.2%, 9.3%) ****	Night Terrors	1.5% (0.0%, 4.1%)
Lack of Focus	2.0% (0.0%, 7.4%)	***Worsening Behavior***	***7.7% (3.5%, 13.3%) ****
Mouthing	6.8% (0.0%, 33.5%)		
Nosebleeds	3.3% (0.0%, 13.7%)		
Rash	2.0% (0.0%, 7.4%)		
Stomach Flu	2.0% (0.0%, 7.4%)		
Trouble Sleeping	***7.6% (2.3%, 15.2%) ****		
Impulsivity	2.0% (0.0%, 7.4%)		

There was a low incidence (<5%) of most AEs for subcutaneously injected mB12 with only three AEs reaching significance: increased irritability (3.4%), trouble sleeping (7.6%) and increased hyperactivity (11.9%), suggesting that for most individuals with ASD, subcutaneously injected mB12 is well tolerated without AEs. There was also a low incidence (<5%) of most AEs for B12 included in an oral MVI. Unlike injected mB12, the oral route was associated with gastrointestinal AEs, although these were also at a low incidence (<5%). Significant AEs for oral formulation included aggression (1.8%) and worsening behavior (7.7%), which is similar in incidence and character to the significant behavioral AEs seen in the injected route. However, again, most participants tolerated the B12 in a MVI without any AEs, suggesting that, in general, it was well tolerated.

4. Discussion

This review identified 17 studies using B12 as a treatment for ASD. Table 6 summarizes the major findings of these studies. Two studies were DBPC controlled studies using mB12 injections and two were DBPC studies using cB12 combined in an MVI. Most studies that specified the type of B12 used mB12 (10/12, 83%). Overall, the treatment was well tolerated with minimal AEs, and the majority of the studies reported positive effects on ASD symptoms, although some studies found that these improvements were limited to a subgroup of children with baseline unfavorable biochemistry.

Table 6. Summary of studies on cobalamin treatment for ASD with clinical outcomes. Childhood Autism Rating Scale (CARS); Clinical Global Impression Scale (CGI); glutathione (GSH); oxidized glutathione (GSSG); intelligence quotient (IQ); multivitamin (MVI); S-adenosylhomocysteine (SAH); S-adenosylmethionine (SAM); methylation capacity (SAM/SAH); subcutaneous (SC); total GSH (tGSH); total glutathione redox ratio (tGSH/GSSG).

Total Studies	Total Participants	Treatment	Outcomes	Adverse Effects
Prospective Double-Blind Placebo Controlled Studies: Subcutaneous Injected Methylcobalamin				
2	87	64.5–75 µg/kg mB12 SC every 3 days	Significant improvement in clinician rated CGI and correlated with increases in methionine and decreases in SAH and improved SAM/SAH	Hyperactivity; mouthing objects
Prospective Double-Blind Placebo Controlled Studies: Oral Cobalamin Combined in Multivitamin				
2	161	MVI containing B12 orally	Improvements in gastrointestinal problems, sleep, hyperactivity, tantrums, and receptive language	Nausea, vomiting, aggression, night terrors, and diarrhea
Prospective Controlled Studies: Oral Cobalamin Combined in Other Vitamin				
1	67	B12 orally with other vitamins	Improved nonverbal IQ, communication, and daily living and social skills.	Worsened behavior
Prospective Uncontrolled Studies: Methylcobalamin Injections or oral B12				
6	218	25–75 µg/kg mB12 2–3x/week	Improved IQ, development and CARS scores. Improved GSH redox status associated with improved expressive communication, personal and domestic daily living skills, and interpersonal, play-leisure, and coping social skills. Improvements in adenosine, methionine, cysteine, tGSH, GSSG, SAM/SAH, tGSH/GSSG, coupling of Complex I and Citrate Synthase mitochondrial enzymes.	Hyperactivity, reduced sleep, and impulsiveness
Retrospective Case Series/Reports: Intramuscular Cobalamin Injections with Type of B12 not specified or oral B12				
6	32	IM B12 Different Forms	Improvements in vision, eye contact, pacing, echolalia, repetitive behaviors and nocturnal enuresis	Anemia on cB12 with improved on mB12

4.1. Improvements in Autism Symptoms with Cobalamin

Cobalamin treatment was found to result in improvements in both core and associated ASD symptoms. Three of the prospective studies examined changes in biochemistry and gave subcutaneously injected mB12 with two of the studies demonstrating overall clinical improvements and all studies suggesting improvements in a subgroup with unfavorable biochemistry. The study that did not show an overall effect used a DBPC crossover design but not a washout period between the crossover, potentially making it more difficult to observe a significant difference between treatment groups [55]. The other DBPC study did not use a crossover design and was able to document improvements as ranked by clinicians compared to placebo [35]. The other prospective study was open-label but differed in two critical ways from the others in its design: first, subcutaneous mB12 was combined with oral folinic acid, and second, only participants with unfavorable biochemical profiles consisting of decreased methylation capacity and decreased GSH redox ratio were entered into the study. This latter study demonstrated significant improvements on all subscales of the VABS with a moderate effect size (0.59) and an average improvement in skills development of 7.7 months during the three-month treatment period. This suggests that mB12 treatment with folinic acid might help some children with ASD "catch up" in development [53]. Other retrospective studies of injected B12 are consistent with these prospective studies, demonstrating improvement in physical health as well as core (e.g., eye contact, echolalia, and repetitive behaviors) and associated (e.g., hyperactivity) ASD behaviors [32,46,47].

Oral B12 combined with a MVI has been studied in several prospective controlled studies with these studies demonstrating improvements in physical medical issues such as gastrointestinal problems and sleep [48], as well as in behaviors such as hyperactivity and tantrums [49], and in cognitive skills, including language [49], non-verbal IQ and social skills [50]. Oral mB12 alone improved nocturnal enuresis in one study [54]. One study in which the route of treatment was not known found that mB12 gave similar improvements in both older and younger children as well as those with lower IQ. This suggests that even older and more severely affected individuals with ASD can improve with mB12 treatment [52].

4.2. Biochemical Effects of Cobalamin

Studies have reported a wide variety of improvements in biochemistry associated with B12 treatment, including improvements in methylation with injected [8,35] and oral [44,49] B12, redox metabolism with injected [8,11] and oral [49] B12 and mitochondrial function with oral [49] or unspecified [45] B12 treatment.

The meta-analysis examined whether there were consistent changes in biochemistry with B12 treatment. Changes in methylation were not found to be consistent when combining studies. However, homocysteine at baseline was markedly lower in the studies that demonstrated an increase in homocysteine with treatment (baseline homocysteine 6.7 ± 0.7 [8] and 4.8 ± 1.8 [11]) as compared to the study that demonstrated a decrease in homocysteine (baseline homocysteine 8.9 ± 1.0 [35]). Furthermore, even after treatment, in the studies where homocysteine started out lower, the post-treatment homocysteine concentrations were still lower than the post-treatment homocysteine in the study where homocysteine started out higher. This was most likely driven by differences in the design of the studies. In the two studies in which homocysteine was low, entry into the study required an unfavorable biochemistry profile [8,11], whereas, in the study with the higher homocysteine, no such criterion was implemented [35]. This may reflect that mB12 can drive homocysteine to an optimal concentration with the direction of change dependent on the starting concentration for the particular participant. Clearly, larger studies, which are sensitive to the baseline biochemical abnormalities, are needed to examine the complexity of the effect of mB12 on methylation. The meta-analysis did demonstrate significant improvements in transsulfuration and redox metabolism across studies with a medium to large effect size, suggesting that mB12 may be important for improving redox metabolism independent of the abnormalities in methylation metabolism.

The strongest evidence that the effect of B12 on biochemistry is clinically important is reflected in the studies which demonstrate that changes in biochemistry are associated with positive changes in clinical symptoms. Although one DBPC study of subcutaneously injected mB12 did not find an overall effect of mB12 on clinical outcomes, it did find that a subgroup of clinical "responders" showed improvements on the clinical global impression scale and at least two additional behavioral measures; these responders had significant improvements in GSH and the GSH redox ratio, suggesting these biomarkers could be used to predict response to mB12 treatment in children with ASD [55]. The second DBPC study of subcutaneously injected mB12 demonstrated that clinician-rated improvements were significantly and positively associated with improvements in methylation metabolism [35]. Finally, in another prospective study of subcutaneously injected mB12, significant improvements in the GSH redox ratio were significantly associated with clinical improvements, including expressive communication, personal and domestic daily living skills, and interpersonal, play-leisure, and coping social skills [53]. These findings further support the notion that certain biochemical abnormalities might predict treatment response to mB12 injections.

4.3. Biological Mechanisms of Actions

There are several potential biological mechanisms of action of B12 treatment. First, as demonstrated by the biochemical meta-analysis, subcutaneously injected mB12 consistently and significantly improves redox metabolism, including increasing Cysteine, GSH, and the GSH redox ratio as well as decreasing GSSG with medium to large effect sizes. A systematic review and meta-analysis have demonstrated that individuals with ASD overall demonstrate low GSH and Cysteine and increased GSSG across multiple research groups in multiple countries [57]. These redox metabolism abnormalities have been documented in multiple tissues in individuals with ASD, including in post-mortem brain [15,58]. In addition, these redox abnormalities have been shown to result in oxidative damage to DNA, protein, and lipids, as well as mitochondrial dysfunction and inflammation in the brain of individuals with ASD [15,59]. Thus, improving redox abnormalities can have widespread positive effects on the physiological function of the brain and other key important organs such as the immune system and GI tract in individuals with ASD.

Second, the brain of individuals with ASD has been repeatedly shown to have an excitatory/inhibitory imbalance such that the cortex is overexcited and underinhibited [60]. Glutamate is the major excitatory neurotransmitter of the cortex, thus decreasing glutamate neurotransmission is believed to be potentially therapeutic in ASD [61]. Glutamate is one of the three key precursors of GSH, along with cysteine and glycine. Thus, improved production of GSH, in part driven by mB12, may have other positive effects in neurotransmitter metabolism by reducing glutamate concentrations in the cortex (See Figure 3).

Third, polymorphisms in TCN2, the cobalamin binding protein, are associated with an increased risk of ASD [9], and ASD is one of the characteristics of some individuals with a mutation in TCN2 [51]. Thus, higher concentrations of B12 may be required in the blood in those with defects in the cobalamin binding protein in order to obtain sufficient levels of B12 into the tissues, including the brain.

Fourth, one controlled study reported a more than 3-fold reduction in mB12 concentration in brain tissue from individuals with ASD [58]. The reason for this finding is not clear but it is very possible that, such as the case with folate, some individuals with ASD may have a defect in the transport mechanism for B12 into the brain. Indeed, in one study, it was found that the folate receptor alpha autoantibody was associated with higher levels of blood cobalamin concentrations [62]. These higher blood concentrations of B12 could potentially be caused by B12 being blocked from uptake into the tissues. If such a transportation mechanism is present, a high blood concentration of B12 may be needed to overcome the blockage in the transportation mechanism, similar to the use of high dose folinic acid as a therapy for dysfunction of the folate receptor alpha [63]. Notably, one study reported that higher than normal serum concentrations of B12 was not associated with any observable adverse effects in individuals with ASD [52].

Fifth, methionine synthase, the key B12 dependent enzyme required for the proper functioning of the methylation cycle may be dysfunctional in the brain of individuals with ASD as one study observed that the mRNA for this enzyme is underexpressed in brain tissue of individuals with ASD [23]. Thus, high concentrations of B12 may be important to allow the limited amount of this enzyme to function optimally in the brain.

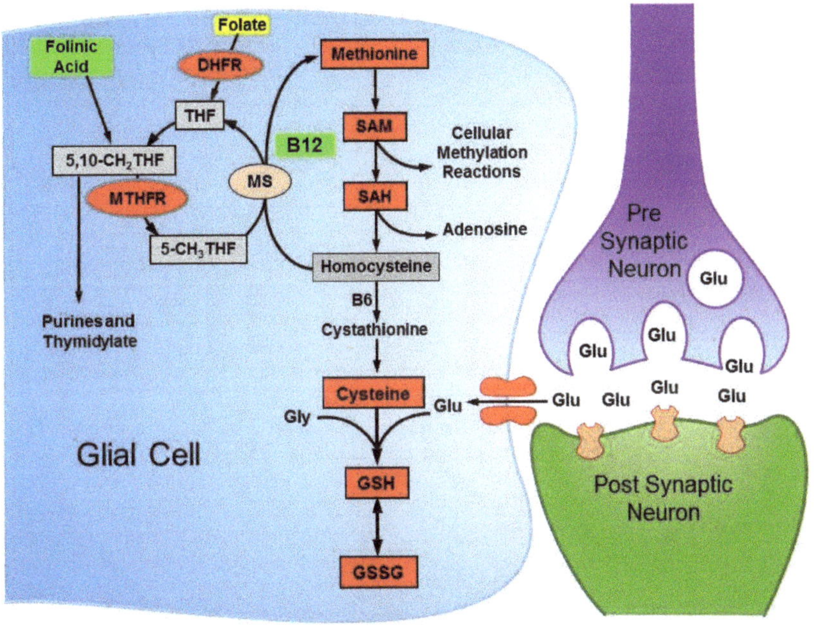

Figure 3. The production of glutathione results in the consumption of glutamate, the major excitatory neurotransmitter of the cortex, thus reducing glutamate in the brain. This diagram shows the connected folate, methylation, and redox metabolic pathways in the brain. Ovals represent enzymes and boxes represent metabolites. Red indicates metabolites and enzymes repeatedly noted to be consistently abnormal in ASD. Green highlights treatments that improve the metabolism of these cycles. Folic acid is shown in yellow as it is a suboptimal treatment because it is oxidized and has to be converted to active forms of folate.

Sixth, B12 could be helpful in improving mitochondrial function. Two studies reported improvements in mitochondrial-related markers in children with ASD. One prospective, controlled, single-blind 12-month study reported improvements in mitochondrial related markers including ATP, NADH, and NADPH with an oral MVI containing 500 mcg of B12 (50% as mB12 and 50% as cB12) along with other nutritional treatments [49]. In another prospective study in 127 children with ASD, B12 treatment was associated with the better coupling of Complex I and Citrate Synthase mitochondrial enzymes [45]. Since mitochondrial dysfunction is a common medical comorbidity in children with ASD [3,4], the use of B12 appears important in treating this problem.

Lastly, some individuals with ASD have lower intake and blood levels of B12 compared to controls. For example, a meta-analysis of 29 studies reported children with ASD had a significantly lower dietary intake of B12 compared to controls [64], while another meta-analysis of 16 studies found plasma B12 concentrations significantly lower in ASD compared to controls, although evidence of potential publication bias was found [5]. These finding may be due to feeding difficulties, which are common in individuals with ASD [65]. Thus, B12 treatment may be correcting a deficiency in some children with ASD. In addition, because the absorption of B12 orally may be dependent on adequate calcium intake [66], future studies examining the effect of calcium intake in conjunction with B12 might be helpful in ASD. Since some patients with ASD take multiple nutritional supplements, the potential interaction between B12 and other nutritional supplements also warrants further studies.

4.4. Formulation

Most studies (67%) that specified the route of administration used an injected form of B12. All studies that used the injected formulation and specified the type of B12 used mB12, except for one study, which initially used cB12 and changed to mB12. All studies that have linked changes in biochemistry with improvements in autism symptoms used subcutaneously injected mB12. The injected formulation is preferred by some practitioners because individuals with ASD may not be able to successfully take B12 orally due to GI disorders. Indeed, gastritis and enterocolitis may prevent optimal absorption while sensory aversions or esophagitis may prevent ASD children from easily swallowing a supplement [67,68]. Furthermore, as mentioned above, if there is a defect in B12 transportation in the blood or across the blood–brain barrier, higher blood concentrations of B12 may be needed to optimally deliver B12 into the organs, particularly the brain. It is possible that the GI tract is not even designed to absorb the necessary quantity of B12 that might be needed if indeed a problem with B12 transportation is present. Injected B12 may help raise the blood level higher than that achieved with oral B12.

A few studies combined B12 with other vitamins and/or minerals, thus these studies may reflect the combination of B12 with other supportive treatments. One study examined changes in biochemical markers of methylation and redox metabolism before and after adding betaine and folinic acid, and then after adding subcutaneously injected mB12 and found that the addition of mB12 to betaine and folinic acid both had a positive effect on methylation and redox metabolism [8]. Thus, in studies that have used other supportive treatments, B12 may have worked in concert with these other treatments. A recent randomized, single-blind study using a combination of various dietary and nutritional treatments in individuals with ASD, including essential fatty acids, Epsom salt baths, digestive enzymes, carnitine, and a MVI containing a combination of mB12 and cB12 reported significant improvements over one year compared to a control group that was not treated, suggesting a combination of treatments, which affect methylation and redox metabolism might lead to more robust improvements [50]. Further research will be needed to understand the optimal combination of treatments.

4.5. Adverse Events

The meta-analysis of AEs demonstrated a low incidence of AEs with most children tolerating the treatment without any AEs. Only one study described a potentially serious AE, anemia when using injected cB12. This AE resolved with changing to injected mB12. mB12 given by injection or orally has not been associated with any severe or serious AEs, perhaps suggesting that it is the preferred form of B12 for individuals with ASD at this time. After the completion of one study, 31/40 (78%) of parents indicated a desire to continue mB12 treatment [11,53]. This suggests that parents observed enough clinical improvements and a low enough rate of adverse effects to continue mB12 injections. Interestingly, although the majority of significant AEs reported pertained to worsening behavior and sleep, some studies have demonstrated significant improvements in such symptoms, including hyperactivity [32,49] and sleep [48], suggesting that overall many children have improvements in these key symptoms, and that having such symptoms at baseline is not necessarily a contraindication for starting B12 treatment. One study reported some individuals with ASD had above normal serum B12 levels with B12 treatment without any apparent AEs [52]. Finally, one retrospective study examined 24 children with ASD who received mB12 injections and compared urinary and plasma cobalt levels to 48 children who did not receive mB12 injections. These children were treated with the standard dose of mB12 used in the SC mB12 studies (75 μg/kg, injected every 1–3 days). The mean plasma cobalt concentration in the mB12 group was significantly elevated (0.82 ± 0.19 μg/L) compared to the untreated group (0.12 ± 0.10). The investigators noted that the study was limited as it could not determine what form of cobalt was present (free or bound in mB12), how the cobalt was distributed in the body, and what the tissue levels would be. Furthermore, no apparent adverse events from this finding were reported in the study [56]. Notably, adverse effects from serum cobalt are unlikely to occur with a blood cobalt concentration under 100 μg/L (using a conservative estimate), which is over 100 times the level reported in this aforementioned study [69]. Furthermore, no study has reported AEs consistent with cobalt toxicity (e.g., iron deficiency, pernicious anemia, cardiomyopathy, and polycythemia).

4.6. Limitation of Published Studies

Many studies demonstrated detection bias as only a few studies used standardized outcomes. This made it impossible to perform a meta-analysis across clinical outcomes. Second, although some studies were prospective, they were uncontrolled and unblinded and not randomized, opening up the possibility of selection and performance bias. Finally, the retrospective studies had the potential drawback of being open to attrition and reporting bias.

5. Conclusions

Overall, B12 appears to have evidence for effectiveness in individuals with ASD, particularly in those who have been identified with unfavorable biochemical profiles. In general, B12 appears to be very well-tolerated and safe. Two types of B12 have been studied in controlled and/or prospective clinical trials: (1) subcutaneously injected mB12 has evidence for improving clinical symptoms of ASD and improving methylation and redox metabolism, especially in those with unfavorable biochemistry and when combined with folinic acid (aka leucovorin) and (2) a mixture of cB12 and mB12 included in a MVI also appears to be associated with improvements in clinical symptoms, biochemistry, and physical medical disorders.

As mentioned above, the current set of studies have their limitations and should be used to design and implement well-controlled blinded randomized clinical trials in the future. Additionally, the ASD population is very heterogeneous, making it important to understand the subset of children with ASD in which B12 treatment may be most effective. There is evidence that B12, particularly subcutaneously injected mB12, may be particularly helpful for a subset of individuals with ASD with unfavorable biomarkers, suggesting that biomarkers need to be studied alongside clinical outcomes with a prior hypothesis regarding subgroups that may optimally respond to treatment. Thus, including reliable biomarkers that can guide treatment will be helpful to optimize this potentially important well-tolerated safe treatment.

Supplementary Materials: The following are available online at https://www.mdpi.com/article/10.3390/jpm11080784/s1, Supplementary Table S1: PRISMA Checklist.

Author Contributions: Conceptualization, methodology, formal analysis, writing—original draft preparation, review and editing, were performed by both D.A.R. and R.E.F. All authors have read and agreed to the published version of the manuscript.

Funding: The review did not receive any financial or grant support from any sources.

Institutional Review Board Statement: Not applicable. This review is not human research.

Informed Consent Statement: Not applicable. This review is not human research.

Data Availability Statement: All data are presented within the article.

Conflicts of Interest: The authors declare no conflict of interest.

References

1. Maenner, M.J.; Shaw, K.A.; Baio, J.; Washington, A.; Patrick, M.; DiRienzo, M.; Christensen, D.L.; Wiggins, L.D.; Pettygrove, S.; Andrews, J.G.; et al. Prevalence of autism spectrum disorder among children aged 8 years—Autism and developmental disabilities monitoring network, 11 sites, United States, 2016. *Morb. Mortal. Wkly. Rep. Surveill. Summ.* **2020**, *69*, 1–12. [CrossRef]
2. Hughes, H.K.; Mills Ko, E.; Rose, D.; Ashwood, P. Immune dysfunction and autoimmunity as pathological mechanisms in autism spectrum disorders. *Front. Cell. Neurosci.* **2018**, *12*, 405. [CrossRef]
3. Rossignol, D.A.; Frye, R.E. Mitochondrial dysfunction in autism spectrum disorders: A systematic review and meta-analysis. *Mol. Psychiatry* **2012**, *17*, 290–314. [CrossRef]

4. Rose, S.; Niyazov, D.M.; Rossignol, D.A.; Goldenthal, M.; Kahler, S.G.; Frye, R.E. Clinical and molecular characteristics of mitochondrial dysfunction in autism spectrum disorder. *Mol. Diagn. Ther.* **2018**, *22*, 571–593. [CrossRef]
5. Chen, L.; Shi, X.J.; Liu, H.; Mao, X.; Gui, L.N.; Wang, H.; Cheng, Y. Oxidative stress marker aberrations in children with autism spectrum disorder: A systematic review and meta-analysis of 87 studies (*N* = 9109). *Transl. Psychiatry* **2021**, *11*, 15. [CrossRef] [PubMed]
6. Lukmanji, S.; Manji, S.A.; Kadhim, S.; Sauro, K.M.; Wirrell, E.C.; Kwon, C.S.; Jette, N. The co-occurrence of epilepsy and autism: A systematic review. *Epilepsy Behav.* **2019**, *98*, 238–248. [CrossRef]
7. Madra, M.; Ringel, R.; Margolis, K.G. Gastrointestinal Issues and autism spectrum disorder. *Child Adolesc. Psychiatr. Clin. N. Am.* **2020**, *29*, 501–513. [CrossRef] [PubMed]
8. James, S.J.; Cutler, P.; Melnyk, S.; Jernigan, S.; Janak, L.; Gaylor, D.W.; Neubrander, J.A. Metabolic biomarkers of increased oxidative stress and impaired methylation capacity in children with autism. *Am. J. Clin. Nutr.* **2004**, *80*, 1611–1617. [CrossRef]
9. James, S.J.; Melnyk, S.; Jernigan, S.; Cleves, M.A.; Halsted, C.H.; Wong, D.H.; Cutler, P.; Bock, K.; Boris, M.; Bradstreet, J.J.; et al. Metabolic endophenotype and related genotypes are associated with oxidative stress in children with autism. *Am. J. Med. Genet. B Neuropsychiatr. Genet.* **2006**, *141B*, 947–956. [CrossRef] [PubMed]
10. Melnyk, S.; Fuchs, G.J.; Schulz, E.; Lopez, M.; Kahler, S.G.; Fussell, J.J.; Bellando, J.; Pavliv, O.; Rose, S.; Seidel, L.; et al. Metabolic imbalance associated with methylation dysregulation and oxidative damage in children with autism. *J. Autism Dev. Disord.* **2012**, *42*, 367–377. [CrossRef]
11. James, S.J.; Melnyk, S.; Fuchs, G.; Reid, T.; Jernigan, S.; Pavliv, O.; Hubanks, A.; Gaylor, D.W. Efficacy of methylcobalamin and folinic acid treatment on glutathione redox status in children with autism. *Am. J. Clin. Nutr.* **2009**, *89*, 425–430. [CrossRef]
12. Melnyk, S.; Jernigan, S.; Savenka, A.; James, S.J. Elevation in S-adenosylhomocysteine and DNA hypomethylation in parents and children with autism. *FASEB J.* **2007**, *21*, A348. [CrossRef]
13. Ladd-Acosta, C.; Hansen, K.D.; Briem, E.; Fallin, M.D.; Kaufmann, W.E.; Feinberg, A.P. Common DNA methylation alterations in multiple brain regions in autism. *Mol. Psychiatry* **2014**, *19*, 862–871. [CrossRef]
14. Nardone, S.; Sams, D.S.; Reuveni, E.; Getselter, D.; Oron, O.; Karpuj, M.; Elliott, E. DNA methylation analysis of the autistic brain reveals multiple dysregulated biological pathways. *Transl. Psychiatry* **2014**, *4*, e433. [CrossRef] [PubMed]
15. Rose, S.; Melnyk, S.; Pavliv, O.; Bai, S.; Nick, T.G.; Frye, R.E.; James, S.J. Evidence of oxidative damage and inflammation associated with low glutathione redox status in the autism brain. *Transl. Psychiatry* **2012**, *2*, e134. [CrossRef]
16. Guo, B.Q.; Ding, S.B.; Li, H.B. Blood biomarker levels of methylation capacity in autism spectrum disorder: A systematic review and meta-analysis. *Acta. Psychiatr. Scand.* **2020**, *141*, 492–509. [CrossRef] [PubMed]
17. Stathopoulos, S.; Gaujoux, R.; Lindeque, Z.; Mahony, C.; Van Der Colff, R.; Van Der Westhuizen, F.; O'Ryan, C. DNA methylation associated with mitochondrial dysfunction in a south african autism spectrum disorder cohort. *Autism Res.* **2020**, *13*, 1079–1093. [CrossRef]
18. Howsmon, D.P.; Kruger, U.; Melnyk, S.; James, S.J.; Hahn, J. Classification and adaptive behavior prediction of children with autism spectrum disorder based upon multivariate data analysis of markers of oxidative stress and DNA methylation. *PLoS Comput. Biol.* **2017**, *13*, e1005385. [CrossRef]
19. Ali, A.; Waly, M.I.; Al-Farsi, Y.M.; Essa, M.M.; Al-Sharbati, M.M.; Deth, R.C. Hyperhomocysteinemia among omani autistic children: A case-control study. *Acta. Biochim. Pol.* **2011**, *58*, 547–551. [CrossRef]
20. Altun, H.; Kurutas, E.B.; Sahin, N.; Gungor, O.; Findikli, E. The levels of vitamin D, vitamin D receptor, homocysteine and complex B vitamin in children with autism spectrum disorders. *Clin. Psychopharmacol. Neurosci.* **2018**, *16*, 383–390. [CrossRef] [PubMed]
21. Fuentes-Albero, M.; Cauli, O. Homocysteine levels in autism spectrum disorder: A clinical update. *Endocr. Metab. Immune Disord. Drug Targets* **2018**, *18*, 289–296. [CrossRef] [PubMed]
22. Guo, B.Q.; Li, H.B.; Ding, S.B. Blood homocysteine levels in children with autism spectrum disorder: An updated systematic review and meta-analysis. *Psychiatry Res.* **2020**, *291*, 113283. [CrossRef]
23. Muratore, C.R.; Hodgson, N.W.; Trivedi, M.S.; Abdolmaleky, H.M.; Persico, A.M.; Lintas, C.; De la Monte, S.; Deth, R.C. Age-dependent decrease and alternative splicing of methionine synthase mRNA in human cerebral cortex and an accelerated decrease in autism. *PLoS ONE* **2013**, *8*, e56927. [CrossRef] [PubMed]
24. Adams, J.B.; Baral, M.; Geis, E.; Mitchell, J.; Ingram, J.; Hensley, A.; Zappia, I.; Newmark, S.; Gehn, E.; Rubin, R.A.; et al. The severity of autism is associated with toxic metal body burden and red blood cell glutathione levels. *J. Toxicol.* **2009**, *2009*, 532640. [CrossRef] [PubMed]
25. James, S.J.; Rose, S.; Melnyk, S.; Jernigan, S.; Blossom, S.; Pavliv, O.; Gaylor, D.W. Cellular and mitochondrial glutathione redox imbalance in lymphoblastoid cells derived from children with autism. *FASEB J.* **2009**, *23*, 2374–2383. [CrossRef] [PubMed]
26. Chauhan, A.; Audhya, T.; Chauhan, V. Brain region-specific glutathione redox imbalance in autism. *Neurochem. Res.* **2012**, *37*, 1681–1689. [CrossRef]
27. Alberti, A.; Pirrone, P.; Elia, M.; Waring, R.H.; Romano, C. Sulphation deficit in "low-functioning" autistic children: A pilot study. *Biol. Psychiatry* **1999**, *46*, 420–424. [CrossRef]
28. Waring, R.H.; Ngong, J.M.; Klovrza, L.; Green, S.; Sharp, H. Biochemical parameters in autistic children. *Dev. Brain Dysfunct.* **1997**, *10*, 40–43.
29. Waring, R.H.; Klovrza, L.V. Sulphur metabolism in autism. *J. Nutr. Environ. Med.* **2000**, *10*, 25–32. [CrossRef]

30. Paul, C.; Brady, D.M. Comparative bioavailability and utilization of particular forms of B12 supplements with potential to mitigate B12-related genetic polymorphisms. *Integr. Med. Clin. J.* **2017**, *16*, 42–49.
31. Stollhoff, K.; Schulte, F.J. Vitamin B12 and brain development. *Eur. J. Pediatr.* **1987**, *146*, 201–205. [CrossRef] [PubMed]
32. Malhotra, S.; Subodh, B.N.; Parakh, P.; Lahariya, S. Brief report: Childhood disintegrative disorder as a likely manifestation of vitamin B12 deficiency. *J. Autism Dev. Disord.* **2013**, *43*, 2207–2210. [CrossRef] [PubMed]
33. Page, M.J.; McKenzie, J.E.; Bossuyt, P.M.; Boutron, I.; Hoffmann, T.C.; Mulrow, C.D.; Shamseer, L.; Tetzlaff, J.M.; Akl, E.A.; Brennan, S.E.; et al. The PRISMA 2020 statement: An updated guideline for reporting systematic reviews. *BMJ* **2021**, *372*, n71. [CrossRef]
34. Higgins, J.P.T.; Altman, D.G.; Sterne, J.A.C. Assessing risk of bias in included studies. In *Cochrane Handbook for Systematic Reviews of Interventions*, 5.1.0 ed.; Higgins, J.P.T., Green, S., Eds.; The Cochrane Collaboration: London, UK, 2011.
35. Hendren, R.L.; James, S.J.; Widjaja, F.; Lawton, B.; Rosenblatt, A.; Bent, S. Randomized, placebo-controlled trial of methyl B12 for children with autism. *J. Child Adolesc. Psychopharmacol.* **2016**, *26*, 774–783. [CrossRef]
36. Lipsey, M.; Wilson, D.B. The way in which intervention studies have "personality" and why it is important to meta-analysis. *Eval. Health Prof.* **2001**, *24*, 236–254.
37. Senn, S. Trying to be precise about vagueness. *Stat. Med.* **2007**, *26*, 1417–1430. [CrossRef] [PubMed]
38. Doi, S.A.; Barendregt, J.J.; Khan, S.; Thalib, L.; Williams, G.M. Advances in the meta-analysis of heterogeneous clinical trials I: The inverse variance heterogeneity model. *Contemp. Clin. Trials* **2015**, *45*, 130–138. [CrossRef]
39. Cohen, J. *Statistical Power Analysis for the Behavioral Sciences*, 2nd ed.; Lawrence Erlbaum Associates: Mahwah, NJ, USA, 2013. [CrossRef]
40. Higgins, J.P.; Thompson, S.G. Quantifying heterogeneity in a meta-analysis. *Stat. Med.* **2002**, *21*, 1539–1558. [CrossRef] [PubMed]
41. Higgins, J.P.; Thompson, S.G.; Deeks, J.J.; Altman, D.G. Measuring inconsistency in meta-analyses. *BMJ* **2003**, *327*, 557–560. [CrossRef]
42. Barendregt, J.J.; Doi, S.A.; Lee, Y.Y.; Norman, R.E.; Vos, T. Meta-analysis of prevalence. *J. Epidemiol. Community Health* **2013**, *67*, 974–978. [CrossRef] [PubMed]
43. Furuya-Kanamori, L.; Barendregt, J.J.; Doi, S.A.R. A new improved graphical and quantitative method for detecting bias in meta-analysis. *Int. J. Evid. Based Healthc.* **2018**, *16*, 195–203. [CrossRef]
44. Kaluzna-Czaplinska, J.; Michalska, M.; Rynkowski, J. Vitamin supplementation reduces the level of homocysteine in the urine of autistic children. *Nutr. Res.* **2011**, *31*, 318–321. [CrossRef] [PubMed]
45. Delhey, L.M.; Nur Kilinc, E.; Yin, L.; Slattery, J.C.; Tippett, M.L.; Rose, S.; Bennuri, S.C.; Kahler, S.G.; Damle, S.; Legido, A.; et al. The effect of mitochondrial supplements on mitochondrial activity in children with autism spectrum disorder. *J. Clin. Med.* **2017**, *6*, 18. [CrossRef]
46. Pineles, S.L.; Avery, R.A.; Liu, G.T. Vitamin B12 optic neuropathy in autism. *Pediatrics* **2010**, *126*, e967–e970. [CrossRef]
47. Duvall, M.G.; Pikman, Y.; Kantor, D.B.; Ariagno, K.; Summers, L.; Sectish, T.C.; Mullen, M.P. Pulmonary hypertension associated with scurvy and vitamin deficiencies in an autistic child. *Pediatrics* **2013**, *132*, e1699–e1703. [CrossRef] [PubMed]
48. Adams, J.B.; Holloway, C. Pilot study of a moderate dose multivitamin/mineral supplement for children with autistic spectrum disorder. *J. Altern. Complementary Med.* **2004**, *10*, 1033–1039. [CrossRef] [PubMed]
49. Adams, J.B.; Audhya, T.; McDonough-Means, S.; Rubin, R.A.; Quig, D.; Geis, E.; Gehn, E.; Loresto, M.; Mitchell, J.; Atwood, S.; et al. Effect of a vitamin/mineral supplement on children and adults with autism. *BMC Pediatr.* **2011**, *11*, 111. [CrossRef]
50. Adams, J.B.; Audhya, T.; Geis, E.; Gehn, E.; Fimbres, V.; Pollard, E.L.; Mitchell, J.; Ingram, J.; Hellmers, R.; Laake, D.; et al. Comprehensive nutritional and dietary intervention for autism spectrum disorder—A randomized, controlled 12-month trial. *Nutrients* **2018**, *10*, 369. [CrossRef]
51. Nashabat, M.; Maegawa, G.; Nissen, P.H.; Nexo, E.; Al-Shamrani, H.; Al-Owain, M.; Alfadhel, M. Long-term outcome of 4 patients with transcobalamin deficiency caused by 2 novel TCN2 mutations. *J. Pediatr. Hematol. Oncol.* **2017**, *39*, e430–e436. [CrossRef]
52. Nakano, K.; Noda, N.; Tachikawa, E.; Urano, M.A.N.; Takazawa, M.; Nakayama, T.; Sasaki, K.; Osawa, M. A preliminary study of methylcobalamin therapy in autism. *J. Tokyo Women's Med. Univ.* **2005**, *75*, 64–69.
53. Frye, R.E.; Melnyk, S.; Fuchs, G.; Reid, T.; Jernigan, S.; Pavliv, O.; Hubanks, A.; Gaylor, D.W.; Walters, L.; James, S.J. Effectiveness of methylcobalamin and folinic acid treatment on adaptive behavior in children with autistic disorder is related to glutathione redox status. *Autism Res. Treat.* **2013**, *2013*, 609705. [CrossRef] [PubMed]
54. Corejova, A.; Janosikova, D.; Pospisilova, V.; Rauova, D.; Kyselovic, J.; Hrabovska, A. Cessation of nocturnal enuresis after intervention with methylcobalamin in an 18-year-old patient with autism. *J. Child. Adolesc. Psychopharmacol.* **2015**, *25*, 821–823. [CrossRef]
55. Bertoglio, K.; Jill James, S.; Deprey, L.; Brule, N.; Hendren, R.L. Pilot study of the effect of methyl B12 treatment on behavioral and biomarker measures in children with autism. *J. Altern. Complementary Med.* **2010**, *16*, 555–560. [CrossRef] [PubMed]
56. Geier, D.A.; Geier, M.R. An autism cohort study of cobalt levels following vitamin B12 injections. *Toxicol. Environ. Chem.* **2010**, *92*, 1025–1037. [CrossRef]
57. Frustaci, A.; Neri, M.; Cesario, A.; Adams, J.B.; Domenici, E.; Dalla Bernardina, B.; Bonassi, S. Oxidative stress-related biomarkers in autism: Systematic review and meta-analyses. *Free Radic. Biol. Med.* **2012**, *52*, 2128–2141. [CrossRef] [PubMed]
58. Zhang, Y.; Hodgson, N.W.; Trivedi, M.S.; Abdolmaleky, H.M.; Fournier, M.; Cuenod, M.; Do, K.Q.; Deth, R.C. Decreased brain levels of vitamin B12 in aging, autism and schizophrenia. *PLoS ONE* **2016**, *11*, e0146797. [CrossRef]

59. Rossignol, D.A.; Frye, R.E. Evidence linking oxidative stress, mitochondrial dysfunction, and inflammation in the brain of individuals with autism. *Front. Physiol.* **2014**, *5*, 150. [CrossRef] [PubMed]
60. Frye, R.E.; Casanova, M.F.; Fatemi, S.H.; Folsom, T.D.; Reutiman, T.J.; Brown, G.L.; Edelson, S.M.; Slattery, J.C.; Adams, J.B. Neuropathological mechanisms of seizures in autism spectrum disorder. *Front. Neurosci.* **2016**, *10*, 192. [CrossRef]
61. Rossignol, D.A.; Frye, R.E. The use of medications approved for alzheimer's disease in autism spectrum disorder: A systematic review. *Front. Pediatrics* **2014**, *2*, 87. [CrossRef]
62. Frye, R.E.; Delhey, L.; Slattery, J.; Tippett, M.; Wynne, R.; Rose, S.; Kahler, S.G.; Bennuri, S.C.; Melnyk, S.; Sequeira, J.M.; et al. Blocking and binding folate receptor alpha autoantibodies identify novel autism spectrum disorder subgroups. *Front. Neurosci.* **2016**, *10*, 80. [CrossRef]
63. Frye, R.E.; Rossignol, D.A.; Scahill, L.; McDougle, C.J.; Huberman, H.; Quadros, E.V. Treatment of folate metabolism abnormalities in autism spectrum disorder. *Semin. Pediatr. Neurol.* **2020**, *35*, 100835. [CrossRef]
64. Esteban-Figuerola, P.; Canals, J.; Fernandez-Cao, J.C.; Arija Val, V. Differences in food consumption and nutritional intake between children with autism spectrum disorders and typically developing children: A meta-analysis. *Autism* **2019**, *23*, 1079–1095. [CrossRef]
65. Sharp, W.G.; Berry, R.C.; McCracken, C.; Nuhu, N.N.; Marvel, E.; Saulnier, C.A.; Klin, A.; Jones, W.; Jaquess, D.L. Feeding problems and nutrient intake in children with autism spectrum disorders: A meta-analysis and comprehensive review of the literature. *J. Autism Dev. Disord.* **2013**, *43*, 2159–2173. [CrossRef] [PubMed]
66. Bauman, W.A.; Shaw, S.; Jayatilleke, E.; Spungen, A.M.; Herbert, V. Increased intake of calcium reverses vitamin B12 malabsorption induced by metformin. *Diabetes Care* **2000**, *23*, 1227–1231. [CrossRef] [PubMed]
67. Walker, S.J.; Langefeld, C.D.; Zimmerman, K.; Schwartz, M.Z.; Krigsman, A. A molecular biomarker for prediction of clinical outcome in children with ASD, constipation, and intestinal inflammation. *Sci. Rep.* **2019**, *9*, 5987. [CrossRef] [PubMed]
68. Esnafoglu, E.; Cirrik, S.; Ayyildiz, S.N.; Erdil, A.; Erturk, E.Y.; Dagli, A.; Noyan, T. Increased serum zonulin levels as an intestinal permeability marker in autistic subjects. *J. Pediatr.* **2017**, *188*, 240–244. [CrossRef]
69. Leyssens, L.; Vinck, B.; Van Der Straeten, C.; Wuyts, F.; Maes, L. Cobalt toxicity in humans—A review of the potential sources and systemic health effects. *Toxicology* **2017**, *387*, 43–56. [CrossRef] [PubMed]

Journal of
Personalized Medicine

MDPI

Article

Ratings of the Effectiveness of Nutraceuticals for Autism Spectrum Disorders: Results of a National Survey

James B. Adams [1,*], Anisha Bhargava [2], Devon M. Coleman [1], Richard E. Frye [3] and Daniel A. Rossignol [4]

1 School of Engineering of Matter, Transport, and Energy, Arizona State University, P.O. Box 876106, Tempe, AZ 85287, USA; devon_marie@live.com
2 Columbia Mailman School of Public Health, 722 W. 168th St., New York, NY 10032, USA; abharg25@asu.edu
3 Section of Neurodevelopmental Disorders, Division of Neurology, Barrow Neurological Institute at Phoenix Children's Hospital, 1919 E Thomas Rd., Phoenix, AZ 85016, USA; rfrye@phoenixchildrens.com
4 Rossignol Medical Center, 24541 Pacific Park Drive, Suite 210, Aliso Viejo, CA 92656, USA; rossignolmd@gmail.com
* Correspondence: jim.adams@asu.edu; Tel.: +1-480-965-3316

Abstract: Autism spectrum disorder (ASD) often involves a wide range of co-occurring medical conditions ("comorbidities") and biochemical abnormalities such as oxidative stress and mitochondrial dysfunction. Nutritional supplements ("Nutraceuticals") are often used to treat both core ASD symptoms and comorbidities, but some have not yet been formally evaluated in ASD. The potential biological mechanisms of nutraceuticals include correction of micronutrient deficiencies due to a poor diet and support for metabolic processes such as redox regulation, mitochondrial dysfunction and melatonin production. This paper reports on the results of the National Survey on Treatment Effectiveness for Autism, focusing on nutraceuticals. The Survey involved 1286 participants from across the United States. Participants rated the overall perceived benefits and adverse effects of each nutraceutical, and also indicated the specific symptoms changed and adverse effects. From these ratings the top-rated nutraceuticals for each of 24 symptoms are listed. Compared to psychiatric and seizure medications rated through the same Survey, on average nutraceuticals had significantly higher ratings of Overall Benefit (1.59 vs. 1.39, $p = 0.01$) and significantly lower ratings of Overall Adverse Effects (0.1 vs. 0.9, $p < 0.001$). Folinic acid and vitamin B12 were two of the top-rated treatments. This study suggests that nutraceuticals may have clinical benefits and favorable adverse effect profiles.

Keywords: autism; autism spectrum disorder; nutraceuticals; survey; vitamins; minerals; B12; folinic acid

Citation: Adams, J.B.; Bhargava, A.; Coleman, D.M.; Frye, R.E.; Rossignol, D.A. Ratings of the Effectiveness of Nutraceuticals for Autism Spectrum Disorders: Results of a National Survey. *J. Pers. Med.* **2021**, *11*, 878. https://doi.org/10.3390/jpm11090878

Academic Editor: Elizabeth B. Torres

Received: 27 July 2021
Accepted: 29 August 2021
Published: 31 August 2021

Publisher's Note: MDPI stays neutral with regard to jurisdictional claims in published maps and institutional affiliations.

Copyright: © 2021 by the authors. Licensee MDPI, Basel, Switzerland. This article is an open access article distributed under the terms and conditions of the Creative Commons Attribution (CC BY) license (https://creativecommons.org/licenses/by/4.0/).

1. Introduction

Autism spectrum disorder (ASD) is a complex neurodevelopmental disorder involving core problems in social communication and repetitive behaviors and affects about 2% of children in the United States [1]. A number of medical conditions cooccur with ASD (termed "comorbidities"), including intellectual disability [2], epilepsy [3], gastrointestinal disorders (such as constipation and diarrhea) [4], sleep disorders [5], attention deficit disorder [5], anxiety [5], and irritability, self-injurious behavior, and depression [6]. Other studies have reported biochemical abnormalities, including problems with methylation pathway insufficiency [7,8], insufficient production of melatonin for sleep [9], mitochondrial dysfunction [10,11] and oxidative stress [12,13]. Currently, there are no FDA-approved medications for treating the core symptoms of ASD (social communication and restricted/repetitive behaviors), although there are two FDA-approved medications for treating the associated symptom of irritability [14].

Compared to typically developing (TD) children, feeding difficulties are common in children with ASD and include food refusal, eating a limited variety of foods and having more problems with mealtime behavior [15], and they may have nutrient-poor diets [16]. One meta-analysis of 17 prospectively controlled studies reported significantly more feeding problems in children with ASD compared to controls (odd ratios 5.11, 95% CI 3.74–6.97) and significantly lower intake of calcium and protein in the ASD group [17]. A systematic review of 29 studies reported that feeding problems were associated with impaired sensory processing, perception, more rigidity and challenging behaviors [18]. A prospective, randomized controlled trial of a comprehensive dietary and nutritional intervention found that a combination of six treatments (vitamins/minerals, essential fatty acids, Epsom salts, carnitine, digestive enzymes, and a healthy low-allergen diet) led to significant improvements over one year in autism symptoms, developmental age, and non-verbal IQ compared to controls [19].

Because of potential deficiencies of nutrients (often related to feeding problems) and biochemical abnormalities (e.g., oxidative stress, mitochondrial dysfunction, methylation problems, among others) reported in individuals with ASD, a number of studies have investigated the use of vitamins, minerals, and other nutritional supplements (hereafter termed "Nutraceuticals"). The use of nutraceuticals is typically considered a form of complementary and alternative medicine (CAM), although many nutraceuticals are based on the science of nutritional biochemistry and target deficiencies and biochemical problems. Owen-Smith et al. (2015) conducted a survey of 42 CAM treatments used in ASD and reported 88% of participants had been treated with at least one CAM treatment [20]. Frye et al. (2011) surveyed the effectiveness of seizure treatments (including nutraceuticals) in 733 children with ASD and seizures compared to 290 controls and reported some CAM treatments (such as vitamin B6, magnesium, taurine, and vitamin B12) were rated as helpful for treating seizures [21]. In addition, a large online survey was conducted by the Autism Research Institute (the "Parent Ratings of Behavioral Effects of Biomedical Interventions Survey") [22]. This survey of 27,000 parents of individuals with ASD rated the effectiveness of 84 various medications, supplements, and diets, using a six-point scale from "made worse" to "made better"; a number of treatments were reported as beneficial, including methylcobalamin (MB12), melatonin, digestive enzymes, fatty acids, cod liver oil, vitamin B6, zinc, magnesium, folic acid, vitamin C, and vitamin A [23]. Although these surveys focused on the overall effectiveness ratings for medications and nutraceuticals used in ASD individuals, most of these studies did not utilize a separate rating scale for the benefits and adverse effects (AEs) and did not obtain information on the effects of these treatments on specific symptoms of ASD.

Some of the medical comorbidities and biochemical abnormalities reported in individuals with ASD might improve with nutraceuticals. For example, randomized clinical trials for ASD have demonstrated the efficacy of melatonin supplementation [9], folinic acid [24–26], vitamin/mineral supplements [27,28], comprehensive nutritional interventions [19], N-acetyl cysteine (NAC) [29], and sulforaphane [30].

This paper presents the results of a national survey (the "National Survey on Treatment Effectiveness for Autism") in individuals with ASD and contains more extensive assessments of the treatment effects on specific behaviors and AEs of nutraceuticals in ASD. A previous paper from this Survey reported on the results for psychiatric and seizure medications [31].

2. Materials and Methods

The research team created the "National Survey on Treatment Effectiveness for Autism" (from now on referred to as "the Survey") and obtained reviews by families of children/adults with ASD and experts in a variety of fields who treat individuals with ASD. This study was approved by the Institutional Review Board of Arizona State University (STUDY00003766). The Survey was advertised to families of individuals with ASD across the country with the assistance of over 50 autism organizations (see Acknowledgements). A full explanation of the Survey creation and distribution can be found in the previous paper [31]. The Survey obtained general medical history and the use of psychiatric and seizure medications, general medications, nutraceuticals, diets, therapies, and information on Kindergarten through grade 12 education. This paper reports data only on the nutraceutical section from Survey responses from 1710 people (of which 1286 (75.2%) rated the effects of nutraceuticals); additional responses were collected since the analysis reported in the previous paper. The exact diagnosis of the individual with ASD was queried using the following categories: autism, Asperger's syndrome, autism spectrum disorder, high-functioning autism, pervasive developmental disorder not otherwise specified (PDD-NOS), no current diagnosis but was previously on the autism spectrum, and "other" in order to capture both DSM-IV and DSM-5 diagnostic categories. These diagnoses were reported by the participant, but not verified in this study since it was an anonymous survey.

The Survey was divided into sub-sections for various types of nutraceuticals (amino acids, vitamins, etc.). At the beginning of each sub-section, the Survey asked what nutraceuticals the participant had taken (from a list of 123 nutraceuticals found in Table S1). For each nutraceutical taken, the Survey asked the participant to rate the overall perceived benefit of the nutraceutical (no benefit = 0, slight benefit = 1, moderate benefit = 2, good benefit = 3, great benefit = 4), the primary symptoms benefited (if any), the overall AE of the nutraceutical (no adverse effect = 0, mild adverse effect = 1, moderate adverse effect = 2, severe adverse effect = 3), and the specific symptoms that were adversely affected (if any). Table 1 shows the symptom list from which participants could select (they could select one or more for each treatment). Finally, the Survey asked for the overall average effect of all nutraceuticals (on a 7-point scale ranging from "much better" to "much worse"). Only treatments with 20 or more responses were included in this analysis. It should be noted that the ratings are the perceived benefit of the evaluator (primarily a caregiver or sometimes the person with ASD), and not ratings by a clinician or physician, which is a limitation of the study.

For each treatment, the top 3 benefits were reported as well as any other benefits with over 20% of participants reporting a benefit. For AEs, the top 3 AEs were reported and any other AEs which were reported by 15% or more of participants. These were arbitrary cut-offs to limit table entries to the most relevant symptoms; a slightly lower cut-off for AEs was chosen since they were so rare.

The top-rated treatments for each symptom were calculated by multiplying the overall net benefit by the percentage of participants who had improvements in that symptom. For each symptom, the three top-rated treatments are reported, as well as any other treatments with a score of 0.2 or higher (equivalent to 10% of participants reporting a moderate benefit).

In order to determine if any of the nutraceuticals were related to changes in ASD severity, two questions were asked on the Survey. Specifically, the ASD severity rated at 3 years of age (which would be close to most patient's diagnosis) was compared to the currently rated ASD severity. The categories of severity were coded on a five-point scale with increasing numeric values corresponding to increasing severity. Specifically, no symptoms (0), very mild symptoms (1), mild symptoms (2), moderate symptoms (3), and severe symptoms (4). The current ASD severity was subtracted from the severity at baseline (3 years of age) such that a decrease in severity would indicate an improvement. The generalized linear model performed in IBM SPSS PASW Release 18.0.0 (Armonk, New York) was used to analyze change in severity. The model included gender (male, female), developmental profile, number of antibiotic treatments in the first 3 years of life (since that has been reported higher in ASD), and baseline ASD severity. In general, only treatments that were used by 100 respondents or more were analyzed to ensure generalizability and a wide range of ASD severity changes. Two different approaches were used. First, it was determined whether use of the nutraceutical was associated with improvements in ASD symptoms by comparing those who used the nutraceutical to those who did not. Second, the association between the perceived benefits of the nutraceutical with the change in ASD symptoms was examined by comparing current ASD severity versus severity at 3 years old. This later analysis including an interaction between treatment and severity at 3 years of age in order to determine whether the change in severity associated with the treatment was affected by the severity of ASD at age 3 years of age. A one-way analysis of variance was also used to determine whether severity at 3 years of age was related to the use of any treatment studied.

Table 1. All Symptom Options.

Benefited Symptom Options	Adverse Symptom Options
General benefit, no one particular symptom	General worsening, no one specific symptom
Aggression/Agitation	Aggression/Agitation
Anxiety	Anxiety
Attention	Bedwetting/Bladder Control
Cognition (ability to think)	Behavior problems
Constipation	Decreased cognition (difficulty thinking/remembering)
Depression	Depression
Diarrhea	Dizziness/Unsteadiness
Eczema/Skin problem	Dry mouth
Health (fewer illnesses and/or less severe illnesses)	Fatigue/Drowsiness
Hyperactivity	Gastrointestinal problems
Irritability	Headache/Migraine
Language/Communication	Hyperactivity
Lethargy (easily tired)	Irritability
OCD	Liver/Kidney problem
Reflux/Vomiting	Loss of appetite
Seizures	Nausea
Self-Injury	Rash
Sensory Sensitivity	Seizures
Sleep (falling asleep)	Self-injury
Sleep (staying asleep)	Sleep Problems
Social Interaction and Understanding	Stimming/Perseveration/Desire for Sameness
Stimming/Perseveration/Desire for Sameness	Tics/Abnormal movements
Tics/Abnormal movements	Weight gain
	Weight loss

3. Results

3.1. Demographics and Medical History

The characteristics of the 1286 participants and their medical history are outlined in Table 2. The majority of the surveys were completed by the primary caregiver of an individual with ASD (85%). More than half of the surveys were for children under 13 years old (54%), with 21% for teenagers and 16% for young adults (18 years or older). Seventy six percent of participants were male, and 24% were female. Autism was the most frequent diagnosis (43%), followed by Autism Spectrum Disorder (22%) and Asperger's syndrome (14%). The most common developmental history was "Abnormal development from early infancy, with no major regression or plateau in development" (32%). Furthermore, most participants received antibiotics during their first 3 years of life, with a median of 3 rounds. Most participants had moderate autism-related symptoms at age 3 years old (38%) and currently (38%).

Table 2. Completion, Age, Gender, Medical Diagnosis, Developmental History, and Antibiotic Use.

	N	%
Survey Completed By		
Primary Caregiver of an Individual with Autism	1094	85%
Adult with High-Functioning Autism 18 years or older who does not have a guardianship	89	7%
Adult with Autism with their Mother/Father/Childhood Guardian	39	3%
Grandparent of an Individual with Autism [1]	58	5%
Other	6	0%
Age of Participant		
Child (under 13 years old)	692	54%
Teenager (13–17 years old)	274	21%
Young Adult (18–30 years old)	202	16%
Adult (over 30 years old)	116	9%
Gender of Participant		
Male	973	76%
Female	305	24%
Other	5	0%
Current Medical Diagnosis		
Autism	548	43%
Asperger's Syndrome	186	14%
Autism Spectrum Disorder	289	22%
High-Functioning Autism	148	12%
Pervasive Developmental Disorder—Not Otherwise Specified (PDD-NOS)	76	6%
No current diagnosis, but he/she was on the autism spectrum previously	18	1%
Other	21	2%
Developmental History		
Abnormal development from early infancy, with no major regression or plateau in development	410	32%
Normal development, followed by a plateau in development that lasted for several months or longer	284	22%
Normal development, followed by major regression	278	22%
Normal development, followed by a major regression and a plateau lasting several months or longer	168	13%
Other	127	10%
Number of Rounds of Antibiotics during the first three years of life		
Average	9.3	
Median	3.0	
None	148	14%
1 Round	183	17%
2 Rounds	138	13%
3 Rounds	163	15%
4 Rounds	67	6%
5 Rounds	63	6%

Table 2. *Cont.*

	N	%
6–7 Rounds	79	7%
8–10 Rounds	90	8%
11–15 Rounds	35	3%
16–20 Rounds	22	2%
21+ Rounds	84	8%
Severity of autism-related symptoms at age 3		
No autistic symptoms	50	4%
Nearly normal, with only very mild symptoms	227	18%
Mild autism	290	23%
Moderate autism	474	38%
Severe autism	222	18%
Severity of autism-related symptoms currently		
No autistic symptoms	14	1%
Nearly normal, with only very mild symptoms	200	16%
Mild autism	390	31%
Moderate autism	475	38%
Severe autism	186	15%

[1]. Grandparents were taken from those responded with "other" and noted they were grandparents. Numbers may not add up to 100% due to rounding.

3.2. Nutraceuticals

Of the 123 nutraceuticals included in the Survey (found in Supplemental Table S1), 58 had 20 or more responses and are reported here. These nutraceuticals are reported in eight general categories—the categories and the number of nutraceuticals for each category are: amino acids (4), essential fatty acids (7), glutathione-related nutraceuticals (4), individual minerals (9), individual vitamins/vitamin-like nutraceuticals (22), multivitamins (3), sleep treatments (3), and others (5). The most commonly used treatments were generic child/adult multivitamin (34%), melatonin (29%), omega 3 fatty acids (15%), vitamin C (14%), krill oil (13%), fish oil (13%), vitamin D (12%), magnesium (12%), Epsom salts (11%), and zinc (10%).

3.2.1. Amino Acids

Amino Acids were rated as having a slight to moderate (1.1 to 1.6) overall perceived benefit with minimal AEs (0.1 to 0.4). For the amino acid blend, glutamine and taurine, the primary benefit was general benefit (43–57%) with small benefits in other symptoms. For tryptophan, the primary benefits were helping with falling asleep and staying asleep (see Table S2 and Figure 1).

3.2.2. Fatty Acids

Fatty Acids (FA) were rated as having a moderate to good benefit (1.2 to 2) with minimal overall AEs (0 to 0.2). For all FAs, the primary benefit was general benefit (32% to 59%), with secondary benefits in attention and cognition. See Table S3 and Figure 2.

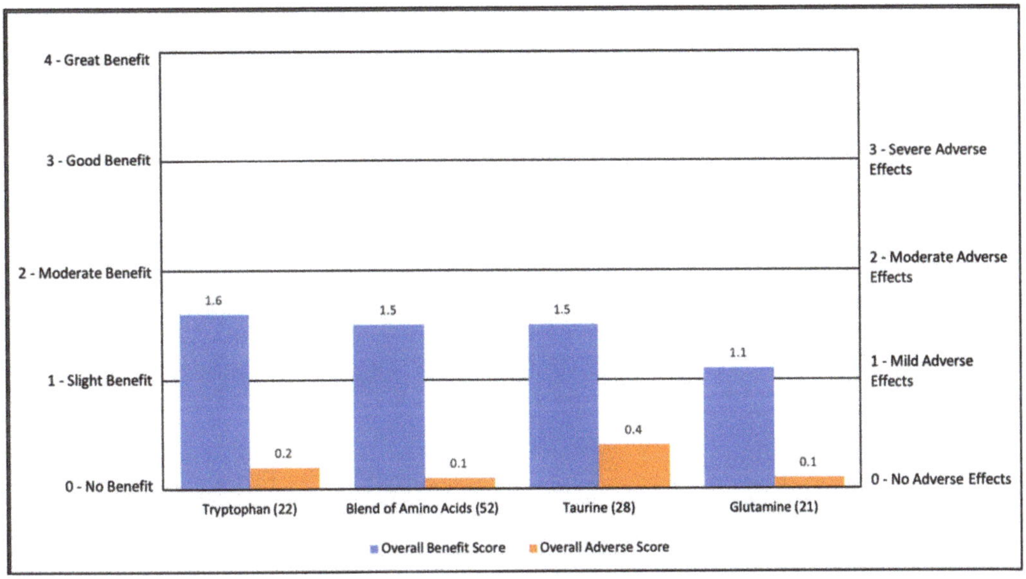

Figure 1. Overall Benefit Score and Adverse Effect Score for Amino Acid Treatments from Highest Overall Benefit to Lowest Overall Benefit.

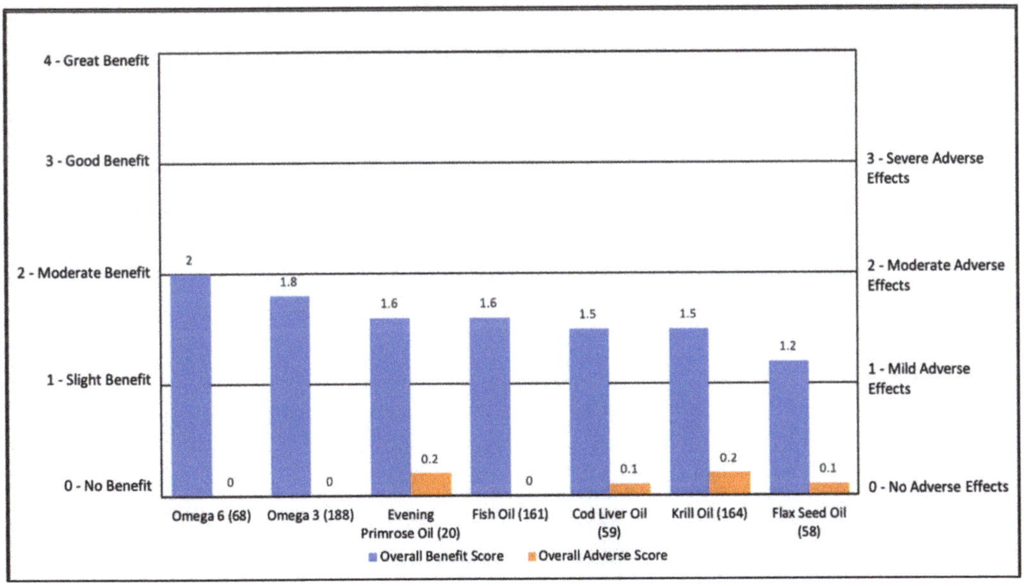

Figure 2. Overall Benefit Score and Adverse Effect Score for Fatty Acid Treatments from Highest Overall Benefit to Lowest Overall Benefit.

3.2.3. Glutathione-Related Nutraceuticals

Glutathione-related nutraceuticals (including NAC) were rated as having a slight to moderate benefit (1.1 to 1.7) with minimal AEs (0 to 0.3). The most common benefit was general benefit (4% to 56%). See Table S3 and Figure 3.

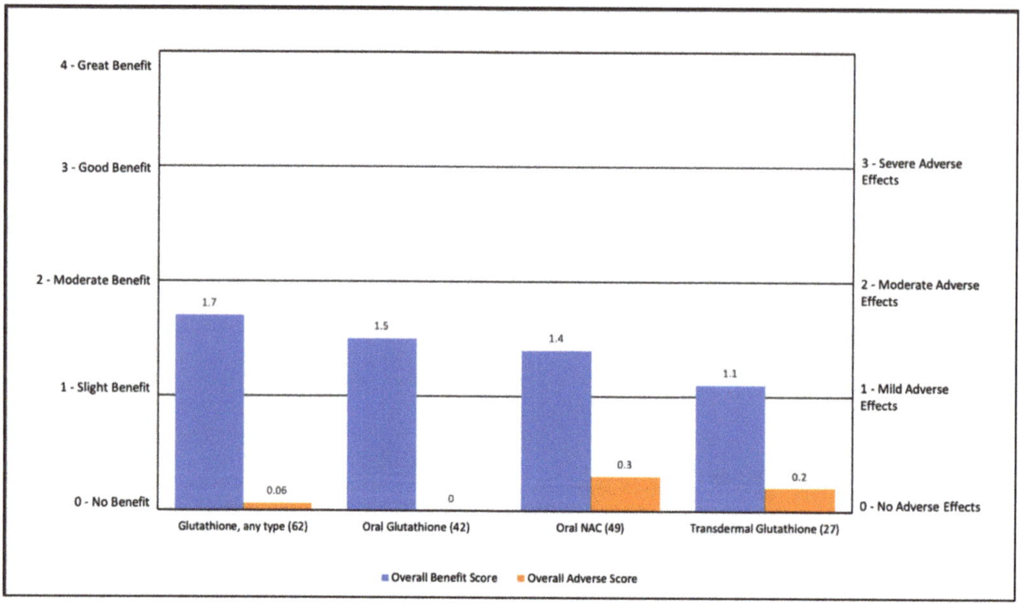

Figure 3. Overall Benefit Score and Adverse Effect Score for Glutathione-Related Treatments from Highest Overall Benefit to Lowest Overall Benefit.

3.2.4. Individual Minerals

Individual minerals were rated as having a slight to moderate benefit (1.3 to 2.1) with minimal AEs (0–0.3). The most common benefit was general benefit (15% to 70%). Lithium also helped with anxiety (24%), and magnesium helped with constipation (27%). Iron caused some gastrointestinal adverse effects in 17%. See Table S4 and Figure 4.

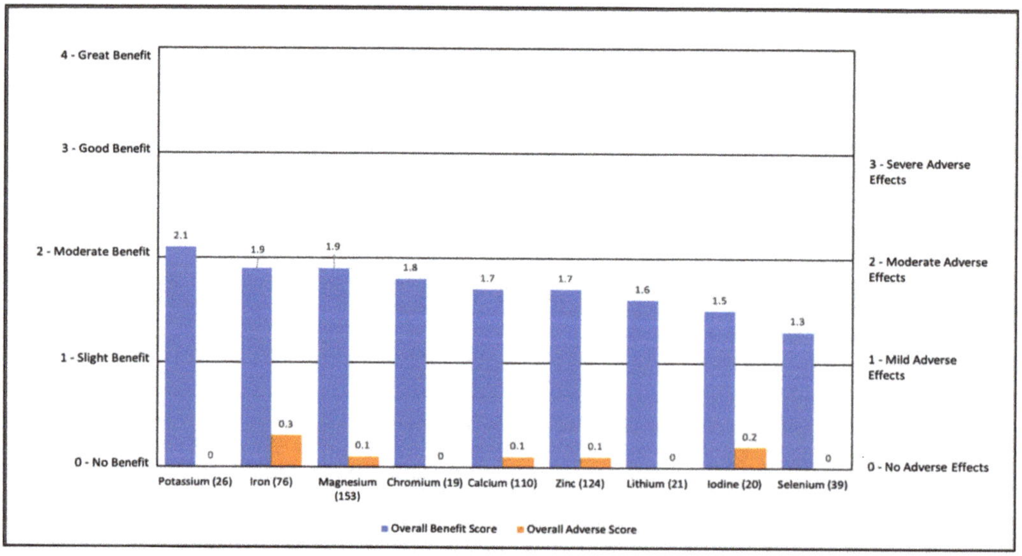

Figure 4. Overall Benefit Score and Adverse Event Score for Individual Minerals from Highest Overall Benefit to Lowest Overall Benefit.

3.2.5. Individual Vitamins/Vitamin-like Nutraceuticals

Individual vitamins and vitamin-like nutraceuticals were rated as having slight to moderate overall benefits (1.0 to 2.2) with minimal AEs (0 to 0.3). The most common benefit was general overall benefit (14% to 62%). High dose folinic acid (above 5 mg/day) improved cognition (33%), attention (29%), and language/communication (24%). Moderate dose folinic acid (below 5 mg/day) also improved language/communication (20%). P5P improved anxiety (20%) and TMG improved language/communication (29%). Injected vitamin B12 improved language/communication (30%), cognition (28%), and attention (20%). Oral vitamin B12 improved cognition (25%) and language/communication (18%). Vitamin C also improved overall health (27%). See Table S6 and Figure 5.

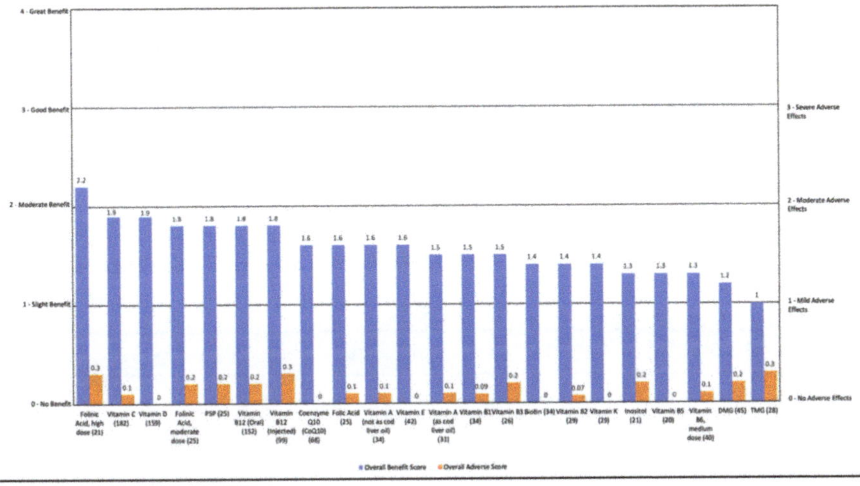

Figure 5. Overall Benefit Score and Adverse Event Score for Individual Vitamins/Vitamin-like Nutraceuticals from Highest Overall Benefit to Lowest Overall Benefit.

3.2.6. Multivitamins

Multivitamins were rated as having a slight to moderate benefit (1.4 to 1.9) with minimal AEs (0.0 to 0.2). The most common benefit was general benefit (50–55%). High dose multivitamin also improved general health (26%), and a high dose multivitamin, specifically designed for ASD, improved cognition (21%). See Table S7 and Figure 6.

3.2.7. Sleep-Related Nutraceuticals

Sleep-related nutraceuticals were rated as having slight to moderate benefit (1.2–2.1), with minimal AEs (0.1 to 0.3). The primary benefit was falling asleep (36–74%), followed by staying asleep (27–35%). For 5-HTP, there was also a general benefit (27%). See Table S8 and Figure 7. It is noteworthy that melatonin had the highest overall benefit score and was used by a very high number of participants.

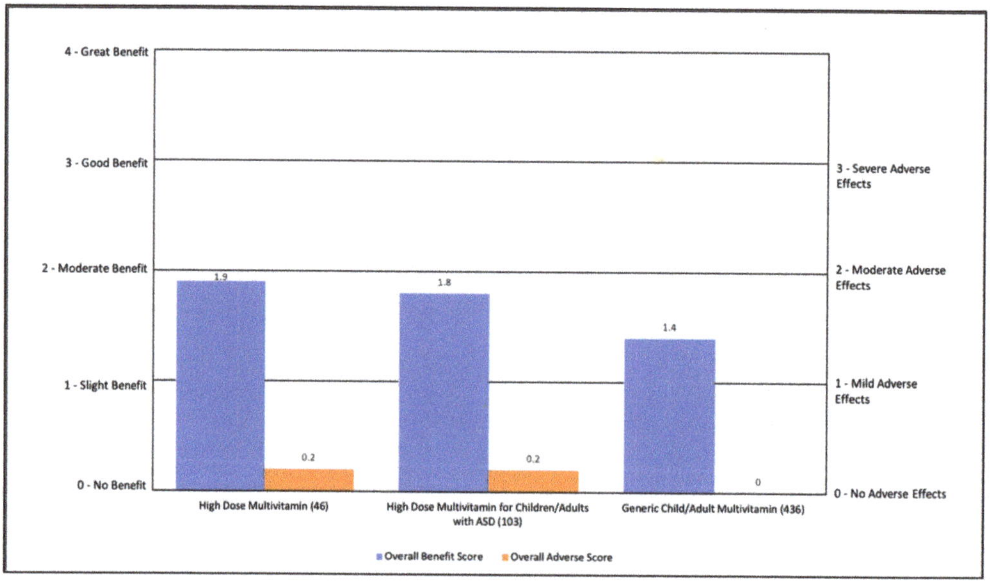

Figure 6. Overall Benefit Score and Adverse Event Score for Multivitamins from Highest Overall Benefit to Lowest Overall Benefit.

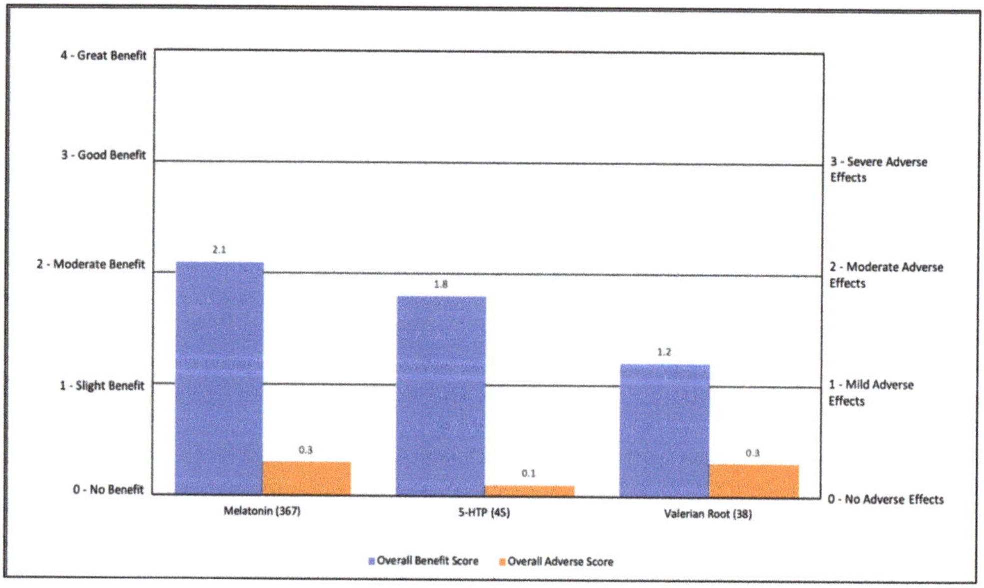

Figure 7. Overall Benefit Score and Adverse Event Score for Sleep Treatments from Highest Overall Benefit to Lowest Overall Benefit.

3.2.8. Other Miscellaneous Nutraceuticals

For other miscellaneous nutraceuticals, the general benefit ranged from 1.3 to 2.2 (slight to moderate benefit) with minimal AEs (0.0 to 0.2). All of these nutraceuticals had improvements in general benefit (22% to 67%). Epsom salts improved aggression/agitation (35%) and attention (26%). A fruit/vegetable powder concentrate also improved constipation (24%) and general health (24%). GABA improved anxiety (26%). See Table S9 and Figure 8.

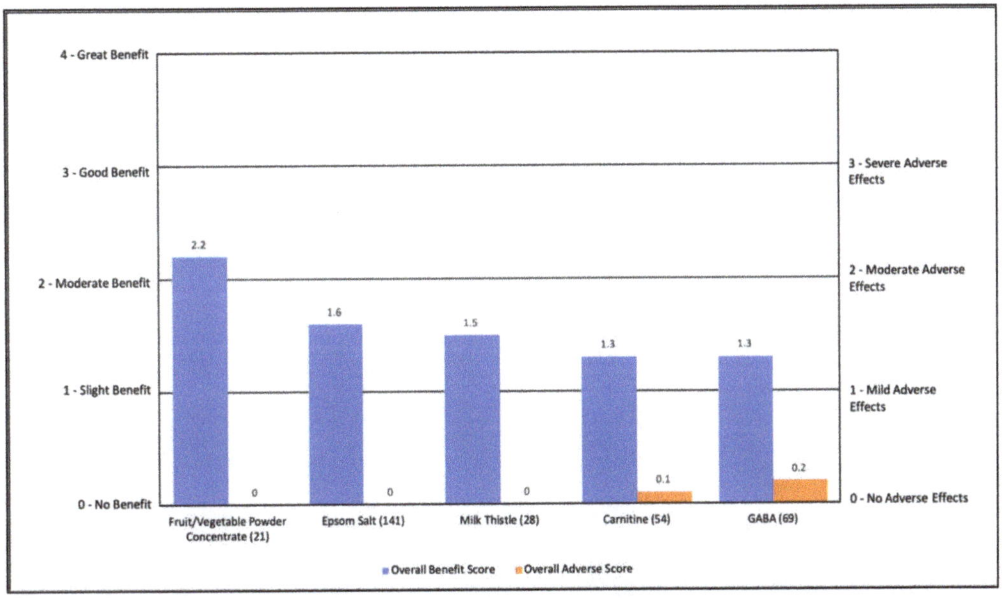

Figure 8. Overall Benefit Score and Adverse Effect Score for Other Miscellaneous Nutraceuticals from Highest Overall Benefit to Lowest Overall Benefit.

3.2.9. Average of All Nutraceuticals

Averaging all the nutraceuticals reported in this paper, the average Overall Benefit and Overall AE was 1.6 (SD = 0.3) and 0.1 (SD = 0.1), respectively, reflecting that participants reported on average slight to moderate benefits with minimal adverse effects.

3.2.10. Top Nutraceuticals by Symptom

Table 3 presents the top-rated nutraceuticals for 24 different symptoms. For most symptoms, nutraceuticals were moderately effective (net benefit scores >0.25), including aggression/agitation, anxiety, attention, cognition, constipation, diarrhea, general benefit, health, hyperactivity, irritability, language/communication, falling asleep, staying asleep, and social interaction/understanding. Other symptoms were only slightly affected (net benefit scores between 0.10 and 0.25) such as depression, eczema/skin problems, lethargy, obsessive-compulsive symptoms, reflux/vomiting, sensory sensitivity, stimming and tics/involuntary movements (Table 3).

It is important to note that less common problems, such as seizures, might receive lower scores since fewer individuals have these problems. These ratings should be interpreted cautiously, as they are averages, but they suggest which treatments families sensed were most helpful for a given symptom, which can potentially help guide treatment selection and future research.

Table 3. Top Nutraceuticals for Symptoms from Highest Overall Net Benefit Rating to Lowest Overall Net Benefit Rating.

Symptoms	Nutraceuticals (Overall Net Benefit Rating)
General benefit, no one particular symptom	Fruit/Vegetable Powder Concentrate (1.49), Potassium (1.30), Omega 6 (1.18), Vitamin C (1.05), Vitamin D (1.00), CoQ10 (1.00), High Dose Folinic Acid (1.00), Chromium (0.97), Vitamin E (0.95), Iodine (0.95), General Glutathione (0.92), Moderate Dose Folinic acid (0.92), High Dose Multivitamin (0.91), Folic Acid (0.89), Vitamin B1 (0.85), Vitamin A (not as cod liver oil) (0.85), High Dose Multivitamin for Children/Adults with ASD (0.83), Vitamin B2 (0.81), Vitamin B3 (0.78), Blend of Amino Acids (0.77), Calcium (0.76), Vitamin A (as cod liver oil) (0.75), Zinc (0.74), Generic Child/Adult Multivitamin (0.75), Omega 3 (0.74), Selenium (0.74), Vitamin B5 (0.72), Iron (0.69), Milk Thistle (0.66), Magnesium (0.66), Krill Oil (0.66), Vitamin K (0.65), PSP (0.64), Oral Vitamin B12 (0.64), Evening Primrose Oil (0.63), Oral Glutathione (0.62), Lithium (0.60), Biotin (0.60), Cod Liver Oil (0.55), Flax Seed Oil (0.52), Medium Dose Vitamin B6 (0.52), Oral NAC (0.51), Fish Oil (0.49), Carnitine (0.49), Injected Vitamin B12 (0.48), Taurine (0.47), 5-HTP (0.46), Transdermal Glutathione (0.44), Epsom Salt (0.34), DMG (0.30), GABA (0.25)
Sleep (falling asleep)	Melatonin (1.33), 5-HTP (0.61), Tryptophan (0.45), Valerian Root (0.44), Magnesium (0.21)
Cognition	High Dose Folinic Acid (0.63), Omega 6 (0.53), Cod Liver Oil (0.43), Omega 3 (0.43), Injected Vitamin B12 (0.42), Oral Vitamin B12 (0.40), Fish Oil (0.39), High Dose Multivitamin for Children/Adults with ASD (0.35), CoQ10 (0.26), High Dose Multivitamin (0.23), Lithium (0.22), Krill Oil (0.21), Moderate Dose Folinic Acid (0.20)
Sleep (staying asleep)	Melatonin (0.63), 5-HTP (0.46), Tryptophan (0.32), Valerian Root (0.24)
Aggression/Agitation	Epsom Salt (0.54), Lithium (0.22), Magnesium (0.20)
Attention	High Dose Folinic Acid (0.54), Omega 6 (0.50), Epsom Salt (0.41), High Dose Multivitamin for Children/Adults with ASD (0.32), Cod Liver Oil (0.30), Omega 3 (0.29), Evening Primrose Oil (0.28), PSP (0.26), Oral Vitamin B12 (0.26), Fish Oil (0.21)
Language/Communication	High Dose Folinic Acid (0.45), Injected Vitamin B12 (0.45), Moderate Dose Folinic Acid (0.33), Omega 6 (0.32), General Glutathione (0.32), Oral Vitamin B12 (0.30), Cod Liver Oil (0.25), Omega 3 (0.25), Epsom Salt (0.24), High Dose Multivitamin (0.23), High Dose Multivitamin for Children/Adults with ASD (0.22), Fish Oil (0.21), TMG (0.20)
Constipation	Fruit/Vegetable Powder Concentrate (0.53), Magnesium (0.48), Vitamin C (0.22)
Health (fewer illnesses and/or less severe illnesses)	Fruit/Vegetable Powder Concentrate (0.53), Vitamin C (0.51), High Dose Multivitamin (0.45), Vitamin D (0.34), Potassium (0.33), Zinc (0.31), High Dose Multivitamin for Children/Adults with ASD (0.29), Vitamin E (0.23)
Anxiety	Lithium (0.37), Magnesium (0.33), PSP (0.32), GABA (0.27), Tryptophan (0.26), High Dose Multivitamin for Children/Adults with ASD (0.22)
Social Interaction and Understanding	High Dose Folinic Acid (0.36), General Glutathione (0.26), Moderate Dose Folinic Acid (0.26), High Dose Multivitamin for Children/Adults with ASD (0.26), Injected Vitamin B12 (0.26), High Dose Multivitamin (0.23), Oral Vitamin B12 (0.22)
Irritability	High Dose Folinic Acid (0.27), Magnesium (0.26), Epsom Salt (0.23), High Dose Multivitamin for Children/Adults with ASD (0.22)
Sensory Sensitivity	High Dose Multivitamin for Children/Adults with ASD (0.22), Lithium (0.15), Injected Vitamin B12 (0.12)
Lethargy (easily tired)	Carnitine (0.21), Chromium (0.19), Injected Vitamin B12 (0.15)
Depression	Epsom Salt (0.18), Tryptophan (0.13), Vitamin D (0.11)
Hyperactivity	High Dose Folinic Acid (0.18), High Dose Multivitamin for Children/Adults with ASD (0.13), Magnesium (0.12)
Stimming/Perseveration/Desire for Sameness	Evening Primrose Oil (0.14), High Dose Multivitamin for Children/Adults with ASD (0.13), Tryptophan (0.13)
OCD	PSP (0.13), Vitamin B3 (0.10), High Dose Folinic Acid (0.09)
Tics/involuntary movements	Tryptophan (0.13), Potassium (0.08), High Dose Multivitamin (0.08)
Eczema/Skin problems	Biotin (0.12), Vitamin E (0.08), Vitamin D (0.07)
Diarrhea	Fruit/Vegetable Powder Concentrate (0.11), Glutamine (0.08), High Dose Multivitamin for Children/Adults with ASD (0.06)
Seizures	High Dose Folinic Acid (0.09), Moderate Dose Folinic Acid (0.07), Oral Vitamin B12 (0.01)
Self-Injurious behaviors	High Dose Folinic Acid (0.09), Oral Glutathione (0.07), High Dose Multivitamin for Children/Adults with ASD (0.06)
Reflux/Vomiting	Epsom Salt (0.06), Milk Thistle (0.05), Vitamin E (0.04)

3.2.11. Overall Effects of Nutraceuticals

As a final part of this Survey, participants were asked to rate the overall effect of nutraceuticals (Table 4). A total of 77% of participants reported that nutraceuticals had a positive effect, ranging from slightly better (24%) to much better (27%), with 23% reporting no effect, and no reports that they generally resulted in worsened symptoms.

Table 4. Rating of the Overall Effects of Nutraceuticals.

	Percentage of Responses
Much Better (3)	27%
Somewhat Better (2)	26%
Slightly Better (1)	24%
No Effect (0)	23%
Mildly Worse (−1)	0%
Somewhat Worse (−2)	0%
Much Worse (−3)	0%
Average	1.6

3.3. Analysis of the Effect on Specific Supplements on Change in Severity

To study the change in ASD severity related to nutraceuticals, nutraceuticals with at least 100 responses were selected in order to ensure there were enough cases to provide an adequate range of change in ASD severity. Since there were multiple categories of Omega 3 fatty acids (Fish Oils, Omega 3 Fatty Acids, Krill Oil) and B12 (oral and injected) these nutraceuticals were combined into categories. Thus, nutraceuticals selected included B12 (n = 170), Omega 3 fatty acids (n = 276), Epsom salt baths (n = 141), calcium (n = 110), magnesium (n = 153), zinc (n = 124), Vitamin C (n = 182), Vitamin D (n = 159), generic multivitamin (MVI) (n = 436), autism specific MVI (n = 103), and melatonin (n = 367). Because two other MVIs were being studied, high dose MVI (n = 45) was also included in the analysis. Because of the interest in the difference between injected vs. oral B12, the analysis was conducted on the separate groups of oral B12 (n = 127) and injected B12 (n = 76) as well as any B12 use. The analysis adjusted for baseline severity at age 3 years of age, developmental profile, number of rounds of antibiotic used in infancy, and gender.

3.3.1. Specific Nutraceutical Use

First, the analysis determined whether the changes in severity from 3 years of age to the current age was related to taking a nutraceutical regardless of the reported specific beneficial response. The uses of any B12 [$\chi(1)^2 = 11.79, p < 0.001$], injected B12 [$\chi(1)^2 = 5.58$, $p = 0.01$] or oral B12 [$\chi(1)^2 = 11.48, p = 0.001$], Calcium [$\chi(1)^2 = 8.29, p < 0.01$], Magnesium [$\chi(1)^2 = 5.83$ $p = 0.01$], Zinc [$\chi(1)^2 = 20.46$ $p < 0.001$], Vitamin D [$\chi(1)^2 = 6.66$ $p = 0.01$], or a multivitamin specifically formulated for ASD [$\chi(1)^2 = 7.00$ $p < 0.01$] were significantly related to a positive improvement in ASD symptoms (a reduction in ASD severity) as seen in Figure 9.

The change in ASD severity was also related to baseline severity at 3 years of age in all of the analyses, which included taking B12 [$\chi(1)^2 = 336, p < 0.001$], B12 injections [$\chi(1)^2 = 332, p < 0.001$], oral B12 [$\chi(1)^2 = 341, p < 0.001$], Omega 3 Fatty Acids [$\chi(1)^2 = 336$, $p < 0.001$], Epsom Salt Baths [$\chi(1)^2 = 329$, $p < 0.001$], Calcium [$\chi(1)^2 = 343$, $p < 0.001$], Magnesium [$\chi(1)^2 = 338, p < 0.001$], Zinc [$\chi(1)^2 = 350, p < 0.001$], Vitamin C [$\chi(1)^2 = 335$, $p < 0.001$], Vitamin D [$\chi(1)^2 = 327, p < 0.001$], Generic MVI [$\chi(1)^2 = 327, p < 0.001$], high dose MVI [$\chi(1)^2 = 337, p < 0.001$], autism specific MVI [$\chi(1)^2 = 321, p < 0.001$], and Melatonin [$\chi(1)^2 = 355$, $p < 0.001$]. In all models, a higher baseline severity was associated with a larger positive change in development as might be expected as higher severity patients have more potential for improvements.

Almost all of the associations shown in Figure 9 demonstrate that treatment was associated with greater improvements. The exceptions were generic multi-vitamin, presumably because that meant participants did not take a multi-vitamin specific for ASD, and melatonin, probably because it treats a specific problem and is given to children with sleep disorders who may require additional non-nutraceutical treatments.

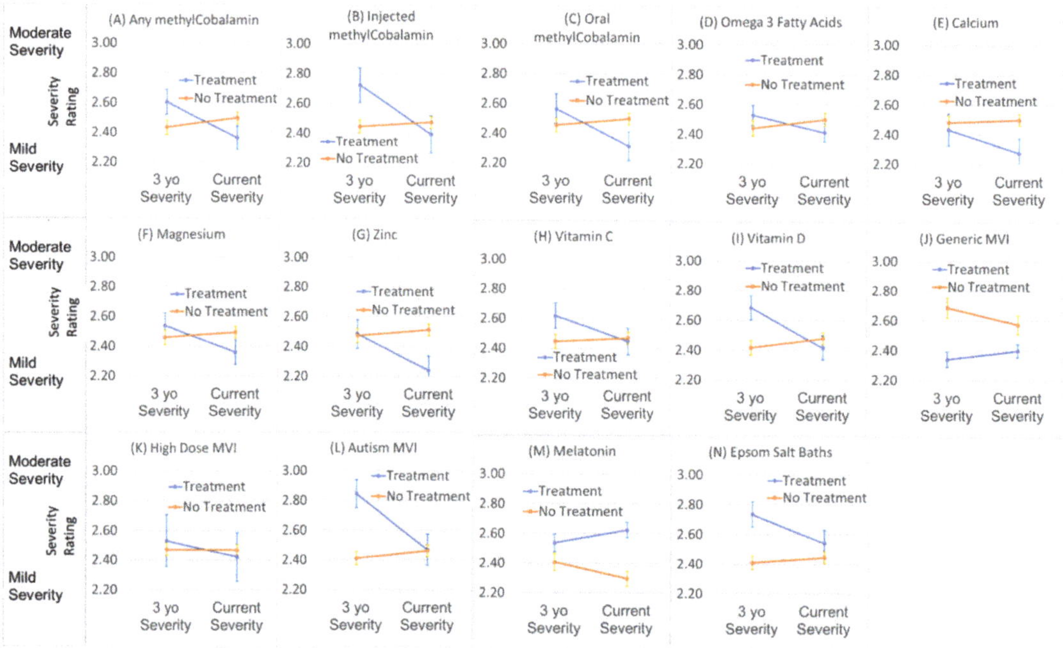

Figure 9. Relationship between nutraceuticals and change in autism severity from 3 years of age to the current age.

3.3.2. Perceived Benefit and Change in Autism Severity

A positive change in ASD severity was associated with the perceived benefit of any B12 supplement [$\chi(1)^2 = 10.14$, $p = 0.001$] and the baseline ASD severity [$\chi(1)^2 = 94.85$, $p < 0.001$] (Figure 10A), as well as the perceived benefit of injected B12 supplement [$\chi(1)^2 = 27.45$, $p < 0.001$] and the baseline ASD severity [$\chi(1)^2 = 61.34$, $p < 0.001$] (Figure 10B). Interestingly, the pattern of the child's development also affected the change in ASD severity when controlling for the benefit of injected B12 [$\chi(1)^2 = 24.32$, $p < 0.001$]. This was due to the children with early onset ASD demonstrating significantly greater benefit (1.5) as compared to those who had a clinical regression and then a developmental plateau (−0.31), those with only a plateau (0.69) or those with a major developmental regression (0.46) when controlling for the perceived benefit of B12 injections.

A positive change in ASD severity was associated with the perceived benefit for Omega 3 Fatty Acids [$\chi(1)^2 = 6.10$, $p = 0.01$] and the baseline ASD severity [$\chi(1)^2 = 148.38$, $p < 0.001$] (Figure 10C). A positive change in ASD severity was associated with the perceived benefit in zinc supplementation [$\chi(1)^2 = 7.25$, $p < 0.01$] and the baseline ASD severity [$\chi(1)^2 = 86.29$, $p < 0.001$]. However, the effect of baseline ASD severity resulted in the perceived benefit only being obvious in the most severely affected patients (Figure 10D). Finally, a positive change in ASD severity was associated with the perceived benefit in Epsom salts [$\chi(1)^2 = 6.59$, $p = 0.01$] and the baseline ASD severity [$\chi(1)^2 = 66.80$, $p < 0.001$] (Figure 10E).

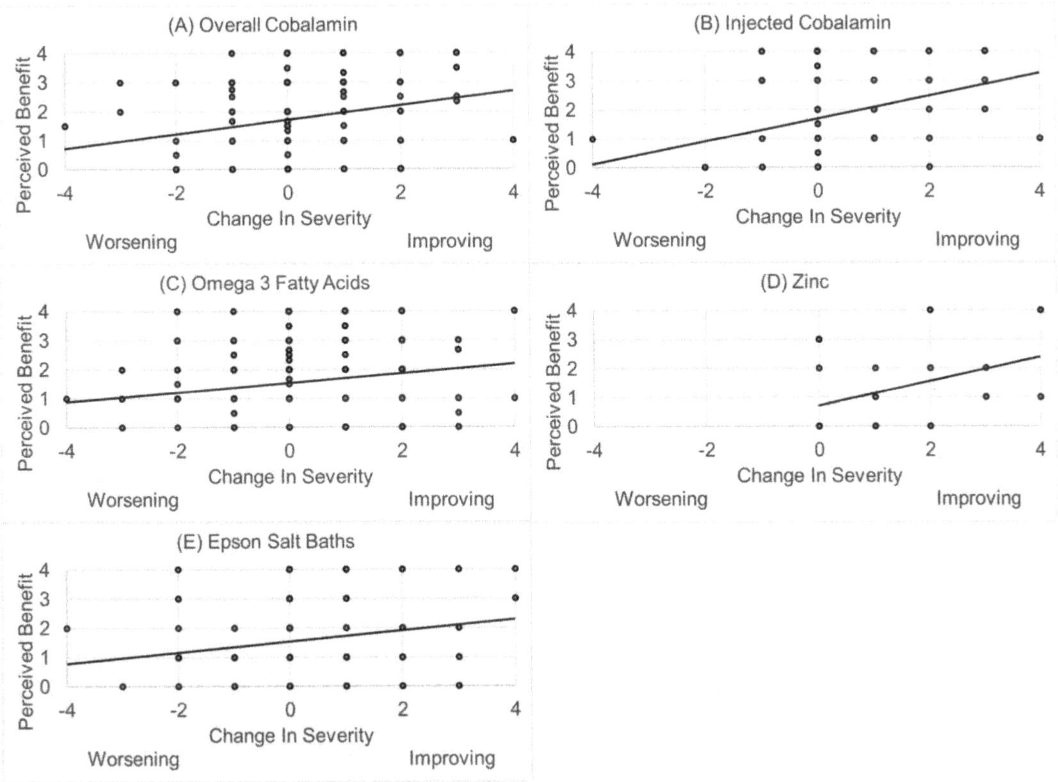

Figure 10. Association between change in ASD severity with the perceived benefit of the nutraceutical (**A**) Overall methylcobalamin; (**B**) Injected methylcobalamin; (**C**) Omega 3 Fatty Acids; (**D**) Zinc; (**E**) Epsom Salt Baths.

We also compared whether the severity of the diagnosis was related to starting any supplement. Those that took injected B12 [$F(1710) = 4.244$, $p = 0.04$], Epsom salt baths [$F(1710) = 9.630$, $p < 0.01$], Vitamin D [$F(1710) = 7.184$, $p < 0.01$], or MVI specific for ASD [$F(1710) = 13.752$, $p < 0.001$] had a higher severity at age 3 years of age whereas those that took a standard MVI [$F(1710) = 16.640$, $p < 0.001$] had a lower severity at age 3 years of age. The interaction with severity at 3 years of age and treatment was included in the linear model to determine if this effected the change in severity with treatment. For injected B12 [$\chi(1)^2 = 7.77$, $p < 0.01$], Oral B12 [$\chi(1)^2 = 3.71$, $p = 0.05$], Epsom salt baths [$\chi(1)^2 = 3.70$, $p = 0.05$], Calcium [$\chi(1)^2 = 4.56$, $p < 0.05$], Magnesium [$\chi(1)^2 = 3.93$, $p < 0.05$], and Zinc [$\chi(1)^2 = 13.16$, $p < 0.001$], the severity of autism at age 3 affected response to the treatment such that more severe individuals demonstrated a slightly lower response to some treatments.

4. Discussion

This study presents the Survey results of participants' reports of the perceived effectiveness and potential AEs of a wide range of nutraceuticals used in individuals with ASD. Nutraceuticals were generally reported to have a higher benefit compared to their AEs, with an average of 1.6 (slight/moderate benefit) and 0.1 (minimal AE), respectively. Reported benefits were generally in the slight/moderate range, and AEs were minimal.

The results of this study found significant benefits for many nutraceuticals with minimal adverse effects and are consistent with the findings of a number of clinical trials studying nutraceuticals in ASD. For example, double-blind, placebo-controlled studies, and/or meta-analyses have reported improvements in children with ASD using L-carnitine [32,33], Coenzyme Q10 (ubiquinone) [34], digestive enzymes [35,36], high dose folinic acid (1–2 mg/kg/day) [24–26], MB12 injections [37], melatonin [9,38–42], a multivitamin/mineral supplement designed specifically for ASD [26,27], NAC [29,43–45], omega 3 fatty acids [46,47], vitamin C [48], vitamin D3 [49,50], and possibly B6/Mg [51,52]. Open-label studies in ASD have also reported benefits for B vitamins [53,54], biotin [55], folic acid [56], an herbal formula [57], glutathione [58], iron [59], vitamin A [60] and zinc [61,62].

Some of the nutraceuticals in this Survey have not been previously studied in ASD including an amino acid blend, glutamine, taurine, tryptophan, evening primrose oil, flax seed oil, krill oil, calcium, chromium, iodine, lithium, potassium, selenium, vitamin E, vitamin K, valerian root, Epsom salts, GABA, and milk thistle. Thus, this Survey provides preliminary data on the effects (both beneficial and adverse) of these unstudied treatments which can help guide researchers to choose the most promising treatments to study in the future.

Some of the treatments reviewed may not only help certain symptoms of ASD but also treat underlying metabolic abnormalities associated with ASD. For example, mitochondrial dysfunction is relatively common in individuals with ASD [10,63] and is potentially treated with carnitine, Coenzyme Q10, B vitamins, and vitamin C [64]. Oxidative stress is also commonly associated with ASD [13] and is potentially treatable with antioxidants such as folinic acid, MB12, vitamin C, vitamin E, glutathione, ribose, and NADH. Melatonin is also an antioxidant and has positive effects on mitochondrial function [65].

Furthermore, children with ASD have been found to have multiple abnormalities related to one-carbon metabolism, including lower plasma levels of methionine, S-adenosylhomocysteine (SAM), homocysteine, cystathionine, cysteine, and total glutathione (GSH), as well as significantly higher concentrations of S-adenosylhomocysteine (SAH), adenosine, and oxidized glutathione (GSSG) [7,8]. Some studies have demonstrated that many children with ASD have a partial blockage in the transportation of folates into the brain due to an autoantibody to the folate receptor alpha, the primary mechanism which transports folate across the blood-brain barrier [66,67]. High dose folinic acid (1–2 mg/kg/day) has been shown to be an effective treatment for children with ASD with primary improvements in language in a double-blind placebo-controlled study [24], consistent with the findings of this Survey. Also consistent with this Survey, an open-label study found that high-dose folinic acid is effective for improving attention in children with ASD who possess the folate receptor alpha antibody [66], and two other placebo-controlled studies have also reported improvements with folinic acid in ASD [25,26]. These positive studies on the benefits of folinic acid are consistent with the results of Table 3, which demonstrates that folinic acid and vitamin B12 are two of the top-rated treatments for many ASD-related symptoms.

These abnormalities in one-carbon metabolism often result in problems in methylation and transsulfuration in ASD, resulting in a reduction in the production of glutathione [68]. In fact, these abnormalities appear to be so prevalent that they may be diagnostic for ASD [69]. Several studies [70,71] have addressed treatment of these linked pathways by providing cobalamin and folate derivatives to supplement the linked methylation-folate pathway in order to enhance the production of glutathione, while other studies have supplemented glutathione directly [58]. The findings of these studies of the benefits of cobalamin, folate, and glutathione are consistent with the results of this Survey.

It is interesting to compare the results of this Survey for nutraceuticals versus the results of this Survey for pharmaceuticals reported previously [31]. Averaging all nutraceuticals and all pharmaceuticals, the nutraceuticals had significantly higher Overall Benefit (1.59 vs. 1.39, $p = 0.01$) and significantly lower Overall Adverse Effect (0.1 vs. 0.9, $p < 0.0001$), based on a 2-sided t-test of the medications that had 20 or more responses [31]. Caution is needed in interpreting these results, since there are substantial variations in ratings for individual treatments. However, in general, these findings suggest that nutraceuticals may be important treatment options for ASD, and more research into nutraceuticals and how they affect metabolism is warranted.

4.1. Strengths of This Study

One strength of this study is that some of these nutraceuticals have not been formally studied to date; therefore, this is the first data available on these treatments for ASD. Another advantage is that a uniform rating scale was used for all treatments, so that direct comparisons between different treatments could be made—this is often not possible for comparing data from clinical trials, since different assessment tools are typically used. Finally, another strength is the large number of participants in this study.

4.2. Limitations of This Study

There are several limitations of this Survey to consider. One limitation is that it is based on survey data, so there may be a significant placebo effect, especially since one of the most common benefits reported was "general benefit—no specific symptom". The ratings are based on perceived benefit (primarily by caregivers) and not by medical professionals. Age at which treatment was administered was not collected, which is a limitation of the study. Furthermore, there was no data collected on the dosages or durations of treatments (other than high versus low dose folinic acid). Therefore, various doses and durations of treatments may have been used by participants. Another limitation is the ASD-related diagnoses were not confirmed with standardized testing but were gathered by participant self-report. Finally, there is the potential for recall bias, where participants may not completely remember the effects of certain treatments. This may be reflected by the fact that no participants listed any of the nutraceuticals as causing worsening in ASD-related symptoms.

5. Conclusions

This Survey provides important information on the overall and specific benefits and adverse effects of 58 of the most commonly used nutraceuticals in ASD. The Overall Benefits were rated slightly higher for the nutraceuticals than for the most commonly used pharmaceuticals reported in the previous paper, with significantly lower ratings of adverse effects. The perception of participants of slight/moderate benefit with minimal adverse effects potentially explains why nutraceuticals were used by 75.2% of individuals with ASD in the Survey. This is consistent with the growing number of positive randomized clinical trials of nutraceuticals in ASD. Further research into nutraceutical treatments for treating biochemical differences and ASD symptoms is warranted.

Supplementary Materials: The following are available online at https://www.mdpi.com/article/10.3390/jpm11090878/s1, Table S1. List of All Nutraceuticals in Survey. Table S2. Amino Acids. Table S3. Fatty Acids. Table S4. Glutathione-related Nutraceuticals. Table S5. Individual Minerals. Table S6. Individual Vitamins/Vitamin-like Nutraceuticals. Table S7. Multivitamins. Table S8. Sleep Treatments. Table S9. Other Miscellaneous Nutraceuticals.

Author Contributions: Conceptualization, J.B.A. and D.M.C.; methodology, J.B.A., D.M.C. and R.E.F. software, D.M.C.; validation, D.M.C. and A.B.; formal analysis, J.B.A., A.B. and R.E.F.; investigation, J.B.A. and D.M.C. resources, J.B.A. data curation, D.M.C. writing—original draft preparation, J.B.A. and A.B.; writing—review and editing, J.B.A., R.E.F. and D.A.R. visualization, A.B.; supervision, J.B.A.; project administration, J.B.A.; funding acquisition, J.B.A. All authors have read and agreed to the published version of the manuscript.

Funding: This research was funded in part by the Autism Research Institute and the Zoowalk for Autism Research.

Institutional Review Board Statement: The study was conducted according to the guidelines of the Declaration of Helsinki and approved by the Institutional Review Board (or Ethics Committee) of Arizona State University (protocol code STUDY00003766 approved 26 January 2016).

Informed Consent Statement: Informed consent was obtained from all subjects involved in the study.

Data Availability Statement: The data presented in this study are available on request from the corresponding author. The data are not publicly available due to plans for additional analysis.

Acknowledgments: We thank the following organizations for helping promote the Survey: Age of Autism, ASU Autism/Asperger's Research Program, Autism Academy for Education and Development, Autism Canada, Autism Conferences of America, Autism File, Autism Free Brain, Autism Nutrition Research Center, Autism Research Institute, Autism Society of Alabama, Autism Society of Bayou, Autism Society of Central Ohio, Autism Society of Central Texas, Autism Society of Dayton, Autism Society of El Paso, Autism Society of Emerald Coast, Autism Society of Greater Akron, Autism Society of Greater Harrisburg, Autism Society of Greater New Orleans, Autism Society of Greater Phoenix, Autism Society of Hawaii, Autism Society of Indiana, Autism Society of Inland Empire, Autism Society of Iowa, Autism Society—Kern Autism Network, Autism Society of Massachusetts, Autism Society of Michigan, Autism Society of Minnesota, Autism Society of Northern Virginia, Autism Society of Northwestern Pennsylvania, Autism Society of Oregon, Autism Society of Pittsburgh, Autism Society of Pennsylvania, Autism Society of San Diego, Autism Society of Southern Arizona, Autism Society of Southeastern Wisconsin, Autism Society of Treasure Valley, Autism Society of Western New York, Autism Society of Westmoreland, Autism Society of West Virginia, Autism Society of Wisconsin, Autism Speaks, Autism Spectrum Therapies, Autism Tennessee, Autism Treatment Network, East Valley Autism Network, Generation Rescue, GOALS for Autism, Inc., Guthrie Mainstream Services, Hope Group, Independent Living Experience, National Autism Association, North Bridge College Success Program, Organization for Autism Research, Southwest Autism Research and Resource Center (SARRC), SEEDs for Autism, S.E.E.K Arizona, STARS, Talking About Curing Autism (TACA), Unlocking Autism, US Autism and Asperger's Association (USAAA). We thank Steve Edelson for his detailed review of the Survey. We especially thank the >1000 participants who participated in the Survey, and those who provided initial feedback on the early versions of the Survey.

Conflicts of Interest: J.B.A. serves as President of the Autism Nutrition Research Center, but does not receive any salary or royalties from them. The other authors declare no conflict of interest. The funders had no role in the design of the study; in the collection, analyses, or interpretation of data; in the writing of the manuscript, or in the decision to publish the results.

References

1. Maenner, M.J.; Shaw, K.A.; Baio, J.; Washington, A.; Patrick, M.; DiRienzo, M.; Christensen, D.L.; Wiggins, L.D.; Pettygrove, S.; Andrews, J.G.; et al. Prevalence of Autism Spectrum Disorder among Children Aged 8 Years—Autism and Developmental Disabilities Monitoring Network, 11 Sites, United States, 2016. *Morb. Mortal. Wkly. Rep. Surveill. Summ.* **2020**, *69*, 1–12. [CrossRef]
2. Dunn, K.; Rydzewska, E.; Fleming, M.; Cooper, S.A. Prevalence of mental health conditions, sensory impairments and physical disability in people with co-occurring intellectual disabilities and autism compared with other people: A cross-sectional total population study in Scotland. *BMJ Open* **2020**, *10*, e035280. [CrossRef]
3. Viscidi, E.W.; Triche, E.W.; Pescosolido, M.F.; McLean, R.L.; Joseph, R.M.; Spence, S.J.; Morrow, E.M. Clinical characteristics of children with autism spectrum disorder and co-occurring epilepsy. *PLoS ONE* **2013**, *8*, e67797. [CrossRef] [PubMed]
4. Holingue, C.; Newill, C.; Lee, L.C.; Pasricha, P.J.; Daniele Fallin, M. Gastrointestinal symptoms in autism spectrum disorder: A review of the literature on ascertainment and prevalence. *Autism Res.* **2018**, *11*, 24–36. [CrossRef] [PubMed]
5. Lai, M.C.; Kassee, C.; Besney, R.; Bonato, S.; Hull, L.; Mandy, W.; Szatmari, P.; Ameis, S.H. Prevalence of co-occurring mental health diagnoses in the autism population: A systematic review and meta-analysis. *Lancet Psychiatry* **2019**, *6*, 819–829. [CrossRef]
6. Hollocks, M.J.; Lerh, J.W.; Magiati, I.; Meiser-Stedman, R.; Brugha, T.S. Anxiety and depression in adults with autism spectrum disorder: A systematic review and meta-analysis. *Psychol. Med.* **2019**, *49*, 559–572. [CrossRef] [PubMed]
7. James, S.J.; Cutler, P.; Melnyk, S.; Jernigan, S.; Janak, L.; Gaylor, D.W.; Neubrander, J.A. Metabolic biomarkers of increased oxidative stress and impaired methylation capacity in children with autism. *Am. J. Clin. Nutr.* **2004**, *80*, 1611–1617. [CrossRef]
8. James, S.J.; Melnyk, S.; Jernigan, S.; Cleves, M.A.; Halsted, C.H.; Wong, D.H.; Cutler, P.; Bock, K.; Boris, M.; Bradstreet, J.J.; et al. Metabolic endophenotype and related genotypes are associated with oxidative stress in children with autism. *Am. J. Med. Genet. Part B Neuropsychiatr. Genet.* **2006**, *141*, 947–956. [CrossRef]
9. Rossignol, D.A.; Frye, R.E. Melatonin in autism spectrum disorders: A systematic review and meta-analysis. *Dev. Med. Child. Neurol.* **2011**, *53*, 783–792. [CrossRef]
10. Rossignol, D.A.; Frye, R.E. Mitochondrial dysfunction in autism spectrum disorders: A systematic review and meta-analysis. *Mol. Psychiatry* **2012**, *17*, 290–314. [CrossRef]
11. Rose, S.; Niyazov, D.M.; Rossignol, D.A.; Goldenthal, M.; Kahler, S.G.; Frye, R.E. Clinical and Molecular Characteristics of Mitochondrial Dysfunction in Autism Spectrum Disorder. *Mol. Diagn. Ther.* **2018**, *22*, 571–593. [CrossRef]

12. Chen, L.; Shi, X.J.; Liu, H.; Mao, X.; Gui, L.N.; Wang, H.; Cheng, Y. Oxidative stress marker aberrations in children with autism spectrum disorder: A systematic review and meta-analysis of 87 studies (N = 9109). *Transl. Psychiatry* **2021**, *11*, 15. [CrossRef] [PubMed]
13. Frustaci, A.; Neri, M.; Cesario, A.; Adams, J.B.; Domenici, E.; Dalla Bernardina, B.; Bonassi, S. Oxidative stress-related biomarkers in autism: Systematic review and meta-analyses. *Free. Radic. Biol. Med.* **2012**, *52*, 2128–2141. [CrossRef]
14. LeClerc, S.; Easley, D. Pharmacological therapies for autism spectrum disorder: A review. *Pharm. Ther.* **2015**, *40*, 389–397.
15. Craig, F.; De Giacomo, A.; Operto, F.F.; Margari, M.; Trabacca, A.; Margari, L. Association between feeding/mealtime behavior problems and internalizing/externalizing problems in autism spectrum disorder (ASD), other neurodevelopmental disorders (NDDs) and typically developing children. *Minerva Pediatr.* **2019**. [CrossRef]
16. Canals-Sans, J.; Esteban-Figuerola, P.; Morales-Hidalgo, P.; Arija, V. Do Children with Autism Spectrum Disorders Eat Differently and Less Adequately than Those with Subclinical ASD and Typical Development? EPINED Epidemiological Study. *J. Autism Dev. Disord.* **2021**. [CrossRef] [PubMed]
17. Sharp, W.G.; Berry, R.C.; McCracken, C.; Nuhu, N.N.; Marvel, E.; Saulnier, C.A.; Klin, A.; Jones, W.; Jaquess, D.L. Feeding problems and nutrient intake in children with autism spectrum disorders: A meta-analysis and comprehensive review of the literature. *J. Autism Dev. Disord.* **2013**, *43*, 2159–2173. [CrossRef]
18. Page, S.D.; Souders, M.C.; Kral, T.V.E.; Chao, A.M.; Pinto-Martin, J. Correlates of Feeding Difficulties among Children with Autism Spectrum Disorder: A Systematic Review. *J. Autism Dev. Disord.* **2021**, 1–20. [CrossRef]
19. Adams, J.B.; Audhya, T.; Geis, E.; Gehn, E.; Fimbres, V.; Pollard, E.L.; Mitchell, J.; Ingram, J.; Hellmers, R.; Laake, D.; et al. Comprehensive Nutritional and Dietary Intervention for Autism Spectrum Disorder-A Randomized, Controlled 12-Month Trial. *Nutrients* **2018**, *10*, 369. [CrossRef]
20. Owen-Smith, A.A.; Bent, S.; Lynch, F.L.; Coleman, K.J.; Yau, V.M.; Pearson, K.A.; Massolo, M.L.; Quinn, V.; Croen, L.A. Prevalence and Predictors of Complementary and Alternative Medicine Use in a Large Insured Sample of Children with Autism Spectrum Disorders. *Res. Autism Spectr. Disord.* **2015**, *17*, 40–51. [CrossRef]
21. Frye, R.E.; Sreenivasula, S.; Adams, J.B. Traditional and non-traditional treatments for autism spectrum disorder with seizures: An on-line survey. *BMC Pediatr.* **2011**, *11*, 37. [CrossRef] [PubMed]
22. ARI. ARI Publ. 34: Parent Ratings of Behavorial Effects of Biomedical Interventions. Available online: https://www.autism.org/treatment-ratings-for-autism/ (accessed on 6 June 2021).
23. Rossignol, D.A. Novel and emerging treatments for autism spectrum disorders: A systematic review. *Ann. Clin. Psychiatry* **2009**, *21*, 213–236. [PubMed]
24. Frye, R.E.; Slattery, J.; Delhey, L.; Furgerson, B.; Strickland, T.; Tippett, M.; Sailey, A.; Wynne, R.; Rose, S.; Melnyk, S.; et al. Folinic acid improves verbal communication in children with autism and language impairment: A randomized double-blind placebo-controlled trial. *Mol. Psychiatry* **2018**, *23*, 247–256. [CrossRef] [PubMed]
25. Batebi, N.; Moghaddam, H.S.; Hasanzadeh, A.; Fakour, Y.; Mohammadi, M.R.; Akhondzadeh, S. Folinic Acid as Adjunctive Therapy in Treatment of Inappropriate Speech in Children with Autism: A Double-Blind and Placebo-Controlled Randomized Trial. *Child. Psychiatry Hum. Dev.* **2021**, *52*, 928–938. [CrossRef]
26. Renard, E.; Leheup, B.; Gueant-Rodriguez, R.M.; Oussalah, A.; Quadros, E.V.; Gueant, J.L. Folinic acid improves the score of Autism in the EFFET placebo-controlled randomized trial. *Biochimie* **2020**, *173*, 57–61. [CrossRef] [PubMed]
27. Adams, J.B.; Holloway, C. Pilot study of a moderate dose multivitamin/mineral supplement for children with autistic spectrum disorder. *J. Altern. Complement. Med.* **2004**, *10*, 1033–1039. [CrossRef]
28. Adams, J.B.; Audhya, T.; McDonough-Means, S.; Rubin, R.A.; Quig, D.; Geis, E.; Gehn, E.; Loresto, M.; Mitchell, J.; Atwood, S.; et al. Effect of a vitamin/mineral supplement on children and adults with autism. *BMC Pediatr.* **2011**, *11*, 1–30. [CrossRef]
29. Lee, T.M.; Lee, K.M.; Lee, C.Y.; Lee, H.C.; Tam, K.W.; Loh, E.W. Effectiveness of N-acetylcysteine in autism spectrum disorders: A meta-analysis of randomized controlled trials. *Aust. N. Z. J. Psychiatry* **2021**, *55*, 196–206. [CrossRef]
30. McGuinness, G.; Kim, Y. Sulforaphane treatment for autism spectrum disorder: A systematic review. *EXCLI J.* **2020**, *19*, 892–903. [CrossRef]
31. Coleman, D.M.; Adams, J.B.; Anderson, A.L.; Frye, R.E. Rating of the Effectiveness of 26 Psychiatric and Seizure Medications for Autism Spectrum Disorder: Results of a National Survey. *J. Child. Adolesc. Psychopharmacol.* **2019**, *29*, 107–123. [CrossRef]
32. Fahmy, S.F.; El-hamamsy, M.H.; Zaki, O.K.; Badary, O.A. l-Carnitine supplementation improves the behavioral symptoms in autistic children. *Res. Autism Spectr. Disord.* **2013**, *7*, 159–166. [CrossRef]
33. Geier, D.A.; Kern, J.K.; Davis, G.; King, P.G.; Adams, J.B.; Young, J.L.; Geier, M.R. A prospective double-blind, randomized clinical trial of levocarnitine to treat autism spectrum disorders. *Med. Sci. Monit.* **2011**, *17*, PI15. [CrossRef]
34. Mousavinejad, E.; Ghaffari, M.A.; Riahi, F.; Hajmohammadi, M.; Tiznobeyk, Z.; Mousavinejad, M. Coenzyme Q10 supplementation reduces oxidative stress and decreases antioxidant enzyme activity in children with autism spectrum disorders. *Psychiatry Res.* **2018**, *265*, 62–69. [CrossRef]
35. Munasinghe, S.A.; Oliff, C.; Finn, J.; Wray, J.A. Digestive enzyme supplementation for autism spectrum disorders: A double-blind randomized controlled trial. *J. Autism Dev. Disord.* **2010**, *40*, 1131–1138. [CrossRef] [PubMed]
36. Saad, K.; Eltayeb, A.A.; Mohamad, I.L.; Al-Atram, A.A.; Elserogy, Y.; Bjorklund, G.; El-Houfey, A.A.; Nicholson, B. A Randomized, Placebo-controlled Trial of Digestive Enzymes in Children with Autism Spectrum Disorders. *Clin. Psychopharmacol. Neurosci.* **2015**, *13*, 188–193. [CrossRef] [PubMed]

37. Hendren, R.L.; James, S.J.; Widjaja, F.; Lawton, B.; Rosenblatt, A.; Bent, S. Randomized, Placebo-Controlled Trial of Methyl B12 for Children with Autism. *J. Child. Adolesc. Psychopharmacol.* **2016**, *26*, 774–783. [CrossRef]
38. Gringras, P.; Nir, T.; Breddy, J.; Frydman-Marom, A.; Findling, R.L. Efficacy and Safety of Pediatric Prolonged-Release Melatonin for Insomnia in Children with Autism Spectrum Disorder. *J. Am. Acad Child. Adolesc. Psychiatry* **2017**, *56*, 948–957.e4. [CrossRef] [PubMed]
39. Gringras, P.; Gamble, C.; Jones, A.P.; Wiggs, L.; Williamson, P.R.; Sutcliffe, A.; Montgomery, P.; Whitehouse, W.P.; Choonara, I.; Allport, T.; et al. Melatonin for sleep problems in children with neurodevelopmental disorders: Randomised double masked placebo controlled trial. *BMJ* **2012**, *345*, e6664. [CrossRef] [PubMed]
40. Cortesi, F.; Giannotti, F.; Sebastiani, T.; Panunzi, S.; Valente, D. Controlled-release melatonin, singly and combined with cognitive behavioural therapy, for persistent insomnia in children with autism spectrum disorders: A randomized placebo-controlled trial. *J. Sleep Res.* **2012**, *21*, 700–709. [CrossRef]
41. Garstang, J.; Wallis, M. Randomized controlled trial of melatonin for children with autistic spectrum disorders and sleep problems. *Child. Care Health Dev.* **2006**, *32*, 585–589. [CrossRef]
42. Wright, B.; Sims, D.; Smart, S.; Alwazeer, A.; Alderson-Day, B.; Allgar, V.; Whitton, C.; Tomlinson, H.; Bennett, S.; Jardine, J.; et al. Melatonin versus placebo in children with autism spectrum conditions and severe sleep problems not amenable to behaviour management strategies: A randomised controlled crossover trial. *J. Autism Dev. Disord.* **2011**, *41*, 175–184. [CrossRef]
43. Hardan, A.Y.; Fung, L.K.; Libove, R.A.; Obukhanych, T.V.; Nair, S.; Herzenberg, L.A.; Frazier, T.W.; Tirouvanziam, R. A randomized controlled pilot trial of oral N-acetylcysteine in children with autism. *Biol. Psychiatry* **2012**, *71*, 956–961. [CrossRef] [PubMed]
44. Ghanizadeh, A.; Moghimi-Sarani, E. A randomized double blind placebo controlled clinical trial of N-Acetylcysteine added to risperidone for treating autistic disorders. *BMC Psychiatry* **2013**, *13*, 196. [CrossRef]
45. Nikoo, M.; Radnia, H.; Farokhnia, M.; Mohammadi, M.R.; Akhondzadeh, S. N-acetylcysteine as an adjunctive therapy to risperidone for treatment of irritability in autism: A randomized, double-blind, placebo-controlled clinical trial of efficacy and safety. *Clin. Neuropharmacol.* **2015**, *38*, 11–17. [CrossRef] [PubMed]
46. Amminger, G.P.; Berger, G.E.; Schafer, M.R.; Klier, C.; Friedrich, M.H.; Feucht, M. Omega-3 fatty acids supplementation in children with autism: A double-blind randomized, placebo-controlled pilot study. *Biol. Psychiatry* **2007**, *61*, 551–553. [CrossRef] [PubMed]
47. Parellada, M.; Llorente, C.; Calvo, R.; Gutierrez, S.; Lazaro, L.; Graell, M.; Guisasola, M.; Dorado, M.L.; Boada, L.; Romo, J.; et al. Randomized trial of omega-3 for autism spectrum disorders: Effect on cell membrane composition and behavior. *Eur. Neuropsychopharmacol.* **2017**, *27*, 1319–1330. [CrossRef] [PubMed]
48. Dolske, M.C.; Spollen, J.; McKay, S.; Lancashire, E.; Tolbert, L. A preliminary trial of ascorbic acid as supplemental therapy for autism. *Prog. Neuropsychopharmacol. Biol. Psychiatry* **1993**, *17*, 765–774. [CrossRef]
49. Li, B.; Xu, Y.; Zhang, X.; Zhang, L.; Wu, Y.; Wang, X.; Zhu, C. The effect of vitamin D supplementation in treatment of children with autism spectrum disorder: A systematic review and meta-analysis of randomized controlled trials. *Nutr. Neurosci.* **2020**, 1–11. [CrossRef]
50. Song, L.; Luo, X.; Jiang, Q.; Chen, Z.; Zhou, L.; Wang, D.; Chen, A. Vitamin D Supplementation is Beneficial for Children with Autism Spectrum Disorder: A Meta-analysis. *Clin. Psychopharmacol. Neurosci.* **2020**, *18*, 203–213. [CrossRef]
51. Adams, J.B.; George, F.; Audhya, T. Abnormally high plasma levels of vitamin B6 in children with autism not taking supplements compared to controls not taking supplements. *J. Altern. Complement. Med.* **2006**, *12*, 59–63. [CrossRef] [PubMed]
52. Pfeiffer, S.I.; Norton, J.; Nelson, L.; Shott, S. Efficacy of vitamin B6 and magnesium in the treatment of autism: A methodology review and summary of outcomes. *J. Autism Dev. Disord.* **1995**, *25*, 481–493. [CrossRef] [PubMed]
53. Ezugha, H.; Goldenthal, M.; Valencia, I.; Anderson, C.E.; Legido, A.; Marks, H. 5q14.3 deletion manifesting as mitochondrial disease and autism: Case report. *J. Child. Neurol.* **2010**, *25*, 1232–1235. [CrossRef] [PubMed]
54. Guevara-Campos, J.; Gonzalez-Guevara, L.; Guevara-Gonzalez, J.; Cauli, O. First Case Report of Primary Carnitine Deficiency Manifested as Intellectual Disability and Autism Spectrum Disorder. *Brain Sci.* **2019**, *9*, 137. [CrossRef] [PubMed]
55. Benke, P.J.; Duchowny, M.; McKnight, D. Biotin and Acetazolamide for Treatment of an Unusual Child with Autism Plus Lack of Nail and Hair Growth. *Pediatr. Neurol.* **2018**, *79*, 61–64. [CrossRef] [PubMed]
56. Sun, C.; Zou, M.; Zhao, D.; Xia, W.; Wu, L. Efficacy of Folic Acid Supplementation in Autistic Children Participating in Structured Teaching: An Open-Label Trial. *Nutrients* **2016**, *8*, 337. [CrossRef]
57. Chan, A.S.; Sze, S.L.; Han, Y.M.Y. An intranasal herbal medicine improves executive functions and activates the underlying neural network in children with autism. *Res. Autism Spectr. Disord.* **2014**, *8*, 681–691. [CrossRef]
58. Kern, J.K.; Geier, D.A.; Adams, J.B.; Garver, C.R.; Audhya, T.; Geier, M.R. A clinical trial of glutathione supplementation in autism spectrum disorders. *Med. Sci. Monit.* **2011**, *17*, CR677–CR682. [CrossRef]
59. Dosman, C.F.; Brian, J.A.; Drmic, I.E.; Senthilselvan, A.; Harford, M.M.; Smith, R.W.; Sharieff, W.; Zlotkin, S.H.; Moldofsky, H.; Roberts, S.W. Children with autism: Effect of iron supplementation on sleep and ferritin. *Pediatr. Neurol.* **2007**, *36*, 152–158. [CrossRef]
60. Guo, M.; Zhu, J.; Yang, T.; Lai, X.; Liu, X.; Liu, J.; Chen, J.; Li, T. Vitamin A improves the symptoms of autism spectrum disorders and decreases 5-hydroxytryptamine (5-HT): A pilot study. *Brain Res. Bull.* **2018**, *137*, 35–40. [CrossRef]

61. Meguid, N.A.; Bjorklund, G.; Gebril, O.H.; Dosa, M.D.; Anwar, M.; Elsaeid, A.; Gaber, A.; Chirumbolo, S. The role of zinc supplementation on the metallothionein system in children with autism spectrum disorder. *Acta Neurol. Belg.* **2019**, *119*, 577–583. [CrossRef]
62. Russo, A.J. Increased Copper in Individuals with Autism Normalizes Post Zinc Therapy More Efficiently in Individuals with Concurrent GI Disease. *Nutr. Metab. Insights* **2011**, *4*, 49–54. [CrossRef] [PubMed]
63. Thorsen, M. Oxidative stress, metabolic and mitochondrial abnormalities associated with autism spectrum disorder. *Prog. Mol. Biol. Transl. Sci.* **2020**, *173*, 331–354. [CrossRef]
64. Delhey, L.M.; Nur Kilinc, E.; Yin, L.; Slattery, J.C.; Tippett, M.L.; Rose, S.; Bennuri, S.C.; Kahler, S.G.; Damle, S.; Legido, A.; et al. The Effect of Mitochondrial Supplements on Mitochondrial Activity in Children with Autism Spectrum Disorder. *J. Clin. Med.* **2017**, *6*, 18. [CrossRef] [PubMed]
65. Rossignol, D.A.; Frye, R.E. Psychotropic Medications for Sleep Disorders in Autism Spectrum Disorders. In *Handbook of Autism and Pervasive Developmental Disorder*; Matson, J.L., Sturmey, P., Eds.; Spring Publishing: Berlin/Heidelberg, Germany, 2020; in press.
66. Frye, R.E.; Sequeira, J.M.; Quadros, E.V.; James, S.J.; Rossignol, D.A. Cerebral folate receptor autoantibodies in autism spectrum disorder. *Mol. Psychiatry* **2013**, *18*, 369–381. [CrossRef] [PubMed]
67. Ramaekers, V.T.; Blau, N.; Sequeira, J.M.; Nassogne, M.C.; Quadros, E.V. Folate receptor autoimmunity and cerebral folate deficiency in low-functioning autism with neurological deficits. *Neuropediatrics* **2007**, *38*, 276–281. [CrossRef]
68. Bjorklund, G.; Tinkov, A.A.; Hosnedlova, B.; Kizek, R.; Ajsuvakova, O.P.; Chirumbolo, S.; Skalnaya, M.G.; Peana, M.; Dadar, M.; El-Ansary, A.; et al. The role of glutathione redox imbalance in autism spectrum disorder: A review. *Free Radic. Biol. Med.* **2020**, *160*, 149–162. [CrossRef]
69. Howsmon, D.P.; Vargason, T.; Rubin, R.A.; Delhey, L.; Tippett, M.; Rose, S.; Bennuri, S.C.; Slattery, J.C.; Melnyk, S.; James, S.J.; et al. Multivariate techniques enable a biochemical classification of children with autism spectrum disorder versus typically-developing peers: A comparison and validation study. *Bioeng. Transl. Med.* **2018**, *3*, 156–165. [CrossRef]
70. Frye, R.E.; Melnyk, S.; Fuchs, G.; Reid, T.; Jernigan, S.; Pavliv, O.; Hubanks, A.; Gaylor, D.W.; Walters, L.; James, S.J. Effectiveness of methylcobalamin and folinic Acid treatment on adaptive behavior in children with autistic disorder is related to glutathione redox status. *Autism Res. Treat.* **2013**, *2013*, 609705. [CrossRef]
71. James, S.J.; Melnyk, S.; Fuchs, G.; Reid, T.; Jernigan, S.; Pavliv, O.; Hubanks, A.; Gaylor, D.W. Efficacy of methylcobalamin and folinic acid treatment on glutathione redox status in children with autism. *Am. J. Clin. Nutr.* **2009**, *89*, 425–430. [CrossRef]

Journal of *Personalized Medicine*

MDPI

Review

A Systematic Review and Meta-Analysis of Immunoglobulin G Abnormalities and the Therapeutic Use of Intravenous Immunoglobulins (IVIG) in Autism Spectrum Disorder

Daniel A Rossignol [1,*] and Richard E Frye [2]

1 Rossignol Medical Center, 24541 Pacific Park Drive, Suite 210, Aliso Viejo, CA 92656, USA
2 Barrow Neurological Institute at Phoenix Children's Hospital, 1919 E Thomas Rd, Phoenix, AZ 85016, USA; rfrye@phoenixchildrens.com
* Correspondence: rossignolmd@gmail.com; Tel.: +321-259-7111

Abstract: Autism spectrum disorder (ASD) is a neurodevelopmental disorder affecting approximately 2% of children in the United States. Growing evidence suggests that immune dysregulation is associated with ASD. One immunomodulatory treatment that has been studied in ASD is intravenous immunoglobulins (IVIG). This systematic review and meta-analysis examined the studies which assessed immunoglobulin G (IgG) concentrations and the therapeutic use of IVIG for individuals with ASD. Twelve studies that examined IgG levels suggested abnormalities in total IgG and IgG 4 subclass concentrations, with concentrations in these IgGs related to aberrant behavior and social impairments, respectively. Meta-analysis supported possible subsets of children with ASD with low total IgG and elevated IgG 4 subclass but also found significant variability among studies. A total of 27 publications reported treating individuals with ASD using IVIG, including four prospective, controlled studies (one was a double-blind, placebo-controlled study); six prospective, uncontrolled studies; 2 retrospective, controlled studies; and 15 retrospective, uncontrolled studies. In some studies, clinical improvements were observed in communication, irritability, hyperactivity, cognition, attention, social interaction, eye contact, echolalia, speech, response to commands, drowsiness, decreased activity and in some cases, the complete resolution of ASD symptoms. Several studies reported some loss of these improvements when IVIG was stopped. Meta-analysis combining the aberrant behavior checklist outcome from two studies demonstrated that IVIG treatment was significantly associated with improvements in total aberrant behavior and irritability (with large effect sizes), and hyperactivity and social withdrawal (with medium effect sizes). Several studies reported improvements in pro-inflammatory cytokines (including TNF-alpha). Six studies reported improvements in seizures with IVIG (including patients with refractory seizures), with one study reporting a worsening of seizures when IVIG was stopped. Other studies demonstrated improvements in recurrent infections, appetite, weight gain, neuropathy, dysautonomia, and gastrointestinal symptoms. Adverse events were generally limited but included headaches, vomiting, worsening behaviors, anxiety, fever, nausea, fatigue, and rash. Many studies were limited by the lack of standardized objective outcome measures. IVIG is a promising and potentially effective treatment for symptoms in individuals with ASD; further research is needed to provide solid evidence of efficacy and determine the subset of children with ASD who may best respond to this treatment as well as to investigate biomarkers which might help identify responsive candidates.

Keywords: autism spectrum disorder; immunoglobulin G; intravenous immunoglobulin

Citation: Rossignol, D.A; Frye, R.E A Systematic Review and Meta-Analysis of Immunoglobulin G Abnormalities and the Therapeutic Use of Intravenous Immunoglobulins (IVIG) in Autism Spectrum Disorder. *J. Pers. Med.* **2021**, *11*, 488. https://doi.org/10.3390/jpm11060488

Academic Editor: Marco Costanzi

Received: 22 April 2021
Accepted: 26 May 2021
Published: 30 May 2021

Publisher's Note: MDPI stays neutral with regard to jurisdictional claims in published maps and institutional affiliations.

Copyright: © 2021 by the authors. Licensee MDPI, Basel, Switzerland. This article is an open access article distributed under the terms and conditions of the Creative Commons Attribution (CC BY) license (https://creativecommons.org/licenses/by/4.0/).

1. Introduction

Autism spectrum disorder (ASD) is a neurodevelopmental disorder which is behaviorally defined by impairments in social communication and the presence of repetitive and restrictive behaviors. ASD affects approximately 2% of children in the United States [1]. Despite decades of research, the etiology and treatment of children with ASD is still very incomplete. This has resulted in a minority of children reaching optimal outcomes with many manifesting symptoms into adulthood and resulting in substantial economic and societal costs [2].

A number of medical comorbidities have been reported in ASD including mitochondrial dysfunction [3], sleep disorders [4], immune related problems [5], gastrointestinal abnormalities [6], inflammation [7], and epilepsy [8]. Addressing these comorbid conditions has the potential to improve the ability to function and the quality of life of children with ASD and their families [9]. One of the more recent promising areas of research is dysfunction of the immune system [10], which is a potential target for treatment.

Several lines of evidence link immune abnormalities to ASD. Family history of atopic [11] and autoimmune [12] disease is associated with ASD. Maternal immune activation during pregnancy has been shown to be associated with an increase in risk of ASD in the offspring in human [13] and animal studies [14]. Individuals with ASD demonstrate specific human leukocyte antigen risk alleles that put them at risk for immune dysfunction [15]. Elevations in specific monocyte cytokine profiles have been associated with ASD [16,17] and specific patterns of inflammatory cytokines have been identified in the cerebrospinal fluid and brain in individuals with ASD [18]. Autoantibodies to the brain [19] and other important proteins such as the folate receptor alpha [20] also appear to be associated with ASD.

Children with ASD also appear to be at increased risk for clinical immune disorders. Some of the immune-related problems reported in ASD include common variable immunodeficiency (CVID), hypogammaglobulinemia (i.e., low total Immunoglobulin G (IgG)) [21] and specific polysaccharide antibody deficiency (SPAD) [22]. One study reported that lower levels of IgG were associated with more severe aberrant behaviors in children with ASD [23]. A number of studies have reported on the use of intravenous immunoglobulin (IVIG) in ASD to treat immune-related problems [21]. Some of the medical comorbidities reported in ASD might also improve with the use of IVIG. For example, IVIG has been shown to have anti-seizure properties [24–26] and anti-inflammatory effects [27–30]. The anti-inflammatory effects of IVIG are observed at higher doses of IVIG (i.e., 2 grams/kg) for inflammatory and autoimmune disorders [31].

This paper is a systematic review and meta-analysis examining the evidence for abnormal IgG concentrations and the therapeutic use of IVIG in ASD. Adverse events (AEs) are also collated. This study demonstrates that IVIG is a promising and potentially effective treatment for symptoms in individuals with ASD, but further research is needed to provide solid evidence of efficacy and determine the subset of children with ASD who may best respond to this treatment, as well as to investigate biomarkers which might help identify responsive candidates.

2. Materials and Methods

2.1. Search Strategy

A prospective protocol for this systematic review was developed a priori, and the search terms and selection criteria were chosen in an attempt to capture all pertinent publications. A computer-aided search of PUBMED, Google Scholar, EmBase, Scopus and ERIC databases from inception through March 2021 was conducted to identify pertinent publications using the search terms 'autism', 'autistic', 'Asperger', 'ASD', 'pervasive', and 'pervasive developmental disorder' in all combinations with the terms 'IVIG', 'IgG', 'immunoglobulin', 'immunoglobulins', 'globulin', 'intravenous immunoglobulin', 'gamma globulin' and 'immunodeficiency.' The references cited in identified publications were also searched to locate additional studies. Supplementary Figure S1 depicts the publications identified during the search process.

2.2. Study Selection and Assessment

This systematic review and meta-analysis followed PRISMA guidelines [32]. The PRISMA Checklist and Flowchart can be found in Supplementary Table S1. One reviewer screened titles and abstracts of all potentially relevant publications. Studies were initially included if they (1) involved individuals with ASD; and (2) reported on the use of IVIG or reported IgG concentrations. Animal models were excluded. Abstracts or posters from conference proceedings were included if published in a journal. Articles were excluded if they: (1) Did not involve humans (for example, cellular models); or (2) did not present new or unique data (such as review articles or letters to the editor). After screening all records, 38 publications met inclusion criteria (see Supplementary Figure S1); two reviewers then independently reviewed these articles for inclusion and assessed factors such as the risk of bias. As per standardized guidelines [33], selection, performance detection, attrition, and reporting biases were considered. One study reported on IgG levels and also treatment with IVIG. Two studies reported on the use of oral immunoglobulin in ASD and were not included in the analysis [34,35]. One manuscript reported an ongoing double-blind placebo controlled (DBPC) crossover study which was never published and not included in the analysis [36].

2.3. Meta-Analysis

MetaXL Version 5.2 (EpiGear International Pty Ltd., Sunrise Beach, Queensland, Australia) was used with Microsoft Excel Version 16.0.12827.20200 (Redmond, WA, USA) to perform the meta-analysis. Mean immunoglobulin titers were pooled across studies using standard methodology [37]. Various manuscripts reported immunoglobulin concentrations in different units. For consistency we report concentrations in mg/dL. In some papers the interquartile intervals were reported rather than standard deviations. In such cases we use the estimator for estimating the standard deviation from interquartile range as defined by the Cochrane Handbook [38]. The data from this meta-analysis is available upon request to the authors.

To compare immunoglobulin titers across groups, pooled mean differences were calculated using the inverse variance heterogeneity model since it has been shown to resolve issues with underestimation of the statistical error and spuriously overconfident estimates with the random effects model when analyzing continuous outcome measures [39]. Cochran's Q was calculated to determine heterogeneity of effects across studies and when significant, the I^2 statistic (Heterogeneity Index) was calculated to determine the percentage of variation across studies that is due to heterogeneity rather than chance [40,41]. The Luis Furuya-Kanamori (LFK) Index derived from Doi plots were reviewed for significant asymmetries ($>\pm 2$) in the prevalence distribution when there were 3 or more studies [42,43].

Few intervention studies used quantitative standardized outcome measures, but two used the Social Responsiveness Scale (SRS) and five used the Aberrant Behavioral Checklist (ABC). Of note, the social withdrawal subscale of the ABC is called lethargy and inadequate eye contact in some studies, but we will refer to it as social withdrawal throughout to be consistent. Only two treatment studies contained enough details to be included in the treatment meta-analysis. Random-effects models, which assume variability in effects from both sampling error and study level differences [44,45], were used to calculate pooled standardized mean effect and pooled effect size. Effect sizes were considered small if Cohen's d' was 0.2; medium for Cohen's d' was 0.5; and large if Cohen's d' was 0.8 or higher [46].

3. Results

3.1. Studies of IgG Concentrations in Autism Spectrum Disorder

Articles examining IgG concentrations in individuals with ASD are first examined followed by studies which have reported therapeutic IVIG use in ASD.

3.1.1. Studies on IgG Concentrations in ASD

Twelve studies were identified that measured IgG concentrations in children with ASD (Table 1). Eight studies examined serum IgG with six using controls and two using standard reference ranges. Two studies examined serum IgG in neonates with both using controls. Two studies examined IgG in cerebrospinal fluid (CSF) with one using controls and one using a standard reference range. Most studies only had a modest number of participants with only four studies having a relatively large number of participants (i.e., 80+).

Table 1. Studies of Immunoglobulin G Concentration in Autism Spectrum Disorder. DD = Developmental Delay, TD = Typical Developing, P = Prospective, R = Retrospective; CSF = Cerebrospinal Fluid; AD = Autistic Disorder; NDR = Neurodevelopmental Regression.

Study	Study Type	Autism Group	Control Group	Outcomes
Studies in Children Using Contemporaneous Control Groups for Comparison				
Croonenberghs et al., 2002 [47]	P	18	22 TD	Total IgG, IgG2 and IgG4 higher in ASD No Difference in IgG1 and IgG3
Trajkovski et al., 2004 [48]	R	35	21 TD Siblings	Total IgG and IgG4 higher in ASD No Difference in IgG1, IgG2 and IgG3
Heuer et al., 2008 [23]	P	166 with AD 27 with ASD	96 TD 32 DD	Total IgG lower in AD Total IgG Inversely Correlated with Behavior
Enstrom et al., 2009 [49]	P	114	96 TD 31 DD	IgG4 higher in ASD No Difference in IgG1, IgG2 and IgG3 IgG4 Correlated with Social Impairment
Spiroski et al., 2009 [50]	R	30	22 TD Sibs 30 Moms 26 Dads	No Difference in Total IgG, IgG1, IgG2, IgG3 or IgG4 between ASD and TD Siblings
Wasilewska et al., 2012 [51]	P	24 NDR	14 TD	No Difference in Total IgG
Studies in Children Using Standard Reference Range as Comparison				
Gupta et al., 1996 [52]	P	25	Standard Reference	20% of ASD had below normal IgG subclasses (IgG1 in 1; IgG2 in 1; IgG3 in 1; IgG4 in 2)
Stern et al., 2005 [53]	P	24 Recurrent Infections	Standard Reference	No Difference in Total IgG
Studies in Neonates Using Contemporaneous Control Groups for Comparison				
Grether et al., 2010 [54]	R	213	265 TD	Neonatal Total IgG lower in ASD Lower IgG Associated with Increased ASD Risk
Grether et al., 2016 [55]	R	84	159 TD 49 DD	Lower IgG Associated with Increased ASD Risk
Studies on Immunoglobulin G Concentrations in the Cerebrospinal Fluid				
Young et al., 1977 [56]	P	5	Standard Reference	IgG in the CSF was normal
Runge et al., 2020 [57]	R	35	39 TD	No Difference in CSF IgG Index

Overall, of the eight studies that examined serum IgG in children with ASD, two reported higher and one reported lower total IgG while the others found no significant difference. One study found increased IgG2 subclass concentrations and three studies reported higher IgG4 concentrations. No studies reports lower IgG subclasses. However, one study found that lower total IgG concentrations was correlated with increased severity of disruptive behaviors as measured by the ABC [23], while another study found that higher IgG 4 concentrations were significantly associated with an increased severity of social interaction impairments as measured by the Autism Diagnostic Observation Schedule (ADOS) [49].

Two studies examined birth samples from archived newborn blood specimens which were obtained from the California Genetic Disease Screening Program and reported that ASD risk was associated with lower total IgG concentrations in the neonatal period [54,55].

The two studies that examined CSF IgG found no significant difference in CSF IgG concentrations or the IgG index as compared to the reference groups [56,57]. However, one study did find increased protein in 33% of ASD cases and oligoclonal bands in one patient (3%) and GAD65 antibodies in two patients (6%) in the CSF.

3.1.2. Meta-Analysis of Immunoglobulin G Concentrations in ASD

Nine studies used control groups as comparisons with two large studies using neonates while the remainder examined children. Seven studies used TD unrelated controls, while two studies used TD sibling controls and three studies used unrelated DD controls. One study divided the ASD groups into those with autistic disorder and those without autistic disorder but with autism features. Because it is not clear how this latter group would map onto the current definition of ASD, it has not been included in the analysis. One of the two studies examining neonates did not provide descriptive statistics of the immunoglobulin concentrations so the studies could not be combined. Only one study used parents as controls and the two studies that used developmentally delayed control groups studied different immunoglobulin measures, so parents and developmentally delayed controls were not included in the meta-analysis.

Table 2 outlines the pooled mean difference when combining studies using non-sibling and sibling controls separately as well as all studies combined (see Supplementary Table S2 for the number of participants per comparison). Both the pooled mean difference for the non-sibling and combined studies found that total IgG was lower in the ASD group with a confidence interval that did not include zero. However, the meta-analysis models for these pooled mean differences were not significant because of large variation among studies, as manifested by the significant Cochran's Q and DOI plots showing major asymmetry with LFK indexes of 8.80 and 8.99, respectively. Pooled mean difference for IgG 4 subclass was significantly elevated in individuals with ASD for all comparisons, with the comparison between ASD and TD siblings demonstrating significant variability across studies. None of the other IgG subclasses were found to be significantly different between ASD and comparisons groups in the meta-analysis.

Table 2. Meta-analysis of Studies on Immunoglobulin G Concentration in Autism Spectrum Disorder. Pooled mean difference (MD) with 95% confidence interval, Cochran's Q (Q), Heterogeneity Index (I^2). Statistics are estimated by inverse variance heterogeneity model. Significant values are Bold. * $p \leq 0.01$; ** $p \leq 0.001$.

	Non-Siblings			**Siblings**			**All Controls**		
	Pooled MD	**Cochran's Q**	**I^2**	**Pooled MD**	**Cochran's Q**	**I^2**	**Pooled MD**	**Cochran's Q**	**I^2**
Total IgG	−231 (−223, −238)	**40 ****	95%	49 (−3, 101)	3.3	70%	−225 (−217, −233)	**153 ****	97%
IgG1	14 (−45, 74)	2.2	54%	17 (−17, 51)	5.5	82%	17 (−13, 46)	7.7	61%
IgG2	9.2 (−1.0, 19.2)	0.0	0%	35.8 (3.5, 68.2)	5.8	83%	11.5 (1.9, 21.2)	8.23	64%
IgG3	-0.3 (−3.2, 2.6)	0.4	0%	0.5 (−3.7, 4.7)	0.4	0%	0.0 (−2.4, 2.4)	0.9	0%
IgG4	***16.6 ** (6.7, 26.4)***	0.7	0%	***19.7 ** (12.8, 26.5)***	**6.5 ***	84%	***18.7 ** (13.1, 24.3)***	7.4	60%

3.1.3. Summary of Immunoglobulin G Concentrations in ASD

Overall, studies on IgG abnormalities in ASD suggest that individuals with ASD may have a wider variation in serum IgG concentrations as compared to non-ASD controls. There appears to be preliminary evidence for both depressed total IgG and elevated IgG 4 subclass, both of which appear to have concentrations related to symptomatology. This may suggest two different immune abnormalities in different subsets of patients. However, with only a few large well-controlled studies, it is difficult to make any firm conclusions.

3.2. The Theraputic Use of IVIG in ASD

A total of 27 publications were identified which examined the use of IVIG in ASD. Four studies were prospective, controlled studies; six were prospective, uncontrolled studies; 2 were retrospective, controlled studies; and 15 were retrospective, uncontrolled studies (case reports and series).

3.2.1. Prospective, Controlled Studies

Four prospective, controlled studies were identified (Table 3). One study used IVIG in children without immune related problems [58] while the children in the other three studies had immune related problems.

Table 3. Prospective Controlled Immunoglobulin G Treatment Studies in Autism Spectrum Disorder. Specific Polysaccharide Antibody Deficiency (SPAD); Common Variable Immunodeficiency (CVID); Aberrant Behavior Checklist (ABC); Not specified (NS).

Study	Medical Indication	Autism Group (N)	IVIG Treatment	Outcomes
Niederhofer, Staffen et al., 2003 [58]	NS	12	400 mg/kg	Improvement in all ABC Subscales and improved drowsiness and activity
Jyonouchi, Geng et al., 2011 [22]	SPAD	10	NR	Decreased pro inflammatory cytokines (IL-6, IL-12 and IL-23) and increased TGF-ß and sTNFRII
Jyonouchi, Geng et al., 2011 [59]	SPAD in 6 CVID in 1	7	NR	NR
Maltsev and Yevtushenko 2016 [60]	NK Cell Deficiency; Reactivated HSV or Measles Infection	78	2g/kg monthly for 6 months	Improvement in all ABC Subscales

The first study was a DBPC crossover study of a one-time dose of IVIG 0.4g/kg or placebo in 12 children with ASD (age range 4.2 to 14.9 years) and reported significant improvements as rated by parents and teachers in ABC irritability, hyperactivity, social withdrawal and inappropriate speech. Improvements were also observed in drowsiness and decreased activity on the Symptom Checklist compared to the placebo group. Significant improvements were not observed by physicians as rated by the Children's Psychiatric Rating Scale (CPRS). Of note, none of the ASD children in this study had abnormalities in IgG or IgM concentrations [58].

Three other studies contained control groups who did not receive a placebo. In the first, 10 children with ASD (age not noted) with specific polysaccharide antibody deficiency (SPAD) and hypogammaglobulinemia were treated with an unspecified IVIG dose and compared to 14 non-ASD children with similar immunodeficiency treated with IVIG and 49 ASD and 39 normal children who did not receive treatment. Pro-inflammatory cytokines (IL-6, IL-12 and IL-23) and productions of IL-12 with exposure to phytohemagglutinin/Concanavalin A and IL-17/IFN-γ with exposure to phytohemagglutinin decreased, while TGF-ß and sTNFR II increased in the children with ASD who received IVIG compared to normal controls. ASD behaviors were not reported in this study [22].

In the second study, seven children with ASD and immunodeficiency (one with CVID and six with SPAD) were treated with any unspecified dose of IVIG, but no effects of IVIG were discussed [59].

Finally, in a third study, 78 children with ASD (ages 2–10 years old, 47 boys, 31 girls) were treated with IVIG 2 g/kg per month for six months. Characteristics of the treated children were compared to characteristics of a control group of 32 ASD children who received conventional therapy without IVIG. Additionally, changes in the ABC scale were compared to baseline measurements in the treatment group. Inclusion criteria for IVIG treatment included the presence of two to four polymorphisms in folate cycle genes, deficiency in natural killer cells, reactivated herpes and/or measles virus infections, or signs of leukoencephalopathy on a brain MRI. The authors reported "complete elimination of the phenotype of autism spectrum disorders" in 21 (27%), "marked improvement" in 33 (42) and mild-to-moderate improvements in 23 (29%). Overall, 77 (99%) had some improvement with IVIG. In the 21 children with the most improvements, one (5%) lost improvements when IVIG was stopped and 12 (50%) who showed mild-to-moderate improvement lost their gains two to four months after completing therapy. Twenty-nine out of 36 patients (81%) with epilepsy had improvement in seizures and 49 out of 68 children (72%) had improvements in gastrointestinal symptoms [60]. Compared to baseline, the treated group improved in ABC irritability, hyperactivity, social withdrawal and inappropriate speech.

3.2.2. Prospective, Uncontrolled Studies

Six prospective, uncontrolled studies were identified (Table 4); five studies administered IVIG to individuals with ASD who had immune related abnormalities whereas one study used IVIG in patients without immune problems [61].

Table 4. Prospective Uncontrolled Immunoglobulin G Treatment Studies in Autism Spectrum Disorder. Specific Polysaccharide Antibody Deficiency (SPAD); Common Variable Immunodeficiency (CVID); Aberrant Behavior Checklist (ABC); Clinical Global Impression Severity (CGI-S); Clinical Global Impression Improvement (CGI-I); Social Responsiveness Scale (SRS); Children's Communication Checklist–2 (CCC-2); Autism Diagnostic Observation Scheduled (ADOS).

Study	Medical Indication	Autism Group	IVIG Treatment	Outcomes
Gupta et al., 1996 [52]	IgG deficiency and others	10	0.4 g/kg every 4 weeks for 6 months	No quantitative outcomes 5 with "marked" or "striking" improvements. 5 with minimal improvements
Plioplys 1998 [61]	None	10	154–375 mg/kg every 6 weeks for 1–6 infusions	No quantitative outcomes 1 remarkable, 4 mild and 5 no improvements
DelGiudice-Asch et al., 1999 [62]	Recurrent infections	7	400 mg/kg every month for 6 months	2 discontinued treatment No significant changes in several quantitative symptom scales
Oleske 2004 [63]	Antibody deficiency	27	0.4–1 g/kg every 3 weeks for 6–18 months	No quantitative outcomes Less recurrent infections ASD symptoms improved in 78%
Melamed et al., 2006 [64]	Humoral and/or cellular immune deficit	12	1 g/kg monthly for 3 years	Non-standard quantitative outcomes Drastic reduction in Infections Improvement in cognition, communication and social skills
Melamed et al. 2018 [65]	Activated CD154 levels <80, recurrent infections or abnormal lymphocyte stimulation test or	14	1 g/kg every 2–4 weeks for 10 doses	Improvement in CGI-S and CGI-S, SRS, CCC–2 and ADOS

In a prospective, open-label study, 10 children (ages three to six years old) with ASD and IgG deficiency or other immune abnormalities were treated with IVIG (0.4 g/kg every four weeks for six months). Four (40%) showed "marked improvements", one (10%) showed "striking improvements" and five (50%) had "minimal improvements". Improvements were noted in social interaction, eye contact, echolalia and better response to commands. Speech improvements included better articulation and improved vocabulary. Younger children had more improvements compared to older patients [52].

In another prospective, open-label study, 10 children with ASD without immune problems (four to 15 years old, mean age eight years) received 0.154–0.375 g/kg IVIG (mean dose 0.27 g/kg) every six weeks. Six children received four infusions, whereas the other four received one, three, five, and six infusions, respectively. Five (50%) did not show improvements, while four (40%) had mild improvements in attention and hyperactivity reported by parents but not confirmed by clinicians; parents of these four children decided not to continue IVIG due to the cost and inconvenience. One child (10%) who received 0.375 g/kg for four infusions had "a very significant amelioration of autistic symptoms"; when the treatment was stopped the improvements were lost over a three-month period [61].

In another prospective, open-label study, seven children with ASD (ages three to six years old) with a history of recurrent infections or seizures were treated with 0.4 g/kg of IVIG every month for six months, with five children completing the study. Children were evaluated with Ritvo-Freeman Real Life Rating Scale (RF), Children Yale-Brown Obsessive-Compulsive Scale, Clinical Global Impression Scale (CGI), and the Autism Modification of the NIMH Global Obsessive-Compulsive Scale. Improvement was noted on the RF sensory responses but was considered not significant after Bonferroni correction [62].

In another prospective, open-label study, 27 children with ASD (ages two to 10 years old, median three years) and immune abnormalities were treated with IVIG 0.4–1.0g/kg every three weeks for six to 18 months. Immune abnormalities included IgG deficiency in five (19%), IgG subclass deficiency in 12 (44%), or recurrent infections that did not respond to conventional therapy with the presence of functional antibody deficiency in 10 (37%). With IVIG treatment, improvements in infections were observed in otitis media in 19 (70%), upper respiratory infections in 11 (41%), and sinopulmonary infections in nine (33%). Parents and physicians reported improvements in ASD symptoms in 21 (78%) [63].

In another prospective study, 12 children with ASD (age not reported) with either a humoral or cellular immune deficit (or both) were treated with 1.0 g/kg of IVIG monthly for three years. All children had a drastic reduction in the number of infections and improvements in cognition, communication, verbal interaction and social skills (1 to 4 point improvements on a scale of 1 to 5) [64].

In a prospective, open-label 30-week study, 14 children with ASD (mean age 7.6 $\pm$ 3.0 years) and immune abnormalities received 1 g/kg of IVIG every two to four weeks for 10 treatments. Immune abnormalities include T or B cell dysfunction, activated CD154 levels <80, or abnormal lymphocyte stimulation test and/or recurrent infections. Outcomes were compared to baseline measurements. Significant improvements were observed in CGI-S total score, CGI-I total score, and SRS total score. Significant improvements on Children's Communication Checklist–2 speech and semantics as well as Autism Diagnostic Observation Schedule (ADOS) stereotyped behaviors and restricted interest, communication plus social interaction total, and reciprocal social interaction were found. Statistically significant improvement on the ABC was only found on the hyperactivity subscale. Significant decreases in TNF-α induced by TLR ligands zymosan, flagellin, and lipopolysaccharide were also reported [65].

3.2.3. Retrospective, Baseline Controlled Case Series with Prospectively Collected Outcomes

Two case series (Table 5) were identified and are reviewed by year published. All studies used IVIG in ASD patients with immune-related problems.

Table 5. Retrospective Case Series Immunoglobulin G Treatment Studies in Autism Spectrum Disorder with Prospectively Baseline Controlled Outcome Measures. Aberrant Behavior Checklist (ABC).

Study	Medical Indication	Autism Group (N)	IVIG Treatment	Outcomes
Boris et al., 2005 [66]	6 with IgG Deficiency	26	400 mg/kg every month for 6 months	Improvements in ABC total and all subscales 22 (85%) lost gains after stopping IVIG
Connery et al., 2018 [19]	Autoimmune encephalopathy	31	0.75–2 g/kg every 2–6 weeks; 77% treated >1 year	Improvements on SRS and ABC scales

In a retrospective case series, 26 children with ASD (ages three to 17 years, mean age 6.8 years) and neurodevelopmental regression (mean age 17 months) were treated with 0.4 g/kg of IVIG monthly for six months. Only 23% of treated patients had low immunoglobulin levels. Total ABC score as well as hyperactivity, inappropriate speech, irritability, social withdrawal and stereotypy subscales showed significant improvement. Twenty-two (85%) lost some improvements when IVIG was stopped [66].

In an open-label study, 31 children with ASD who had evidence of autoimmune encephalopathy (presence of various brain autoantibodies) were treated with 0.75–2g/kg IVIG every two to six weeks; 77% were treated for more than one year. Significant improvements were observed in SRS total score and cognition and mannerisms subscales and ABC total score and irritability, lethargy, hyperactivity and inappropriate speech subscales [19]. Of interest, this study also found that the anti-Dopamine D2L and anti-tubulin antibodies of the Cunningham panel (Moleculera, Oklahoma City, OK, USA) were predictive of response to IVIG.

3.2.4. Retrospective, Uncontrolled Case Series

Three case series (Table 6) were identified and are reviewed by year published. All studies used IVIG in ASD patients with immune-related problems.

Table 6. Retrospective Uncontrolled Case Series. Specific Polysaccharide Antibody Deficiency (SPAD); Aberrant Behavior Checklist (ABC).

Study	Medical Indication	Autism Group (N)	IVIG Treatment	Outcomes
Knutsen and Fenton 1998 [67]	1 with IgG deficiency 3 with intractable epilepsy	3	1.0–1.7 g/kg up to 11 months	No quantitative outcomes 2 seizure free, 1 with seizure improved ASD symptoms improved in 2 and worsened in 1
Jyonouchi et al., 2012 [68]	SPAD 4 with intractable epilepsy	8	0.6–1g/kg every 3 weeks for 1–6 years	No quantitative outcomes Four with seizure improvement One with cognitive improvements
Fadeyi and Li 2018 [69]	IgG deficiency	3	NR	No quantitative outcomes Improvements in ASD symptoms and IgG and IgM levels

Three children with ASD and intractable epilepsy defined as at least three seizures per day were treated with 1.0–1.7 g/kg of IVIG for up to 11 months. One child had low total IgG and the others had normal IgG levels. Two patients became seizure-free and the third had a reduction in seizures. Two children had improvement in social interaction, communication and behavior. In one child, seizures and ASD symptoms worsened when IVIG was discontinued [67].

Eight children with ASD and SPAD (ages six to 16 years old) who had worsening of cognitive skills and behavioral symptoms with "immune insults" were treated with 0.6–1 g/kg of IVIG every three weeks for one to six years. Three children had below normal total IgG. Treatment improved recurrent infections. In the four patients with treatment resistant epilepsy, seizures were significantly improved. Overall ASD symptoms were not reported to improve but behavioral exacerbations associated with infections did improve. Parents reported improvement in cognitive skills in one child but standardized clinical outcome measures did not confirm this [68].

Finally, in a retrospective case series, three children with ASD who had IgG deficiency were treated with an unspecified dose of IVIG over five to eight years. Serum IgG and IgM concentrations improved with improvement in immunoglobulin concentrations believed to correlated with an improvement in ASD symptoms [69].

3.2.5. Retrospective, Uncontrolled Case Reports

Twelve studies were case reports (Table 7) and described patients with ASD treated with IVIG for mostly immune-mediated conditions, with two publications reporting on the same case [70,71]. Indications for IVIG ranged from purely immune conditions to immune related neurological conditions, as well as one case report for neuroleptic malignant syndrome which is not usually believe to be an immune related condition.

Table 7. Retrospective Uncontrolled Case Studies of Immunoglobulin G Treatment in Autism Spectrum Disorder. Chronic inflammatory Demyelinating Polyneuropathy (CIDP); Common Variable Immunodeficiency (CVID); N-Methyl-D-Aspartic Acid (NMDA); Nicotinic Acetylcholine Receptor (nAChR); Not Reported (NR), month old (mo), years old (yo).

Study	Medical Indication	Participant	IVIG Treatment	Outcomes (Non-Quantitative)
		Immune Abnormality		
Suez and Scharnwebber 1997 [72]	CVID	15 yo boy	NR	Significant improvement in ASD symptoms
Wang et al., 2005 [73]	CVID	22 yo man	Monthly Dose NR	Significant improvements in appetite, weight gain, and serious infections
Salehi Sadaghiani et al., 2013 [74]	CVID	13 yo boy	NR	No improvements reported
		Inflammatory Neuropathy		
Sommerville et al., 2007 [75]	CIDP Epilepsy	8 yo boy	0.4 g/kg/d for 5 day	No improvements reported
Kamata et al., 2017 [76]	Inflammatory Neuropathy	6 yo girl	0.4 g/kg/d for 5 day	Neuropathy improved No mention of changes in ASD symptoms
		Immune Mediated Encephalopathy		
Scott et al., 2014 [77]	anti-NMDA receptor encephalitis	33 mo boy	0.4 g/kg/d for 5 day	Language and social skills improved
Menon et al., 2014 [79]	anti-nAChR receptor encephalitis	5 yo boy	w/plasmapheresis	Improvements in hyperactivity, agitation, speech, and social interaction
Akcakaya et al., 2015, 2016 [70,71]	Enterovirus Encephalitis, Seizures	14 yo girl	0.02 g/kg	Improvements in eye contact, speech, communication, and seizures
Gonzalez-Toro et al., 2013 [78]	anti-NMDA receptor encephalitis	5 yo boy	0.4 g/kg/day for 5 days	Improvements in ASD symptoms and language
Bouboulis and Mast 2016 [80]	Autoimmune Encephalopathy	5 yo boy	1.6 g/kg every 8 weeks for 2 years	Improvements in ASD symptoms, language, learning, and memory
		Other Conditions		
Xu et al., 2017 [81]	Neuroleptic malignant syndrome	32 yo man	NR	Seizures and dysautonomia improved No mention of changes in ASD symptoms

Three case reports describe individuals with ASD and immune conditions. A 15-year-old boy with ASD and CVID treated with IVIG was reported to have resolution of recurrent infections and marked improvement in ASD symptoms [72]. A 22-year-old man with ASD with a large mesenteric granulomatous mass and CVID was treated with monthly IVIG. Appetite, weight and serious infections improved but no changes in ASD behaviors were mentioned [73]. Finally, a 13-year-old boy with ASD and CVID with recurrent infections was treated with IVIG but he continued to have infections and no note was made of changes in ASD behaviors [74].

Two cases of patients with inflammatory neuropathies were reported. An eight-year-old boy with ASD, epilepsy and chronic inflammatory demyelinating polyneuropathy (CIDP) was treated with IVIG and IV methylprednisolone, but weakness progressed. No mention was made of any changes in ASD symptoms with IVIG [75]. A six-year-old girl with ASD and right upper arm weakness due to a demyelinating neuropathy was treated with one course of IVIG with resolution of the neuropathy symptoms but no mention if ASD symptoms improved [76].

Five cases of immune mediated encephalopathy were reported with four of the cases being autoimmune encephalopathy. A 33-month-old boy with ASD and neurodevelopmental regression was diagnosed with anti-N-Methyl-D-aspartic acid (NMDA) receptor encephalitis by lumbar puncture. Treatment with 2 g/kg of IVIG over five days resulted in improvements in language and social skills on the third treatment day [77]. A five-year-old ASD girl diagnosed with anti-NMDA receptor encephalitis by lumbar puncture was treated with 20 mg/kg/day of IV steroids for five days, 0.4 g/kg of IVIG for five days and 0.375 g/kg of rituximab weekly for four weeks. Improvements were noted in seizures and language with this combination [78]. A five-year-old boy experiencing neurodevelopmental regression with the emergence of ASD symptoms including social isolation and repetitive behaviors was diagnosed with autoimmune encephalitis due to alpha-3 subunit nicotinic acetylcholine receptor autoantibodies. Treatment with plasmapheresis followed by monthly IVIG resulted in significant improvements after five months with the child being able to attend a regular classroom, resolution of hyperactivity and improvements in social interaction [79]. A five-year-old ASD boy with infection-induced autoimmune encephalopathy was treated with 1.6 g/kg of IVIG every eight weeks for two years, resulting in marked improvements in social interaction, language, learning and memory; he maintained the cognitive improvements when IVIG was stopped [80]. Lastly, a 14-year-old previously healthy girl with neurodevelopmental regression and the development of ASD symptoms including lack of eye contact, impaired communication, and social withdrawal with the onset of seizures was found to have enterovirus encephalitis as well as a low IgG index in the CSF. Treatment with 20 mg/kg of IVIG for five days resulted in improvements in eye contact, speech, and communication, as well as a resolution of her seizures [70,71].

Finally, a 32-year-old man with ASD and mental retardation diagnosed with neuroleptic malignant syndrome and seizures was treated with IVIG after he failed multiple anti-epileptics. Two weeks later, his seizures and dysautonomia resolved; no mention was made if ASD symptoms improved [81].

3.2.6. Meta-Analysis of Behavioral Responses to Intravenous Immunoglobulin

Five studies used the ABC instrument as an outcome measure, but only two studies provided information to obtain means and standard deviations before and after the treatments to combine outcome measures. Both retrospective studies obtained data prospectively with baseline measurements [19,66]. Two other studies also observed changes in ABC scores from baseline but one did not report any variation measure [60] and the other reported range as a measure of variation [65]. The DBPC crossover study [58] is not appropriate to combine with the open-label studies because of the differences in methodology. Thus, two studies with a total of 46 participants with two sets of measurements for each participant (baseline and treatment) were included in the meta-analysis.

ABC irritability and total score were found to significantly improve with IVIG with a large effect size [total: $d' = 0.80$ (0.37, 1.23), $p < 0.001$; irritability: $d' = 0.87$ (0.44, 1.31), $p < 0.0001$]. ABC social Withdrawal and hyperactivity were found to significantly improve with IVIG treatment with a medium effect size [social withdrawal: d′ = 0.54 (0.12, 0.95), $p = 0.01$; hyperactivity: d′ = 0.67 (0.25, 1.09), $p = 0.001$]. ABC stereotyped movements and inappropriate speech were not found to significantly improve when the studies were combined.

Two studies [19,65] used the SRS as an outcome measure but one study reported range as a variation measure [65], so these studies could not be combined.

3.3. Adverse Effects

Most studies did not report any AEs. One case series specifically reported that no AEs were observed. None of the prospective controlled studies reported AEs. Two prospective uncontrolled studies reported AEs. Melamed et al. (2018) reported that four (29%) had infusion site reactions and three (21%) had a headache. Connery et al. (2018) reported AEs, mostly during the infusion, with headaches in 39%, vomiting in 29%, worsening behaviors in 16%, anxiety in 13%, fever in 13%, nausea in 10%, fatigue in 10%, and rash in 5%; two (6%) patients discontinued IVIG because of AEs. One case report reported agitation, combative behavior, and fearfulness [80]. None of the other case reports reported AEs. Thus, the majority of studies did not report AEs, but most studies were not specifically designed to follow AEs as outcome measurements and none of the studies were designed to measure safety. As most of the AEs of IVIG are well known, many AEs may have been considered part of the standard treatment. Most of the AEs reported are consistent with standard IVIG treatment.

4. Discussion

This systemic review aimed to identify studies examining IgG concentrations and the use of IVIG in individuals with ASD. We identified 12 studies which examined IgG concentrations and 27 studies that described the use of IVIG in ASD (one study fell into both categories). We found limited evidence for changes in immunoglobulin concentrations in children with ASD, suggesting this might be present in subgroups of children with more severe ASD. Evidence for the effectiveness of IVIG treatment was also found but studies demonstrated many limitations. In most cases, IVIG was used to treat immune abnormalities in individuals with ASD as IVIG is a common, safe and well-tolerated treatment for immune disorders.

Nine of the 12 studies examining IgG concentrations included controls, with two using sibling controls and seven using non-related controls; one study used parents as comparisons and three used non-ASD developmentally delayed controls as a comparison group. One study found that total IgG and IgG4 concentrations were higher in ASD as compared to sibling controls, while the other sibling study demonstrated no differences between those with and without ASD. In studies with non-related control children, two studies demonstrated elevated IgG and IgG4 concentrations in ASD as compared to controls, with one study finding that higher IgG4 concentrations were associated with more severe social interaction impairments in those with ASD. Three studies demonstrated lower IgG in ASD as compared to non-related controls; one study demonstrated a significantly lowered median IgG concentration in ASD as compared to controls, with the depression in IgG concentration related to more severe aberrant behaviors. One study demonstrated that 20% of children with ASD had subclass deficiency, including two with IgG4 deficiency, and another study demonstrated a lower IgG concentration in the neonatal period for those who went on to be diagnosed with ASD, with neonatal IgG concentration significantly related to the risk of developing ASD. Two studies demonstrated no differences in serum IgG concentrations between ASD and control participants, while another study demonstrated no difference in the CSF IgG index between ASD and control individuals.

Overall, immunoglobulin studies in ASD reveal two patterns of IgG alterations. Three studies demonstrate depressed total IgG levels and three studies demonstrated elevated IgG concentrations which were primary driven by elevated IgG4 concentrations. Interesting, both abnormalities were correlated with more severe ASD-related symptoms. The meta-analysis was consistent with this pattern but also demonstrated significant variability among studies which would be expected if there are subgroups of children with different immunological profiles.

Meta-analysis demonstrated a trend toward lower total IgG concentrations in children with ASD as a group with a large variation in this finding across studies. Several lines of evidence support the notion that this finding is driven by a subgroup of children with ASD and hypogammaglobulinemia rather than simple biological variability. First, a lower total IgG concentration has been found to be correlated with more severe aberrant behaviors in the only large study to examine this relationship [23]. Second, studies on neonates suggest that lower IgG levels were associated with an increased risk for developing ASD [54,55]. Third, treatment studies have suggested that treatment of children with ASD and hypogammaglobulinemia results in improved ASD symptoms [52,63,64,66,67,69].

The fact that low total IgG levels in the neonatal period is associated with the development of ASD may suggest that the humoral immune system may be depressed early in life. Consistent with humoral immune system abnormalities, children with ASD are more likely to have recurrent viral and bacterial infections. For example, a history of otitis media (OM) and antibiotic use is associated with increased risk of ASD [82]; children with ASD are more likely to have OM, especially complicated OM, suggesting more severe OM infections [83], as compared to non-ASD siblings; children with ASD are more likely to have recurrent OM and upper respiratory and other infections [5,84]; and those children with ASD who have recurrent infections are found to be more medically complex and lower functioning [84]. Recurrent infections could be linked to depressed immune response. Studies have suggested that children with ASD and recurrent infections and other immune abnormalities have associated abnormal Toll-like receptor responses [85], dysregulation of inflammatory and counterregulatory cytokines [86], changes in regulatory microRNA [17], and atypical mitochondrial respiration [16].

Meta-analysis has demonstrated that elevation in IgG 4 subclass is related to ASD. Although commonly associated IgG4-related disease, such as fibro-inflammatory changes in the salivary and lacrimal glands, orbit, pancreas, and kidneys [87] is not common for children with ASD, elevated IgG4 is associated with eosinophilic esophagitis [88], a disorder that is under diagnosed and associated with restricted feeding in ASD [89]. This raises the possibility that IgG4 could potentially be used to help differentiate children with feeding disorders due to eosinophilic esophagitis and behavioral issues. Clearly this is an important and promising area of research.

Interestingly, eosinophilic esophagitis is associated with IgE-mediated food allergies which is associated with enteric microbiome alterations in non-ASD children [90,91]. As microbiome imbalances have been associated with ASD [92] and may have important consequences in immune regulation [93], microbiome alterations may be playing a role in immune dysregulation in ASD. The fact that chronic gastrointestinal symptoms have also been linked to non-IgE-mediated food allergies [94] and immune dysregulation [85] in children with ASD demonstrates the complex relationship between gastrointestinal symptoms and immune dysfunction in ASD and the complicated nature of management and treatment of ongoing symptoms in ASD.

Studies which have been conducted on measuring IgG in ASD have been innovative in examining IgG concentrations prior to symptom onset to help understand the role of immune dysfunction in the etiology of ASD and in examining their parents given the research that suggests a transgenerational effect in the etiology of ASD. Clearly, further studies will be needed to better understand the potential subgroups of children with ASD and immune abnormalities, especially with respect to the developmental nature of IgG concentrations. These studies point to the possibility of subsets of children with ASD with different immune profiles, but further studies are needed to verify these abnormalities.

There were four prospective controlled studies of IVIG but only one of these was a DBPC study [58] and only two examined changes in ASD symptoms, with both studies reporting improvements. One of these aforementioned studies enrolled children with immune abnormalities while the other did not. One of the other two studies which did not examine changes in symptoms instead measured changes in cytokines with IVIG. The limited number of controlled and placebo-controlled studies is disappointing but given the risk-benefit of an intravenous treatment in children, a high level of certainty of the efficacy is needed before such studies are launched, so the lack of such studies is understandable at this time. More studies will be necessary for future evaluation of this treatment.

Six studies were prospective without a control group with five of the studies enrolling children with ASD and immune problems. Immune problems varied widely from recurrent infections to quantitatively diagnosed immune deficiencies. All studies reported improvements but in one study the improvements were not statistically significant after correction for multiple comparisons. Unfortunately, only two of the six studies used standardized clinical outcome measures to document improvements.

Two studies were retrospective case series of prospectively collected outcomes with both studies using the ABC questionnaire, allowing the combining of these studies in a meta-analysis, which demonstrated improvements on the ABC scale including significant improvements in irritability, hyperactivity, and social withdrawal, as well as total aberrant behaviors (all with medium to large effect sizes).

Three case series and twelve case reports described treatment of children with ASD with IVIG. Only one study used standardized quantitative clinical outcome measures and all studies which reported changes in ASD symptoms reported improvements. Only one case report and one case series enrolled patients without immune-related problems.

One of the major limitations of the IVIG treatment studies was the lack of standardized outcome measures. The most commonly used standardized outcome measure was the ABC, which was used in five studies, all of which demonstrated improvement in aberrant behaviors. The next most commonly used standardized outcome measure was the SRS in two studies, both of which demonstrated improvements in social function. Other studies noted clinical improvements in communication, irritability, hyperactivity, cognition, attention, social interaction, eye contact, echolalia, speech, and responsiveness, although standardized measures were not always used to collect these observations. Besides improvements in ASD symptoms, other benefits were seen from IVIG. Six studies reported improvements in seizures with IVIG [60,67,68,76,78,81], with one study reporting a worsening of seizures when IVIG was stopped [67]. Other studies demonstrated improvements in recurrent infections [64,73], appetite [73], weight gain [73], neuropathy [76], dysautonomia [81], pro-inflammatory cytokines [22], and gastrointestinal symptoms [60].

The dose of IVIG varied widely from 20 mg/kg to 2 g/kg and the treatment duration varied from one total IVIG treatment to recurrent treatment for many years, but most studies did not document the exact dose and frequency of the treatment. Overall, most studies did not report if AEs occurred, and for the four studies that did, the AEs were of limited duration and severity [19,65,67,80].

The biological mechanism by which IVIG has its therapeutic effect was investigated in a limited number of studies. One prospective controlled study [22] and one prospective uncontrolled study [65] found a decrease in inflammatory cytokines, and one case series demonstrated an improvement in IgG and IgM concentrations [69] with IVIG treatment. Given that IgG and IgM [23] and inflammatory cytokine [17] concentrations have been associated with ASD behaviors, modulation of these factors could play a role in the therapeutic effect of IVIG. Two prospective uncontrolled studies [63,64] and two case series [72,73] noted a substantial decrease in the number of infections with IVIG treatment, and one case series noted an improvement in behavioral exacerbations associated with infections [68]. Given that a subgroup of children with ASD have been described with immune abnormalities who have behavioral exacerbation with infections [86], simply improving the number of infections may improve the ability to function and quality of life for some individuals with ASD. The therapeutic effect of IVIG for modulating autoantibodies may have been effective in the case-series [19] and case-studies [70,71,77–80] of patients with ASD and autoimmune encephalopathy caused by anti-NMDA receptor [77,78], anti-nAChR receptor [79], anti-dopamine receptor [19], and anti-tubulin [19] autoantibodies. Finally, the therapeutic effect of IVIG on seizures may have been therapeutic in the cases described with refractory seizures [67,68,70,71].

Thus, these studies suggest IVIG treatment can be effective for some individuals with ASD, particularly those with underlying immune-related problems. However, many studies had substantial limitations, including a lack of a control group, only qualitative outcomes reported, no standardized reporting of details of dosing and duration of treatment, and no standardized reporting of AEs. Indeed, this does suggest that the majority of the studies are open to bias. Additionally, several studies did not report commonly used measures of variance such as standard deviation or interquartile range, making their data difficult to include in a meta-analysis. Thus, future studies will need to address these limitations in order to provide high quality evidence for the use of IVIG in ASD.

5. Conclusions

ASD is a prevalent and life-long neurodevelopmental disorder with no known cure. Standard of care treatments are effective in some individuals but leave many with incomplete recovery. A better understanding of the underlying physiological abnormalities is beginning to emerge with evidence supporting abnormalities in immune function, making the immune system a potential target for treatment. Several common treatments for children with ASD also have effects on the immune system, suggesting that their efficacy in ASD may in part be linked to their effects on modulating immune function [95]. This review provide support for the notion that at least a subset of children with ASD have immune abnormalities, particularly in humoral immunity characterized by abnormal concentrations of immunoglobulins and may respond to the immune modulating effect of IVIG therapy. This study has found that there is limited evidence that some children with ASD have abnormal IgG concentrations, but this may be driven by a subgroup with abnormalities. The other major finding in this meta-analysis was an elevation in IgG4 subclass. Variations in IgG concentration were perhaps related to ASD symptom severity, suggesting that for some individuals with abnormal IgG concentrations, IVIG may be a directly targeted treatment.

Still IVIG has many other clinical effects aside from replacing endogenous IgG. Indeed, IVIG can modulate the immune system and is commonly used in neurological disorders to treat pathophysiological processes involving inappropriate activation of the immune system. IVIG is a common treatment because it is usually well tolerated with minimal and non-serious AEs. Additionally, as compared to other treatments which modulate the immune system, IVIG modulates immune function while also providing immune protection, so concerns for immune suppression and opportunistic infections are minimized.

Overall, IVIG appears to be effective in many children with ASD, particularly in those with identified immune problems. It also appears to be well tolerated. However, the quality of the evidence for the use of IVIG is still below what is commonly accepted for a routinely used treatment with the bulk of the studies being uncontrolled. Many studies demonstrated bias, including selection bias (lack of randomization), performance bias (lack of blinding), detection bias (lack of standardized outcomes), attrition bias (retrospective studies are prone to losing patients to follow-up), and reporting bias (case studies tend to report positive rather than negative outcomes). Thus, the current set of studies presented should be used to design and implement well-controlled, blinded randomized clinical trials in the future. Additionally, the populations used in these studies are very heterogeneous with many different immune system abnormalities, making it hard to determine if there is a particular subset of children with ASD in which the treatment may be most effective. Thus, further identification of biomarkers that can guide treatment will be helpful.

6. Patents

No patents to report.

Supplementary Materials: Following are available online at https://www.mdpi.com/article/10.3390/jpm11060488/s1, Figure S1: PRISMA 2020 flow diagram for new systematic reviews which included searches of databases, registers and other sources, Table S1: PRISMA 2020 Checklist, Table S2: Number of Participants for Meta-analysis of studies on immunoglobulin G Concentration in Autism Spectrum Disorder.

Author Contributions: D.A.R. and R.E.F. has drafted and reviewed this manuscript. All authors have read and agreed to the published version of the manuscript.

Funding: This research received no external funding.

Institutional Review Board Statement: Not applicable.

Informed Consent Statement: Not applicable.

Conflicts of Interest: The authors declare no conflict of interest.

References

1. Maenner, M.J.; Shaw, K.A.; Baio, J.; Washington, A.; Patrick, M.; DiRienzo, M.; Christensen, D.L.; Wiggins, L.D.; Pettygrove, S. Prevalence of Autism Spectrum Disorder Among Children Aged 8 Years—Autism and Developmental Disabilities Monitoring Network, 11 Sites, United States, 2016. *Mmwr. Surveill Summ.* **2020**, *69*, 1–12. [CrossRef]
2. Cakir, J.; Frye, R.E.; Walker, S.J. The lifetime social cost of autism: 1990–2029. *Res. Autism Spectr. Disord.* **2020**, *72*, 101502. [CrossRef]
3. Rossignol, D.A.; Frye, R.E. Mitochondrial dysfunction in autism spectrum disorders: A systematic review and meta-analysis. *Mol. Psychiatry* **2012**, *17*, 290–314. [CrossRef]
4. Rossignol, D.A.; Frye, R.E. Psychotropic Medications for Sleep Disorders in Autism Spectrum Disorders. In *Handbook on Autism and Pervasive Developmental Disorde—Assessment, Diagnosis and Treatmeny*; Matson, J.L., Sturmey, P., Eds.; Springer Nature: Cham, Switzerland, 2020.
5. Vargason, T.; Frye, R.E.; McGuinness, D.L.; Hahn, J. Clustering of co-occurring conditions in autism spectrum disorder during early childhood: A retrospective analysis of medical claims data. *Autism Res. Off. J. Int. Soc. Autism Res.* **2019**, *12*, 1272–1285. [CrossRef] [PubMed]
6. Holingue, C.; Newill, C.; Lee, L.C.; Pasricha, P.J.; Daniele Fallin, M. Gastrointestinal symptoms in autism spectrum disorder: A review of the literature on ascertainment and prevalence. *Autism Res. Off. J. Int. Soc. Autism Res.* **2018**, *11*, 24–36. [CrossRef] [PubMed]
7. Liao, X.; Yang, J.; Wang, H.; Li, Y. Microglia mediated neuroinflammation in autism spectrum disorder. *J. Psychiatr. Res.* **2020**, *130*, 167–176. [CrossRef] [PubMed]
8. Anukirthiga, B.; Mishra, D.; Pandey, S.; Juneja, M.; Sharma, N. Prevalence of Epilepsy and Inter-Ictal Epileptiform Discharges in Children with Autism and Attention-Deficit Hyperactivity Disorder. *Indian J. Pediatr.* **2019**, *86*, 897–902. [CrossRef] [PubMed]
9. Tilford, J.M.; Payakachat, N.; Kuhlthau, K.A.; Pyne, J.M.; Kovacs, E.; Bellando, J.; Williams, D.K.; Brouwer, W.B.; Frye, R.E. Treatment for Sleep Problems in Children with Autism and Caregiver Spillover Effects. *J. Autism Dev. Disord.* **2015**, *45*, 3613–3623. [CrossRef]
10. Rossignol, D.A.; Frye, R.E. A review of research trends in physiological abnormalities in autism spectrum disorders: Immune dysregulation, inflammation, oxidative stress, mitochondrial dysfunction and environmental toxicant exposures. *Mol. Psychiatry* **2012**, *17*, 389–401. [CrossRef]
11. Croen, L.A.; Qian, Y.; Ashwood, P.; Daniels, J.L.; Fallin, D.; Schendel, D.; Schieve, L.A.; Singer, A.B.; Zerbo, O. Family history of immune conditions and autism spectrum and developmental disorders: Findings from the study to explore early development. *Autism Res. Off. J. Int. Soc. Autism Res.* **2019**, *12*, 123–135. [CrossRef]
12. Wu, S.; Ding, Y.; Wu, F.; Li, R.; Xie, G.; Hou, J.; Mao, P. Family history of autoimmune diseases is associated with an increased risk of autism in children: A systematic review and meta-analysis. *Neurosci. Biobehav. Rev.* **2015**, *55*, 322–332. [CrossRef] [PubMed]
13. Ramirez-Celis, A.; Becker, M.; Nuño, M.; Schauer, J.; Aghaeepour, N.; Van de Water, J. Risk assessment analysis for maternal autoantibody-related autism (MAR-ASD): A subtype of autism. *Mol. Psychiatry* **2021**. [CrossRef]
14. Gumusoglu, S.B.; Stevens, H.E. Maternal Inflammation and Neurodevelopmental Programming: A Review of Preclinical Outcomes and Implications for Translational Psychiatry. *Biol. Psychiatry* **2019**, *85*, 107–121. [CrossRef]
15. Harville, T.; Rhodes-Clark, B.; Bennuri, S.C.; Delhey, L.; Slattery, J.; Tippett, M.; Wynne, R.; Rose, S.; Kahler, S.; Frye, R.E. Inheritance of HLA-Cw7 Associated With Autism Spectrum Disorder (ASD). *Front. Psychiatry* **2019**, *10*, 612. [CrossRef]
16. Jyonouchi, H.; Geng, L.; Rose, S.; Bennuri, S.C.; Frye, R.E. Variations in Mitochondrial Respiration Differ in IL-1ß/IL-10 Ratio Based Subgroups in Autism Spectrum Disorders. *Front. Psychiatry* **2019**, *10*, 71. [CrossRef]
17. Jyonouchi, H.; Geng, L.; Streck, D.L.; Dermody, J.J.; Toruner, G.A. MicroRNA expression changes in association with changes in interleukin-1ß/interleukin10 ratios produced by monocytes in autism spectrum disorders: Their association with neuropsychiatric symptoms and comorbid conditions (observational study). *J. Neuroinflamm.* **2017**, *14*, 229. [CrossRef] [PubMed]

18. Vargas, D.L.; Nascimbene, C.; Krishnan, C.; Zimmerman, A.W.; Pardo, C.A. Neuroglial activation and neuroinflammation in the brain of patients with autism. *Ann. Neurol.* **2005**, *57*, 67–81. [CrossRef] [PubMed]
19. Connery, K.; Tippett, M.; Delhey, L.M.; Rose, S.; Slattery, J.C.; Kahler, S.G.; Hahn, J.; Kruger, U.; Cunningham, M.W.; Shimasaki, C.; et al. Intravenous immunoglobulin for the treatment of autoimmune encephalopathy in children with autism. *Transl. Psychiatry* **2018**, *8*, 148. [CrossRef] [PubMed]
20. Frye, R.E.; Sequeira, J.M.; Quadros, E.V.; James, S.J.; Rossignol, D.A. Cerebral folate receptor autoantibodies in autism spectrum disorder. *Mol. Psychiatry* **2013**, *18*, 369–381. [CrossRef] [PubMed]
21. Gupta, S.; Samra, D.; Agrawal, S. Adaptive and Innate Immune Responses in Autism: Rationale for Therapeutic Use of Intravenous Immunoglobulin. *J. Clin. Immunol.* **2010**, *30* (Suppl. S1), S90–S96. [CrossRef]
22. Jyonouchi, H.; Geng, L.; Kapoor, S.; Streck, D.; Toruner, G.J.J.o.A.; Immunology, C. Characterization Of Children With Autism Spectrum Disorders (asd) Requiring Intravenous Immunoglobulin (ivig) For Specific Polysaccharide Antibody Deficiency (spad)/hypogammaglobulinemia-Distinct Patterns Of Cytokine Production And Gene Expression Profiles. *J. Allergy Clin. Immunol.* **2011**, *127*, AB231. [CrossRef]
23. Heuer, L.; Ashwood, P.; Schauer, J.; Goines, P.; Krakowiak, P.; Hertz-Picciotto, I.; Hansen, R.; Croen, L.A.; Pessah, I.N.; Van de Water, J. Reduced levels of immunoglobulin in children with autism correlates with behavioral symptoms. *Autism Res. Off. J. Int. Soc. Autism Res.* **2008**, *1*, 275–283. [CrossRef]
24. Hausman-Kedem, M.; Menascu, S.; Greenstein, Y.; Fattal-Valevski, A. Immunotherapy for GRIN2A and GRIN2D-related epileptic encephalopathy. *Epilepsy Res.* **2020**, *163*, 106325. [CrossRef]
25. Geva-Dayan, K.; Shorer, Z.; Menascu, S.; Linder, I.; Goldberg-Stern, H.; Heyman, E.; Lerman-Sagie, T.; Ben Zeev, B.; Kramer, U. Immunoglobulin treatment for severe childhood epilepsy. *Pediatr. Neurol.* **2012**, *46*, 375–381. [CrossRef]
26. Gross-Tsur, V.; Shalev, R.S.; Kazir, E.; Engelhard, D.; Amir, N. Intravenous high-dose gammaglobulins for intractable childhood epilepsy. *Acta Neurol. Scand.* **1993**, *88*, 204–209. [CrossRef]
27. Schwab, I.; Nimmerjahn, F. Intravenous immunoglobulin therapy: How does IgG modulate the immune system? *Nat. Rev. Immunol.* **2013**, *13*, 176–189. [CrossRef] [PubMed]
28. Tha-In, T.; Bayry, J.; Metselaar, H.J.; Kaveri, S.V.; Kwekkeboom, J. Modulation of the cellular immune system by intravenous immunoglobulin. *Trends Immunol.* **2008**, *29*, 608–615. [CrossRef] [PubMed]
29. Kaneko, Y.; Nimmerjahn, F.; Ravetch, J.V. Anti-inflammatory activity of immunoglobulin G resulting from Fc sialylation. *Science* **2006**, *313*, 670–673. [CrossRef]
30. Kazatchkine, M.D.; Kaveri, S.V. Immunomodulation of autoimmune and inflammatory diseases with intravenous immune globulin. *N. Engl. J. Med.* **2001**, *345*, 747–755. [CrossRef]
31. Negi, V.S.; Elluru, S.; Siberil, S.; Graff-Dubois, S.; Mouthon, L.; Kazatchkine, M.D.; Lacroix-Desmazes, S.; Bayry, J.; Kaveri, S.V. Intravenous immunoglobulin: An update on the clinical use and mechanisms of action. *J. Clin. Immunol.* **2007**, *27*, 233–245. [CrossRef] [PubMed]
32. Page, M.J.; McKenzie, J.E.; Bossuyt, P.M.; Boutron, I.; Hoffmann, T.C.; Mulrow, C.D.; Shamseer, L.; Tetzlaff, J.M.; Akl, E.A.; Brennan, S.E.; et al. The PRISMA 2020 statement: An updated guideline for reporting systematic reviews. *BMJ (Clin. Res. Ed.)* **2021**, *372*, n71. [CrossRef]
33. Higgins, J.P.T.; Altman, D.G.; Sterne, J.A.C. Assessing risk of bias in included studies. In *Cochrane Handbook for Systematic Reviews of Interventions*, Version 5.1.0 ed.; Higgins, J.P.T., Green, S., Eds.; The Cochrane Collaboration: London, UK, 2011.
34. Schneider, C.K.; Melmed, R.D.; Barstow, L.E.; Enriquez, F.J.; Ranger-Moore, J.; Ostrem, J.A. Oral human immunoglobulin for children with autism and gastrointestinal dysfunction: A prospective, open-label study. *J. Autism Dev. Disord.* **2006**, *36*, 1053–1064. [CrossRef]
35. Handen, B.L.; Melmed, R.D.; Hansen, R.L.; Aman, M.G.; Burnham, D.L.; Bruss, J.B.; McDougle, C.J. A double-blind, placebo-controlled trial of oral human immunoglobulin for gastrointestinal dysfunction in children with autistic disorder. *J. Autism Dev. Disord.* **2009**, *39*, 796–805. [CrossRef]
36. Gupta, S. Immunological treatments for autism. *J. Autism Dev. Disord.* **2000**, *30*, 475–479. [CrossRef] [PubMed]
37. Altman, D.G.; Machin, D.; Bryant, T.N.; Gardner, M.J. *Statistics with Confidence*, 2nd ed.; BMJ Books: Oxford, UK, 2000.
38. Higgins, J.P.T.; Green, S. *Cochrane Handbook for Systematic Reviews of Interventions*; Wiley Online Library: Hoboken, NJ, USA, 2008.
39. Doi, S.A.; Barendregt, J.J.; Khan, S.; Thalib, L.; Williams, G.M. Advances in the meta-analysis of heterogeneous clinical trials I: The inverse variance heterogeneity model. *Contemp. Clin. Trials* **2015**, *45*, 130–138. [CrossRef] [PubMed]
40. Higgins, J.P.; Thompson, S.G. Quantifying heterogeneity in a meta-analysis. *Stat. Med.* **2002**, *21*, 1539–1558. [CrossRef]
41. Higgins, J.P.; Thompson, S.G.; Deeks, J.J.; Altman, D.G. Measuring inconsistency in meta-analyses. *BMJ* **2003**, *327*, 557–560. [CrossRef]
42. Barendregt, J.J.; Doi, S.A.; Lee, Y.Y.; Norman, R.E.; Vos, T. Meta-analysis of prevalence. *J. Epidemiol. Community Health* **2013**, *67*, 974–978. [CrossRef]
43. Furuya-Kanamori, L.; Barendregt, J.J.; Doi, S.A.R. A new improved graphical and quantitative method for detecting bias in meta-analysis. *Int. J. Evid. Based Healthc.* **2018**, *16*, 195–203. [CrossRef]
44. Lipsey, M.; Wilson, D.B. The way in which intervention studies have "personality" and why it is important to meta-analysis. *Eval. Health Prof.* **2001**, *24*, 236–254.
45. Senn, S. Trying to be precise about vagueness. *Stat Med.* **2007**, *26*, 1417–1430. [CrossRef] [PubMed]

46. Cohen, J. *Statistical Power Analysis for the Behavioral Sciences*, 2nd ed.; Lawrence Erlbaum Associates: New York, NY, USA, 1988. [CrossRef]
47. Croonenberghs, J.; Wauters, A.; Devreese, K.; Verkerk, R.; Scharpe, S.; Bosmans, E.; Egyed, B.; Deboutte, D.; Maes, M. Increased serum albumin, gamma globulin, immunoglobulin IgG, and IgG2 and IgG4 in autism. *Psychol. Med.* **2002**, *32*, 1457–1463. [CrossRef]
48. Trajkovski, V.; Ajdinski, L.; Spiroski, M. Plasma concentration of immunoglobulin classes and subclasses in children with autism in the Republic of Macedonia: Retrospective study. *Croat. Med. J.* **2004**, *45*, 746–749. [PubMed]
49. Enstrom, A.; Krakowiak, P.; Onore, C.; Pessah, I.N.; Hertz-Picciotto, I.; Hansen, R.L.; Van de Water, J.A.; Ashwood, P. Increased IgG4 levels in children with autism disorder. *Brain Behav. Immun.* **2009**, *23*, 389–395. [CrossRef]
50. Spiroski, M.; Trajkovski, V.; Trajkov, D.; Petlichkovski, A.; Efinska-Mladenovska, O.; Hristomanova, S.; Djulejic, E.; Paneva, M.; Bozhikov, J. Family analysis of immunoglobulin classes and subclasses in children with autistic disorder. *Bosn. J. Basic Med. Sci.* **2009**, *9*, 283–289. [CrossRef] [PubMed]
51. Wasilewska, J.; Kaczmarski, M.; Stasiak-Barmuta, A.; Tobolczyk, J.; Kowalewska, E. Low serum IgA and increased expression of CD23 on B lymphocytes in peripheral blood in children with regressive autism aged 3-6 years old. *Arch. Med. Sci.* **2012**, *8*, 324–331. [CrossRef] [PubMed]
52. Gupta, S.; Aggarwal, S.; Heads, C. Dysregulated immune system in children with autism: Beneficial effects of intravenous immune globulin on autistic characteristics. *J. Autism Dev. Disord.* **1996**, *26*, 439–452. [CrossRef]
53. Stern, L.; Francoeur, M.J.; Primeau, M.N.; Sommerville, W.; Fombonne, E.; Mazer, B.D. Immune function in autistic children. *Ann. Allergy Asthma Immunol.* **2005**, *95*, 558–565. [CrossRef]
54. Grether, J.K.; Croen, L.A.; Anderson, M.C.; Nelson, K.B.; Yolken, R.H. Neonatally measured immunoglobulins and risk of autism. *Autism Res. Off. J. Int. Soc. Autism Res.* **2010**, *3*, 323–332. [CrossRef]
55. Grether, J.K.; Ashwood, P.; Van de Water, J.; Yolken, R.H.; Anderson, M.C.; Torres, A.R.; Westover, J.B.; Sweeten, T.; Hansen, R.L.; Kharrazi, M.; et al. Prenatal and Newborn Immunoglobulin Levels from Mother-Child Pairs and Risk of Autism Spectrum Disorders. *Front. Neurosci.* **2016**, *10*, 218. [CrossRef]
56. Young, J.G.; Caparulo, B.K.; Shaywitz, B.A.; Johnson, W.T.; Cohen, D.J. Childhood autism. Cerebrospinal fluid examination and immunoglobulin levels. *J. Am. Acad. Child Psychiatry* **1977**, *16*, 174–179. [CrossRef]
57. Runge, K.; Tebartz van Elst, L.; Maier, S.; Nickel, K.; Denzel, D.; Matysik, M.; Kuzior, H.; Robinson, T.; Blank, T.; Dersch, R.; et al. Cerebrospinal Fluid Findings of 36 Adult Patients with Autism Spectrum Disorder. *Brain Sci.* **2020**, *10*, 355. [CrossRef]
58. Niederhofer, H.; Staffen, W.; Mair, A. Immunoglobulins as an alternative strategy of psychopharmacological treatment of children with autistic disorder. *Neuropsychopharmacology* **2003**, *28*, 1014–1015. [CrossRef]
59. Jyonouchi, H.; Geng, L.; Streck, D.L.; Toruner, G.A. Children with autism spectrum disorders (ASD) who exhibit chronic gastrointestinal (GI) symptoms and marked fluctuation of behavioral symptoms exhibit distinct innate immune abnormalities and transcriptional profiles of peripheral blood (PB) monocytes. *J. Neuroimmunol.* **2011**, *238*, 73–80. [CrossRef] [PubMed]
60. Maltsev, D.; Yevtushenko, S.J.I.N.J. High-Dose Intravenous Immunoglobulin Therapy Efficiency in Children with Autism Spectrum Disorders Associated with Genetic Deficiency of Folate Cycle Enzymes. *Int. Neurol. J.* **2016**, *2*, 35–48. [CrossRef]
61. Plioplys, A.V. Intravenous immunoglobulin treatment of children with autism. *J. Child Neurol.* **1998**, *13*, 79–82. [CrossRef] [PubMed]
62. DelGiudice-Asch, G.; Simon, L.; Schmeidler, J.; Cunningham-Rundles, C.; Hollander, E. Brief report: A pilot open clinical trial of intravenous immunoglobulin in childhood autism. *J. Autism. Dev. Disord.* **1999**, *29*, 157–160. [CrossRef]
63. Oleske, J. Another view of autism. *UMDNJ Res.* **2004**, *Winter*, 22–23.
64. Melamed, I.; McDonald, A.; Gonzalez, M.J.C.I. Sa. 46. Autism as a Neuro-Immune Disease-the Benefit Effect of IVIG. *Clin. Immunol.* **2006**, *119*, S121. [CrossRef]
65. Melamed, I.R.; Heffron, M.; Testori, A.; Lipe, K. A pilot study of high-dose intravenous immunoglobulin 5% for autism: Impact on autism spectrum and markers of neuroinflammation. *Autism Res. Off. J. Int. Soc. Autism Res.* **2018**, *11*, 421–433. [CrossRef] [PubMed]
66. Boris, M.; Goldblatt, A.; Edelson, S.M. Improvement in children with autism treated with intravenous gamma globulin. *J. Nutr. Environ. Med.* **2005**, *15*, 169–176. [CrossRef]
67. Knutsen, A.P.; Fenton, G. High-dose intravenous immunoglobulin therapy in three children with seizure disorders and autistic features. *Pediatr. Asthma Allergy Immunol.* **1998**, *12*, 213–216. [CrossRef]
68. Jyonouchi, H.; Geng, L.; Streck, D.L.; Toruner, G.A. Immunological characterization and transcription profiling of peripheral blood (PB) monocytes in children with autism spectrum disorders (ASD) and specific polysaccharide antibody deficiency (SPAD): Case study. *J. Neuroinflamm.* **2012**, *9*, 4. [CrossRef]
69. Fadeyi, M.; Li, T.J.J.o.D.A. Evaluating possible use of IVIG in autism spectrum disorder (ASD). *J. Drug Assess.* **2018**, *7*, 14. [CrossRef]
70. Akcakaya, N.H.; Tekturk, P.; Cagatay, A.; Tur, E.K.; Yapici, Z. Atypical enterovirus encephalitis causing behavioral changes and autism-like clinical manifestations: Case report. *Acta Neurol. Belg.* **2016**, *116*, 679–681. [CrossRef]
71. Akcakaya, H.; Tekturk, P.; Tur, E.K.; Eraksoy, M.; Yapici, Z. P103—2340: Atypical enterovirus encephalitis causing behavioral changes and autism-like clinical manifestations: Case report. *Eur. J. Paediatr. Neurol.* **2015**, *19*, S123. [CrossRef]

72. Suez, D.; Scharnwebber, K. Intravenous Immunoglobulin (IVIG) Therapy in an Autistic Child with Common Variable Immune Deficiency (CVID)-Case Report. *J. Allergy Clin. Immunol.* **1997**, *99*, S2.
73. Wang, J.; Rodriguez-Davalos, M.; Levi, G.; Sauter, B.; Gondolesi, G.E.; Cunningham-Rundles, C. Common variable immunodeficiency presenting with a large abdominal mass. *J. Allergy Clin. Immunol.* **2005**, *115*, 1318–1320. [CrossRef] [PubMed]
74. Salehi Sadaghiani, M.; Aghamohammadi, A.; Ashrafi, M.R.; Hosseini, F.; Abolhassani, H.; Rezaei, N. Autism in a child with common variable immunodeficiency. *Iran J. Allergy Asthma Immunol.* **2013**, *12*, 287–289. [PubMed]
75. Sommerville, L.; Cordeiro, N.; McHenry, P.; O'Regan, M. CBP012 Chronic demyelinating neuropathy with multiple vitamin deficiencies in a child with autism. *Eur. J. Paediatr. Neurol.* **2007**, *11*, 89. [CrossRef]
76. Kamata, A.; Muramatsu, K.; Sawaura, N.; Makioka, N.; Ogata, T.; Kuwashima, M.; Arakawa, H. Demyelinating neuropathy in a 6-year-old girl with autism spectrum disorder. *Pediatr. Int. Off. J. Jpn. Pediatr. Soc.* **2017**, *59*, 951–954. [CrossRef]
77. Scott, O.; Richer, L.; Forbes, K.; Sonnenberg, L.; Currie, A.; Eliyashevska, M.; Goez, H.R. Anti-N-methyl-D-aspartate (NMDA) receptor encephalitis: An unusual cause of autistic regression in a toddler. *J. Child Neurol.* **2014**, *29*, 691–694. [CrossRef]
78. Gonzalez-Toro, M.C.; Jadraque-Rodriguez, R.; Sempere-Perez, A.; Martinez-Pastor, P.; Jover-Cerda, J.; Gomez-Gosalvez, F. [Anti-NMDA receptor encephalitis: Two paediatric cases]. *Rev. Neurol.* **2013**, *57*, 504–508. [PubMed]
79. Menon, D.U.; Garg, A.; Chedrawi, A.K.; Pardo, C.A.; Johnston, M.V. Subacute encephalitis in a child seropositive for alpha-3 subunit of neuronal nicotinic acetylcholine receptors antibody. *J. Pediatr. Neurol.* **2014**, *12*, 161–166.
80. Bouboulis, D.A.; Mast, P.A. Infection-Induced Autoimmune Encephalopathy: Treatment with Intravenous Immune Globulin Therapy. A Report of Six Patients. *Int. J. Neurol. Res.* **2016**, *2*, 256–258. [CrossRef]
81. Xu, Z.; Prasad, K.; Yeo, T. Progressive Encephalomyelitis with Rigidity and Myoclonus in an Intellectually Disabled Patient Mimicking Neuroleptic Malignant Syndrome. *J. Mov. Disord.* **2017**, *10*, 99–101. [CrossRef] [PubMed]
82. Wimberley, T.; Agerbo, E.; Pedersen, C.B.; Dalsgaard, S.; Horsdal, H.T.; Mortensen, P.B.; Thompson, W.K.; Köhler-Forsberg, O.; Yolken, R.H. Otitis media, antibiotics, and risk of autism spectrum disorder. *Autism Res. Off. J. Int. Soc. Autism Res.* **2018**, *11*, 1432–1440. [CrossRef]
83. Adams, D.J.; Susi, A.; Erdie-Lalena, C.R.; Gorman, G.; Hisle-Gorman, E.; Rajnik, M.; Elrod, M.; Nylund, C.M. Otitis Media and Related Complications Among Children with Autism Spectrum Disorders. *J. Autism Dev. Disord.* **2016**, *46*, 1636–1642. [CrossRef]
84. Mason-Brothers, A.; Ritvo, E.R.; Freeman, B.J.; Jorde, L.B.; Pingree, C.C.; McMahon, W.M.; Jenson, W.R.; Petersen, P.B.; Mo, A. The UCLA-University of Utah epidemiologic survey of autism: Recurrent infections. *Eur. Child Adolesc. Psychiatry* **1993**, *2*, 79–90. [CrossRef]
85. Jyonouchi, H.; Geng, L.; Cushing-Ruby, A.; Quraishi, H. Impact of innate immunity in a subset of children with autism spectrum disorders: A case control study. *J. Neuroinflamm.* **2008**, *5*, 52. [CrossRef]
86. Jyonouchi, H.; Geng, L.; Davidow, A.L. Cytokine profiles by peripheral blood monocytes are associated with changes in behavioral symptoms following immune insults in a subset of ASD subjects: An inflammatory subtype? *J. Neuroinflamm.* **2014**, *11*, 187. [CrossRef]
87. Maritati, F.; Peyronel, F.; Vaglio, A. IgG4-related disease: A clinical perspective. *Rheumatol. Oxf. Engl.* **2020**, *59*, iii123–iii131. [CrossRef]
88. Lim, A.H.; Wong, S.; Nguyen, N.Q. Eosinophilic Esophagitis and IgG4: Is There a Relationship? *Dig. Dis. Sci.* **2021**. [CrossRef]
89. Heifert, T.A.; Susi, A.; Hisle-Gorman, E.; Erdie-Lalena, C.R.; Gorman, G.; Min, S.B.; Nylund, C.M. Feeding Disorders in Children With Autism Spectrum Disorders Are Associated With Eosinophilic Esophagitis. *J. Pediatr. Gastroenterol. Nutr.* **2016**, *63*, e69–e73. [CrossRef]
90. Goldberg, M.R.; Mor, H.; Magid Neriya, D.; Magzal, F.; Muller, E.; Appel, M.Y.; Nachshon, L.; Borenstein, E.; Tamir, S.; Louzoun, Y.; et al. Microbial signature in IgE-mediated food allergies. *Genome Med.* **2020**, *12*, 92. [CrossRef]
91. Lee, K.H.; Guo, J.; Song, Y.; Ariff, A.; O'Sullivan, M.; Hales, B.; Mullins, B.J.; Zhang, G. Dysfunctional Gut Microbiome Networks in Childhood IgE-Mediated Food Allergy. *Int. J. Mol. Sci.* **2021**, *22*, 79. [CrossRef]
92. Andreo-Martínez, P.; Rubio-Aparicio, M.; Sánchez-Meca, J.; Veas, A.; Martínez-González, A.E. A Meta-analysis of Gut Microbiota in Children with Autism. *J. Autism Dev. Disord.* **2021**. [CrossRef] [PubMed]
93. Roussin, L.; Prince, N.; Perez-Pardo, P.; Kraneveld, A.D.; Rabot, S.; Naudon, L. Role of the Gut Microbiota in the Pathophysiology of Autism Spectrum Disorder: Clinical and Preclinical Evidence. *Microorganisms* **2020**, *8*, 1369. [CrossRef] [PubMed]
94. Jyonouchi, H. Food allergy and autism spectrum disorders: Is there a link? *Curr. Allergy Asthma Rep.* **2009**, *9*, 194–201. [CrossRef]
95. Thom, R.P.; McDougle, C.J. Immune Modulatory Treatments for Autism Spectrum Disorder. *Semin. Pediatr. Neurol.* **2020**, *35*, 100836. [CrossRef] [PubMed]

Journal of *Personalized Medicine*

MDPI

Review

Ways to Address Perinatal Mast Cell Activation and Focal Brain Inflammation, including Response to SARS-CoV-2, in Autism Spectrum Disorder

Theoharis C. Theoharides [1,2,3,4]

[1] Laboratory of Molecular Immunopharmacology and Drug Discovery, Department of Immunology, Tufts University School of Medicine, 136 Harrison Avenue, Suite 304, Boston, MA 02111, USA; theoharis.theoharides@tufts.edu; Tel.: +1-(617)-636-6866; Fax: +1-(617)-636-2456
[2] School of Graduate Biomedical Sciences, Tufts University School of Medicine, Boston, MA 02111, USA
[3] Department of Internal Medicine, Tufts University School of Medicine and Tufts Medical Center, Boston, MA 02111, USA
[4] Department of Psychiatry, Tufts University School of Medicine and Tufts Medical Center, Boston, MA 02111, USA

Abstract: The prevalence of autism spectrum disorder (ASD) continues to increase, but no distinct pathogenesis or effective treatment are known yet. The presence of many comorbidities further complicates matters, making a personalized approach necessary. An increasing number of reports indicate that inflammation of the brain leads to neurodegenerative changes, especially during perinatal life, "short-circuiting the electrical system" in the amygdala that is essential for our ability to feel emotions, but also regulates fear. Inflammation of the brain can result from the stimulation of mast cells—found in all tissues including the brain—by neuropeptides, stress, toxins, and viruses such as SARS-CoV-2, leading to the activation of microglia. These resident brain defenders then release even more inflammatory molecules and stop "pruning" nerve connections, disrupting neuronal connectivity, lowering the fear threshold, and derailing the expression of emotions, as seen in ASD. Many epidemiological studies have reported a strong association between ASD and atopic dermatitis (eczema), asthma, and food allergies/intolerance, all of which involve activated mast cells. Mast cells can be triggered by allergens, neuropeptides, stress, and toxins, leading to disruption of the blood–brain barrier (BBB) and activation of microglia. Moreover, many epidemiological studies have reported a strong association between stress and atopic dermatitis (eczema) during gestation, which involves activated mast cells. Both mast cells and microglia can also be activated by SARS-CoV-2 in affected mothers during pregnancy. We showed increased expression of the proinflammatory cytokine IL-18 and its receptor, but decreased expression of the anti-inflammatory cytokine IL-38 and its receptor IL-36R, only in the amygdala of deceased children with ASD. We further showed that the natural flavonoid luteolin is a potent inhibitor of the activation of both mast cells and microglia, but also blocks SARS-CoV-2 binding to its receptor angiotensin-converting enzyme 2 (ACE2). A treatment approach should be tailored to each individual patient and should address hyperactivity/stress, allergies, or food intolerance, with the introduction of natural molecules or drugs to inhibit mast cells and microglia, such as liposomal luteolin.

Keywords: amygdala; autism spectrum disorder; brain; COVID-19; children; cytokines; flavonoids; inflammation; luteolin; mast cells; microglia; SARS-CoV-2; stress

Citation: Theoharides, T.C. Ways to Address Perinatal Mast Cell Activation and Focal Brain Inflammation, including Response to SARS-CoV-2, in Autism Spectrum Disorder. *J. Pers. Med.* **2021**, *11*, 860. https://doi.org/10.3390/jpm11090860

Academic Editors: Richard E. Frye, Richard Boles, Shannon Rose and Daniel Rossignol

Received: 27 June 2021
Accepted: 24 August 2021
Published: 29 August 2021

Publisher's Note: MDPI stays neutral with regard to jurisdictional claims in published maps and institutional affiliations.

Copyright: © 2021 by the author. Licensee MDPI, Basel, Switzerland. This article is an open access article distributed under the terms and conditions of the Creative Commons Attribution (CC BY) license (https://creativecommons.org/licenses/by/4.0/).

1. Introduction

ASD is characterized by difficulties in communication and apparently purposeless repetitive movements [1–5]. The prevalence is estimated to be 1 in 54 children in the United States [6,7] and is associated with enormous economic burden [8–11]. However, ASD pathogenesis is still unknown. Moreover, most children with ASD have a number of comorbidities such as hyperactivity, gastrointestinal problems, allergies, and seizures [12–14], making the development of effective treatments difficult and prompting the need for a personalized approach [15].

A number of risk factors during gestation [16], especially pre-eclampsia [17–19], preterm birth, and low birth weight [20–22], as well as atopic conditions, autoimmune diseases, [23–25] infection, and psychological stress, have been increasingly associated with higher risk of ASD in the offspring (Table 1) [26,27]. There have been many reports of different aspects of immune dysfunction in ASD [28–32]. In fact, maternal antibodies have been implicated in brain pathology in ASD [33], especially autoantibodies against proteins in the developing fetal brain [34–36]. We had proposed that focal inflammation in the amygdala may contribute to ASD [37–39] via activation of microglia [40–43]. The present manuscript is organized in different parts, stressing certain risk factors such as SARS-CoV2 infection, psychological stress, atopic conditions, and finally, treatment approaches.

Table 1. Conditions Associated with Higher Risk of ASD.

• Autoimmunity	[24,25,44]
• Allergies	[45–52]
• Asthma	[50,53]
• Atopic dermatitis	[54,55]
• COVID-19	[56,57]
• High fever	[58,59]
• Hypothyroidism	[24]
• Infection	[58,60,61]
• Inflammation	[38,39]
• Low birth weight/preterm birth	[16,20–22,62]
• Pre-eclampsia	[17–19]
• Mastocytosis	[63]
• Psoriasis	[23–25]
• Rheumatoid arthritis	[24]
• Stress	[16,62,64–72]

2. Infections and COVID-19

Infections [58,60,61] and high fever [58,59] during gestation have been associated with higher risk for ASD. However, there is very little information available on the effect of viruses, especially SARS-CoV-2, on the fetus. Viral proteins can interact with placenta cells [73]. One recent paper that reviewed findings from 101 women infected with SARS-CoV-2 reported that there is vertical transmission of SARS-CoV-2 from the mother to the infant, with adverse effects on the newborn [74]. However, two other papers reported negligible transmission [75,76]. However, transmission may not be required for the virus to induce neuroinflammation, as it may affect peripheral nerves [77] or the developing brain via the Spike protein directly affecting brain cells [78].

Recent publications reported increased perinatal complications in mothers infected with SARS-CoV-2 [56,79], especially pre-eclampsia [79] and premature birth [56,79], associated with inflammatory responses [80,81]. Pre-eclampsia is characterized by high levels of corticotropin-releasing hormone (CRH) [82,83], which is typically secreted from the hypothalamus under stress [84]. With respect to children infected with SARS-CoV-2, even though they have milder pulmonary symptoms than adults [85–91], a number of papers have reported the presence of Multisystem Inflammatory Syndrome in children (MIS-C) [92–94] and adolescents [95]. In such cases, symptoms typically occur 4–6 weeks after infection and are reminiscent of Kawasaki disease [96] but also include neurologic involvement [97]. Moreover, the clinical presentation is associated with elevated markers of inflammation and the presence of multiple autoantibodies [98], and one paper suggested that MIS may be a form of mast cell activation syndrome (MCAS) presenting with neuropsychiatric symptoms and brain fog [57]. In fact, perinatal brain inflammation [99] can contribute to the pathogenesis of neuropsychiatric disorders [100,101], including ASD [16,38,102]. A recent NIH study reported blood vessel damage and perivascular inflammation in brains of deceased patients with COVID-19 [103].

COVID-19 has been associated with neurological [104–112], neurodegenerative [107,113], and mental [114–124] disorders, including ASD [125]. Moreover, it is now recognized that as many as 50% of those infected with SARS-CoV-2 [126] develop a post-acute syndrome known as "long-COVID syndrome" [127–129]. This syndrome is particularly associated with neurologic and psychiatric symptoms, especially brain fog, [128,130–132], as well as persistent fatigue apparently independent of the severity of the initial symptoms [133]. In fact, the Simons Fnd. (New York, NY, USA) recently announced the funding of longitudinal studies of mothers infected with maternal COVID-19 for increased risk for ASD. (https://www.sfari.org/grant/maternal-covid-19-as-a-potential-risk-for-autism-supplemental-funding-for-ongoing-pregnancy-cohorts-request-for-applications/ (accessed on 1 June 2021).

The detrimental effects of stress, inflammation, and auto-immunity were discussed recently [134], especially with respect to COVID-19 [113] and mast cells [135]. A number of subsequent reviews have discussed neurobiological aspects [136] and neuroinflammation in the context of ASD [137–139]. In this paper, we discuss how environmental and stress stimuli trigger fetal or neonatal mast cells to secrete proinflammatory mediators, leading to focal inflammation in the amygdala, regulating emotions and fear (Figure 1) [140] and contributing to ASD [38,45,141]. We further propose a set of laboratory tests and approaches to better identify comorbidities and help each individual to be the best they can be.

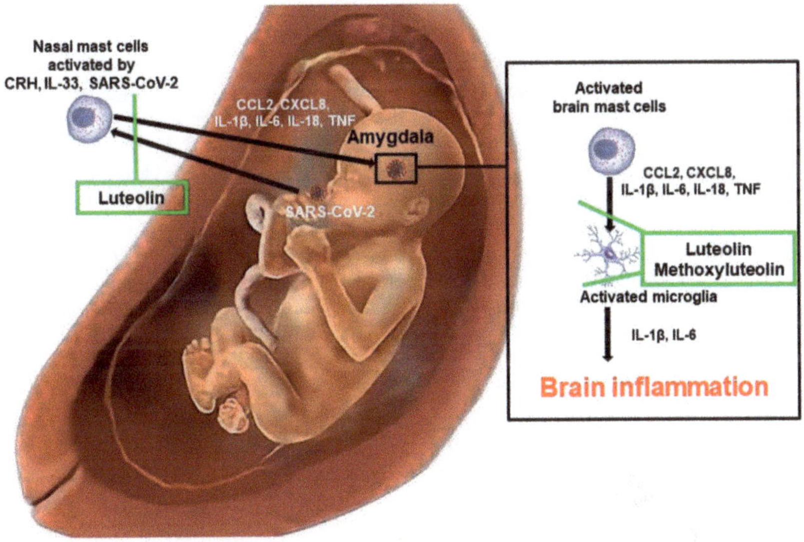

Figure 1. Diagrammatic representation of how SARS-CoV-2 could stimulate fetal mast cells and result in inflammation of the brain. SARS-CoV-2 could stimulate fetal or neonatal mast cells especially in the nose and enter the brain via the olfactory nerve tract, reaching the amygdala. There, it could further activate mast cells and microglia to release pro-inflammatory mediators, thus contributing to brain inflammation and ASD. Luteolin could block these processes.

3. Psychological Stress

Psychological stress can have pro-inflammatory effects [64,134] via CRH [142] stimulating mast cells [135]. One study showed that prenatal and early postnatal stress were associated with elevated serum levels of IL-6 in humans [143]. Another study reported that acute psychological stress increased the circulating levels of proinflammatory cytokines [144]. A longitudinal study of mothers' serum measurements during gestation linked IL-6 to decreased executive function in their offspring [145]. We had shown that acute restraint stress significantly increased serum IL-6 in mice, which was entirely dependent on mast cells [146]. It is interesting that IL-6 has also been reported to promote human mast cell production and reactivity [147]. Moreover, prenatal stress or exposure to IL-6 resulted in increased microglia ramification in mice and was prevented by IL-6 blockade [148].

Psychological stress could also lead to increased vascular permeability [135]. This process also contributes to the disruption of the blood–brain barrier (BBB) [149,150] via release of CRH [151] and IL-6 [152], permitting entry into the brain of viral particles, cytokines, or other toxic substances, thus further exacerbating brain inflammation. Breakdown of the BBB has been reported in the developing brain following inflammation [153]. We further showed that restraint stress in rodents increased BBB permeability [149,150,154,155] via CRH stimulating mast cells [154,156,157]. The BBB typically prevents circulating toxic substances, but also immune cells, from entering the brain. The BBB is not fully developed until the third trimester [158–160] and is more vulnerable to toxins and drugs [161]. It was recently shown that common drugs such as acetaminophen (paracetamol) and cimetidine can enter the fetal brain in higher amounts than the adult brain [162]. Moreover, umbilical cord blood biomarkers indicative of acetaminophen exposure were significantly associated with the risk of ASD in childhood [163]. Hence, many atopic or pathogenic conditions, including exposure to certain drugs, could influence brain development during pregnancy or even lactation.

Stress associated with COVID-19 [134] can further affect the emotional state of individuals [118,119,164–167], especially social isolation, loneliness, and anxiety [168]. One study reported that prenatal stress was linked to higher risk of newborns developing attention-deficit hyperactivity disorder (ADHD) [65,66] and ASD [67–72]. A more recent study of 1638 pregnant women concluded that a high level of perceived stress through pregnancy, especially during the second trimester, was associated with an increased risk of the offspring developing ASD at 6 months of age [62]. Prenatal stress may lead to maternal immune dysregulation, thus contributing to ASD [70]. It is interesting that maternal psychological stress during pregnancy increased cord blood levels of IgE [169], suggesting that it could contribute to an increased risk in the fetus of developing allergic reactions or sensitivity to postnatal exposure to allergens. Psychological stress also increased the risk of childhood atopic dermatitis (AD) [170,171] and asthma [172–174]. To make matters worse, children with ASD cannot handle stress [175,176] and have an exacerbated sense of fear [39].

4. Mast Cell Activation

Infection with SARS-CoV-2 is primarily characterized by the release of a storm of pro-inflammatory cytokines [177–185], especially IL-6 [186–189] and IL-1β [190,191]. Mast cells are a key source of such cytokines in COVID-19 [192–195] and could contribute to interstitial lung edema and immunothromboses [196].

We reported that children born to mothers with systemic mastocytosis [63], which is characterized by a greater number of hyperactive mast cells than in the general population [197], had a higher risk of developing ASD [1,2,7,198,199]. The word atopy is commonly used to denote a tendency, usually early in life, to become sensitized to and produce immune IgE to environmental antigens. Many epidemiological studies reported a strong association between atopic diseases and behavioral problems in general [200] and in ASD in particular [46,47]. Other epidemiological studies showed a strong association between risk for developing ASD and allergies [45,46,48–50], especially asthma [50,53] and atopic dermatitis (AD) [54], but also food hypersensitivity [12,201–205]. In fact, the presence of allergies was associated with elevated serum levels of autoantibodies against brain antigens in children with ASD [206]. Parental history of AD was strongly associated with children developing AD [207]. It was reported that maternal immune activation [208] and autoimmune diseases [209], especially psoriasis, but also allergies and asthma, were associated with a higher risk of ASD [23]. In another study, almost 50% of children with ASD had relatives with rheumatoid diseases as compared to 26% in the control group [210]. In a recent large study, mothers who suffered from asthma, allergy, atopy, or eczema during pregnancy were associated with a higher risk of neuropsychiatric problems in children [55]. Three recent studies reported strong associations with ASD and food allergy [211] and food intolerance [202] that could lead to brain inflammation and cognitive impairment [212].

A recent publication showed that the mother's circulating immune IgE resulted in vertical transmission of AD in the newborn via stimulation of fetal mast cells [213]; both passive and active prenatal sensitization conferred allergen sensitivity [213]. This important paper indicated that fetal mast cells were functional and could be stimulated by specific IgE and allergens present in the mother during gestation. Even though these studies were limited to pulmonary and skin mast cells, reactivity could also extend to brain mast cells. In fact, prenatal allergen exposure was even shown to program lifelong changes in adults rats' social and sexual behavior, including effects on microglia activation and neonatal dendritic spine density [214]. Fetal mast cells could potentially respond to other stimuli such as neuropeptides and toxins, including the alarmin IL-33 [215,216], with detrimental effects on brain development, especially in premature babies [16].

Activated brain mast cells have been shown to contribute to cognitive dysfunction via microglia activation and neuronal apoptosis [217]. Mast cells are ubiquitous in the body [218] and are critical for allergic diseases [219], including mastocytosis [197]. However, mast cells also participate in inflammation [220,221] by secreting histamine and multiple pro-inflammatory cytokines and chemokines [222,223], including IL-1β [224], IL-6 [225], and TNF [226]. Mast cells are also present in the brain, especially the meninges [227,228] and the median eminence [229], where they are located perivascularly, close to nerve endings positive for CRH [227]. We showed that stress stimulates mast cells via CRH [135] leading to increased dura vascular permeability, an effect that was absent in mast cell-deficient mice [230]. Moreover, mast cells can activate the hypothalamic–pituitary–adrenal (HPA) axis [142,231–233] via the release of histamine [234], IL-6 [152], and CRH [151]. Moreover, neurotensin [235] and substance P (SP) [236], neuropeptides implicated in inflammation, induced CRHR-1, thus creating an autocrine loop. Moreover, SP induced the ST2 receptor for IL-33 [226], further exacerbating mast cell activation by the combined action of neuropeptides and IL-33.

Mast cells respond not only to allergic but also to many other stimuli that can act alone or increase mast cell reactivity [197]. Mast cells can also be triggered by viruses [237] including SARS-CoV-2 [192,195]. In fact, gene expression of the coronavirus surface receptor angiotensin-converting enzyme 2 (ACE2) was recently shown to be induced by interferon [238], and mast cells can elicit strong pro-inflammatory and Type I interferon responses in the presence of viruses [239], implying an autocrine action on ACE2 expression. Following stimulation, mast cells release large amounts of pro-inflammatory mediators [222] such as histamine, tryptase, chemokines (e.g., CCL2, CCXL8) [240], and cytokines (IL-6, [225] IL-1β [224], TNF [226]), especially when primed by IL-33 [216,241]. Histamine can stimulate macrophages to release IL-1 [242], which in turn stimulates mast cells to release IL-6 [225]. Mast cells can also secrete mitochondrial DNA (mtDNA) extracellularly [243], which serves as an alarmin and can stimulate pro-inflammatory mediator secretion from immune cells [244,245]. We reported elevated extracellular mtDNA in the serum of children with ASD [246]. In fact, it was recently reported that mtDNA may mediate prenatal environmental influences in ASD [247], was increased in the serum of COVID-19 patients, and correlated with disease severity [248]. Moreover, mast cells synthesize and release platelet-activating factor (PAF), which has been implicated in inflammation [249] and microthromboses [250] characterizing COVID-19. In fact, a recent paper reported a strong association across the globe with SARS-CoV-2 infection rates and levels of pollen known to be involved in upper respiratory system allergies, thus implicating mast cell activation [251]

5. Mast Cells and Microglia

Microglia are specialized resident macrophages of the Central Nervous System (CNS) with important functions in both health and disease. They are especially implicated in neuroinflammation [252–254] and neurodegenerative [252,255–257] diseases. Activation of microglia has been reported in ASD [41–43,258], as documented by the release of the pro-inflammatory mediators IL-1β and CXCL8 [259]. Microglia were recently implicated in COVID-19 [260] and were also associated with neuroinflammation [261]. The transition of microglia from the resting to the activated proinflammatory phase is regulated by several intrinsic and extrinsic factors. Microglia can be activated by numerous molecules including pathogen-associated molecular patterns (PAMPs) and endogenous damage-associated patterns (DAMPs) acting on Toll-like receptors (TLRs), but also in response to molecules released from mast cells, such as histamine and tryptase (Table 2) [39]. It was recently reported that elevated protein synthesis in microglia resulted in autism-like synaptic and behavioral changes in mice [262]. A dysfunctional neuroimmune cross-talk may result in a state of chronic fetal microglial activation leading to a disruption of neurogenesis and synaptic pruning [263], processes critical for the development of ASD.

Table 2. Molecules Activating Microglia.

- Chemokines (CCL2, CxCl8)
- Cytokines (IL-1β, IL-6, IL-18, TNF)
- Histamine
- Lipopolysaccharide (LPS)
- Neuropeptides (CRH, HK-1, Neurotensin, SP)
- Neurotransmitters
- Pathogens (SARS-CoV-2)
- Potassium
- Prostaglandin D2
- Proteases (MMP-3, Thrombin, Tryptase)

Mast cells interact with microglia in the brain [264], leading to their activation [264–267] and to neuroinflammation [266,268]. This effect is absent in mast cell-deficient mice [39,269]. Activation of mast cells [270,271] and microglia [272], especially in the hypothalamus [273], could lead to cognitive dysfunction [274]. Microglia express receptors for CRH [275] and could be further activated by stress, especially in association with COVID-19 [276]. Microglia also express receptors for neurotensin (NT) (Table 2) [277]. We reported that NT is increased in the serum of patients with ASD [278,279] and can activate human microglia to secrete pro-inflammatory molecules [259]. We also reported increased gene expression of the pro-inflammatory microRNA-155 (miR-155) in the amygdala of children with ASD [280], as well as reduced expression of the anti-inflammatory cytokine IL-38 [281]. Microglia also express TLRs [282] and were recently implicated in COVID-19 [260,283].

6. Treatment Approaches

It is critical to identify the presence of any atopy or allergies and food intolerance, especially the presence of Mast Cell Activation Syndrome (MCAS) [284,285] or systemic mastocytosis (SM) [197], by measuring the levels of the molecules listed in Table 3. Of note is IgG4 because it is involved in food intolerance and has been reported to be elevated in the plasma of children with ASD [286].

Table 3. Laboratory Tests for Diagnosis of Atopic Diseases.

Blood
- IgA, IgG_1, IgG_4, IgE
- Immune IgE (RAST for alpha-gal, casein, dust, dust mites, egg, fungi, grass, gluten, pollen)
- Anti-IgE receptor antibody (basophil activation or histamine release test)
- CCL2, CXCL8 (IL-8)
- Chromogranin A *
- Eosinophilic cationic protein (ECP)
- Food Intolerance Panel
- Heparin
- IL-4, IL-6, IL-31, IL-33
- Prostaglandin D_2 (PGD_2)
- Tryptase

Urine collected for 24 h or first morning void (must be kept and sent cold)
- N-methylhistamine (NMH) or methylimidazole acetic acid (MIA)
- PGD_2
- 23BPG=2,3-Dinor-11β-$PGF_{2\alpha}$

* Should be measured after one week of NO antacids, otherwise there is a high chance of false positive results. Elevated chromogranin A is not indicative of atopy, but of a somewhat similar condition called carcinoid syndrome associated with activated enterochromaffin cells in the gut.

It is also important to avoid histamine-rich foods, especially ripe tomatoes and avocados, cheeses, spinach, tangerines, spices, and sardines, which have been associated with histamine intolerance [287]. In this context, it is useful to conduct gene analysis for metabolizing enzymes, especially diamine oxidase (DAO), which breaks down histamine, and enzymes that break down phenols such as monoamine oxidase (MAO), catecholamine-ortho-methyl transferase (COMT), and phenol sulfur transferase (PST) to ascertain phenol intolerance that can contribute to hyperactivity. If DAO gene expression is defective and/or its activity in the blood is low, DAO supplements can be added about 30 min before meals, but one should be careful to avoid the common dyes and preservatives mentioned below.

Unfortunately, many medications, supplements, and vitamins contain "inactive" ingredients that are not tolerated by many children with ASD, leading to unexpected or worsening of behaviors. Such ingredients to be avoided include dyes, preservatives, gluten, monosodium glutamate (MSG), polyethylene glycol (PGE), galactosaccharide (GOS), salicylates, silicum, soy talc, and Twin 80. In addition, herbicides such as glyphosate and atrazine should be avoided, as they have been reported to stimulate mast cells and promote inflammation [288], besides their known neurotoxic effects.

One should choose the best tolerated antihistamine [289,290] from the list shown in Table 4, especially rupatadine, which also blocks mast cells, [291–293], and avoid large doses that may lead to confusion [294]. In fact, the Food and Drug Administration (FDA) recently warned that taking higher-than-recommended doses of diphenhydramine (Benadryl) can lead to serious heart problems, seizures, coma, or even death. https://www.fda.gov/drugs/drug-safety-and-availability/fda-warns-about-serious-problems-high-doses-allergy-medicine-diphenhydramine-benadryl (accessed on 1 June 2021).

Table 4. Different histamine-1 receptor antagonists.

Generic Drug	(Trade Name)
Bilastine *	Nonsedating, non-metabolized
Cetirizine	Nonsedating
Cyproheptadine	Antiserotonergic
Diphenhydramine	Sedating
Hydroxyzine	Anxiolytic
Ketotifen *	Anti-eosinophilic
Loratadine	Nonsedating
Rupatadine *	Anti-PAF (Platelet activating factor), mast cell inhibitor
Tricyclic Antidepressants	
Amitriptyline	Weight gain
Doxepin	Also histamine-2 receptor antagonist
Phenothiazines	
Promethazine	Antiemetic
Prochlorperazine	Antiemetic, mast cell inhibitor

* Available only via compounding in the United States.

As discussed, anxiety, fear, and stress are major factors leading to hyperactivity. This should be investigated (by measuring total blood catecholamines and glutamate) and addressed with the use of a chamomile/passiflora/valerian extract or Ashwagandha [295,296]. If these are not sufficient, one should consider the beta-blocker propranolol that has good anti-anxiety properties without clouding the mental abilities and has also been reported to improve language in children with ASD [297]. Alternatively, one may recommend the use of alpha 2-receptor agonists [298] such as clonidine [299,300] and guanfacine [301,302], usually administered at bedtime especially since clonidine reduces sleep initiation latency and night awakening [303]. Moreover, caution should be exercised because such adrenergic blocking drugs may cause bradycardia and a drop in blood pressure. Cannabidiol (CBD) oil may be useful but it should be used with caution in individuals with atopic problems, because it has been reported to trigger the activation of cultured leukemic mast cells [304].

There has been considerable progress in defining drugs that block tyrosine kinases (TK) that are involved in mast cell proliferation [305]. The use of biologics for TNF [306,307] and IL-1β, [308]; has significantly improved the treatment of inflammatory skin diseases. However, these agents have a number of limitations as they may cause paradoxical inflammation, reduced ability to fight infection, and cancer development [309]. In spite of such advances, there is no clinically effective inhibitor of human mast cell mediator secretion. Moreover, inhibitors of the tyrosine kinase c-kit receptor that reduce MC proliferation [310] do not inhibit mast cell activation [311]. There are still no clinically effective mast cell inhibitors [221,312]. Disodium cromoglycate (cromolyn), known as a "mast cell stabilizer," had originally been shown to inhibit rat peritoneal MC histamine release [313]. However, cromolyn does not effectively inhibit either murine MC [314] or human MC [315–317] and has even been reported to potentiate histamine release from mast cells [318].

Instead of cromolyn, one should choose the best purity, source, and formulation of the flavonoids luteolin and quercetin [319–323]. These flavonoids are readily available and are generally considered safe [45,324–326]. Luteolin has broad anti-viral properties [327–329] and inhibits the entry of the corona virus into host cells [237,330,331]. Furthermore, luteolin better penetrates into the brain, inhibits both microglia [259,332–334] and mast cells [317,335], is neuroprotective [336–339], and has been reported to reduce neuroinflammation [337,340–342] and cognitive dysfunction [61,343–345], especially brain fog [346]. In fact, flavonoids were recently shown to improve cerebral cortical oxygenation and cognition in healthy adults. [347,348] Moreover, flavonoids induce the synthesis and secretion of neurotrophic factors, including brain-derived neurotrophic factor (BDNF) [77,349,350], known to be deficient in certain conditions associated with ASD, such as RETT syndrome [351]. The beneficial actions of luteolin are summarized in Table 5.

Table 5. Beneficial Actions of Luteolin *.

• Antagonizes SARS-CoV-2 Spike protein binding	[237,330,331,352]
• Has broad antiviral properties	[327–329]
• Improves cerebral cortical oxygenation and cognition	[347,348]
• Induces the synthesis and secretion of BDNF	[77,349–351]
• Inhibits serine proteases required for Spike protein processing	[353,354]
• Inhibits neuroinflammation	[340–342]
• Inhibits the release and action of PAF	[249,250]
• Inhibits mast cell stimulation by different triggers	[317,335]
• Inhibits microglia activation	[259,332–334]
• Interferes with coronavirus replication	[355]
• Is neuroprotective	[336–339]
• Reduces cognitive decline	[61,343–346]
• Reduces oxidative stress	[320]
• Regulates inflammasome activation	[356]

* Methoxyluteolin is more potent, metabolically stable, enters the brain more efficiently, and is better tolerated due to the absence of phenolic groups.

Luteolin and quercetin are not water-soluble and are difficult to absorb in powder form after oral administration [357], but their intestinal uptake can be greatly improved [358] in liposomal preparations using olive pomace oil [358]. In fact, such a luteolin formulation in olive pomace oil (NeuroProtek®) has been reported to improve ASD [359,360], while another one (BrainGain®) reduced brain fog [344]. The latter formulation also provided the additional neuroprotective [361–366] and anti-inflammatory [367,368] actions of olive pomace oil polyphenols, as well as the increase in memory induced by the olive oil component hydroxytyrosol [365,369].

The beneficial actions of these supplements could be combined with that of a unique, hypoallergenic skin lotion containing tetramethoxyflavone (GentleDerm®) [305], which can be applied on the forehead for direct absorption by temporal blood vessels. Tetramethoxyflavone (methoxyluteolin, methlut) is a more potent inhibitor of human mast cells than either quercetin of luteolin [317,335] and also inhibits human microglia [259,333].

The natural molecule berberine may be particularly useful in cases of PANS/PANDAS because of its antibacterial properties, but also because it can inhibit mast cells [370,371] and improve brain circulation [372]. In addition, high doses of Vitamin D3 are recommended, because this vitamin has been found to be present at low levels in mothers and/or children with ASD [371,373–375] and also decreases atopic responses [376]. When all fails, intravenous Ig may be administered [289].

7. Conclusions

It is critical to try to address each child individually (Table 6) [377] by first identifying any comorbidity, especially atopic diseases and hyperactivity, as well as any metabolic issue especially related to vitamins B1, B6, B12, folic acid/MTHFR, thyroid, or vitamin D3 deficiency, since these may be easily overcome. Inflammation of the brain may be reduced with the use of the natural flavonoid luteolin, especially when formulated in liposomal form in olive pomace oil that significantly increases oral absorption (BrainGain®, PureLut®, NeuroProtek® with FDA Certificate of Free Sale). The beneficial actions of these supplements could be augmented by the use of a unique, hypoallergenic skin lotion (GentleDerm®), which contains the more potent methoxyluteolin and can be applied on the temples for direct absorption by brain blood vessels. Thus, inhibiting the activation of mast cells and microglia not only would prevent vertical transmission of atopic disorders, but also may prevent inflammation of the brain and reduce the risk of the offspring developing neuropsychiatric disorders, especially ASD (US patents US 7,906,153; 8,268,365; 9050275).

Table 6. Treatment Approaches.

Hyperactivity
- Ashwagandha
- Chamomile/Passiflora/Valerian extract
- Clonidine or guanfacine
- C-Acetyl cysteine (NAC)
- Hydroxyzine
- Propranolol

Allergic Inflammation
- Berberine
- Luteolin *
- Rupatadine
- Vitamin D3

Neuronal fatigue
- Folinate calcium or methylfolate
- Glutathione
- Methyl B12
- S-Adenosylmethionine (SAMe)

OCD
- Aripiprazole
- Risperidone

* Children with phenol intolerance: PureLut®; NeuroProtek-Low Phenol®, Adults with Brain Fog: BrainGain®; NeuroProtek®, Adults also with allergies: FibroProtek®, Adults also with interstitial cystitis: CystoProtek®.

Funding: This research received no external funding.

Institutional Review Board Statement: Not applicable.

Informed Consent Statement: Not applicable.

Data Availability Statement: Not applicable.

Acknowledgments: Many thanks are due to Maria Theoharides for help drawing the figure.

Conflicts of Interest: The author declares no conflict of interest. The author is the recipient of US Patents 8,268,365, 9,050,275 and 9,176,146 covering brain inflammation and ASD. He is also the Scientific Director of Algonot, LLC (Florida, USA) that develops unique dietary supplements containing flavonoids.

Abbreviations

ACE2	Angiotensin-converting enzyme 2
ADHD	Attention Deficit Hyperactivity Disorder
BBB	Blood–brain barrier
BDNF	Brain-derived neurotrophic factor
CNS	Central nervous system
CRH	Corticotropin-releasing hormone
DAMPs	Damage-associated molecular patterns
HPA	Hypothalamic–pituitary–adrenal
MCAS	Mast Cell Activation Syndrome
MCI	Mild cognitive impairment
mtDNA	Mitochondrial DNA
MIS	Multisystem Inflammatory Syndrome
NT	Neurotensin
PANS	Pediatric Acute Neuropsychiatric Syndrome
PAMPs	Pathogen-associated molecular patterns
PAF	Platelet-activating factor
SP	Substance P
TLR	Toll-like receptor

References

1. Johnson, C.P.; Myers, S.M. Identification and evaluation of children with autism spectrum disorders. *Pediatrics* **2007**, *120*, 1183–1215. [CrossRef]
2. Lai, M.C.; Lombardo, M.V.; Baron-Cohen, S. Autism. *Lancet* **2014**, *383*, 896–910. [CrossRef]
3. Howes, O.D.; Rogdaki, M.; Findon, J.L.; Wichers, R.H.; Charman, T.; King, B.H.; Loth, E.; McAlonan, G.M.; McCracken, J.T.; Parr, J.; et al. Autism spectrum disorder: Consensus guidelines on assessment, treatment and research from the British Association for Psychopharmacology. *J. Psychopharmacol.* **2018**, *32*, 3–29. [CrossRef] [PubMed]
4. Braconnier, M.L.; Siper, P.M. Neuropsychological assessment in autism spectrum disorder. *Curr. Psychiatry Rep.* **2021**, *23*, 63. [CrossRef] [PubMed]
5. Iles, A. Autism spectrum disorders. *Prim. Care* **2021**, *48*, 461–473. [CrossRef]
6. Maenner, M.J.; Shaw, K.A.; Baio, J.; Washington, A.; Patrick, M.; DiRienzo, M.; Christensen, D.L.; Wiggins, L.D.; Pettygrove, S.; Andrews, J.G.; et al. Prevalence of autism spectrum disorder among children aged 8 years—Autism and developmental disabilities monitoring network, 11 sites, United States, 2016. *MMWR Surveill. Summ.* **2020**, *69*, 1–12. [CrossRef]
7. Xu, G.; Strathearn, L.; Liu, B.; Bao, W. Prevalence of autism spectrum disorder among US children and adolescents, 2014–2016. *JAMA* **2018**, *319*, 81–82. [CrossRef]
8. Baxter, A.J.; Brugha, T.S.; Erskine, H.E.; Scheurer, R.W.; Vos, T.; Scott, J.G. The epidemiology and global burden of autism spectrum disorders. *Psychol. Med.* **2015**, *45*, 601–613. [CrossRef]
9. Leigh, J.P.; Du, J. Brief report: Forecasting the economic burden of autism in 2015 and 2025 in the United States. *J. Autism Dev. Disord.* **2015**, *12*, 4135–4139. [CrossRef] [PubMed]
10. Buescher, A.V.; Cidav, Z.; Knapp, M.; Mandell, D.S. Costs of autism spectrum disorders in the United Kingdom and the United States. *JAMA Pediatr.* **2014**, *168*, 721–728. [CrossRef] [PubMed]
11. Rogge, N.; Janssen, J. The economic costs of autism spectrum disorder: A literature review. *J. Autism Dev. Disord.* **2019**, *49*, 2873–2900. [CrossRef]
12. Xue, M.; Brimacombe, M.; Chaaban, J.; Zimmerman-Bier, B.; Wagner, G.C. Autism spectrum disorders: Concurrent clinical disorders. *J. Child Neurol.* **2008**, *23*, 6–13.
13. Bauman, M.L. Medical comorbidities in autism: Challenges to diagnosis and treatment. *Neurotherapeutics* **2010**, *7*, 320–327. [CrossRef]
14. Underwood, J.F.G.; Kendall, K.M.; Berrett, J.; Lewis, C.; Anney, R.; Van den Bree, M.B.; Hall, J. Autism spectrum disorder diagnosis in adults: Phenotype and genotype findings from a clinically derived cohort. *Br. J. Psychiatry* **2019**, *215*, 647–653. [CrossRef]
15. Mesleh, A.G.; Abdulla, S.A.; El-Agnaf, O. Paving the way toward personalized medicine: Current advances and challenges in Multi-OMICS approach in autism spectrum disorder for biomarkers discovery and patient stratification. *J. Pers. Med.* **2021**, *11*, 41. [CrossRef]
16. Angelidou, A.; Asadi, S.; Alysandratos, K.D.; Karagkouni, A.; Kourembanas, S.; Theoharides, T.C. Perinatal stress, brain inflammation and risk of autism—Review and proposal. *BMC Pediatr.* **2012**, *12*, 89. [CrossRef]
17. Wang, H.; Laszlo, K.D.; Gissler, M.; Li, F.; Zhang, J.; Yu, Y.; Li, J. Maternal hypertensive disorders and neurodevelopmental disorders in offspring: A population-based cohort in two Nordic countries. *Eur. J. Epidemiol.* **2021**, *36*, 519–530. [CrossRef]
18. Barron, A.; McCarthy, C.M.; O'Keeffe, G.W. Preeclampsia and neurodevelopmental outcomes: Potential pathogenic roles for inflammation and oxidative stress? *Mol. Neurobiol.* **2021**, *58*, 2734–2756. [CrossRef] [PubMed]
19. Katz, J.; Reichenberg, A.; Kolevzon, A. Prenatal and perinatal metabolic risk factors for autism: A review and integration of findings from population-based studies. *Curr. Opin. Psychiatry* **2021**, *34*, 94–104. [CrossRef] [PubMed]
20. Crump, C.; Sundquist, J.; Sundquist, K. Preterm or early term birth and risk of autism. *Pediatrics* **2021**, *148*, e2020032300. [CrossRef] [PubMed]
21. Stephens, B.E.; Bann, C.M.; Watson, V.E.; Sheinkopf, S.J.; Peralta-Carcelen, M.; Bodnar, A.; Yolton, K.; Goldstein, R.F.; Dusick, A.M.; Wilson-Costello, D.E.; et al. Screening for autism spectrum disorders in extremely preterm infants. *J. Dev. Behav. Pediatr.* **2012**, *33*, 535–541. [CrossRef]
22. McGowan, E.C.; Sheinkopf, S.J. Autism and preterm birth: Clarifying risk and exploring mechanisms. *Pediatrics* **2021**, *148*, e2021051978. [CrossRef]
23. Croen, L.A.; Grether, J.K.; Yoshida, C.K.; Odouli, R.; Van de Water, J. Maternal autoimmune diseases, asthma and allergies, and childhood autism spectrum disorders: A case-control study. *Arch. Pediatr. Adolesc. Med.* **2005**, *159*, 151–157. [CrossRef] [PubMed]
24. Wu, S.; Ding, Y.; Wu, F.; Li, R.; Xie, G.; Hou, J.; Mao, P. Family history of autoimmune diseases is associated with an increased risk of autism in children: A systematic review and meta-analysis. *Neurosci. Biobehav. Rev.* **2015**, *55*, 322–332. [CrossRef]
25. Lee, H.; Hsu, J.W.; Tsai, S.J.; Huang, K.L.; Bai, Y.M.; Su, T.P.; Chen, T.J.; Chen, M.H. Risk of attention deficit hyperactivity and autism spectrum disorders among the children of parents with autoimmune diseases: A nationwide birth cohort study. *Eur. Child Adolesc. Psychiatry* **2021**, 1–9. [CrossRef]
26. Matelski, L.; van de Water, J. Risk factors in autism: Thinking outside the brain. *J. Autoimmun.* **2016**, *67*, 1–7. [CrossRef]
27. Muhle, R.A.; Reed, H.E.; Stratigos, K.A.; Veenstra-Vanderweele, J. The emerging clinical neuroscience of autism spectrum disorder: A review. *JAMA Psychiatry* **2018**, *75*, 514–523. [CrossRef]

28. Zimmerman, A.W.; Jyonouchi, H.; Comi, A.M.; Connors, S.L.; Milstien, S.; Varsou, A.; Heyes, M.P. Cerebrospinal fluid and serum markers of inflammation in autism. *Pediatr. Neurol.* **2005**, *33*, 195–201. [CrossRef]
29. Estes, M.L.; McAllister, A.K. Immune mediators in the brain and peripheral tissues in autism spectrum disorder. *Nat. Rev. Neurosci.* **2015**, *16*, 469–486. [CrossRef] [PubMed]
30. Meltzer, A.; van de Water, J. The role of the immune system in autism spectrum disorder. *Neuropsychopharmacology* **2017**, *42*, 284–298. [CrossRef] [PubMed]
31. Matta, S.M.; Hill-Yardin, E.L.; Crack, P.J. The influence of neuroinflammation in autism spectrum disorder. *Brain Behav. Immun.* **2019**, *79*, 75–90. [CrossRef]
32. Hughes, H.K.; Mills, K.E.; Rose, D.; Ashwood, P. Immune dysfunction and autoimmunity as pathological mechanisms in autism spectrum disorders. *Front. Cell Neurosci.* **2018**, *12*, 405. [CrossRef]
33. Kowal, C.; Athanassiou, A.; Chen, H.; Diamond, B. Maternal antibodies and developing blood-brain barrier. *Immunol. Res.* **2015**, *63*, 18–25. [CrossRef]
34. Edmiston, E.; Ashwood, P.; van de Water, J. Autoimmunity, autoantibodies, and autism spectrum disorder. *Biol. Psychiatry* **2017**, *81*, 383–390. [CrossRef] [PubMed]
35. Jones, K.L.; van de Water, J. Maternal autoantibody related autism: Mechanisms and pathways. *Mol. Psychiatry* **2019**, *24*, 252–265. [CrossRef] [PubMed]
36. Mazon-Cabrera, R.; Vandormael, P.; Somers, V. Antigenic targets of patient and maternal autoantibodies in autism spectrum disorder. *Front. Immunol.* **2019**, *10*, 1474. [CrossRef] [PubMed]
37. Theoharides, T.C.; Zhang, B. Neuro-inflammation, blood-brain barrier, seizures and autism. *J. Neuroinflamm.* **2011**, *8*, 168. [CrossRef] [PubMed]
38. Theoharides, T.C.; Asadi, S.; Patel, A.B. Focal brain inflammation and autism. *J. Neuroinflamm.* **2013**, *10*, 46. [CrossRef] [PubMed]
39. Theoharides, T.C.; Kavalioti, M.; Tsilioni, I. Mast cells, stress, fear and autism spectrum disorder. *Int. J. Mol. Sci.* **2019**, *20*, 3611. [CrossRef] [PubMed]
40. Rodriguez, J.I.; Kern, J.K. Evidence of microglial activation in autism and its possible role in brain underconnectivity. *Neuron Glia Biol.* **2011**, *7*, 205–213. [CrossRef] [PubMed]
41. Gupta, S.; Ellis, S.E.; Ashar, F.N.; Moes, A.; Bader, J.S.; Zhan, J.; West, A.B.; Arking, D.E. Transcriptome analysis reveals dysregulation of innate immune response genes and neuronal activity-dependent genes in autism. *Nat. Commun.* **2014**, *5*, 5748. [CrossRef]
42. Koyama, R.; Ikegaya, Y. Microglia in the pathogenesis of autism spectrum disorders. *Neurosci. Res.* **2015**, *100*, 1–5. [CrossRef]
43. Takano, T. Role of microglia in autism: Recent advances. *Dev. Neurosci.* **2015**, *37*, 195–202. [CrossRef]
44. Theoharides, T.C.; Asadi, S.; Panagiotidou, S.; Weng, Z. The "missing link" in autoimmunity and autism: Extracellular mitochondrial components secreted from activated live mast cells. *Autoimmun. Rev.* **2013**, *12*, 1136–1142. [CrossRef] [PubMed]
45. Theoharides, T.C.; Tsilioni, I.; Patel, A.B.; Doyle, R. Atopic diseases and inflammation of the brain in the pathogenesis of autism spectrum disorders. *Transl. Psychiatry* **2016**, *6*, e844. [CrossRef]
46. Liao, T.C.; Lien, Y.T.; Wang, S.; Huang, S.L.; Chen, C.Y. Comorbidity of atopic disorders with autism spectrum disorder and attention deficit/hyperactivity disorder. *J. Pediatr.* **2016**, *171*, 248–255. [CrossRef] [PubMed]
47. Theoharides, T.C. Is a subtype of autism an "allergy of the brain"? *Clin. Ther.* **2013**, *35*, 584–591. [CrossRef]
48. Magalhaes, E.S.; Pinto-Mariz, F.; Bastos-Pinto, S.; Pontes, A.T.; Prado, E.A.; Deazevedo, L.C. Immune allergic response in Asperger syndrome. *J. Neuroimmunol.* **2009**, *216*, 108–112. [CrossRef] [PubMed]
49. Jyonouchi, H. Autism spectrum disorders and allergy: Observation from a pediatric allergy/immunology clinic. *Expert. Rev. Clin. Immunol.* **2010**, *6*, 397–411. [CrossRef] [PubMed]
50. Lyall, K.; van de Water, J.; Ashwood, P.; Hertz-Picciotto, I. Asthma and allergies in children with autism spectrum disorders: Results from the charge study. *Autism Res.* **2015**, *8*, 567–574. [CrossRef] [PubMed]
51. Angelidou, A.; Alysandratos, K.D.; Asadi, S.; Zhang, B.; Francis, K.; Vasiadi, M.; Kalogeromitros, D.; Theoharides, T.C. Brief Report: "Allergic Symptoms" in children with Autism Spectrum Disorders. More than meets the eye? *J. Autism Dev. Disord.* **2011**, *41*, 1579–1585. [CrossRef] [PubMed]
52. Saitoh, B.Y.; Tanaka, E.; Yamamoto, N.; Kruining, D.V.; Iinuma, K.; Nakamuta, Y.; Yamaguchi, H.; Yamasaki, R.; Matsumoto, K.; Kira, J.I. Early postnatal allergic airway inflammation induces dystrophic microglia leading to excitatory postsynaptic surplus and autism-like behavior. *Brain Behav Immun.* **2021**, *95*, 362–380. [CrossRef] [PubMed]
53. Kotey, S.; Ertel, K.; Whitcomb, B. Co-occurrence of autism and asthma in a nationally-representative sample of children in the United States. *J. Autism Dev. Disord.* **2014**, *44*, 3083–3088. [CrossRef] [PubMed]
54. Billeci, L.; Tonacci, A.; Tartarisco, G.; Ruta, L.; Pioggia, G.; Gangemi, S. Association between atopic dermatitis and autism spectrum disorders: A systematic review. *Am. J. Clin. Dermatol.* **2015**, *16*, 371–388. [CrossRef]
55. Patel, S.; Cooper, M.N.; Jones, H.; Whitehouse, A.J.O.; Dale, R.C.; Guastella, A.J. Maternal immune-related conditions during pregnancy may be a risk factor for neuropsychiatric problems in offspring throughout childhood and adolescence. *Psychol. Med.* **2020**, 1–11. [CrossRef]
56. Angelidou, A.; Sullivan, K.; Melvin, P.R.; Shui, J.E.; Goldfarb, I.T.; Bartolome, R.; Chaudhary, N.; Vaidya, R.; Culic, I.; Singh, R.; et al. Association of maternal perinatal SARS-CoV-2 infection with neonatal outcomes during the COVID-19 pandemic in Massachusetts. *JAMA Netw. Open* **2021**, *4*, e217523. [CrossRef]

57. Theoharides, T.C.; Conti, P. COVID-19 and multisystem inflammatory syndrome, or is it mast cell activation syndrome? *J. Biol. Regul. Homeost. Agents* **2020**, *34*, 1633–1636.
58. Holingue, C.; Brucato, M.; Ladd-Acosta, C.; Hong, X.; Volk, H.; Mueller, N.T.; Wang, X.; Fallin, M.D. Interaction between maternal immune activation and antibiotic use during pregnancy and child risk of autism spectrum disorder. *Autism Res.* **2020**, *13*, 2230–2241. [CrossRef]
59. Wilkerson, D.S.; Volpe, A.G.; Dean, R.S.; Titus, J.B. Perinatal complications as predictors of infantile autism. *Int. J. Neurosci.* **2002**, *112*, 1085–1098. [CrossRef]
60. Tioleco, N.; Silberman, A.E.; Stratigos, K.; Banerjee-Basu, S.; Spann, M.N.; Whitaker, A.H.; Turner, J.B. Prenatal maternal infection and risk for autism in offspring: A meta-analysis. *Autism Res.* **2021**, *14*, 1296–1316. [CrossRef]
61. Yao, Z.H.; Yao, X.L.; Zhang, Y.; Zhang, S.F.; Hu, J.C. Luteolin could improve cognitive dysfunction by inhibiting neuroinflammation. *Neurochem. Res.* **2018**, *43*, 806–820. [CrossRef]
62. Shen, Q.; Zhang, Q.; Zhao, J.; Huang, Z.; Wang, X.; Ni, M.; Tang, Z.; Liu, Z. Association between maternal perceived stress in all trimesters of pregnancy and infant atopic dermatitis: A prospective birth cohort study. *Front. Pediatr.* **2020**, *8*, 526994. [CrossRef] [PubMed]
63. Theoharides, T.C. Autism spectrum disorders and mastocytosis. *Int. J. Immunopathol. Pharmacol.* **2009**, *22*, 859–865. [CrossRef]
64. Theoharides, T.C. Effect of stress on neuroimmune processes. *Clin. Ther.* **2020**, *42*, 1007–1014. [CrossRef]
65. Ronald, A.; Pennell, C.E.; Whitehouse, A.J. Prenatal maternal stress associated with ADHD and autistic traits in early childhood. *Front. Psychol.* **2010**, *1*, 223. [CrossRef]
66. Okano, L.; Ji, Y.; Riley, A.W.; Wang, X. Maternal psychosocial stress and children's ADHD diagnosis: A prospective birth cohort study. *J. Psychosom. Obstet. Gynaecol.* **2019**, *40*, 217–225. [CrossRef] [PubMed]
67. MacKinnon, N.; Kingsbury, M.; Mahedy, L.; Evans, J.; Colman, I. The association between prenatal stress and externalizing symptoms in childhood: Evidence from the avon longitudinal study of parents and children. *Biol. Psychiatry* **2018**, *83*, 100–108. [CrossRef] [PubMed]
68. Beversdorf, D.Q.; Manning, S.E.; Hillier, A.; Anderson, S.L.; Nordgren, R.E.; Walters, S.E.; Nagaraja, H.N.; Cooley, W.C.; Gaelic, S.E.; Bauman, M.L. Timing of prenatal stressors and autism. *J. Autism. Dev. Disord.* **2005**, *35*, 471–478. [CrossRef]
69. Crafa, D.; Warfa, N. Maternal migration and autism risk: Systematic analysis. *Int. Rev. Psychiatry* **2015**, *27*, 64–71. [CrossRef] [PubMed]
70. Beversdorf, D.Q.; Stevens, H.E.; Margolis, K.G.; van de Water, J. Prenatal stress and maternal immune dysregulation in autism spectrum disorders: Potential points for intervention. *Curr. Pharm. Des.* **2019**, *25*, 4331–4343. [CrossRef]
71. Evans, D.W.; Canavera, K.; Kleinpeter, F.L.; Maccubbin, E.; Taga, K. The fears, phobias and anxieties of children with autism spectrum disorders and Down syndrome: Comparisons with developmentally and chronologically age matched children. *Child Psychiatry Hum. Dev.* **2005**, *36*, 3–26. [CrossRef] [PubMed]
72. Beversdorf, D.Q.; Stevens, H.E.; Jones, K.L. Prenatal stress, maternal immune dysregulation, and their association with autism spectrum disorders. *Curr. Psychiatry Rep.* **2018**, *20*, 76. [CrossRef] [PubMed]
73. Fuentes-Zacarias, P.; Murrieta-Coxca, J.M.; Gutierrez-Samudio, R.N.; Schmidt, A.; Markert, U.R.; Morales-Prieto, D.M. Pregnancy and pandemics: Interaction of viral surface proteins and placenta cells. *Biochim. Biophys. Acta Mol. Basis. Dis.* **2021**, *1867*, 166218. [CrossRef] [PubMed]
74. Facchetti, F.; Bugatti, M.; Drera, E.; Tripodo, C.; Sartori, E.; Cancila, V.; Papaccio, M.; Castellani, R.; Casola, S.; Boniotti, M.B.; et al. SARS-CoV2 vertical transmission with adverse effects on the newborn revealed through integrated immunohistochemical, electron microscopy and molecular analyses of Placenta. *EBioMedicine* **2020**, *59*, 102951. [CrossRef] [PubMed]
75. Sharma, R.; Seth, S.; Sharma, R.; Yadav, S.; Mishra, P.; Mukhopadhyay, S. Perinatal outcome and possible vertical transmission of coronavirus disease 2019: Experience from North India. *Clin. Exp. Pediatr.* **2021**, *64*, 239–246. [CrossRef] [PubMed]
76. Kaklamanos, E.G.; Menexes, G.; Makrygiannakis, M.A.; Topitsoglou, V.; Kalfas, S. Tooth wear in a sample of community-dwelling elderly Greeks. *Oral Health Prev. Dent.* **2020**, *18*, 133–138.
77. Moosavi, F.; Hosseini, R.; Saso, L.; Firuzi, O. Modulation of neurotrophic signaling pathways by polyphenols. *Drug Des. Devel. Ther.* **2016**, *10*, 23–42.
78. Theoharides, T.C.; Conti, P. Be aware of SARS-CoV-2 spike protein: There is more than meets the eye. *J. Biol. Regul. Homeost. Agents* **2021**, *35*, 833–838.
79. Villar, J.; Ariff, S.; Gunier, R.B.; Thiruvengadam, R.; Rauch, S.; Kholin, A.; Roggero, P.; Prefumo, F.; do Vale, M.S.; Cardona-Perez, J.A. Maternal and neonatal morbidity and mortality among pregnant women with and without COVID-19 infection: The INTERCOVID multinational cohort study. *JAMA Pediatr.* **2021**, *175*, 817–826. [CrossRef]
80. Lu-Culligan, A.; Chavan, A.R.; Vijayakumar, P.; Irshaid, L.; Courchaine, E.M.; Milano, K.M.; Tang, Z.; Pope, S.D.; Song, E.; Vogels, C.F. SARS-CoV-2 infection in pregnancy is associated with robust inflammatory response at the maternal-fetal interface. *medRxiv* **2021**. [CrossRef]
81. Narang, K.; Enninga, E.A.L.; Gunaratne, M.D.S.K.; Ibirogba, E.R.; Trad, A.T.A.; Elrefaei, A.; Theiler, R.N.; Ruano, R.; Szymanski, L.M.; Chakraborty, R. SARS-CoV-2 infection and COVID-19 during pregnancy: A multidisciplinary review. *Mayo Clin. Proc.* **2020**, *95*, 1750–1765. [CrossRef]
82. Grammatopoulos, D.K.; Hillhouse, E.W. Role of corticotropin-releasing hormone in onset of labour. *Lancet* **1999**, *354*, 1546–1549. [CrossRef]

83. Ng, E.K.; Leung, T.N.; Tsui, N.B.; Lau, T.K.; Panesar, N.S.; Chiu, R.W.; Lo, Y.M. The concentration of circulating corticotropin-releasing hormone mRNA in maternal plasma is increased in preeclampsia. *Clin. Chem.* **2003**, *49*, 727–731. [CrossRef]
84. Chrousos, G.P. The hypothalamic-pituitary-adrenal axis and immune-mediated inflammation. *N. Engl. J. Med.* **1995**, *332*, 1351–1362. [CrossRef] [PubMed]
85. She, J.; Liu, L.; Liu, W. COVID-19 epidemic: Disease characteristics in children. *J. Med. Virol.* **2020**, *92*, 747–754. [CrossRef] [PubMed]
86. Dong, Y.; Mo, X.; Hu, Y.; Qi, X.; Jiang, F.; Jiang, Z.; Tong, S. Epidemiology of COVID-19 among Children in China. *Pediatrics* **2020**, *145*, e20200702. [CrossRef] [PubMed]
87. Ludvigsson, J.F. Systematic review of COVID-19 in children shows milder cases and a better prognosis than adults. *Acta Paediatr.* **2020**, *109*, 1088–1095. [CrossRef]
88. Tian, S.; Hu, N.; Lou, J.; Chen, K.; Kang, X.; Xiang, Z.; Chen, H.; Wang, D.; Liu, N.; Liu, D. Characteristics of COVID-19 infection in Beijing. *J. Infect.* **2020**, *80*, 401–406. [CrossRef]
89. Ciotti, M.; Angeletti, S.; Minieri, M.; Giovannetti, M.; Benvenuto, D.; Pascarella, S.; Sagnelli, C.; Bianchi, M.; Bernardini, S.; Ciccozzi, M. COVID-19 outbreak: An overview. *Chemotherapy* **2019**, *64*, 215–223. [CrossRef] [PubMed]
90. Hong, H.; Wang, Y.; Chung, H.T.; Chen, C.J. Clinical characteristics of novel coronavirus disease 2019 (COVID-19) in newborns, infants and children. *Pediatr. Neonatol.* **2020**, *61*, 131–132. [CrossRef]
91. Castagnoli, R.; Votto, M.; Licari, A.; Brambilla, I.; Bruno, R.; Perlini, S.; Rovida, F.; Baldanti, F.; Marseglia, G.L. Severe acute respiratory syndrome Coronavirus 2 (SARS-CoV-2) infection in children and adolescents: A systematic review. *JAMA Pediatr.* **2020**, *174*, 882–889. [CrossRef] [PubMed]
92. Greene, A.G.; Saleh, M.; Roseman, E.; Sinert, R. Toxic shock-like syndrome and COVID-19: A case report of multisystem inflammatory syndrome in children (MIS-C). *Am. J. Emerg. Med.* **2020**, *38*, 30492–30497. [CrossRef] [PubMed]
93. Levin, M. Childhood multisystem inflammatory syndrome—A new challenge in the pandemic. *N. Engl. J. Med.* **2020**, *383*, 393–395. [CrossRef]
94. Feldstein, L.R.; Rose, E.B.; Horwitz, S.M.; Collins, J.P.; Newhams, M.M.; Son, M.B.F.; Newburger, J.W.; Kleinman, L.C.; Heidemann, S.M.; Martin, A.A. Multisystem inflammatory syndrome in U.S. children and adolescents. *N. Engl. J. Med.* **2020**, *383*, 334–346. [CrossRef] [PubMed]
95. Jiang, L.; Tang, K.; Levin, M.; Irfan, O.; Morris, S.K.; Wilson, K.; Klein, J.D.; Bhutta, Z.A. COVID-19 and multisystem inflammatory syndrome in children and adolescents. *Lancet Infect. Dis.* **2020**, *20*, e276–e288. [CrossRef]
96. Rowley, A.H. Understanding SARS-CoV-2-related multisystem inflammatory syndrome in children. *Nat. Rev. Immunol.* **2020**, *20*, 453–454. [CrossRef] [PubMed]
97. Schwartz, L.B.; Bradford, T.R.; Littman, B.H.; Wintroub, B.U. The fibrinogenolytic activity of purified tryptase from human lung mast cells. *J. Immunol.* **1985**, *135*, 2762–2767.
98. Consiglio, C.R.; Cotugno, N.; Sardh, F.; Pou, C.; Amodio, D.; Rodriguez, L.; Tan, Z.; Zicari, S.; Ruggiero, A.; Pascucci, G.R. The immunology of multisystem inflammatory syndrome in children with COVID-19. *Cell* **2020**, *183*, 968–981. [CrossRef]
99. Hagberg, H.; Gressens, P.; Mallard, C. Inflammation during fetal and neonatal life: Implications for neurologic and neuropsychiatric disease in children and adults. *Ann. Neurol.* **2012**, *71*, 444–457. [CrossRef] [PubMed]
100. Jones, K.A.; Thomsen, C. The role of the innate immune system in psychiatric disorders. *Mol. Cell Neurosci.* **2013**, *53*, 52–62. [CrossRef]
101. Chavarria, A.; Alcocer-Varela, J. Is damage in central nervous system due to inflammation? *Autoimmun. Rev.* **2004**, *3*, 251–260. [CrossRef] [PubMed]
102. Le Belle, J.E.; Sperry, J.; Ngo, A.; Ghochani, Y.; Laks, D.R.; Lopez-Aranda, M.; Silva, A.J.; Kornblum, H.I. Maternal inflammation contributes to brain overgrowth and autism-associated behaviors through altered redox signaling in stem and progenitor cells. *Stem Cell Rep.* **2014**, *3*, 725–734. [CrossRef] [PubMed]
103. Lee, M.H.; Perl, D.P.; Nair, G.; Li, W.; Maric, D.; Murray, H.; Dodd, S.J.; Koretsky, A.P.; Watts, J.A.; Cheung, V.; et al. Microvascular injury in the brains of patients with Covid-19. *N. Engl. J. Med.* **2020**, *384*, 481–483. [CrossRef]
104. Helms, J.; Kremer, S.; Merdji, H.; Clere-Jehl, R.; Schenck, M.; Kummerlen, C.; Collange, O.; Boulay, C.; Fafi-Kremer, S.; Ohana, M. Neurologic features in severe SARS-CoV-2 infection. *N. Engl. J. Med.* **2020**, *382*, 2268–2270. [CrossRef] [PubMed]
105. Fotuhi, M.; Mian, A.; Meysami, S.; Raji, C.A. Neurobiology of COVID-19. *J. Alzheimers Dis.* **2020**, *76*, 3–19. [CrossRef]
106. Najjar, S.; Najjar, A.; Chong, D.J.; Pramanik, B.K.; Kirsch, C.; Kuzniecky, R.I.; Pacia, S.V.; Azhar, S. Central nervous system complications associated with SARS-CoV-2 infection: Integrative concepts of pathophysiology and case reports. *J. Neuroinflamm.* **2020**, *17*, 231. [CrossRef]
107. Singh, A.K.; Bhushan, B.; Maurya, A.; Mishra, G.; Singh, S.K.; Awasthi, R. Novel coronavirus disease 2019 (COVID-19) and neurodegenerative disorders. *Dermatol. Ther.* **2020**, *33*, e13591. [CrossRef]
108. Liotta, E.M.; Batra, A.; Clark, J.R.; Shlobin, N.A.; Hoffman, S.C.; Orban, Z.S.; Koralnik, I.J. Frequent neurologic manifestations and encephalopathy-associated morbidity in Covid-19 patients. *Ann.Clin. Transl. Neurol.* **2020**, *7*, 2221–2230. [CrossRef]
109. Koralnik, I.J.; Tyler, K.L. COVID-19: A global threat to the nervous system. *Ann. Neurol.* **2020**, *88*, 1–11. [CrossRef]
110. Nepal, G.; Rehrig, J.H.; Shrestha, G.S.; Shing, Y.K.; Yadav, J.K.; Ojha, R.; Pokhrel, G.; Tu, Z.L.; Huang, D.Y. Neurological manifestations of COVID-19: A systematic review. *Crit. Care* **2020**, *24*, 421. [CrossRef] [PubMed]

111. Favas, T.T.; Dev, P.; Chaurasia, R.N.; Chakravarty, K.; Mishra, R.; Joshi, D.; Mishra, V.N.; Kumar, A.; Singh, V.K.; Pandey, M.; et al. Neurological manifestations of COVID-19: A systematic review and meta-analysis of proportions. *Neurol. Sci.* **2020**, *41*, 3437–3470. [CrossRef] [PubMed]
112. Nazari, S.; Azari, J.A.; Mirmoeeni, S.; Sadeghian, S.; Heidari, M.E.; Assarzadegan, F.; Puormand, S.M.; Ebadi, H.; Fathi, D. Central nervous system manifestations in COVID-19 patients: A systematic review and meta-analysis. *Brain Behav.* **2021**, *11*, e02025. [CrossRef]
113. Kempuraj, D.; Selvakumar, G.P.; Ahmed, M.E.; Raikwar, S.P.; Thangavel, R.; Khan, A.; Zaheer, S.A.; Iyer, S.S.; Burton, C.; James, D.; et al. COVID-19, mast cells, cytokine storm, psychological stress, and neuroinflammation. *Neuroscientist* **2020**, *26*, 402–414. [CrossRef]
114. Schirinzi, T.; Landi, D.; Liguori, C. COVID-19: Dealing with a potential risk factor for chronic neurological disorders. *J. Neurol.* **2020**, *268*, 1171–1178. [CrossRef] [PubMed]
115. Ongur, D.; Perlis, R.; Goff, D. Psychiatry and COVID-19. *JAMA* **2020**, *324*, 1149–1150. [CrossRef]
116. Vindegaard, N.; Benros, M.E. COVID-19 pandemic and mental health consequences: Systematic review of the current evidence. *Brain Behav. Immun.* **2020**, *89*, 531–542. [CrossRef]
117. Pfefferbaum, B.; North, C.S. Mental health and the Covid-19 pandemic. *N. Engl. J. Med.* **2020**, *383*, 510–512. [CrossRef]
118. Xiang, Y.-T.; Yang, Y.; Li, W.; Zhang, L.; Zhang, Q.; Cheung, T.; Ng, C. Timely mental health care for the 2019 novel coronavirus outbreak is urgently needed. *Lancet Psychiatry* **2020**, *7*, 228–229. [CrossRef]
119. Gordon, J.A.; Borja, S.E. The COVID-19 pandemic: Setting the mental health research agenda. *Biol. Psychiatry* **2020**, *88*, 130–131. [CrossRef] [PubMed]
120. Taquet, M.; Luciano, S.; Geddes, J.R.; Harrison, P.J. Bidirectional associations between COVID-19 and psychiatric disorder: Retrospective cohort studies of 62,354 COVID-19 cases in the USA. *Lancet Psychiatry* **2021**, *8*, 130–140. [CrossRef]
121. Steardo, L., Jr.; Steardo, L.; Verkhratsky, A. Psychiatric face of COVID-19. *Transl. Psychiatry* **2020**, *10*, 261. [CrossRef]
122. Shader, R.I. COVID-19 and depression. *Clin. Ther.* **2020**, *42*, 962–963. [CrossRef]
123. Smith, C.M.; Komisar, J.R.; Mourad, A.; Kincaid, B.R. COVID-19-associated brief psychotic disorder. *BMJ Case Rep.* **2020**, *13*, e236940. [CrossRef]
124. Druss, B.G. Addressing the COVID-19 pandemic in populations with serious mental illness. *JAMA Psychiatry* **2020**, *77*, 891–892. [CrossRef] [PubMed]
125. Steinman, G. COVID-19 and autism. *Med. Hypotheses* **2020**, *142*, 109797. [CrossRef]
126. Baig, A.M. Chronic COVID syndrome: Need for an appropriate medical terminology for long-COVID and COVID long-haulers. *J. Med. Virol.* **2020**, *93*, 2555–2556. [CrossRef]
127. Moreno-Perez, O.; Merino, E.; Leon-Ramirez, J.M.; Andres, M.; Ramos, J.M.; renas-Jimenez, J.; Asensio, S.; Sanchez, R.; Ruiz-Torregrosa, P.; Galan, I. Post-acute COVID-19 Syndrome. Incidence and risk factors: A Mediterranean cohort study. *J. Infect.* **2021**, *82*, 378–383. [CrossRef]
128. Nalbandian, A.; Sehgal, K.; Gupta, A.; Madhavan, M.V.; McGroder, C.; Stevens, J.S.; Cook, J.R.; Nordvig, A.S.; Shalev, D.; Sehrawat, T.S.; et al. Post-acute COVID-19 syndrome. *Nat. Med.* **2021**, *27*, 601–615. [CrossRef]
129. Montagne, A.; Nation, D.A.; Sagare, A.P.; Barisano, G.; Sweeney, M.D.; Chakhoyan, A.; Pachicano, M.; Joe, E.; Nelson, A.R.; D'Orazio, L.M.; et al. APOE4 leads to blood-brain barrier dysfunction predicting cognitive decline. *Nature* **2020**, *581*, 71–76. [CrossRef] [PubMed]
130. Baig, A.M. Deleterious outcomes in long-hauler COVID-19: The effects of SARS-CoV-2 on the CNS in chronic COVID syndrome. *ACS Chem. Neurosci.* **2020**, *11*, 4017–4020. [CrossRef] [PubMed]
131. Huang, C.; Huang, L.; Wang, Y.; Li, X.; Ren, L.; Gu, X.; Kang, L.; Guo, L.; Liu, M.; Zhou, X.; et al. 6-month consequences of COVID-19 in patients discharged from hospital: A cohort study. *Lancet* **2021**, *397*, 220–232. [CrossRef]
132. Higgins, V.; Sohaei, D.; Diamandis, E.P.; Prassas, I. COVID-19: From an acute to chronic disease? Potential long-term health consequences. *Crit. Rev.Clin. Lab. Sci.* **2020**, *58*, 297–310. [CrossRef]
133. Townsend, L.; Dyer, A.H.; Jones, K.; Dunne, J.; Mooney, A.; Gaffney, F.; O'Connor, L.; Leavy, D.; O'Brien, K.; Dowds, J. Persistent fatigue following SARS-CoV-2 infection is common and independent of severity of initial infection. *PLoS ONE* **2020**, *15*, e0240784. [CrossRef]
134. Theoharides, T.C. Stress, inflammation, and autoimmunity: The 3 modern erinyes. *Clin. Ther.* **2020**, *42*, 742–744. [CrossRef] [PubMed]
135. Theoharides, T.C. The impact of psychological stress on mast cells. *Ann. Allergy Asthma Immunol. Off. Publ. Am. Coll. Allergy Asthma Immunol.* **2020**, *125*, 388–392. [CrossRef]
136. Keller, F.; Persico, A.M. The neurobiological context of autism. *Mol. Neurobiol.* **2003**, *28*, 1–22. [CrossRef]
137. El-Ansary, A.; Al-Ayadhi, L. Neuroinflammation in autism spectrum disorders. *J. Neuroinflamm.* **2012**, *9*, 265. [CrossRef] [PubMed]
138. Young, A.M.; Chakrabarti, B.; Roberts, D.; Lai, M.C.; Suckling, J.; Baron-Cohen, S. From molecules to neural morphology: Understanding neuroinflammation in autism spectrum condition. *Mol. Autism* **2016**, *7*, 9. [CrossRef]
139. Prata, J.; Machado, A.S.; von Doellinger, O.; Almeida, M.I.; Barbosa, M.A.; Coelho, R.; Santos, S.G. The contribution of inflammation to autism spectrum disorders: Recent clinical evidence. *Methods Mol. Biol.* **2019**, *2011*, 493–510.
140. Platt, M.P.; Agalliu, D.; Cutforth, T. Hello from the other side: How autoantibodies circumvent the blood-brain barrier in autoimmune encephalitis. *Front. Immunol.* **2017**, *8*, 442. [CrossRef]

141. Theoharides, T.C.; Angelidou, A.; Alysandratos, K.D.; Zhang, B.; Asadi, S.; Francis, K.; Toniato, E.; Kalogeromitros, D. Mast cell activation and autism. *Biochim. Biophys. Acta* **2012**, *1822*, 34–41. [CrossRef]
142. Theoharides, T.C.; Donelan, J.M.; Papadopoulou, N.; Cao, J.; Kempuraj, D.; Conti, P. Mast cells as targets of corticotropin-releasing factor and related peptides. *Trends Pharmacol. Sci.* **2004**, *25*, 563–568. [CrossRef] [PubMed]
143. Pedersen, J.M.; Mortensen, E.L.; Christensen, D.S.; Rozing, M.; Brunsgaard, H.; Meincke, R.H.; Petersen, G.L.; Lund, R. Prenatal and early postnatal stress and later life inflammation. *Psychoneuroendocrinology* **2018**, *88*, 158–166. [CrossRef]
144. Marsland, A.L.; Walsh, C.; Lockwood, K.; John-Henderson, N.A. The effects of acute psychological stress on circulating and stimulated inflammatory markers: A systematic review and meta-analysis. *Brain Behav. Immun.* **2017**, *64*, 208–219. [CrossRef] [PubMed]
145. Rudolph, M.D.; Graham, A.M.; Feczko, E.; Miranda-Dominguez, O.; Rasmussen, J.M.; Nardos, R.; Entringer, S.; Wadhwa, P.D.; Buss, C.; Fair, D.A. Maternal IL-6 during pregnancy can be estimated from newborn brain connectivity and predicts future working memory in offspring. *Nat. Neurosci.* **2018**, *21*, 765–772. [CrossRef]
146. Huang, M.; Pang, X.; Karalis, K.; Theoharides, T.C. Stress-induced interleukin-6 release in mice is mast cell-dependent and more pronounced in Apolipoprotein E knockout mice. *Cardiovasc. Res.* **2003**, *59*, 241–249. [CrossRef]
147. Desai, A.; Jung, M.Y.; Olivera, A.; Gilfillan, A.M.; Prussin, C.; Kirshenbaum, A.S.; Beaven, M.A.; Metcalfe, D.D. IL-6 promotes an increase in human mast cell numbers and reactivity through suppression of suppressor of cytokine signaling 3. *J. Allergy Clin. Immunol.* **2016**, *137*, 1863–1871. [CrossRef]
148. O'Keeffe, G.W. A new role for placental IL-6 signalling in determining neurodevelopmental outcome. *Brain Behav. Immun.* **2017**, *62*, 9–10. [CrossRef] [PubMed]
149. Theoharides, T.C.; Konstantinidou, A. Corticotropin-releasing hormone and the blood-brain-barrier. *Front. Biosci.* **2007**, *12*, 1615–1628. [CrossRef] [PubMed]
150. Fiorentino, M.; Sapone, A.; Senger, S.; Camhi, S.S.; Kadzielski, S.M.; Buie, T.M.; Kelly, D.L.; Cascella, N.; Fasano, A. Blood-brain barrier and intestinal epithelial barrier alterations in autism spectrum disorders. *Mol. Autism* **2016**, *7*, 49. [CrossRef]
151. Kempuraj, D.; Papadopoulou, N.G.; Lytinas, M.; Huang, M.; Kandere-Grzybowska, K.; Madhappan, B.; Boucher, W.; Christodoulou, S.; Athanassiou, A.; Theoharides, T.C. Corticotropin-releasing hormone and its structurally related urocortin are synthesized and secreted by human mast cells. *Endocrinology* **2004**, *145*, 43–48. [CrossRef]
152. Mastorakos, G.; Chrousos, G.P.; Weber, J.S. Recombinant interleukin-6 activates the hypothalamic-pituitary-adrenal axis in humans. *J. Clin. Endocrinol. Metab.* **1993**, *77*, 1690–1694.
153. Stolp, H.B.; Dziegielewska, K.M.; Ek, C.J.; Habgood, M.D.; Lane, M.A.; Potter, A.M.; Saunders, N.R. Breakdown of the blood-brain barrier to proteins in white matter of the developing brain following systemic inflammation. *Cell Tissue Res.* **2005**, *320*, 369–378. [CrossRef]
154. Esposito, P.; Chandler, N.; Kandere-Grzybowska, K.; Basu, S.; Jacobson, S.; Connolly, R.; Tutor, D.; Theoharides, T.C. Corticotropin-releasing hormone (CRH) and brain mast cells regulate blood-brain-barrier permeability induced by acute stress. *J. Pharmacol. Exp. Ther.* **2002**, *303*, 1061–1066. [CrossRef]
155. Theoharides, T.C.; Doyle, R. Autism, gut-blood-brain barrier and mast cells. *J. Clin. Psychopharm.* **2008**, *28*, 479–483. [CrossRef] [PubMed]
156. Rozniecki, J.J.; Sahagian, G.G.; Kempuraj, D.; Tao, K.; Jocobson, S.; Zhang, B.; Theoharides, T.C. Brain metastases of mouse mammary adenocarcinoma is increased by acute stress. *Brain Res.* **2010**, *1366*, 204–210. [CrossRef] [PubMed]
157. Theoharides, T.C.; Rozniecki, J.J.; Sahagian, G.; Jocobson, S.; Kempuraj, D.; Conti, P.; Kalogeromitros, D. Impact of stress and mast cells on brain metastases. *J. Neuroimmunol.* **2008**, *205*, 1–7. [CrossRef] [PubMed]
158. Saunders, N.R. Ontogeny of the blood-brain barrier. *Exp. Eye Res.* **1977**, *25*, 523–550. [CrossRef]
159. Saunders, N.R.; Liddelow, S.A.; Dziegielewska, K.M. Barrier mechanisms in the developing brain. *Front Pharmacol.* **2012**, *3*, 46. [CrossRef]
160. Bueno, D.; Parvas, M.; Hermelo, I.; Garcia-Fernandez, J. Embryonic blood-cerebrospinal fluid barrier formation and function. *Front. Neurosci.* **2014**, *8*, 343. [CrossRef]
161. Saunders, N.R.; Dziegielewska, K.M.; Mollgard, K.; Habgood, M.D. Recent developments in understanding barrier mechanisms in the developing brain: Drugs and drug transporters in pregnancy, susceptibility or protection in the fetal brain? *Annu. Rev. Pharmacol. Toxicol.* **2019**, *59*, 487–505. [CrossRef] [PubMed]
162. Koehn, L.; Habgood, M.; Huang, Y.; Dziegielewska, K.; Saunders, N. Determinants of drug entry into the developing brain. *F1000 Res.* **2019**, *8*, 1372. [CrossRef] [PubMed]
163. Ji, Y.; Azuine, R.E.; Zhang, Y.; Hou, W.; Hong, X.; Wang, G.; Riley, A.; Pearson, C.; Zuckerman, B.; Wang, X. Association of cord plasma biomarkers of in utero acetaminophen exposure with risk of attention-deficit/hyperactivity disorder and autism spectrum disorder in childhood. *JAMA Psychiatry* **2019**, *77*, 180–189. [CrossRef] [PubMed]
164. Li, Z.; Ge, J.; Yang, M.; Feng, J.; Qiao, M.; Jiang, R.; Bi, J.; Zhan, G.; Xu, X.; Wang, L.; et al. Vicarious traumatization in the general public, members, and non-members of medical teams aiding in COVID-19 control. *Brain Behav. Immun.* **2020**, *88*, 916–919. [CrossRef]
165. Zhang, K.; Zhou, X.; Liu, H.; Hashimoto, K. Treatment concerns for psychiatric symptoms in patients with COVID-19 with or without psychiatric disorders. *Br. J. Psychiatry* **2020**, *217*, 351. [CrossRef]

166. Walton, M.; Murray, E.; Christian, M.D. Mental health care for medical staff and affiliated healthcare workers during the COVID-19 pandemic. *Eur. Heart, J. Acute Cardiovasc. Care* **2020**, *9*, 241–247. [CrossRef]
167. Ren, Y.; Zhou, Y.; Qian, W.; Li, Z.; Liu, Z.; Wang, R.; Qi, L.; Yang, J.; Song, X.; Zeng, L.; et al. Letter to the Editor "A longitudinal study on the mental health of general population during the COVID-19 epidemic in China". *Brain Behav. Immunol.* **2020**, *87*, 132–133. [CrossRef]
168. Loades, M.E.; Chatburn, E.; Higson-Sweeney, N.; Reynolds, S.; Shafran, R.; Brigden, A.; Linney, C.; McManus, M.N.; Borwick, C.; Crawley, E. Rapid systematic review: The impact of social isolation and loneliness on the mental health of children and adolescents in the context of COVID-19. *J. Am. Acad. Child Adolesc. Psychiatry* **2020**, *59*, 1218–1239. [CrossRef]
169. Peters, J.L.; Cohen, S.; Staudenmayer, J.; Hosen, J.; Platts-Mills, T.A.; Wright, R.J. Prenatal negative life events increases cord blood IgE: Interactions with dust mite allergen and maternal atopy. *Allergy* **2012**, *67*, 545–551. [CrossRef]
170. Wang, I.J.; Wen, H.J.; Chiang, T.L.; Lin, S.J.; Guo, Y.L. Maternal psychologic problems increased the risk of childhood atopic dermatitis 1. *Pediatr. Allergy Immunol.* **2016**, *27*, 169–176. [CrossRef]
171. Andersson, N.W.; Hansen, M.V.; Larsen, A.D.; Hougaard, K.S.; Kolstad, H.A.; Schlunssen, V. Prenatal maternal stress and atopic diseases in the child: A systematic review of observational human studies. *Allergy* **2016**, *71*, 15–26. [CrossRef] [PubMed]
172. Medsker, B.; Forno, E.; Simhan, H.; Celedon, J.C. Prenatal stress, prematurity, and asthma. *Obstet. Gynecol. Surv.* **2015**, *70*, 773–779. [CrossRef] [PubMed]
173. Rosa, M.J.; Lee, A.G.; Wright, R.J. Evidence establishing a link between prenatal and early-life stress and asthma development. *Curr. Opin. Allergy Clin. Immunol.* **2018**, *18*, 148–158. [CrossRef] [PubMed]
174. Van de Loo, K.F.; van Gelder, M.M.; Roukema, J.; Roeleveld, N.; Merkus, P.J.; Verhaak, C.M. Prenatal maternal psychological stress and childhood asthma and wheezing: A meta-analysis. *Eur. Respir. J.* **2016**, *47*, 133–146. [CrossRef]
175. Postorino, V.; Kerns, C.M.; Vivanti, G.; Bradshaw, J.; Siracusano, M.; Mazzone, L. Anxiety disorders and obsessive-compulsive disorder in individuals with autism spectrum disorder. *Curr. Psychiatry Rep.* **2017**, *19*, 92. [CrossRef]
176. Cai, R.Y.; Richdale, A.L.; Uljarevic, M.; Dissanayake, C.; Samson, A.C. Emotion regulation in autism spectrum disorder: Where we are and where we need to go. *Autism Res.* **2018**, *11*, 962–978. [CrossRef]
177. Ye, Q.; Wang, B.; Mao, J. The pathogenesis and treatment of the 'Cytokine Storm' in COVID-19. *J. Infect.* **2020**, *80*, 607–613. [CrossRef] [PubMed]
178. Chen, G.; Wu, D.; Guo, W.; Cao, Y.; Huang, D.; Wang, H.; Wang, T.; Zhang, X.; Chen, H.; Yu, H.; et al. Clinical and immunological features of severe and moderate coronavirus disease 2019. *J. Clin. Investig.* **2020**, *130*, 2620–2629. [CrossRef]
179. Conti, P.; Ronconi, G.; Caraffa, A.; Gallenga, C.E.; Ross, R.; Frydas, I.; Kritas, S.K. Induction of pro-inflammatory cytokines (IL-1 and IL-6) and lung inflammation by Coronavirus-19 (COVI-19 or SARS-CoV-2): Anti-inflammatory strategies. *J. Biol. Regul. Homeost. Agents* **2020**, *34*, 327–331.
180. Giamarellos-Bourboulis, E.J.; Netea, M.G.; Rovina, N.; Akinosoglou, K.; Antoniadou, A.; Antonakos, N.; Damoraki, G.; Gkavogianni, T.; Adami, M.-E.; Katsaounou, P.; et al. Complex immune dysregulation in COVID-19 patients with severe respiratory failure. *Cell Host. Microbe* **2020**, *27*, 992–1000. [CrossRef]
181. Tang, Y.; Liu, J.; Zhang, D.; Xu, Z.; Ji, J.; Wen, C. Cytokine storm in COVID-19: The current evidence and treatment strategies. *Front. Immunol.* **2020**, *11*, 1708. [CrossRef]
182. Paces, J.; Strizova, Z.; Smrz, D.; Cerny, J. COVID-19 and the immune system. *Physiol. Res.* **2020**, *69*, 379–388. [CrossRef]
183. Ragab, D.; Salah, E.H.; Taeimah, M.; Khattab, R.; Salem, R. The COVID-19 cytokine storm; What we know so far. *Front. Immunol.* **2020**, *11*, 1446. [CrossRef]
184. Brodin, P. Immune determinants of COVID-19 disease presentation and severity. *Nat. Med.* **2021**, *27*, 28–33. [CrossRef] [PubMed]
185. Canna, S.W.; Cron, R.Q. Highways to hell: Mechanism-based management of cytokine storm syndromes. *J. Allergy Clin. Immunol.* **2020**, *146*, 949–959. [CrossRef]
186. Herold, T.; Jurinovic, V.; Arnreich, C.; Lipworth, B.J.; Hellmuth, J.C.; von Bergwelt-Baildon, M.; Klein, M.; Weinberger, T. Elevated levels of IL-6 and CRP predict the need for mechanical ventilation in COVID-19. *J. Allergy Clin. Immunol.* **2020**, *146*, 128–136. [CrossRef] [PubMed]
187. Han, H.; Ma, Q.; Li, C.; Liu, R.; Zhao, L.; Wang, W.; Zhang, P.; Liu, X.; Gao, G.; Liu, F. Profiling serum cytokines in COVID-19 patients reveals IL-6 and IL-10 are disease severity predictors. *Emerg. Microbes. Infect.* **2020**, *9*, 1123–1130. [CrossRef]
188. Mazzoni, A.; Salvati, L.; Maggi, L.; Capone, M.; Vanni, A.; Spinicci, M.; Mencarini, J.; Caporale, R.; Peruzzi, B.; Antonelli, A.; et al. Impaired immune cell cytotoxicity in severe COVID-19 is IL-6 dependent. *J. Clin. Investig.* **2020**, *130*, 4694–4703. [CrossRef]
189. Liu, F.; Li, L.; Xu, M.; Wu, J.; Luo, D.; Zhu, Y.; Li, B.; Song, X.; Zhou, X. Prognostic value of interleukin-6, C-reactive protein, and procalcitonin in patients with COVID-19. *J. Clin. Virol.* **2020**, *127*, 104370. [CrossRef] [PubMed]
190. Copaescu, A.; Smibert, O.; Gibson, A.; Phillips, E.J.; Trubiano, J.A. The role of IL-6 and other mediators in the cytokine storm associated with SARS-CoV-2 infection. *J. Allergy Clin. Immunol.* **2020**, *146*, 518–534. [CrossRef] [PubMed]
191. Conti, P.; Caraffa, A.; Gallenga, C.E.; Ross, R.; Kritas, S.K.; Frydas, I.; Younes, A.; Ronconi, G. Coronavirus-19 (SARS-CoV-2) induces acute severe lung inflammation via IL-1 causing cytokine storm in COVID-19: A promising inhibitory strategy. *J. Biol. Regul. Homeost. Agents* **2020**, *34*, 1971–1975.
192. Kritas, S.K.; Ronconi, G.; Caraffa, A.; Gallenga, C.E.; Ross, R.; Conti, P. Mast cells contribute to coronavirus-induced inflammation: New anti-inflammatory strategy. *J. Biol. Regul. Homeost. Agents* **2020**, *34*, 9–14.

193. Theoharides, T.C. COVID-19, pulmonary mast cells, cytokine storms, and beneficial actions of luteolin. *Biofactors* **2020**, *46*, 306–308. [CrossRef] [PubMed]
194. Afrin, L.B.; Weinstock, L.B.; Molderings, G.J. Covid-19 hyperinflammation and post-Covid-19 illness may be rooted in mast cell activation syndrome. *Int. J. Infect. Dis.* **2020**, *100*, 327–332. [CrossRef] [PubMed]
195. Theoharides, T.C. Potential association of mast cells with COVID-19. *Ann. Allergy Asthma Immunol.* **2020**, *126*, 217–218. [CrossRef] [PubMed]
196. Motta, J.D.S., Jr.; Miggiolaro, A.F.R.D.S.; Nagashima, S.; de Paula, C.B.V.; Baena, C.P.; Scharfstein, J.; de Noronha, L. Mast cells in alveolar septa of COVID-19 patients: A pathogenic pathway that may link interstitial edema to immunothrombosis. *Front. Immunol.* **2020**, *11*, 574862. [CrossRef]
197. Theoharides, T.C.; Valent, P.; Akin, C. Mast cells, mastocytosis, and related disorders. *N. Engl. J. Med.* **2015**, *373*, 163–172. [CrossRef]
198. Fombonne, E. Epidemiology of pervasive developmental disorders. *Pediatr. Res.* **2009**, *65*, 591–598. [CrossRef]
199. McPartland, J.; Volkmar, F.R. Autism and related disorders. *Handb. Clin. Neurol.* **2012**, *106*, 407–418. [PubMed]
200. Chang, H.Y.; Seo, J.H.; Kim, H.Y.; Kwon, J.W.; Kim, B.J.; Kim, H.B.; Lee, S.Y.; Jang, G.C.; Song, D.J.; Kim, W.K. Allergic diseases in preschoolers are associated with psychological and behavioural problems. *Allergy Asthma Immunol. Res.* **2013**, *5*, 315–321. [CrossRef]
201. Jyonouchi, H. Food allergy and autism spectrum disorders: Is there a link? *Curr. Allergy Asthma Rep.* **2009**, *9*, 194–201. [CrossRef] [PubMed]
202. Li, H.; Liu, H.; Chen, X.; Zhang, J.; Tong, G.; Sun, Y. Association of food hypersensitivity in children with the risk of autism spectrum disorder: A meta-analysis. *Eur. J. Pediatr.* **2021**, *180*, 999–1008. [CrossRef] [PubMed]
203. Xu, G.; Snetselaar, L.G.; Jing, J.; Liu, B.; Strathearn, L.; Bao, W. Association of food allergy and other allergic conditions with autism spectrum disorder in children. *JAMA Netw. Open* **2018**, *1*, e180279. [CrossRef] [PubMed]
204. Tan, Y.; Thomas, S.; Lee, B.K. Parent-reported prevalence of food allergies in children with autism spectrum disorder: National health interview survey, 2011–2015. *Autism Res.* **2019**, *12*, 802–805. [CrossRef]
205. Peretti, S.; Mariano, M.; Mazzocchetti, C.; Mazza, M.; Pino, M.C.; Verrotti Di, P.A.; Valenti, M. Diet: The keystone of autism spectrum disorder? *Nutr. Neurosci.* **2019**, *22*, 825–839. [CrossRef]
206. Mostafa, G.A.; Al-Ayadhi, L.Y. The possible relationship between allergic manifestations and elevated serum levels of brain specific auto-antibodies in autistic children. *J. Neuroimmunol.* **2013**, *261*, 77–81. [CrossRef]
207. Ravn, N.H.; Halling, A.S.; Berkowitz, A.G.; Rinnov, M.R.; Silverberg, J.I.; Egeberg, A.; Thyssen, J.P. How does parental history of atopic disease predict the risk of atopic dermatitis in a child? A systematic review and meta-analysis. *J. Allergy Clin. Immunol.* **2020**, *145*, 1182–1193. [CrossRef]
208. Estes, M.L.; McAllister, A.K. Maternal immune activation: Implications for neuropsychiatric disorders. *Science* **2016**, *353*, 772–777. [CrossRef] [PubMed]
209. Zerbo, O.; Leong, A.; Barcellos, L.; Bernal, P.; Fireman, B.; Croen, L.A. Immune mediated conditions in autism spectrum disorders. *Brain Behav. Immun.* **2015**, *46*, 232–236. [CrossRef]
210. Comi, A.M.; Zimmerman, A.W.; Frye, V.H.; Law, P.A.; Peeden, J.N. Familial clustering of autoimmune disorders and evaluation of medical risk factors in autism. *J. Child Neurol.* **1999**, *14*, 388–394. [CrossRef]
211. Jarmołowska, B.; Bukało, M.; Fiedorowicz, E.; Cieślińska, A.; Kordulewska, N.K.; Moszyńska, M.; Świątecki, A.; Kostyra, E. Role of Milk-Derived Opioid Peptides and Proline Dipeptidyl Peptidase-4 in Autism Spectrum Disorders. *Nutrients* **2019**, *11*, 87. [CrossRef]
212. Zhou, L.; Chen, L.; Li, X.; Li, T.; Dong, Z.; Wang, Y.T. Food allergy induces alteration in brain inflammatory status and cognitive impairments. *Behav. Brain Res.* **2019**, *364*, 374–382. [CrossRef] [PubMed]
213. Msallam, R.; Balla, J.; Rathore, A.P.S.; Kared, H.; Malleret, B.; Saron, W.A.A.; Liu, Z.; Hang, J.W.; Dutertre, C.A.; Larbi, A.; et al. Fetal mast cells mediate postnatal allergic responses dependent on maternal IgE. *Science* **2020**, *370*, 941–950. [CrossRef]
214. Lenz, K.M.; Pickett, L.A.; Wright, C.L.; Davis, K.T.; Joshi, A.; McCarthy, M.M. Mast cells in the developing brain determine adult sexual behavior. *J. Neurosci.* **2018**, *38*, 8044–8059. [CrossRef]
215. Theoharides, T.C.; Petra, A.I.; Taracanova, A.; Panagiotidou, S.; Conti, P. Targeting IL-33 in autoimmunity and inflammation. *J. Pharmacol. Exp. Ther.* **2015**, *354*, 24–31. [CrossRef]
216. Theoharides, T.C.; Leeman, S.E. Effect of IL-33 on de novo synthesized mediators from human mast cells. *J. Allergy Clin. Immunol.* **2019**, *143*, 451. [CrossRef] [PubMed]
217. Zhang, X.; Dong, H.; Li, N.; Zhang, S.; Sun, J.; Zhang, S.; Qian, Y. Activated brain mast cells contribute to postoperative cognitive dysfunction by evoking microglia activation and neuronal apoptosis. *J. Neuroinflamm.* **2016**, *13*, 127. [CrossRef]
218. Gurish, M.F.; Austen, K.F. Developmental origin and functional specialization of mast cell subsets. *Immunity* **2012**, *37*, 25–33. [CrossRef]
219. Olivera, A.; Beaven, M.A.; Metcalfe, D.D. Mast cells signal their importance in health and disease. *J. Allergy Clin. Immunol.* **2018**, *142*, 381–393. [CrossRef]
220. Galli, S.J.; Tsai, M.; Piliponsky, A.M. The development of allergic inflammation. *Nature* **2008**, *454*, 445–454. [CrossRef] [PubMed]
221. Theoharides, T.C.; Alysandratos, K.D.; Angelidou, A.; Delivanis, D.A.; Sismanopoulos, N.; Zhang, B.; Asadi, S.; Vasiadi, M.; Weng, Z.; Miniati, A.; et al. Mast cells and inflammation. *Biochim. Biophys. Acta* **2012**, *1822*, 21–33. [CrossRef]

222. Mukai, K.; Tsai, M.; Saito, H.; Galli, S.J. Mast cells as sources of cytokines, chemokines, and growth factors. *Immunol. Rev.* **2018**, *282*, 121–150. [CrossRef] [PubMed]
223. Theoharides, T.C.; Alysandratos, K.D.; Angelidou, A.; Delivanis, D.A.; Sismanopoulos, N.; Zhang, B.; Asadi, S.; Vasiadi, M.; Weng, Z.; Miniati, A. Interleukin-1 family cytokines and mast cells: Activation and inhibition. *J. Biol. Regul. Homeost. Agents* **2019**, *33*, 1–6.
224. Taracanova, A.; Tsilioni, I.; Conti, P.; Norwitz, E.R.; Leeman, S.E.; Theoharides, T.C. Substance P and IL-33 administered together stimulate a marked secretion of IL-1beta from human mast cells, inhibited by methoxyluteolin. *Proc. Natl. Acad. Sci. USA* **2018**, *115*, e9381–e9390. [CrossRef]
225. Kandere-Grzybowska, K.; Letourneau, R.; Kempuraj, D.; Donelan, J.; Poplawski, S.; Boucher, W.; Athanassiou, A.; Theoharides, T.C. IL-1 induces vesicular secretion of IL-6 without degranulation from human mast cells. *J. Immunol.* **2003**, *171*, 4830–4836. [CrossRef] [PubMed]
226. Taracanova, A.; Alevizos, M.; Karagkouni, A.; Weng, Z.; Norwitz, E.; Conti, P.; Leeman, S.E.; Theoharides, T.C. SP and IL-33 together markedly enhance TNF synthesis and secretion from human mast cells mediated by the interaction of their receptors. *Proc. Natl. Acad. Sci. USA* **2017**, *114*, e4002–e4009. [CrossRef] [PubMed]
227. Rozniecki, J.J.; Dimitriadou, V.; Lambracht-Hall, M.; Pang, X.; Theoharides, T.C. Morphological and functional demonstration of rat dura mast cell-neuron interactions in vitro and in vivo. *Brain Res.* **1999**, *849*, 1–15. [CrossRef]
228. Polyzoidis, S.; Koletsa, T.; Panagiotidou, S.; Ashkan, K.; Theoharides, T.C. Mast cells in meningiomas and brain inflammation. *J. Neuroinflammation* **2015**, *12*, 170. [CrossRef] [PubMed]
229. Pang, X.; Letourneau, R.; Rozniecki, J.J.; Wang, L.; Theoharides, T.C. Definitive characterization of rat hypothalamic mast cells. *Neuroscience* **1996**, *73*, 889–902. [CrossRef]
230. Kandere-Grzybowska, K.; Gheorghe, D.; Priller, J.; Esposito, P.; Huang, M.; Gerard, N.; Theoharides, T.C. Stress-induced dura vascular permeability does not develop in mast cell-deficient and neurokinin-1 receptor knockout mice. *Brain Res.* **2003**, *980*, 213–220. [CrossRef]
231. Matsumoto, I.; Inoue, Y.; Shimada, T.; Aikawa, T. Brain mast cells act as an immune gate to the hypothalamic-pituitary-adrenal axis in dogs. *J. Exp. Med.* **2001**, *194*, 71–78. [CrossRef] [PubMed]
232. Bugajski, A.J.; Chlap, Z.; Gadek-Michalska, A.; Borycz, J.; Bugajski, J. Degranulation and decrease in histamine levels of thalamic mast cells coincides with corticosterone secretion induced by compound 48/80. *Inflamm. Res.* **1995**, *44*, S50–S51. [CrossRef] [PubMed]
233. Kalogeromitros, D.; Syrigou, E.I.; Makris, M.; Kempuraj, D.; Stavrianeas, N.G.; Vasiadi, M.; Theoharides, T.C. Nasal provocation of patients with allergic rhinitis and the hypothalamic-pituitary-adrenal axis. *Ann. Allergy Asthma Immunol.* **2007**, *98*, 269–273. [CrossRef]
234. Scaccianoce, S.; Lombardo, K.; Nicolai, R.; Affricano, D.; Angelucci, L. Studies on the involvement of histamine in the hypothalamic-pituitary-adrenal axis activation induced by nerve growth factor. *Life Sci.* **2000**, *67*, 3143–3152. [CrossRef]
235. Alysandratos, K.; Asadi, S.; Angelidou, A.; Zhang, B.; Sismanopoulos, N.; Yang, H.; Critchfield, A.; Theoharides, T.C. Neurotensin and CRH interactions augment human mast cell activation. *PLoS ONE* **2012**, *7*, e48934. [CrossRef] [PubMed]
236. Asadi, S.; Alysandratos, K.-D.; Angelidou, A.; Miniati, A.; Sismanopoulos, N.; Vasiadi, M.; Zhang, B.; Kalogeromitros, D.; Theoharides, T.C. Substance P (SP) induces expression of functional corticotropin-releasing hormone receptor-1 (CRHR-1) in human mast cells. *J. Investig. Dermatol.* **2012**, *132*, 324–329. [CrossRef]
237. Marshall, J.S.; Portales-Cervantes, L.; Leong, E. Mast cell responses to viruses and pathogen products. *Int. J. Mol. Sci.* **2019**, *20*, 4241. [CrossRef]
238. Ziegler, C.G.K.; Allon, S.J.; Nyquist, S.K.; Mbano, I.M.; Miao, V.N.; Tzouanas, C.N.; Cao, Y.; Yousif, A.S.; Bals, J.; Hauser, B.M. SARS-CoV-2 receptor ACE2 is an interferon-stimulated gene in human airway epithelial cells and is detected in specific cell subsets across tissues. *Cell* **2020**, *181*, 1016–1035. [CrossRef]
239. Dietrich, N.; Rohde, M.; Geffers, R.; Kroger, A.; Hauser, H.; Weiss, S.; Gekara, N.O. Mast cells elicit proinflammatory but not type I interferon responses upon activation of TLRs by bacteria. *Proc. Natl. Acad. Sci. USA* **2010**, *107*, 8748–8753. [CrossRef]
240. Bawazeer, M.A.; Theoharides, T.C. IL-33 stimulates human mast cell release of CCL5 and CCL2 via MAPK and NF-kappaB, inhibited by methoxyluteolin. *Eur. J. Pharmacol.* **2019**, *865*, 172760. [CrossRef]
241. Saluja, R.; Khan, M.; Church, M.K.; Maurer, M. The role of IL-33 and mast cells in allergy and inflammation. *Clin. Transl. Allergy* **2015**, *5*, 33. [CrossRef] [PubMed]
242. Conti, P.; Caraffa, A.; Tete, G.; Gallenga, C.E.; Ross, R.; Kritas, S.K.; Frydas, I.; Younes, A.; Di, E.P.; Ronconi, G. Mast cells activated by SARS-CoV-2 release histamine which increases IL-1 levels causing cytokine storm and inflammatory reaction in COVID-19. *J. Biol. Regul. Homeost. Agents* **2020**, *34*, 1629–1632.
243. Zhang, B.; Asadi, S.; Weng, Z.; Sismanopoulos, N.; Theoharides, T.C. Stimulated human mast cells secrete mitochondrial components that have autocrine and paracrine inflammatory actions. *PLoS ONE* **2012**, *7*, e49767. [CrossRef]
244. Collins, L.V.; Hajizadeh, S.; Holme, E.; Jonsson, I.M.; Tarkowski, A. Endogenously oxidized mitochondrial DNA induces in vivo and in vitro inflammatory responses. *J. Leukoc. Biol.* **2004**, *75*, 995–1000. [CrossRef] [PubMed]
245. Sun, S.; Sursal, T.; Adibnia, Y.; Zhao, C.; Zheng, Y.; Li, H.; Otterbein, L.E.; Hauser, C.J.; Itagaki, K. Mitochondrial DAMPs increase endothelial permeability through neutrophil dependent and independent pathways. *PLoS ONE* **2013**, *8*, e59989. [CrossRef] [PubMed]

246. Zhang, B.; Angelidou, A.; Alysandratos, K.D.; Vasiadi, M.; Francis, K.; Asadi, S.; Theoharides, A.; Sideri, K.; Lykouras, L.; Kalogeromitros, D. Mitochondrial DNA and anti-mitochondrial antibodies in serum of autistic children. *J. Neuroinflammation* **2010**, *7*, 80. [CrossRef]
247. Frye, R.E.; Cakir, J.; Rose, S.; Palmer, R.F.; Austin, C.; Curtin, P.; Arora, M. Mitochondria may mediate prenatal environmental influences in autism spectrum disorder. *J. Pers. Med.* **2021**, *11*, 218. [CrossRef] [PubMed]
248. Scozzi, D.; Cano, M.; Ma, L.; Zhou, D.; Zhu, J.H.; O'Halloran, J.A.; Goss, C.W.; Rauseo, A.M.; Liu, Z.; Sahu, S.K.; et al. Circulating mitochondrial DNA is an early indicator of severe illness and mortality from COVID-19. *JCI Insight* **2021**, *6*, e143299.
249. Demopoulos, C.; Antonopoulou, S.; Theoharides, T.C. COVID-19, microthromboses, inflammation, and platelet activating factor. *Biofactors* **2020**, *46*, 927–933. [CrossRef]
250. Theoharides, T.C.; Antonopoulou, S.; Demopoulos, C.A. Coronavirus 2019, microthromboses, and platelet activating factor. *Clin. Ther.* **2020**, *42*, 1850–1852. [CrossRef]
251. Damialis, A.; Gilles, S.; Sofiev, M.; Sofieva, V.; Kolek, F.; Bayr, D.; Plaza, M.P.; Leier-Wirtz, V.; Kaschuba, S.; Ziska, L.H. Higher airborne pollen concentrations correlated with increased SARS-CoV-2 infection rates, as evidenced from 31 countries across the globe. *Proc. Natl. Acad. Sci. USA* **2021**, *118*, e2019034118. [CrossRef]
252. Subhramanyam, C.S.; Wang, C.; Hu, Q.; Dheen, S.T. Microglia-mediated neuroinflammation in neurodegenerative diseases. *Semin. Cell Dev. Biol.* **2019**, *94*, 112–120. [CrossRef] [PubMed]
253. Colonna, M.; Butovsky, O. Microglia function in the central nervous system during health and neurodegeneration. *Annu. Rev. Immunol.* **2017**, *35*, 441–468. [CrossRef]
254. Voet, S.; Prinz, M.; van Loo, G. Microglia in central nervous system inflammation and multiple sclerosis pathology. *Trends Mol. Med.* **2019**, *25*, 112–123. [CrossRef]
255. Perry, V.H.; Nicoll, J.A.; Holmes, C. Microglia in neurodegenerative disease. *Nat. Rev. Neurol.* **2010**, *6*, 193–201. [CrossRef]
256. Ransohoff, R.M. How neuroinflammation contributes to neurodegeneration. *Science* **2016**, *353*, 777–783. [CrossRef]
257. Hickman, S.; Izzy, S.; Sen, P.; Morsett, L.; El, K.J. Microglia in neurodegeneration. *Nat. Neurosci.* **2018**, *21*, 1359–1369. [CrossRef] [PubMed]
258. Xu, Z.X.; Kim, G.H.; Tan, J.W.; Riso, A.E.; Sun, Y.; Xu, E.Y.; Liao, G.Y.; Xu, H.; Lee, S.H.; Do, N.Y. Elevated protein synthesis in microglia causes autism-like synaptic and behavioral aberrations. *Nat. Commun.* **2020**, *11*, 1797. [CrossRef] [PubMed]
259. Patel, A.B.; Tsilioni, I.; Leeman, S.E.; Theoharides, T.C. Neurotensin stimulates sortilin and mTOR in human microglia inhibitable by methoxyluteolin, a potential therapeutic target for autism. *Proc. Natl. Acad. Sci. USA* **2016**, *113*, e7049–e7058. [CrossRef]
260. Vargas, G.; Medeiros Geraldo, L.H.; Gedeao, S.N.; Viana, P.M.; Regina Souza, L.F.; Carvalho Alcantara, G.F. Severe acute respiratory syndrome coronavirus 2 (SARS-CoV-2) and glial cells: Insights and perspectives. *Brain Behav. Immun. Health* **2020**, *7*, 100127. [CrossRef]
261. Tremblay, M.E.; Madore, C.; Bordeleau, M.; Tian, L.; Verkhratsky, A. Neuropathobiology of COVID-19: The role for glia. *Front. Cell Neurosci.* **2020**, *14*, 592214. [CrossRef]
262. Lee, N.; Chan, P.K.; Ip, M.; Wong, E.; Ho, J.; Ho, C.; Cockram, C.S.; Hui, D.S. Anti-SARS-CoV IgG response in relation to disease severity of severe acute respiratory syndrome. *J. Clin. Virol.* **2006**, *35*, 179–184. [CrossRef]
263. Sotgiu, S.; Manca, S.; Gagliano, A.; Minutolo, A.; Melis, M.C.; Pisuttu, G.; Scoppola, C.; Bolognesi, E.; Clerici, M.; Guerini, F.R.; et al. Immune regulation of neurodevelopment at the mother-foetus interface: The case of autism. *Clin. Transl. Immunol.* **2020**, *9*, e1211. [CrossRef] [PubMed]
264. Hendriksen, E.; van Bergeijk, D.; Oosting, R.S.; Redegeld, F.A. Mast cells in neuroinflammation and brain disorders. *Neurosci. Biobehav. Rev.* **2017**, *79*, 119–133. [CrossRef]
265. Skaper, S.D.; Facci, L.; Giusti, P. Neuroinflammation, microglia and mast cells in the pathophysiology of neurocognitive disorders: A review. *CNS Neurol. Disord. Drug Targets* **2014**, *13*, 1654–1666. [CrossRef]
266. Skaper, S.D.; Facci, L.; Zusso, M.; Giusti, P. Neuroinflammation, mast cells, and glia: Dangerous liaisons. *Neuroscientist* **2017**, *23*, 478–498. [CrossRef] [PubMed]
267. Zhang, X.; Wang, Y.; Dong, H.; Xu, Y.; Zhang, S. Induction of microglial activation by mediators released from mast cells. *Cell Physiol. Biochem.* **2016**, *38*, 1520–1531. [CrossRef]
268. Theoharides, T.C.; Stewart, J.M.; Panagiotidou, S.; Melamed, I. Mast cells, brain inflammation and autism. *Eur. J. Pharmacol.* **2015**, *778*, 96–102. [CrossRef] [PubMed]
269. Dong, H.; Zhang, X.; Wang, Y.; Zhou, X.; Qian, Y.; Zhang, S. Suppression of brain mast cells degranulation inhibits microglial activation and central nervous system inflammation. *Mol. Neurobiol.* **2017**, *54*, 997–1007. [CrossRef]
270. Shaik-Dasthagirisaheb, Y.B.; Conti, P. The role of mast cells in Alzheimer's disease. *Adv. Clin. Exp. Med.* **2016**, *25*, 781–787. [CrossRef]
271. Kempuraj, D.; Mentor, S.; Thangavel, R.; Ahmed, M.E.; Selvakumar, G.P.; Raikwar, S.P.; Dubova, I.; Zaheer, S.; Iyer, S.S.; Zaheer, A. Mast cells in stress, pain, blood-brain barrier, neuroinflammation and Alzheimer's disease. *Front. Cell Neurosci.* **2019**, *13*, 54. [CrossRef]
272. Hansen, D.V.; Hanson, J.E.; Sheng, M. Microglia in Alzheimer's disease. *J. Cell Biol.* **2018**, *217*, 459–472. [CrossRef] [PubMed]
273. Hatziagelaki, E.; Adamaki, M.; Tsilioni, I.; Dimitriadis, G.; Theoharides, T.C. Myalgic encephalomyelitis/chronic fatigue syndrome-metabolic disease or disturbed homeostasis due to focal inflammation in the hypothalamus? *J. Pharmacol. Exp. Ther.* **2018**, *367*, 155–167. [CrossRef] [PubMed]

274. Breach, M.R.; Dye, C.N.; Joshi, A.; Platko, S.; Gilfarb, R.A.; Krug, A.R.; Franceschelli, D.V.; Galan, A.; Dodson, C.M.; Lenz, K.M. Maternal allergic inflammation in rats impacts the offspring perinatal neuroimmune milieu and the development of social play, locomotor behavior, and cognitive flexibility. *Brain Behav Immun.* **2021**, *95*, 269–286. [CrossRef] [PubMed]
275. Wang, W.; Ji, P.; Riopelle, R.J.; Dow, K.E. Functional expression of corticotropin-releasing hormone (CRH) receptor 1 in cultured rat microglia. *J. Neurochem.* **2002**, *80*, 287–294. [CrossRef]
276. Podlesek, A.; Komidar, L.; Kavcic, V. The relationship between perceived stress and subjective cognitive decline during the COVID-19 epidemic. *Front Psychol.* **2021**, *12*, 647971. [CrossRef]
277. Martin, S.; Dicou, E.; Vincent, J.P.; Mazella, J. Neurotensin and the neurotensin receptor-3 in microglial cells. *J. Neurosci. Res.* **2005**, *81*, 322–326. [CrossRef]
278. Angelidou, A.; Francis, K.; Vasiadi, M.; Alysandratos, K.-D.; Zhang, B.; Theoharides, A.; Lykouras, L.; Sideri, K.; Kalogeromitros, D.; Theoharides, T.C. Neurotensin is increased in serum of young children with autistic disorder. *J. Neuroinflam.* **2010**, *7*, 48. [CrossRef] [PubMed]
279. Tsilioni, I.; Dodman, N.; Petra, A.I.; Taliou, A.; Francis, K.; Moon-Fanelli, A.; Shuster, L.; Theoharides, T.C. Elevated serum neurotensin and CRH levels in children with autistic spectrum disorders and tail-chasing Bull Terriers with a phenotype similar to autism. *Transl. Psychiatry* **2014**, *4*, e466. [CrossRef]
280. Almehmadi, K.A.; Tsilioni, T.T.C. Increased expression of miR-155p5 in amygdala of children with Autism Spectrum Disorder. *Autism Res.* **2019**, *13*, 18–23. [CrossRef] [PubMed]
281. Tsilioni, I.; Pantazopoulos, H.; Conti, P.; Leeman, S.E.; Theoharides, T.C. IL-38 inhibits microglial inflammatory mediators and is decreased in amygdala of children with autism spectrum disorder. *Proc. Natl. Acad. Sci. USA* **2020**, *117*, 16475–16480. [CrossRef] [PubMed]
282. Jack, C.S.; Arbour, N.; Manusow, J.; Montgrain, V.; Blain, M.; McCrea, E.; Shapiro, A.; Antel, J.P. TLR signaling tailors innate immune responses in human microglia and astrocytes. *J. Immunol.* **2005**, *175*, 4320–4330. [CrossRef]
283. Murta, V.; Villarreal, A.; Ramos, A.J. Severe acute respiratory syndrome Coronavirus 2 impact on the central nervous system: Are astrocytes and microglia main players or merely bystanders? *ASN Neuro.* **2020**, *12*, 1759091420954960. [CrossRef] [PubMed]
284. Akin, C.; Valent, P.; Metcalfe, D.D. Mast cell activation syndrome: Proposed diagnostic criteria. *J. Allergy Clin. Immunol.* **2010**, *126*, 1099–1104. [CrossRef]
285. Theoharides, T.C.; Tsilioni, I.; Ren, H. Recent advances in our understanding of mast cell activation—Or should it be mast cell mediator disorders? *Expert. Rev. Clin. Immunol.* **2019**, *15*, 639–656. [CrossRef] [PubMed]
286. Enstrom, A.; Krakowiak, P.; Onore, C.; Pessah, I.N.; Hertz-Picciotto, I.; Hansen, R.L.; Van de Water, J.A.; Ashwood, P. Increased IgG4 levels in children with autism disorder. *Brain Behav. Immun.* **2009**, *23*, 389–395. [CrossRef] [PubMed]
287. Maintz, L.; Novak, N. Histamine and histamine intolerance. *Am. J. Clin. Nutr.* **2007**, *85*, 1185–1196. [CrossRef]
288. Kumar, S.; Khodoun, M.; Kettleson, E.M.; McKnight, C.; Reponen, T.; Grinshpun, S.A.; Adhikari, A. Glyphosate-rich air samples induce IL-33, TSLP and generate IL-13 dependent airway inflammation. *Toxicology* **2014**, *325*, 42–51. [CrossRef]
289. Rossignol, D.A.; Frye, R.E. A systematic review and meta-analysis of immunoglobulin g abnormalities and the therapeutic use of Intravenous Immunoglobulins (IVIG) in autism spectrum disorder. *J. Pers. Med.* **2021**, *11*, 488. [CrossRef]
290. Church, M.K. Allergy, histamine and antihistamines. *Handb. Exp. Pharmacol.* **2017**, *241*, 321–331.
291. Vasiadi, M.; Kalogeromitros, D.; Kempuraj, D.; Clemons, A.; Zhang, B.; Chliva, C.; Makris, M.; Wolfberg, A.; House, M.; Theoharides, T.C. Rupatadine inhibits proinflammatory mediator secretion from human mast cells triggered by different stimuli. *Int. Arch. Allergy Immunol.* **2010**, *151*, 38–45. [CrossRef]
292. Alevizos, M.; Karagkouni, A.; Vasiadi, M.; Sismanopoulos, N.; Makris, M.; Kalogeromitros, D.; Theoharides, T.C. Rupatadine inhibits inflammatory mediator release from human LAD2 cultured mast cells stimulated by PAF. *Ann. Allergy Asthma Immunol.* **2013**, *111*, 524–527. [CrossRef] [PubMed]
293. Siebenhaar, F.; Förtsch, A.; Krause, K.; Weller, K.; Metz, M.; Magerl, M.; Martus, P.; Church, M.K.; Maurer, M. Rupatadine improves quality of life in mastocytosis: A randomized, double-blind, placebo-controlled trial. *Allergy* **2013**, *68*, 949–952. [CrossRef] [PubMed]
294. Theoharides, T.C.; Stewart, J.M. Antihistamines and mental status. *J. Clin. Psychopharmacol.* **2016**, *36*, 195–197. [CrossRef] [PubMed]
295. Zahiruddin, S.; Basist, P.; Parveen, A.; Parveen, R.; Khan, W.; Gaurav; Ahmad, S. Ashwagandha in brain disorders: A review of recent developments. *J. Ethnopharmacol.* **2020**, *257*, 112876. [CrossRef] [PubMed]
296. Ng, Q.X.; Loke, W.; Foo, N.X.; Tan, W.J.; Chan, H.W.; Lim, D.Y.; Yeo, W.S. A systematic review of the clinical use of Withania somnifera (Ashwagandha) to ameliorate cognitive dysfunction. *Phytother. Res.* **2020**, *34*, 583–590. [CrossRef]
297. Beversdorf, D.Q.; Saklayen, S.; Higgins, K.F.; Bodner, K.E.; Kanne, S.M.; Christ, S.E. Effect of propranolol on word fluency in autism. *Cogn. Behav. Neurol.* **2011**, *24*, 11–17. [CrossRef]
298. Beversdorf, D.Q.; Saklayen, S.; Higgins, K.F.; Bodner, K.E.; Kanne, S.M.; Christ, S.E. alpha2-adrenergic agonists or stimulants for preschool-age children with attention-deficit/hyperactivity disorder. *JAMA* **2021**, *325*, 2067–2075.
299. Banas, K.; Sawchuk, B. Clonidine as a treatment of behavioural disturbances in autism spectrum disorder: A systematic literature review. *J. Can. Acad. Child Adolesc. Psychiatry* **2020**, *29*, 110–120.

300. Reichow, B.; Volkmar, F.R.; Bloch, M.H. Systematic review and meta-analysis of pharmacological treatment of the symptoms of attention-deficit/hyperactivity disorder in children with pervasive developmental disorders. *J. Autism Dev. Disord.* **2013**, *43*, 2435–2441. [CrossRef]
301. Politte, L.C.; Scahill, L.; Figueroa, J.; McCracken, J.T.; King, B.; McDougle, C.J. A randomized, placebo-controlled trial of extended-release guanfacine in children with autism spectrum disorder and ADHD symptoms: An analysis of secondary outcome measures. *Neuropsychopharmacology* **2018**, *43*, 1772–1778. [CrossRef] [PubMed]
302. Okazaki, K.; Yamamuro, K.; Iida, J.; Kishimoto, T. Guanfacine monotherapy for ADHD/ASD comorbid with Tourette syndrome: A case report. *Ann. Gen. Psychiatry* **2019**, *18*, 2. [CrossRef] [PubMed]
303. Ming, X.; Gordon, E.; Kang, N.; Wagner, G.C. Use of clonidine in children with autism spectrum disorders. *Brain Dev.* **2008**, *30*, 454–460. [CrossRef]
304. Del Giudice, E.; Rinaldi, L.; Passarotto, M.; Facchinetti, F.; D'Arrigo, A.; Guiotto, A.; Carbonare, M.D.; Battistin, L.; Leon, A. Cannabidiol, unlike synthetic cannabinoids, triggers activation of RBL-2H3 mast cells. *J. Leukoc. Biol.* **2007**, *81*, 1512–1522. [CrossRef] [PubMed]
305. Caslin, H.; Kiwanuka, K.N.; Haque, T.T.; Taruselli, M.; Macknight, H.P.; Paranjape, A.; Ryan, J.J. Controlling mast cell activation and homeostasis: Work Influenced by Bill Paul that continues today. *Front. Immunol.* **2018**, *9*, 868. [CrossRef]
306. Noda, S.; Krueger, J.G.; Guttman-Yassky, E. The translational revolution and use of biologics in patients with inflammatory skin diseases. *J. Allergy Clin. Immunol.* **2015**, *135*, 324–336. [CrossRef]
307. Leonardi, C.L.; Powers, J.L.; Matheson, R.T.; Goffe, B.S.; Zitnik, R.; Wang, A.; Gottlieb, A.B. Etanercept as monotherapy in patients with psoriasis. *N. Engl. J. Med.* **2003**, *349*, 2014–2022. [CrossRef]
308. Ruzicka, T.; Mihara, R. Anti-interleukin-31 receptor a antibody for atopic dermatitis. *N. Engl. J. Med.* **2017**, *376*, 2093. [CrossRef]
309. Olivieri, I.; D'Angelo, S.; Palazzi, C.; Padula, A. Treatment strategies for early psoriatic arthritis. *Expert. Opin. Pharmacother.* **2009**, *10*, 271–282. [CrossRef]
310. Heinrich, M.C.; Griffith, D.J.; Druker, B.J.; Wait, C.L.; Ott, K.A.; Zigler, A.J. Inhibition of c-kit receptor tyrosine kinase activity by STI 571, a selective tyrosine kinase inhibitor. *Blood* **2000**, *96*, 925–932. [CrossRef] [PubMed]
311. Gotlib, J.; Kluin-Nelemans, J.C.; George, T.I.; Akin, C.; Sotlar, K.; Hermine, O.; Awan, F.T.; Hexner, E.; Mauro, M.J.; Sternberg, D.W.; et al. Efficacy and safety of midostaurin in advanced systemic mastocytosis. *N. Engl. J. Med.* **2016**, *374*, 2530–2541. [CrossRef]
312. Finn, D.F.; Walsh, J.J. Twenty-first century mast cell stabilizers. *Br. J. Pharmacol.* **2013**, *170*, 23–37. [CrossRef]
313. Theoharides, T.C.; Sieghart, W.; Greengard, P.; Douglas, W.W. Antiallergic drug cromolyn may inhibit histamine secretion by regulating phosphorylation of a mast cell protein. *Science* **1980**, *207*, 80–82. [CrossRef]
314. Oka, T.; Kalesnikoff, J.; Starkl, P.; Tsai, M.; Galli, S.J. Evidence questioning cromolyn's effectiveness and selectivity as a 'mast cell stabilizer' in mice. *Lab. Investig.* **2012**, *92*, 1472–1482. [CrossRef] [PubMed]
315. Weng, Z.; Zhang, B.; Asadi, S.; Sismanopoulos, N.; Butcher, A.; Fu, X.; Katsarou-Katsari, A.; Antoniou, C.; Theoharides, T.C. Quercetin is more effective than cromolyn in blocking human mast cell cytokine release and inhibits contact dermatitis and photosensitivity in humans. *PLoS ONE* **2012**, *7*, e33805-k. [CrossRef]
316. Dos Santos, R.V.; Magerl, M.; Martus, P.; Zuberbier, T.; Church, M.; Escribano, L.; Maurer, M. Topical sodium cromoglicate relieves allergen- and histamine-induced dermal pruritus. *Br. J. Dermatol.* **2010**, *162*, 674–676. [CrossRef] [PubMed]
317. Weng, Z.; Patel, A.B.; Panagiotidou, S.; Theoharides, T.C. The novel flavone tetramethoxyluteolin is a potent inhibitor of human mast cells. *J. Allergy Clin. Immunol.* **2015**, *135*, 1044–1052. [CrossRef] [PubMed]
318. Church, M.K.; Gradidge, C.F. Potentiation of histamine release by sodium cromoglycate. *Life Sci.* **1978**, *23*, 1899–1904. [CrossRef]
319. Kempuraj, D.; Madhappan, B.; Christodoulou, S.; Boucher, W.; Cao, J.; Papadopoulou, N.; Cetrulo, C.L.; Theoharides, T.C. Flavonols inhibit proinflammatory mediator release, intracellular calcium ion levels and protein kinase C theta phosphorylation in human mast cells. *Br. J. Pharmacol.* **2005**, *145*, 934–944. [CrossRef]
320. Seelinger, G.; Merfort, I.; Schempp, C.M. Anti-oxidant, anti-inflammatory and anti-allergic activities of luteolin. *Planta Med.* **2008**, *74*, 1667–1677. [CrossRef]
321. Calis, Z.; Mogulkoc, R.; Baltaci, A.K. The roles of flavonoles/flavonoids in neurodegeneration and neuroinflammation. *Mini. Rev. Med. Chem.* **2020**, *20*, 1475–1488. [CrossRef] [PubMed]
322. Jager, A.K.; Saaby, L. Flavonoids and the CNS. *Molecules* **2011**, *16*, 1471–1485. [CrossRef]
323. Leyva-Lopez, N.; Gutierrez-Grijalva, E.P.; Ambriz-Perez, D.L.; Heredia, J.B. Flavonoids as cytokine modulators: A possible therapy for inflammation-related diseases. *Int. J. Mol. Sci.* **2016**, *17*, 921. [CrossRef]
324. Harwood, M.; Nielewska-Nikiel, B.; Borzelleca, J.F.; Flamm, G.W.; Williams, G.M.; Lines, T.C. A critical review of the data related to the safety of quercetin and lack of evidence of in vivo toxicity, including lack of genotoxic/carcinogenic properties. *Food Chem. Toxicol.* **2007**, *45*, 2179–2205. [CrossRef]
325. Okamoto, T. Safety of quercetin for clinical application (Review). *Int. J. Mol. Med.* **2005**, *16*, 275–278. [CrossRef]
326. Andres, S.; Pevny, S.; Ziegenhagen, R.; Bakhiya, N.; Schäfer, B.; Hirsch-Ernst, K.; Lampen, A. Safety aspects of the use of quercetin as a dietary supplement. *Mol. Nutr. Food Res.* **2018**, *62*, 1700447. [CrossRef] [PubMed]
327. Xu, L.; Su, W.; Jin, J.; Chen, J.; Li, X.; Zhang, X.; Sun, M.; Sun, S.; Fan, P.; An, D.; et al. Identification of luteolin as enterovirus 71 and coxsackievirus A16 inhibitors through reporter viruses and cell viability-based screening. *Viruses* **2014**, *6*, 2778–2795. [CrossRef]

328. Fan, W.; Qian, S.; Qian, P.; Li, X. Antiviral activity of luteolin against Japanese encephalitis virus. *Virus Res.* **2016**, *220*, 112–116. [CrossRef] [PubMed]
329. Yan, H.; Ma, L.; Wang, H.; Wu, S.; Huang, H.; Gu, Z.; Jiang, J.; Li, Y. Luteolin decreases the yield of influenza A virus in vitro by interfering with the coat protein I complex expression. *J. Nat. Med.* **2019**, *73*, 487–496. [CrossRef]
330. Russo, M.; Moccia, S.; Spagnuolo, C.; Tedesco, I.; Russo, G.L. Roles of flavonoids against coronavirus infection. *Chem. Biol. Interact.* **2020**, *328*, 109211. [CrossRef]
331. Derosa, G.; Maffioli, P.; D'Angelo, A.; Di, P.F. A role for quercetin in coronavirus disease 2019 (COVID-19). *Phytother. Res.* **2020**, *35*, 1230–1236. [CrossRef]
332. Rezai-Zadeh, K.; Ehrhart, J.; Bai, Y.; Sanberg, P.R.; Bickford, P.; Tan, J.; Shytle, R.D. Apigenin and luteolin modulate microglial activation via inhibition of STAT1-induced CD40 expression. *J. Neuroinflammation* **2008**, *5*, 41. [CrossRef] [PubMed]
333. Jang, S.; Kelley, K.W.; Johnson, R.W. Luteolin reduces IL-6 production in microglia by inhibiting JNK phosphorylation and activation of AP-1. *Proc. Natl. Acad. Sci. USA* **2008**, *105*, 7534–7539. [CrossRef] [PubMed]
334. Burton, M.D.; Rytych, J.L.; Amin, R.; Johnson, R.W. Dietary luteolin reduces proinflammatory microglia in the brain of senescent mice. *Rejuvenation. Res.* **2016**, *19*, 286–292. [CrossRef] [PubMed]
335. Patel, A.B.; Theoharides, T.C. Methoxyluteolin inhibits neuropeptide-stimulated proinflammatory mediator release via mTOR activation from human mast cells. *J. Pharmacol. Exp. Ther.* **2017**, *361*, 462–471. [CrossRef]
336. Dajas, F.; Rivera-Megret, F.; Blasina, F.; Arredondo, F.; Abin-Carriquiry, J.; Costa, G.; Echeverry, C.; Lafon, L.; Heizen, H.; Ferreira, M.; et al. Neuroprotection by flavonoids. *Braz. J. Med. Biol. Res.* **2003**, *36*, 1613–1620. [CrossRef]
337. Kempuraj, D.; Thangavel, R.; Kempuraj, D.D.; Ahmed, M.E.; Selvakumar, G.P.; Raikwar, S.P.; Zaheer, S.A.; Iyer, S.S.; Govindarajan, R.; Chandrasekaran, P.N. Neuroprotective effects of flavone luteolin in neuroinflammation and neurotrauma. *Biofactors* **2020**, *47*, 190–197. [CrossRef]
338. Lin, T.Y.; Lu, C.W.; Wang, S.J. Luteolin protects the hippocampus against neuron impairments induced by kainic acid in rats. *Neuro Toxicol.* **2016**, *55*, 48–57. [CrossRef]
339. Ashaari, Z.; Hassanzadeh, G.; Alizamir, T.; Yousefi, B.; Keshavarzi, Z.; Mokhtari, T. The flavone luteolin improves central nervous system disorders by different mechanisms: A review. *J. Mol. Neurosci.* **2018**, *65*, 491–506. [CrossRef]
340. Bernatoniene, J.; Kazlauskaite, J.A.; Kopustinskiene, D.M. Pleiotropic Effects of Isoflavones in Inflammation and Chronic Degenerative Diseases. *Int J Mol Sci.* **2021**, *22*, 5656. [CrossRef]
341. Theoharides, T.C.; Conti, P.; Economu, M. Brain inflammation, neuropsychiatric disorders, and immunoendocrine effects of luteolin. *J. Clin. Psychopharmacol.* **2014**, *34*, 187–189. [CrossRef]
342. Silva Dos Santos, J.; Gonçalves Cirino, J.P.; de Oliveira Carvalho, P.; Ortega, M.M. The Pharmacological Action of Kaempferol in Central Nervous System Diseases: A Review. *Front Pharmacol.* **2021**, *11*, 565700. [CrossRef] [PubMed]
343. Devi, S.A.; Chamoli, A. Polyphenols as an effective therapeutic intervention against cognitive decline during normal and pathological brain aging. *Adv. Exp. Med. Biol.* **2020**, *1260*, 159–174. [PubMed]
344. Theoharides, T.C.; Stewart, J.M.; Hatziagelaki, E.; Kolaitis, G. Brain "fog", inflammation and obesity: Key aspects of 2 neuropsychiatric disorders improved by luteolin. *Front. Neurosci.* **2015**, *9*, 225. [CrossRef] [PubMed]
345. Rezai-Zadeh, K.; Douglas, S.R.; Bai, Y.; Tian, J.; Hou, H.; Mori, T.; Zeng, J.; Obregon, D.; Town, T.; Tan, J. Flavonoid-mediated presenilin-1 phosphorylation reduces Alzheimer's disease beta-amyloid production. *J. Cell Mol. Med.* **2009**, *13*, 574–588. [CrossRef]
346. Theoharides, T.C.; Cholevas, C.; Polyzoidis, K.; Politis, A. Long-COVID syndrome-associated brain fog and chemofog: Luteolin to the rescue. *Biofactors* **2021**, *47*, 232–241. [CrossRef]
347. Gratton, G.; Weaver, S.R.; Burley, C.V.; Low, K.A.; Maclin, E.L.; Johns, P.W.; Pham, Q.S.; Lucas, S.J.E.; Fabiani, M.; Rendeiro, C. Dietary flavanols improve cerebral cortical oxygenation and cognition in healthy adults. *Sci. Rep.* **2020**, *10*, 19409. [CrossRef]
348. Yeh, T.S.; Yuan, C.; Ascherio, A.; Rosner, B.; Willett, W.; Blacker, D. Long-term dietary flavonoid intake and subjective cognitive decline in US men and women. *Neurology* **2021**. [CrossRef]
349. Du, X.; Hill, R.A. 7,8-Dihydroxyflavone as a pro-neurotrophic treatment for neurodevelopmental disorders. *Neurochem. Int.* **2015**, *89*, 170–180. [CrossRef]
350. Xu, S.L.; Bi, C.W.; Choi, R.C.; Zhu, K.Y.; Miernisha, A.; Dong, T.T.; Tsim, K.W. Flavonoids induce the synthesis and secretion of neurotrophic factors in cultured rat astrocytes: A signaling response mediated by estrogen receptor. *Evid. Based Complement Alternat. Med.* **2013**, *2013*, 127075. [CrossRef]
351. Theoharides, T.C.; Athanassiou, M.; Panagiotidou, S.; Doyle, R. Dysregulated brain immunity and neurotrophin signaling in Rett syndrome and autism spectrum disorders. *J. Neuroimmunol.* **2015**, *279*, 33–38. [CrossRef] [PubMed]
352. Yi, L.; Li, Z.; Yuan, K.; Qu, X.; Chen, J.; Wang, G.; Zhang, H.; Luo, H.; Zhu, L.; Jiang, P.; et al. Small molecules blocking the entry of severe acute respiratory syndrome coronavirus into host cells. *J. Virol.* **2004**, *78*, 11334–11339. [CrossRef] [PubMed]
353. Jo, S.; Kim, S.; Shin, D.H.; Kim, M.S. Inhibition of SARS-CoV 3CL protease by flavonoids. *J. Enzyme Inhib. Med. Chem.* **2020**, *35*, 145–151. [CrossRef] [PubMed]
354. Xue, G.; Gong, L.; Yuan, C.; Xu, M.; Wang, X.; Jiang, L.; Huang, M. A structural mechanism of flavonoids in inhibiting serine proteases. *Food Funct.* **2017**, *8*, 2437–2443. [CrossRef]
355. Richman, S.; Morris, M.C.; Broderick, G.; Craddock, T.J.A.; Klimas, N.G.; Fletcher, M.A. Pharmaceutical interventions in chronic fatigue syndrome: A literature-based commentary. *Clin. Ther.* **2019**, *41*, 798–805. [CrossRef] [PubMed]

356. Yi, Y.S. Regulatory roles of flavonoids on inflammasome activation during inflammatory responses. *Mol. Nutr. Food Res.* **2018**, *62*, e1800147. [CrossRef] [PubMed]
357. Fu, X.; Zhang, J.; Guo, L.; Xu, Y.; Sun, L.; Wang, S.; Feng, Y.; Gou, L.; Zhang, L.; Liu, Y. Protective role of luteolin against cognitive dysfunction induced by chronic cerebral hypoperfusion in rats. *Pharmacol. Biochem. Behav.* **2014**, *126*, 122–130. [CrossRef]
358. Theoharides, T.C. Luteolin supplements: All that glitters is not gold. *Biofactors* **2020**, *47*, 242–244. [CrossRef] [PubMed]
359. Taliou, A.; Zintzaras, E.; Lykouras, L.; Francis, K. An open-label pilot study of a formulation containing the anti-inflammatory flavonoid luteolin and its effects on behavior in children with autism spectrum disorders. *Clin. Ther.* **2013**, *35*, 592–602. [CrossRef]
360. Tsilioni, I.; Taliou, A.; Francis, K.; Theoharides, T.C. Children with Autism Spectrum Disorders, who improved with a luteolin containing dietary formulation, show reduced serum levels of TNF and IL-6. *Transl. Psychiatry* **2015**, *5*, e647. [CrossRef]
361. Beauchamp, G.K.; Keast, R.S.; Morel, D.; Lin, J.; Pika, J.; Han, Q.; Lee, C.H.; Smith, A.B.; Breslin, P.A. Phytochemistry: Ibuprofen-like activity in extra-virgin olive oil. *Nature* **2005**, *437*, 45–46. [CrossRef] [PubMed]
362. Angeloni, C.; Malaguti, M.; Barbalace, M.C.; Hrelia, S. Bioactivity of olive oil phenols in neuroprotection. *Int. J. Mol. Sci.* **2017**, *18*, 2230. [CrossRef] [PubMed]
363. Casamenti, F.; Stefani, M. Olive polyphenols: New promising agents to combat aging-associated neurodegeneration. *Expert. Rev. Neurother.* **2017**, *17*, 345–358. [CrossRef] [PubMed]
364. Omar, S.H.; Scott, C.J.; Hamlin, A.S.; Obied, H.K. Olive biophenols reduces Alzheimer's pathology in SH-SY5Y cells and appswe mice. *Int. J. Mol. Sci.* **2018**, *20*, 125. [CrossRef]
365. Calahorra, J.; Shenk, J.; Wielenga, V.H.; Verweij, V.; Geenen, B.; Dederen, P.J.; Peinado, M.A.; Siles, E.; Wiesmann, M.; Kiliaan, A.J. Hydroxytyrosol, the major phenolic compound of olive oil, as an acute therapeutic strategy after ischemic stroke. *Nutrients* **2019**, *11*, 2430. [CrossRef]
366. Khalatbary, A.R. Olive oil phenols and neuroprotection. *Nutr. Neurosci.* **2013**, *16*, 243–249. [CrossRef]
367. Marquez-Martin, A.; de La, P.R.; Fernandez-Arche, A.; Ruiz-Gutierrez, V.; Yaqoob, P. Modulation of cytokine secretion by pentacyclic triterpenes from olive pomace oil in human mononuclear cells. *Cytokine* **2006**, *36*, 211–217. [CrossRef] [PubMed]
368. Hornedo-Ortega, R.; Cerezo, A.B.; De Pablos, R.M.; Krisa, S.; Richard, T.; García-Parrilla, M.C.; Troncoso, A.M. Phenolic compounds characteristic of the mediterranean diet in mitigating microglia-mediated neuroinflammation. *Front. Cell Neurosci.* **2018**, *12*, 373. [CrossRef]
369. Bertelli, M.; Kiani, A.K.; Paolacci, S.; Manara, E.; Kurti, D.; Dhuli, K.; Bushati, V.; Miertus, J.; Pangallo, D.; Baglivo, M.; et al. Hydroxytyrosol: A natural compound with promising pharmacological activities. *J. Biotechnol.* **2020**, *309*, 29–33. [CrossRef]
370. Li, W.; Yin, N.; Tao, W.; Wang, Q.; Fan, H.; Wang, Z. Berberine suppresses IL-33-induced inflammatory responses in mast cells by inactivating NF-kappaB and p38 signaling. *Int. Immunopharmacol.* **2019**, *66*, 82–90. [CrossRef]
371. Fu, S.; Ni, S.; Wang, D.; Fu, M.; Hong, T. Berberine suppresses mast cell-mediated allergic responses via regulating FcvarepsilonRI-mediated and MAPK signaling. *Int. Immunopharmacol.* **2019**, *71*, 1–6. [CrossRef]
372. Zhu, J.; Cao, D.; Guo, C.; Liu, M.; Tao, Y.; Zhou, J.; Wang, F.; Zhao, Y.; Wei, J.; Zhang, Y.; et al. Berberine facilitates angiogenesis against ischemic stroke through modulating microglial polarization via AMPK signaling. *Cell Mol. Neurobiol.* **2019**, *39*, 751–768. [CrossRef] [PubMed]
373. Sengenc, E.; Kiykim, E.; Saltik, S. Vitamin D levels in children and adolescents with autism. *J. Int. Med. Res.* **2020**, *48*, 300060520934638. [CrossRef] [PubMed]
374. Petruzzelli, M.G.; Marzulli, L.; Margari, F.; De Giacomo, A.; Gabellone, A.; Giannico, O.V.; Margari, L. Vitamin D Deficiency in Autism Spectrum Disorder: A Cross-Sectional Study. *Dis. Markers* **2020**, *2020*, 9292560. [CrossRef] [PubMed]
375. Wang, Z.; Ding, R.; Wang, J. The association between vitamin D status and Autism Spectrum Disorder (ASD): A systematic review and meta-analysis. *Nutrients* **2020**, *13*, 86. [CrossRef] [PubMed]
376. Theoharides, T.C. Vitamin D and atopy. *Clin. Ther.* **2017**, *39*, 880–883. [CrossRef]
377. Chen, D.; Jia, T.; Zhang, Y.; Cao, M.; Loth, E.; Lo, C.Z.; Cheng, W.; Liu, Z.; Gong, W.; Sahakian, B.J.; et al. Neural Biomarkers Distinguish Severe from Mild Autism Spectrum Disorder Among High-Functioning Individuals. *Front Hum Neurosci.* **2021**, *15*, 657857. [CrossRef]

Journal of Personalized Medicine

MDPI

Article

Transdermal Electrical Neuromodulation for Anxiety and Sleep Problems in High-Functioning Autism Spectrum Disorder: Feasibility and Preliminary Findings

Stephen T. Foldes [1,2,3,4], Amanda R. Jensen [5], Austin Jacobson [1], Sarah Vassall [6], Emily Foldes [7], Ann Guthery [8], Danni Brown [1], Todd Levine [8], William James Tyler [3] and Richard E. Frye [4,5,*]

1 Division of Research, Barrow Neurologic Institute at Phoenix Children's Hospital, Phoenix, AZ 85016, USA; stephen.foldes@dignityhealth.org (S.T.F.); ajacobson2@phoenixchildrens.com (A.J.); dbrown4@phoenixchildrens.com (D.B.)
2 Division of Neurology, Barrow Neurologic Institute, Phoenix, AZ 85013, USA
3 School of Biological and Health Sciences, Arizona State University, Tempe, AZ 85287, USA; wtyler@asu.edu
4 Department of Child Health, University of Arizona College of Medicine Phoenix, Phoenix, AZ 85004, USA
5 Section on Neurodevelopmental Disorders, Division of Neurology, Barrow Neurologic Institute at Phoenix Children's Hospital, Phoenix, AZ 85016, USA; ajensen1@phoenixchildrens.com
6 Division of Psychology, Vanderbilt University, Nashville, TN 37240, USA; sarah.g.vassall@Vanderbilt.Edu
7 Speech and Hearing Science, Arizona State University, Tempe, AZ 85287, USA; elfoldes@gmail.com
8 Division of Psychiatry, Barrow Neurologic Institute at Phoenix Children's Hospital, Phoenix, AZ 85016, USA; aguthery@phoenixchildrens.com (A.G.); tlevine2@phoenixchildrens.com (T.L.)
* Correspondence: rfrye@phoenixchildrens.com; Tel.: +1-602-933-0970

Citation: Foldes, S.T.; Jensen, A.R.; Jacobson, A.; Vassall, S.; Foldes, E.; Guthery, A.; Brown, D.; Levine, T.; Tyler, W.J.; Frye, R.E. Transdermal Electrical Neuromodulation for Anxiety and Sleep Problems in High-Functioning Autism Spectrum Disorder: Feasibility and Preliminary Findings. *J. Pers. Med.* **2021**, *11*, 1307. https://doi.org/10.3390/jpm11121307

Academic Editor: Guido Krenning

Received: 17 September 2021
Accepted: 22 November 2021
Published: 6 December 2021

Publisher's Note: MDPI stays neutral with regard to jurisdictional claims in published maps and institutional affiliations.

Copyright: © 2021 by the authors. Licensee MDPI, Basel, Switzerland. This article is an open access article distributed under the terms and conditions of the Creative Commons Attribution (CC BY) license (https://creativecommons.org/licenses/by/4.0/).

Abstract: Background: Autism spectrum disorder (ASD) is associated with anxiety and sleep problems. We investigated transdermal electrical neuromodulation (TEN) of the cervical nerves in the neck as a safe, effective, comfortable and non-pharmacological therapy for decreasing anxiety and enhancing sleep quality in ASD. Methods: In this blinded, sham-controlled study, seven adolescents and young adults with high-functioning ASD underwent five consecutive treatment days, one day of the sham followed by four days of subthreshold TEN for 20 min. Anxiety-provoking cognitive tasks were performed after the sham/TEN. Measures of autonomic nervous system activity, including saliva α-amylase and cortisol, electrodermal activity, and heart rate variability, were collected from six participants. Results: Self-rated and caretaker-rated measures of anxiety were significantly improved with TEN treatment as compared to the sham, with effect sizes ranging from medium to large depending on the rating scale. Sleep scores from caretaker questionnaires also improved, but not significantly. Performance on two of the three anxiety-provoking cognitive tasks and heart rate variability significantly improved with TEN stimulation as compared to the sham. Four of the seven (57%) participants were responders, defined as a $\geq$ 30% improvement in self-reported anxiety. Salivary α-amylase decreased with more TEN sessions and decreased from the beginning to the end of the session on TEN days for responders. TEN was well-tolerated without significant adverse events. Conclusions: This study provides preliminary evidence that TEN is well-tolerated in individuals with ASD and can improve anxiety.

Keywords: α-amylase; autism spectrum disorder; anxiety; cortisol; heart rate variability; neuromodulation; sleep anxiety; transdermal electrical neuromodulation; neurostimulation

1. Introduction

Autism spectrum disorder (ASD) is a behaviorally defined neurodevelopmental disorder with lifelong consequences that affects children during critical times in their lives [1]. The Centers for Disease Control and Prevention (CDC) estimates that ASD affects about 2% of children (1 in 54) in the United States (US) [2]. The only standard treatment for core ASD symptoms is behavioral therapy. Although behavioral therapy can be effective if started early in life [3,4], only a minority of children obtain optimal outcomes [5,6] and most require lifelong supportive care [7]. The economic burden of intense and continuous educational, medical and social support is impressive [8], with the lifetime social costs to date in the US estimated to be more than $7 trillion [9]. In addition, the child's disability creates a spillover effect that decreases the quality of life of the entire family [10–12].

1.1. Co-Occurring Conditions Can Interfere with Daily Function

ASD is associated with many co-occurring medical conditions, including intellectual disability [13], epilepsy [14], gastrointestinal disorders [15], sleep disorders [16], ADHD [16], anxiety [16], irritability, self-injurious behavior and depression [17]. While these conditions are not considered core symptoms of ASD, they can limit the functional ability of the individual, preventing them from gaining optimal benefit from therapies. Anxiety [18,19] and sleep problems [20,21] are difficult-to-treat lifelong conditions that commonly start in childhood and continue into adolescence and adulthood. These conditions commonly result in difficultly with the transition into independence, as well as significantly decreasing the ability to function optimally in everyday life.

Anxiety disorders are estimated to affect 40% of children and adolescents with ASD [19], which is consistently higher than the prevalence in neurotypical (NT) children [22,23]. Anxiety results in the avoidance of social situations, further worsening social isolation, which is commonly associated with ASD [24]. This is particularly problematic during adolescence and young adulthood, when high-functioning individuals with ASD are expected to interact with others independently. For individuals with ASD who are low-functioning with limited communication, anxiety commonly drives aberrant behaviors, such as aggression and self-injurious behavior. These behaviors are commonly refractory to treatment and can lead to institutionalization, making finding effective treatments extremely important. Anxiety also has detrimental physical effects on health beyond affecting daily activities. For example, studies on the NT population have shown that unmanaged anxiety can breakdown biological functions, such as the immune [25,26] and cardiovascular [27] systems.

Sleep problems are more common in children and adolescents with ASD compared to the NT population, with a prevalence up to of 82% and persistent across their lifespan [28]. Sleep problems commonly start in early life and are potentially an early warning sign of ASD [29,30]. In young adulthood they reduce quality of life [31] and are associated with unemployment [20]. As discussed in our recent review, sleep problems in individuals with ASD are associated with worse ASD symptom severity, communication and social function, and increased irritability, stereotypy, hyperactive, anxiety, aggression and inattention [32]. Poor sleep in individuals with ASD results in a spillover effect which decreases quality of life for both the individual and the family [12]. Successful treatment of sleep problems improves a wide variety of ASD symptoms, including daytime behavior and function [32] as well as quality of life [12].

1.2. Treatment Approaches to Modulate Physiological Drivers of Symptoms

Standard treatments for core and associated ASD symptoms in addition to co-occurring conditions usually include psychopharmacological management, which tends to provide a suboptimal result in many cases. Indeed, pharmacological approaches borrowed from the treatment of the NT population do not translate well regarding both efficacy and AE profile. This leaves a large knowledge gap in the efficacious and safe treatment for these detrimental co-morbidities.

While there are many effective ways to manage anxiety in the NT population, these approaches are limited in effectiveness in ASD. Pharmacological approaches suffer from AEs, such as drowsiness, blunting general affect, impairing attention and dependence. In fact, a Cochrane review found that the standard treatment for anxiety in NT individuals, SSRIs, were not only not effective for individuals with ASD but may do more harm than good [33]. Relaxation-based treatments [34] and exercise [35] can be beneficial but require investments of time and training that often prohibit compliance and can be challenging for young adults, especially with ASD. Thus, alternative approaches to treat anxiety are needed for children and adolescents with ASD.

Sleep problems may be refractory to treatment in many individuals with ASD. Although standard behavioral therapy is the first line for treatment, it tends to be ineffective in children with ASD [36]. Melatonin has good clinical trial evidence for use in children with ASD for sleep initiation, but not for sleep maintenance [32,36]. Good evidence for other pharmaceutical treatments is lacking [32]. In fact, in individuals with ASD, especially adolescents and young adults, sleep initiation and maintenance are often refractory to standard treatments and can interfere with their ability to function.

Perhaps the greatest limitation of many ASD treatments is that most medical interventions focus on symptomatic relief rather than targeting underlying pathophysiological mechanisms. Thus, a safe, effective and well-tolerated treatment that addresses underlying pathophysiological abnormalities in ASD could accelerate the achievement of optimal outcomes for a greater proportion of individuals with ASD. New approaches to managing anxiety and sleep quality could greatly enhance the quality of life and activities of daily living for children with ASD as they transition into adulthood and age out of services.

Multiple studies have documented autonomic nervous system (ANS) imbalances in individuals with ASD with relative sympathetic overactivation, leading to hyper-arousal, anxiety [37] and poor sleep [38]. ANS imbalances are linked to clinical symptoms associated with ASD. For example, heart rate variability (HRV) is associated with gastrointestinal symptoms [39], and an atypical pupillary light reflex is linked to sensory symptoms [40].

1.3. An Alternative Treatment Approach to Modulate the Physiological Drivers of Anxiety and Sleep Disruption

Based on evidence from NT individuals with anxiety [41], and plausible biological mechanisms of action, we hypothesized that transdermal electrical neuromodulation (TEN) of the cervical nerves is a safe, effective, comfortable and non-pharmacological therapy to modulate the central nervous system for decreasing anxiety and enhancing sleep quality, leading to an improved quality of life for people with ASD. Most importantly, TEN has the potential to improve many symptoms associated with ASD by correcting underlying dysregulated pathways which modulate anxiety, wakefulness and autonomic dysregulation. In contrast to pharmacological treatments which modulate general neurotransmitter pathways, potentially leading to unnecessary off-target, non-specific effects that can cause AEs, TEN modulates specific dysregulation pathways and provides targeted neuromodulation to alter endogenous neurotransmitter pathways.

Using noninvasive electrical activation of peripheral, cervical or cranial nerves, TEN regulates the activity of several deep-brain nuclei within the ascending reticular activating system (RAS) [42,43] (Figure 1). RAS nuclei modulate the sympathetic nervous system by regulating norepinephrine (NE) from the locus coeruleus (LC), acetylcholine (Ach) from pedunculopontine nuclei (PPN) and serotonin (5-HT) from raphe nuclei (RN) [44,45]. These pathways have wide-ranging effects on cortical and subcortical brain regions, resulting in modulation of attention, awareness, arousal and sleep.

TEN applied to the trigeminal or vagus nerves is therapeutic for ADHD [46], migraine headache [47], major depressive disorder [42], post-traumatic stress disorder [48] and generalized anxiety disorder [49], among others. Furthermore, it is consistently reported to be well-tolerated without any AEs.

1.4. TEN May Be an Excellent Treatment for Anxiety and Sleep in ASD

Although TEN has not been used in ASD, the related technique of transcutaneous electrical acupoint stimulation was found to improve anxiety, general ASD and sensory symptoms in two controlled studies, with one study demonstrating improvement in plasma arginine-vasopressin levels [50,51]. Similarly, this technique has been shown to improve behaviors in valproic acid rodent models of ASD [52]. Interestingly, there is significant interest for the use of TEN in ASD [53]. This may lead to clinicians recommending these devices to children with ASD off-label, without any evidence for their effectiveness or best practices. It is therefore important to study TEN in order to provide evidence for effectiveness and define an optimal protocol. Given the unique nature of ASD, it is first important to assess the feasibility of TEN for this specific population, including sensitivity to electrodes and co-operation, as well as to confirm its safety.

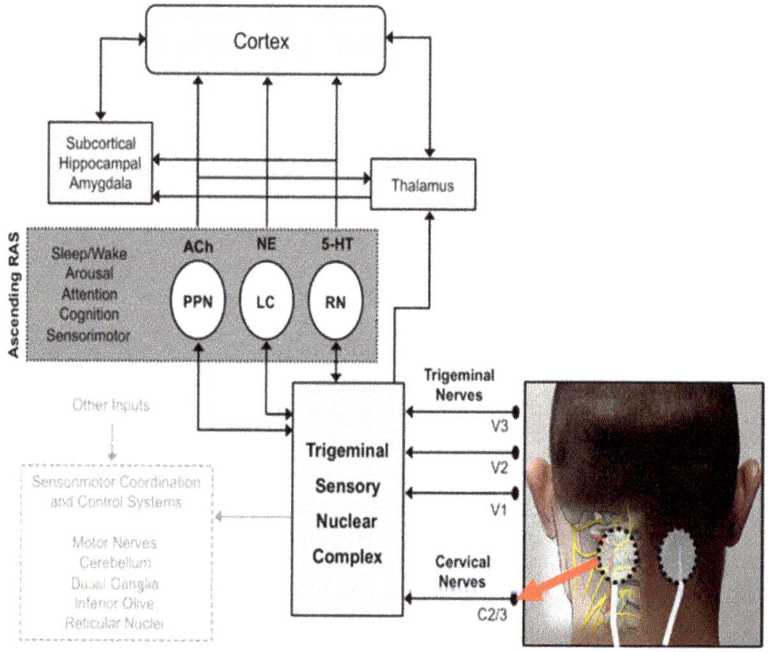

Figure 1. Mechanisms of electrical stimulation to improve anxiety and sleep. Cervical nerves are stimulated using a wearable transdermal neurostimulator placed on the back of the neck at the C2/C3 level, as shown. This modulates the ascending reticular activating system (RAS) via the trigeminal sensory nuclear complex. The ascending RAS includes the pedunculopontine nucleus (PPN), the locus coeruleus (LC) and raphe nuclei (RN), and modulates acetylcholine (Ach), norepinephrine (NE) and serotonin (5-HT) to higher-order brain structures to modulate attention and regulate awareness, arousal and sleep.

In our previous study [41], as compared to the sham, TEN significantly suppressed basal sympathetic tone, as measured by functional infrared thermography of facial temperatures, and lowered anxiety on the Profile of Mood States scale in healthy adults. With experimental stress, TEN produced a significant suppression of HRV, electrodermal activation (EDA) and salivary α-amylase levels compared to the sham. Thus, here we extended this treatment to individuals with ASD and anxiety.

2. Materials and Methods

This trial was registered on ClinicalTrials.gov as NCT03859336 and approved by the Phoenix Children's Hospital (PCH) Institutional Review Board #19.265 (Phoenix, AZ). All parents of participants provided written informed consent. Those under 18 years of age also provided assent, and those older than 18 years of age provided consent. This study followed the CONSORT guidelines for pilot and feasibility trials [54]. The CONSORT checklist is available as Supplementary Table S1. This was planned as a one-year study, but was extended 6 months to facilitate recruitment because of COVID-19 restrictions put in place by Phoenix Children's Hospital.

2.1. Participants

Seven children and adolescents with high-functioning ASD and anxiety participated in this study (mean (SD) ages: 14.1 (4.5), 71% (5) males) (Table 1). They were recruited from the PCH Precision Medicine Autism Clinic, as well as social media advertisements.

Table 1. Participant characteristics. Baseline Kaufman Brief Intelligence Test-2 (KBIT-2), child-rated Screen for Child Anxiety Related Disorders (C-SCARED), parent-rated Screen for Child Anxiety Related Disorders (P-SCARED), Parent-Rated Anxiety Scale (PRAS) and Total and Sleep Anxiety Score of the Children's Sleep Health Questionnaire (CSHQ).

					Baseline			
Study ID	**Age (Years)**	**Gender**	**KBIT-2 Score**	**SCARED—Child**	**SCARED—Parent**	**PRAS**	**Total CSHQ**	**Sleep Anxiety**
TEN-01	12	Female	103	14	25	43	46	4
TEN-03	13	Male	83	12	25	38	63	6
TEN-05	10	Male	116	25	46	48	64	8
TEN-06	21	Male	109	26	33	32	54	5
TEN-07	20	Male	104	28	29	42	59	6
TEN-08	10	Male	96	18	36	38	52	5
TEN-09	13	Female	109	37	50	45	53	4

Inclusion criteria: (1) previous diagnosis of ASD confirmed by the gold-standard instrument the Autism Diagnostic Interview–Revised (ADI-R) by a research reliable examiner; (2) age of 10–25 years old; (3) intellectual quotient > 80 on the Kaufman Brief Intelligence Test (KBIT-2); (4) Self- or parent-reported complaints of anxiety; (5) Screen for Child Anxiety Related Disorders–Parent (SCARED-P) form score $\geq$ 25; (6) able to follow directions in English; (7) ability to maintain all ongoing complementary, traditional and behavioral treatments during the study; and (8) no changes to any therapies for at least two months prior to time of participation.

Exclusion criteria: (1) implanted device; (2) history of electroconvulsive therapy; (3) history of significant face, head or neck injury, or surgery including metal plate or screw implants; (4) current or chronic neck pain; (5) pregnant or planning to become pregnant during the study period; (6) history of migraines or frequent headaches (more than once a week); (7) fainting (vasovagal syncope or neurocardiogenic syncope); (8) diagnosis of Raynaud's disease; (9) temporomandibular joint disorder or other facial neuropathy; (10) poor vision or hearing that is uncorrectable; (11) epilepsy or seizures in the last 2 years; or (12) evidence of skin disease or skin abnormalities affecting the neck or upper back.

2.2. Study Design

This was a single-blinded sham-controlled study. Participants who qualified underwent 5 consecutive visits at the same time each day, receiving 20 min of the sham on day 1 and TEN on the next 4 consecutive days (See Figure 2). The participants and their parents were blinded to if or when they would receive the sham, only being told that they might receive the sham as part of the study. On day 1, screening procedures occurred in which the eligibility criteria, medical history and concomitant medications and therapies were reviewed. A urine hCG test was performed if the participant was female. Participants completed the KBIT-2. If their score was $\geq$ 80 they qualified to continue on to the baseline session, as well as the 4 following sessions.

Daily sessions began with the parent completing parent-rated questionnaires while the participant supplied a saliva sample and answered a pre-treatment AE questionnaire. TEN electrodes were taped to the back of the participant's neck before a 5 min quiet physiological baseline period. Twenty minutes of the sham or TEN followed. After treatment, participants completed the ~15 min cognitive battery to stimulate anxiety, similar to that of a school test. The participant then answered the post-stimulation questionnaires to measure anxiety and any adverse events, as well as provided a second saliva sample. Saliva was collected on days 1, 2, 4 and 5. Sleep questionnaires were only performed on days 1 and 5. Parent-rated anxiety scales were completed every day of participation. During a follow-up phone call one week after study completion, anxiety and sleep symptoms were queried and a CSHQ was collected.

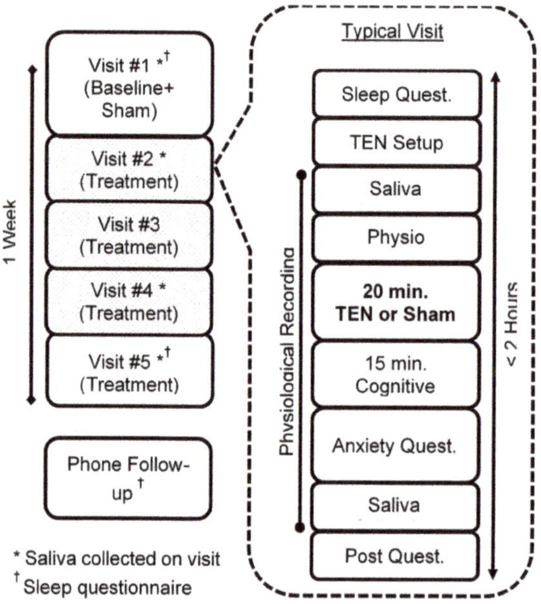

Figure 2. Study design.

2.3. TEN Treatment

During treatment, bipolar electrical stimulation was delivered to the cervical plexus (C2-C4) on the back of the neck (see Figure 1). The stimulation electrodes were 1.25″ (3.2 cm) round hydrogel PALS electrodes from Axelgaard Manufacturing Co., Ltd. (Fallbrook, CA, USA). Stimulation was delivered at a frequency of 300 Hz, pulse width of 350 ms and a duty cycle of 50% using a custom-made stimulation device. Stimulation amplitude was determined at every visit to ensure the current was just below the sensory threshold (see Table 2). To do this, the current amplitude was gradually increased until the participant's sensation threshold was met, then the amplitude was set 0.5 mA lower, where the participant could not feel the stimulation. Stimulation was delivered at this amplitude for 20 min. For the day 1 sham, the same procedure was performed to determine the stimulation threshold, but no stimulation occurred for the 20 min.

Table 2. TEN parameters.

Study ID	Frequency (Hz)	Duty Cycle	Pulse Width (ms)	Daily Threshold (Milliamps)				
				Day 1	Day 2	Day 3	Day 4	Day 5
TENS-01	300	50%	350	2.5	2.0	3.5	3.0	3.0
TENS-03	300	50%	350	4.5	4.0	5.5	6.5	5.5
TENS-05	300	50%	350	2.5	2.0	2.0	2.5	2.5
TENS-06	300	50%	350	2.5	3.5	3.5	2.5	4.5
TENS-07	300	50%	350	0.5	3.0	1.5	1.0	1.5
TENS-08	300	50%	350	3.5	13.5	13.5	12.5	8.5
TENS-09	300	50%	350	2.0	3.0	1.0	1.0	1.0

2.4. Outcome Measures

2.4.1. Anxiety Measures

There are few adequate measures of anxiety for ASD, but the SCARED has excellent performance for the measurement of anxiety in ASD [55–57] with strong psychometrics, measurement invariance, test–retest reliability and external validity [58]. The PRAS-ASD is a recently developed tool for assessing anxiety in ASD [59]. In contrast to the parent-reported SCARED, there is no currently established thresholds for anxiety with the PRAS-ASD; therefore, the parent-reported SCARED was used in screening.

2.4.2. Sleep Measures

The CSHQ, the standard tool for assessing sleep problems in ASD [60], was given to parents at baseline, visit #5 and at one-week follow-up.

2.4.3. Cognitive Battery

A ~15 min time-pressured cognitive battery was performed after stimulation/sham to replicate the anxiety in a test-taking situation, which is a common cause for anxiety in adolescents and young adults with ASD. The battery included three tests, given in the same order each day but with different question sequences depending on the day. The tests were explained to the participants before any stimulation on the first visit, and they were allowed to practice until they were comfortable. To account for cognitive differences, the task speed was faster for those with a high IQ (KBIT-2 score $\geq$ 100) and slower for those with a lower IQ (KBIT-2 score > 80–< 100).

The first test was the Paced Auditory Serial Addition Test (PASAT) [61] where the participant listened to random single-digit numbers being spoken in increasingly rapid succession, added the two most recent numbers heard and verbally responded to the administrator with the sum. The test presented 91 numbers ranging from 0 to 9 with an interstimulus interval (ISI) that started at 4 s and decreased to 2 s for participants with a KBIT-2 score > 80–< 100, or started at 3 s and decreased to 1 s for participants with a KBIT-2 score $\geq$ 100. This task is well-known to increase anxiety [62] and has been used as an experimental inducer of psychological stress [63].

The next test was the symbol search task (SST), which required a participant to identify and count the number of target shapes found within a grid of shapes presented on a screen. The task consisted of 49 image grids made from 5 different shapes with similar features. The image grid started with a size of 3 $\times$ 3 and increased to 8 $\times$ 8 throughout the task. Image grids were presented in 6 blocks. Each block consisted of 8 image grids presented for n seconds each, where n was related to the size of the grid and the baseline IQ of the participant. For the easier version, a $n \times n$ shape array was shown for n seconds (e.g., at the end of the study an 8 $\times$ 8 grid was shown for 8 s), while for the harder version the array is shown for n-1 s (e.g., at the end of the study an 8 $\times$ 8 grid was shown for 7 s). Participants verbally reported their responses.

The final test was the n-back task (NBT), where a participant determined if a presented shape matched the shape presented 2 shapes earlier (2-back). The task consists of 50 sequential shapes chosen from 5 different shapes with similar features. Shapes were shown for 3 s with a 2 s ISI for participants with a lower IQ and 2 s with a 1 s ISI for participants with a higher IQ. This test is widely used to assess working memory, which is commonly impaired in ASD [64]

Tasks were created using PsychoPy [65] and presented on a screen or speaker in front of the participant. A study coordinator sat behind the participant and scored their performance using prepared scoring sheets with the correct answers already indicated on them.

2.4.4. Autonomic Assessments

Several outcome measures were evaluated to investigate the effect of TEN on the ANS. Salivary was collected by a study coordinator at the beginning and end of day 1 (sham) as well as days 2, 4 and 5. Samples were blindly analyzed by Salimetrics Laboratory (Carlsbad, CA, USA) for α-amylase and cortisol levels. Saliva was collected by passive drool. Participants were instructed to not brush their teeth within 45 min, eat within one hour, consume caffeine or alcohol within 12 h or have dental work performed within 24 h of their scheduled appointment. Participants were also rinsed their mouths before saliva collection. Samples were immediately stored at −20 °C, where they stayed until shipment to the laboratory for analysis.

Electrical activity across the heart was collected by bio-medical engineers using a Polar H10 device with a chest strap (Polar USA, Bethpage, NY, USA). This system has been evaluated in children [66]. The system calculated HRV from the R-R intervals using a proprietary algorithm. Data were streamed to our custom-coded data acquisition system and collated with other data sources. The changes in the average HRV were calculated during TEN/sham and during each test compared to the last 4 min of the baseline period. HRV is known to be associated with anxiety [67], and was quantified as the standard deviation of the normal-to-normal heartbeat interval.

EDA data were also gathered by bio-medical engineers; they were measured at the base or tip of the index and middle fingers using the Shimmer-3 GSR+ Unit (Dublin, Ireland). The phasic component of the EDA was computed using LedaLab with adaptive smoothing and continuous decomposition [68]. After processing with LedaLab, the maximum EDA values were extracted around each cognitive battery question (−2 to +2 s of question onset). The median EDA value across each test type was then computed as the overall EDA response to a test. During the cognitive battery, it was noted that participants' anxiety levels were different for different tests, and during some challenging tests they would quit their effort early. To account for this, we considered only the first half of the questions (i.e., up to question 45, 24 and 25 for PASAT, SST and NBT, respectively). We also assessed the change in EDA across the day for the test that elicited the strongest EDA response for each individual on their initial visit. This represented the most stressful test for the individual. Several studies have used EDA to quantify the sympathetic response resulting from anxiety in ASD [37,38].

2.4.5. Measurement of Adverse Events

In addition to daily parent interviews, adverse events were monitored by using pre- and post-treatment questionnaires. These questions included potential symptoms, including headache, neck pain, tingling, itchiness, sleepiness, difficulty paying attention, unusual feelings/attitudes/emotions, nausea, tense muscles, dizziness, anxious/worried/nervous, forgetful, heart beating loudly, sweating, abnormal sleep or seizures. These symptoms were reviewed both at the beginning and end of every session.

2.5. Statistical Analysis

All variables were examined for normality using probability–probability plots, and link functions were adjusted to account for variables which deviated from normality. Ordinal questionnaire data were best represented by a Poisson loglinear link function, while other outcome variables were best represented by a normal distribution.

In general, a generalized linear model (GLM) was used for analysis as implemented in SPSS PASW release 18.0.0 (IBM, Armonk, NY, USA), using the appropriate link function as mentioned above. The GLM is calculated using maximal likelihood estimation with 100 maximum interactions and 5 maximal step-having, absolute convergence criteria of 10^{-5} for a change in parameter estimates and a singularity tolerance of 10^{-11}. The GLM calculates parameter significance by determining the change in the variance of the model as a parameter is added, essentially determining if adding the parameter to the model significantly increases the variance accounted for by the model. This is represented by the chi-square statistic. The effect size, φ, is calculated from the chi-square statistic as $\sqrt{x^2/n}$, where n is the number of observations. Given that χ^2 is a one-sided asymmetric distribution, only the lower bound of the effect size is calculated, which is provided in parathesis after the effect size. This was calculated using the chisq_to_phi function provided by the 'effectsize' library in R version 4.1.1 (The R Foundation for Statistical Computing, Vienna, Austria). For φ 0.1 is consider a small effect, 0.3 is considered a medium effect and 0.5 is considered a large effect.

Analysis using the GLM followed two approaches. First, a continuous variable that represented a linear increase in effect over treatment days was used to represent a change in effect with additional treatment days in order to identify a dose effect. Second, a dichotomous treatment effect (no treatment vs. treatment) represented whether treatment of all days combined was different than the sham. For salivary measures that were collected before and after the testing session, a dichotomous effect (before vs. after) factor was added to examine the change over the experimental session as well as the interaction of this factor with the treatment effect variable. For the responder analysis, the interaction of the dichotomous responder factor (responder vs. non-responder) with the treatment effect was examined. For a further illustration of individual measures as treatment progresses, please refer to Supplemental Figure S1 and Supplemental Figure S2.

3. Results

Thirteen individuals were screened for participation from January 2020 to July 2021. Six individuals did not pass the screening. Three did not meet the anxiety threshold, one's IQ was too low, one had changed anxiety medication with <6 weeks prior to the study and one could not be contacted when starting the study. Of the participants that started the study, none discontinued the study. A CONSORT flow diagram is presented as Supplementary Figure S1.

3.1. Adverse Effects

There were no significant AEs reported during the trial. Participants were specifically asked about the comfort of electrode placement and stimulation. No participant reported discomfort from the study procedures, including the electrodes. After completing the trial, one participant who had a history of precocious puberty and periodic oligomenorrhea experienced oligomenorrhea. The participant had stopped her medication to suppress menses 3 months prior to the study. It is not known whether TEN triggered the recurrent oligomenorrhea.

3.2. Anxiety

In general, the three anxiety questionnaires demonstrated progressive improvement in overall anxiety over 4 days of TEN treatment as compared to the sham. Over the group, the C-SCARED improved from a median of 25 to 19 (i.e., 24%), while the P-SCARED improved from a median of 33 to 31 (i.e., 7%). As seen in Supplemental Figure S1A, all participants demonstrated an improvement in the C-SCARED score at the last TEN day, with all ending with scores below the clinical cutoff (i.e., <25). The C-SCARED demonstrated a dose effect with a progressive reduction in score with increasing days of TEN ($\chi^2(1) = 9.86$, $p < 0.01$; $\varphi = 0.53$ (0.25)), and was reduced for all treatment days combined ($\chi^2(1) = 7.39$, $p < 0.01$; $\varphi = 0.45$ (0.18)) (Figures 3 and 4A).

As seen in Supplemental Figure S1B, six of the seven (86%) participants demonstrated an improvement on the P-SCARED, with three (43%) ending with scores below the clinical cutoff (i.e., <25). The P-SCARED also demonstrated a dose effect with a progressive reduction in score with increasing days of TEN ($\chi^2(1) = 7.69$, $p < 0.01$; $\varphi = 0.47$ (0.19)), and was reduced for all treatment days combined ($\chi^2(1) = 5.70$, $p = 0.02$; $\varphi = 0.40$ (0.12)) (Figure 4B).

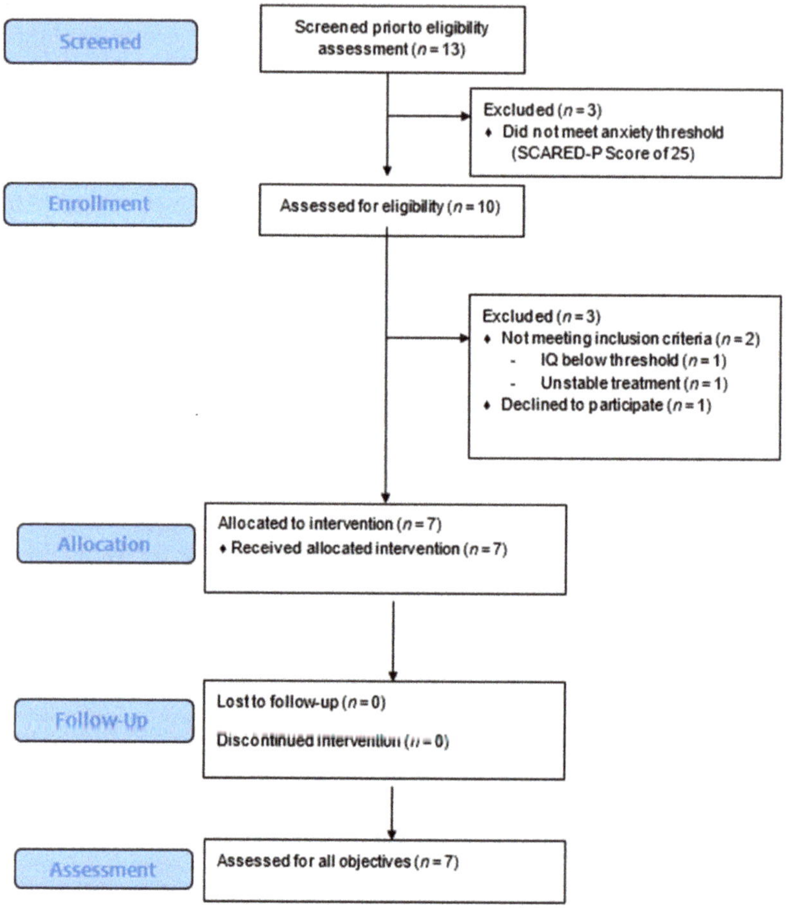

Figure 3. CONSORT flow diagram illustrating the allocation of each subject. Thirteen subjects were screened and 7 underwent treatment and assessment for all objectives.

As seen in Supplemental Figure S1C, the PRAS decreased in five of the seven participants (71%) and, as a group, demonstrated a significantly greater effect with increasing days of TEN treatment ($\chi^2(1) = 4.09$, $p < 0.05$; $\varphi = 0.34$ (0.04)), but was not significantly different for overall effect of all days combined (Figure 4C).

3.3. Sleep

As seen in Supplemental Figure S1D–E, five of the seven (71%) participants improved in total CSHQ score, and five of the seven (71%) participants improved in CSHQ anxiety score. From the CSHQ, sleep anxiety and total score decreased the week following TEN although these changes did not reach statistical significance (Figure 4D,E). The CSHQ decreased from a median of 54 to 51 (5%) in overall symptoms, and the sleep anxiety subscale decreased from 6 to 4 (33%) one week following TEN treatment. These findings are consistent with unsolicited feedback from multiple parents reporting improved sleep following the study.

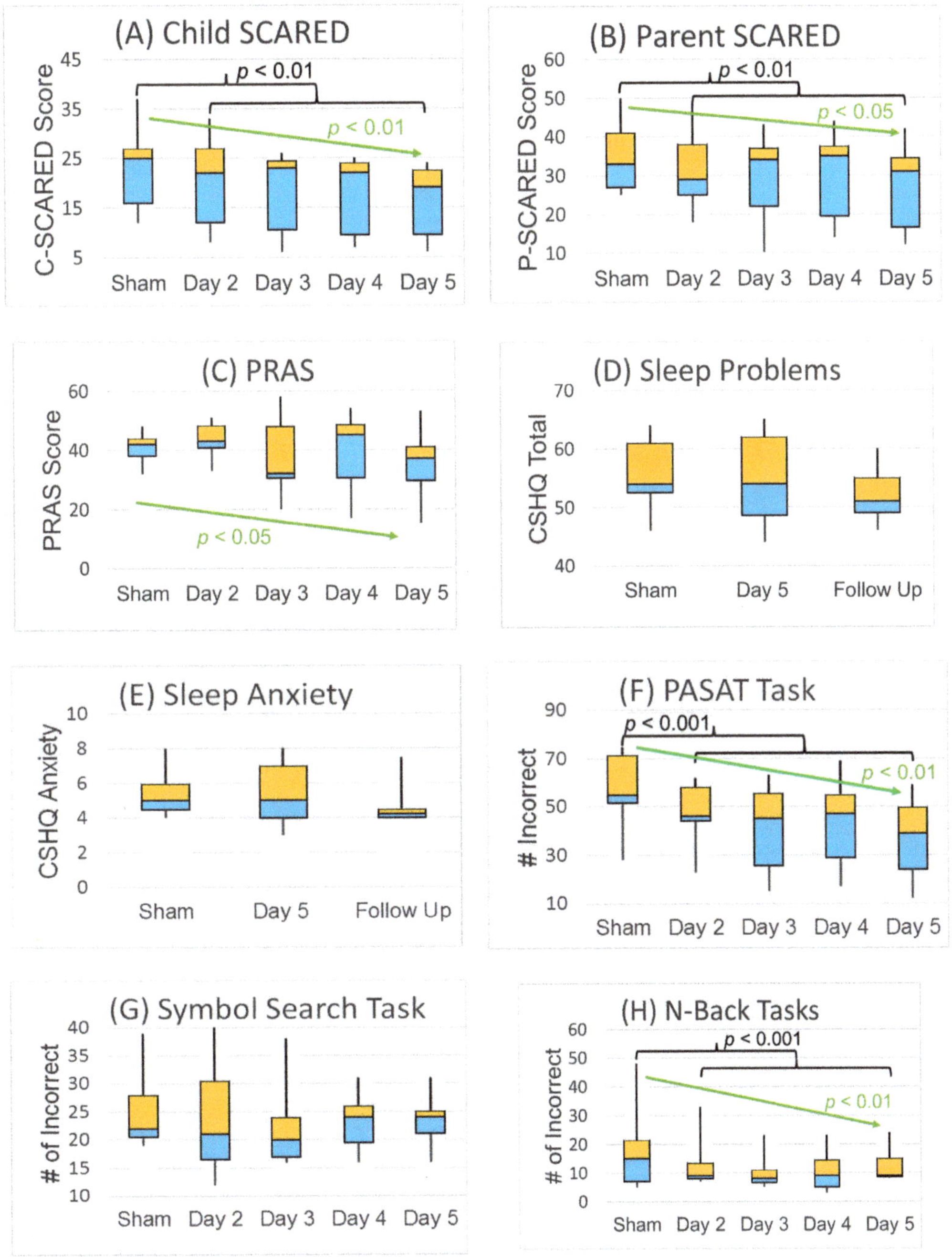

Figure 4. Effects of TEN treatment on (**A–C**) anxiety, (**D**,**E**) sleep and (**F–H**) cognitive performance ($n = 7$). Median, quartiles and min and max are shown. Black brackets represent significant differences between the sham day and TEN days (days 2–5). Green arrows represent significant trends in outcome with more treatment days.

3.4. Anxiety-Provoking Task Performance

As seen in Supplementary Figure S1F, all of the participants demonstrated improvement on the PASAT, with the median number of incorrect responses declining from 55 to 39 for the PASAT, a 29% improvement with a very large effect size. PASAT performance significantly improved with an increasing number of TEN sessions ($\chi^2(1) = 39.57$, $p < 0.001$; $\varphi = 1.06$ (0.79)), and was better on the days with TEN as compared to the sham ($\chi^2(1) = 29.91$, $p < 0.001$; $\varphi = 0.92$ (0.65)) (Figure 4F). As can be seen in Supplementary Figure S1G, six of the seven (86%) improved performance on the SST, with the median number of incorrect answers declining from 22 to 24. There was no significant change in the number of incorrect answers on the SST (Figure 4G). As can be seen in Supplementary Figure S1H, only three of the seven (43%) showed improvement and one of the seven (14%) demonstrated no change on the NBT. However, given the large improvements in one particular participant, the median number of incorrect answers declined from 15 to 9, a 40% improvement with a large effect size. NBT performance significantly improved with more TEN sessions (dose effect) ($\chi^2(1) = 9.43$, $p < 0.01$; $\varphi = 0.52$ (0.24)), and was better on the days with TEN as compared to the sham ($\chi^2(1) = 16.75$, $p < 0.001$; $\varphi = 0.69$ (0.41)) (Figure 4H).

3.5. Salivary Biomarkers

As can be seen in Supplementary Figure S2A-B, across the group salivary α-amylase and cortisol levels varied considerably, and were not significantly different between the sham and TEN days, did not significantly change with more TEN and did not significantly change over each experimental day (Figure 5).

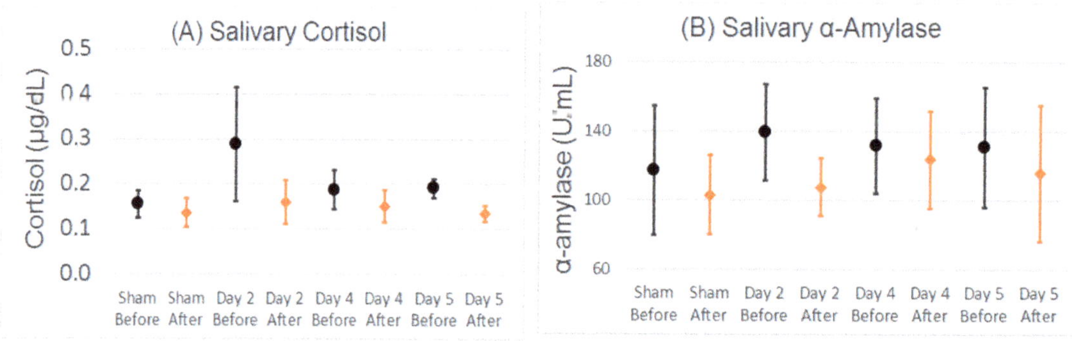

Figure 5. Salivary (**A**) cortisol and (**B**) α-amylase changes before and after TEN/sham and anxiety-provoking tasks. Mean and standard error bars are shown. There were no statistically significant differences between the sham and TEN days, or before as compared to after TEN/sham and anxiety-provoking tasks for the whole group.

3.6. Heart Rate Variability

Figure 6A demonstrates the HRV changes over experimental sessions for one example participant. From this figure it is obvious that the change in HRV is different for the sham vs. the experimental sessions. During sham stimulation (red line) HRV decreases (becomes more pathologic), and then continues to decrease during the anxiety-inducing tasks, demonstrating the stressful effects of the cognitive battery. On the first day of TEN treatment (dark blue; day two), the HRV increases with TEN (improved autonomic balance). Individual responses for HRV variability are shown in Supplementary Figure S2C–F. HRV was significantly higher on TEN treatment days as compared to the sham during the stimulation period ($\chi^2(1) = 6.37$, $p = 0.01$, $\varphi = 0.46$ (0.16); Figure 6B) and the PASAT ($\chi^2(1) = 4.74$, $p < 0.05$, $\varphi = 0.40$ (0.09); Figure 6C). Although this trend was also seen during SST (Figure 6D) and the NBT (Figure 6E), the difference was not statistically significant. The effect of TEN on HRV did not appear to progressively change across days of stimulation.

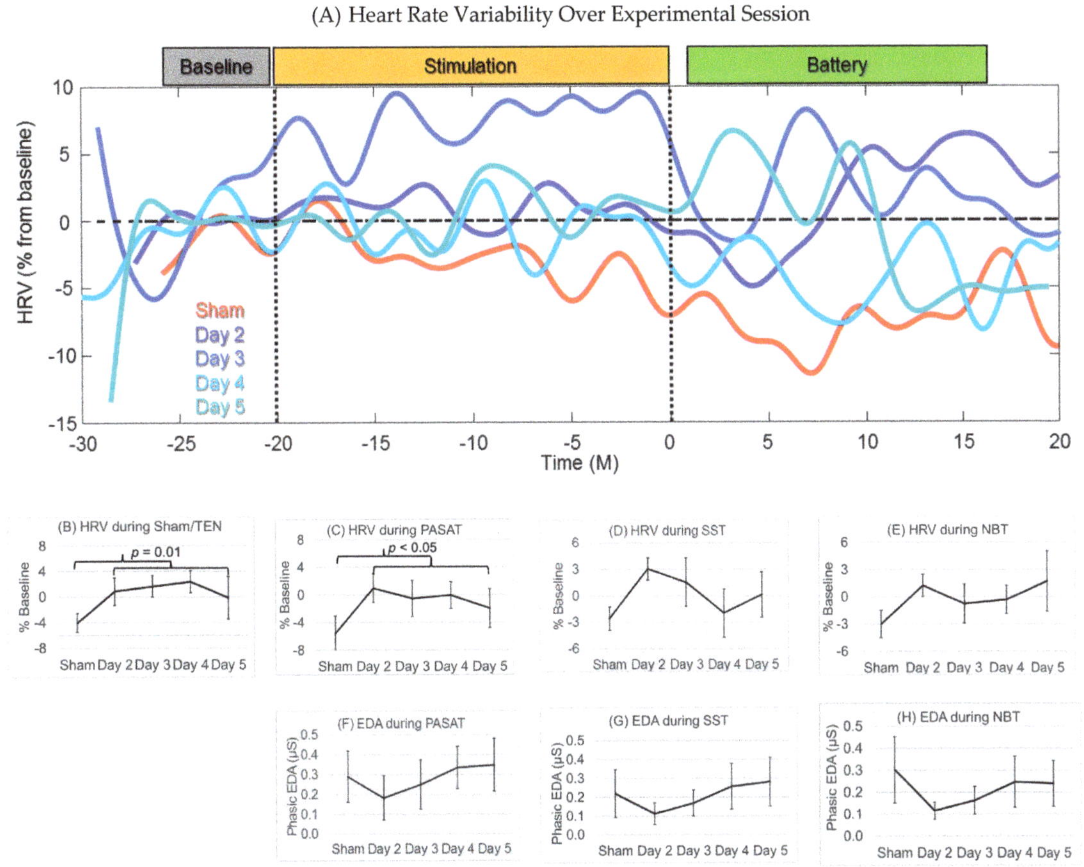

Figure 6. The effect of TEN on HRV and EDA. Mean and standard error bars are shown. The increase in HRV is shown for (**A**) an example individual, (**B**) across the group for the time period of the sham/TEN and (**C**–**E**) and for the anxiety-provoking tasks. HRV was significantly higher (improved) during TEN sessions as compared to the sham during the (**B**) stimulation and (**C**) the PASAT (shown as black brackets). EDA during (**F**–**H**) anxiety-provoking tasks decreased after the sham, but did not reach significance at the group level. No EDA was computed during the sham/TEN.

3.7. Electrodermal Activity

We have compared the phasic EDA response during the anxiety-provoking tasks between the sham and TEN treatment days. Individual responses for EDA are shown in Supplementary Figure S2G,H. Overall, there was a consistent pattern to the effect of TEN on EDA. On the first day there was a decrease in phasic EDA response (Figure 6F–H). However, the EDA appeared to return to baseline levels after the first stimulation day. There was no significant difference for treatment vs. the sham, and no progressive effect over increasing days of treatment.

3.8. Effect of Intelligence

The effect of IQ on baseline measures was evaluated. A higher IQ was associated with higher anxiety scores on the baseline C-SCARED ($\chi^2(1) = 9.76$, $p < 0.01$, $\varphi = 1.18$ (0.56)) and P-SCARED ($\chi^2(1) = 4.16$, $p < 0.05$, $\varphi = 0.77$ (0.11)), but not PRAS. A higher IQ was associated with better baseline performance on the PASAT ($\chi^2(1) = 7.06$, $p < 0.01$, $\varphi = 1.00$ (0.38)), but was not related to performance on the NBT or SST. A higher IQ was related to a higher overall salivary α-amylase ($\chi^2(1) = 7.29$, $p < 0.01$, $\varphi = 1.10$ (0.43)) at baseline, but not related to salivary a-amylase change or cortisol. IQ was not associated with changes in the C-SCARED, CSHQ or task performance across sessions, but it was related to improvements in anxiety rated with the P-SCARED ($\chi^2(1) = 6.38$, $p = 0.01$, $\varphi = 0.43$ (0.15)) and PRAS ($\chi^2(1) = 8.40$, $p < 0.01$, $\varphi = 0.49$ (0.21)) such that higher IQ was associated with more moderate ratings of improvement in anxiety on these parent-rated scales.

3.9. Responder Analysis

Results for participants who responded well to the TEN treatments compared to the sham (responders) were compared to the results from non-responders. Responders were defined as participants with an average of $\geq$ 30% improvement in C-SCARED with treatment compared to the sham. Four participants (57%) were categorized as responders and three (43%) as non-responders. There were no significant differences in the anxiety or sleep questionnaires at baseline between responders and non-responders, but responders performed worse on the SST ($\chi^2(1) = 5.04$, $p < 0.05$, $\varphi = 0.85$ (0.22)) and the PASAT ($\chi^2(1) = 13.05$, $p < 0.001$, $\varphi = 1.37$ (0.74)) during the baseline (sham) day. There were no differences in salivary cortisol or a-amylase between responders and non-responders.

Unsurprisingly, responders demonstrated a greater improvement (i.e., decrease) in the C-SCARED ($\chi^2(2) = 11.25$, $p < 0.01$, $\varphi = 0.57$ (0.29)) than non-responders. This difference increased with more treatments ($\chi^2(1) = 9.99$, $p < 0.01$, $\varphi = 0.53$ (0.26)). For those considered responders, the median C-SCARED dropped from 23 to 15 (35%), whereas the median C-SCARED dropped from 12 to 8 (4%) for the non-responders. For responders, the change in the improvement in the C-SCARED ranged from a minimum drop from 12 to 8, a 33% drop, to a maximum drop from 18 to 6, a 67% drop. For non-responders, the change in the C-SCARED ranged from a minimum drop from 25 to 24, a 4% drop, to a maximum drop from 14 to 11, a 21% drop. The median P-SCARED dropped from 32.5 to 24 (27%) for responders, but only dropped from 33 to 31 (6%) for non-responders. For responders, the change in the improvement in the P-SCARED ranged from a minimum increase from 29 to 34, a 17% increase, to a maximum drop from 36 to 14, a 61% drop. For non-responders, the change in the P-SCARED ranged from a minimum drop from 33 to 31, a 6% drop, to a maximum drop from 46 to 35, a 24% drop. However, there were no significant differences between groups in the PRAS-ASD or sleep questionnaires. The median PRAS-ASD dropped from 40 to 33 (18%) for responders, but only dropped from 43 to 38 (12%) for non-responders. For responders, the change in the improvement in the PRAS-ASD ranged from a minimum increase from 42 to 53, a 27% increase, to a maximum drop from 38 to 15, a 61% drop. For non-responders, the change in the PRAS-ASD ranged from a minimum increase from 32 to 38, a 19% increase, to a maximum drop from 43 to 30, a 30% drop. The median total CSHQ sleep score dropped from 56 to 53 (16%) for responders, and dropped from 54 to 47 (13%) for non-responders. For responders, the change in the improvement in the total CSHQ sleep score ranged from a minimum increase from 52 to 56, an 8% increase, to a maximum drop from 63 to 51, a 19% drop. For non-responders, the change in the total CSHQ sleep score ranged from a minimum unchanged score of 46, a 0% change, to a maximum drop from 54 to 47, a 13% drop. The median total CSHQ sleep anxiety score dropped from 5.5 to 4 (17%) for responders, and dropped from 5 to 4 (20%) for non-responders. For responders, the change in the improvement in the total CSHQ sleep anxiety score ranged from a minimum of unchanged at 4, a 0% increase, to a maximum drop from 6 to 4, a 33% drop. For non-responders, the change in the total CSHQ sleep anxiety score ranged from a minimum unchanged score of 4, a 0% change, to a maximum drop from 5 to 4, a 20% drop.

Average daily salivary α-amylase became progressively higher across days in two of the non-responders, while it stayed stable and then decreased for the four responders ($\chi^2(2) = 27.02$, $p < 0.001$, $\varphi = 0.67$ (0.46)). In the responders salivary α-amylase within the day decreased after TEN treatment, as compared to before TEN treatment, whereas in non-responders it did not show a consistent change and even increased during day four of the study ($\chi^2(2) = 26.73$, $p < 0.001$, $\varphi = 0.67$ (0.46)) (Figure 7). There was no difference in change in cortisol for responders and non-responders.

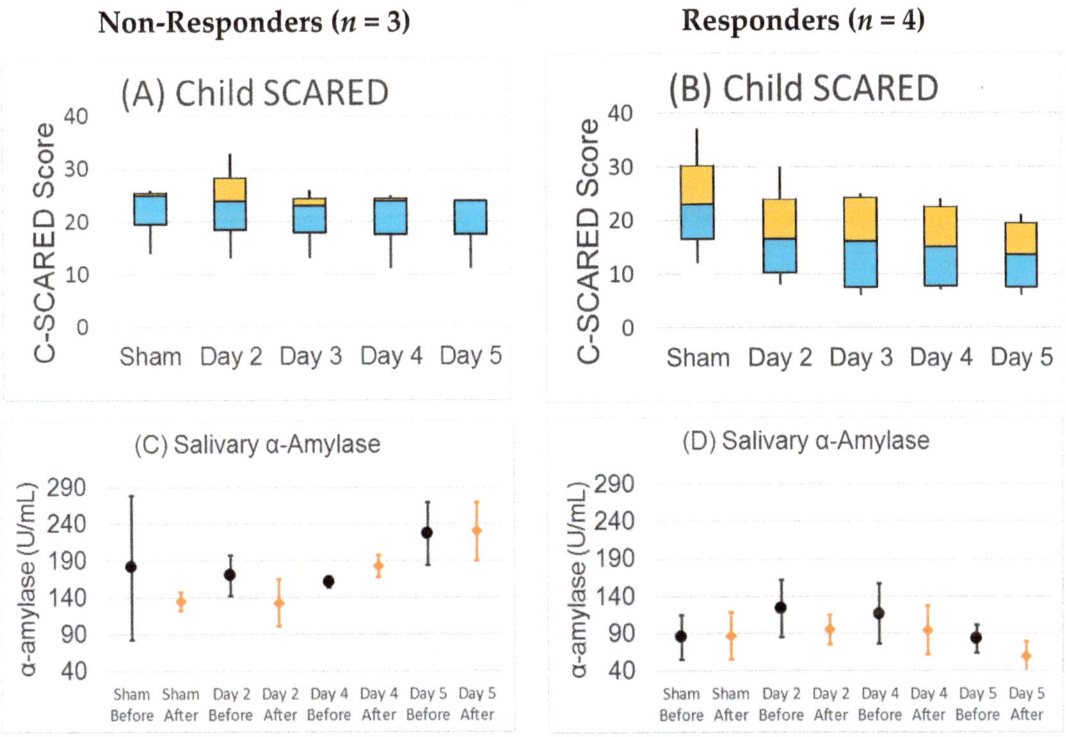

Figure 7. Responder analysis. Responders were defined as participants with an average of ≥30% improvement in the child-rated SCARED with treatment compared to the sham. In non-responders, the (**A**) child-rated SCARED did not change over sessions and (**C**) salivary α-amylase increased with more TEN sessions. In contrast, in responders the (**B**) child-rated SCARED markedly decreased and (**D**) α-amylase not only decreased with more TEN stimulation across multiple sessions, but also decreased from the beginning of the session to the end of the session on days the participants received TEN. For the child-rated SCARED median, quartiles and min and max are shown. For salivary α-amylase mean and standard error bars are shown.

4. Discussion

TEN is a well-tolerated method for subthreshold neurostimulation that is FDA-approved for brain-based disorders such as ADHD [46] and migraines [47], and also appears to have some effectiveness in major depressive disorder [42], post-traumatic stress disorder [48] and generalized anxiety disorder [49]. This is the first study to investigate the tolerability and effectiveness of TEN therapy in ASD, a disorder with many co-morbidities including anxiety and sleep disruption. In this study, adolescents with high-functioning ASD and anxiety underwent four daily TEN treatments following an initial sham run-in treatment day. Anxiety was monitored using standardized participant and caregiver questionnaires, sleep was monitored with caregiver questionnaires and multiple measures of ANS activity were collected including salivary cortisol and α-amylase, HRV and EDA during anxiety-provoking tasks and HRV during TEN.

The treatment was well-tolerated with no reported AEs, consistent with studies of transcutaneous electrical acupoint stimulation in which children with ASD find the treatment tolerable, without AEs [50,51]. This study demonstrates the feasibility of TEN for individuals with ASD. This is reassuring as many suffer from hypersensitivity to tactile stimuli, making them unable to tolerate electrodes placed on their skin, as well as have symptoms of ADHD, which makes them unable to sit still for prolonged periods of time. These data suggest that TEN is a promising treatment for individuals with ASD that can be tolerated for a typical stimulation period.

4.1. TEN Improved Rating of Anxiety in ASD

Across the group, anxiety scores were improved on treatment days as compared to the sham when considering both the participant- and caregiver-rated SCARED. Similarly, more days of stimulation had greater improvement in anxiety in all three anxiety questionnaires. The C-SCARED improved by 24% (from 25 to 19) across days, while the P-SCARED improved by 7% (from 33 to 31). Given the cutoff for anxiety is 25 for the SCARED, these results demonstrate that TEN had a clinically significant improvement in anxiety on the group level. In fact, all of the seven participants had a C-SCARED below the threshold for symptoms of an anxiety disorder after TEN treatment. This impact was even stronger for those considered responders, where the C-SCARED dropped 35% from 23 to 15 and the P-SCARED dropped 27% from 32.5 to 24. The PRAS drop in total score from 42 at baseline to 37 on day five. The effect sizes varied from a large effect of 0.53 for the C-SCARED to a medium effect of 0.34 for the PRAS.

Previous studies suggest that a 55% decrease in the P-SCARED and a 50% decrease in the C-SCARED optimally predicted treatment response in a 6 month study of the SSRI sertraline and/or cognitive behavior therapy in NT youths [69]. Although this study did not demonstrate this level of treatment response, the 4-day treatment period was much shorter in duration. Thus, assessing a longer term treatment will be necessary to understand if the effect of TEN is cumulative. The results suggest TEN treatment could have a cumulative effect on improving anxiety in ASD. Although the questionnaire demonstrated a positive response to treatment, questionnaires are subjective, and studies have shown that they do not capture anxiety differences equivalently for all individuals with ASD [70]. More objective measurements of anxiety would improve future studies.

4.2. Possible Effect of TEN on Sleep in ASD

Though the improvements in sleep questionnaire scores did not reach significance, the findings were promising. We were especially encouraged by several participants' unsolicited feedback, reporting improvement in sleep after TEN treatment. We did find that the CSHQ decreased three points (5%) in overall symptoms and two points (33%) in the sleep anxiety subscale one week following TEN treatment. These improvements in CSHQ scores are similar to those reported in other studies of sleep treatment in ASD. For example, three weeks of transcranial direct current stimulation to the left dorsal lateral prefrontal cortex was associated with a statistically significant 2.7-point drop in the total CSHQ score in the treatment group of a single-blinded, randomized, parallel clinical study of children with ASD [71], and a meta-analysis found that non-pharmacological interventions for insomnia in children with ASD was associated with a 4.71-point improvement in the CSHQ [72]. In contrast, one-month of controlled-release melatonin in children with ASD is associated with a 20-point improvement in the total CSHQ score and a 3.5-point improvement on the sleep anxiety scale in an open-label study [73].

Sleep problems are complicated to treat and may require prolonged treatment to measure improvements. These results are encouraging following only 5 days of treatment; a longer follow-up may be necessary to determine the full effect of treatment. An additional limitation of our sleep analysis is the use of the well-validated, but subjective, CSHQ. As a secondary reporter measure, it may not accurately capture the sleep quality of the participant. The addition of more objective measures of sleep, such as actigraphy, would provide a reliable index of sleep quality and quantity. Actigraphy utilizes established technology and algorithms to measure sleep onset and duration, as well as the number and duration of nighttime wakings.

4.3. TEN Improved Performance on Anxiety-Provoking Tasks

To test cognitive performance, we utilized three anxiety-provoking tasks. These tasks involve executive function, which is not only commonly impaired in high-functioning adolescents with ASD but is also a key deficit that impedes performance in a wide variety of everyday tasks. It should be noted that this is the first time anxiety-provoking tasks have been used in a treatment trial of anxiety for individuals with ASD. Such assays should be considered as part of the assessment for anxiety treatments in other studies, given the importance of executive function skills in performance in academia, social interactions and general skills of daily living.

TEN was associated with a substantial improvement in performance for two of the three anxiety-provoking tasks. The median number of incorrect responses declined from 55 to 39 for the PASAT, a 29% improvement with a very large effect size, and declined from 15 to 9 for the NBT, a 40% improvement with a large effect size. The PASAT has been used in clinical trials for multiple sclerosis, traumatic brain injury and gerontology where the score improvements with treatment were smaller than seen in this study [61,74].

For the SST, the only anxiety-provoking task without a significant improvement in performance, the median number of incorrect answers increased from 22 to 24, an actual worsening of performance over the week. Analysis of the individual scores indicated that several of the participants performed worse on day four and five as compared to day three, which parallels the feedback provided from participants who reported they became uninterested with the task after performing it several times. This could indicate a complete lack of anxiety to successfully complete the task. Future studies might integrate other techniques, such as eye tracking, to help monitor performance and engagement.

4.4. Cortisol Response to Social Paradigms as a Bio-Marker for Stress in ASD

Cortisol is considered a measure of stress, commonly used to measure levels of general stress in many studies. However, in our study we did not find that it was a reliable biomarker of anxiety. This may be related to the ASD population, as other studies have also not found it to be a reliable measure of stress with those with ASD. Studies examining the responsiveness of cortisol in ASD also demonstrate an overall under-reactivity involving social threats [75–77], with this hyporeactive cortisol response to a social stressor greater in those with ASD and anxiety than compared to those with ASD and controls [78]. Some studies have shown greater cortisol reactivity in those with ASD as compared to controls to a nonsocial stressor [79], but not others [80,81]. Thus, a blunted cortisol response is not completed unexpected for the ASD group, especially those with anxiety. In addition, cortisol levels might be less likely to change with TEN as it is regulated through the hypothalamic–pituitary–adrenal axis which has multiple levels of potential dysregulation not directly linked to immediate sympathetic and parasympathetic neuromodulation.

4.5. α-Amylase Response to Social Paradigms as a Bio-Marker for Stress in ASD

As α-amylase levels are directly related to sympathetic nervous system activation, it was expected that TEN would modulate α-amylase as a marker of ANS sympathetic activity. Although changes in α-amylase were not significant across the entire group of participants, it did seem to be different for those that responded to the treatment as compared to those that did not respond. For the responders to TEN, the α-amylase salivary concentrations showed a steady decrease across days of treatment, with the α-amylase salivary concentration decreasing following TEN treatment with each day of treatment. This decrease in α-amylase suggests a decrease in sympathetic activity with TEN treatment for the responder group. In contrast, those that did not respond to TEN had α-amylase levels that increased progressively on each successive day of stimulation, and the measured change within each day did not correlate with treatment. While we interpret this as an indication of decreased anxiety due to TEN treatment, this biomarker may be representing something more basic about modulation of the ANS. Indeed, the increase in α-amylase in the non-responders may have indicated that the TEN treatment parameters used in this study are not tuned to positively modulating the ANS in these specific participants, and that other TEN parameters may be needed for these participants to respond. Further research is needed to validate α-amylase as a potential biomarker of response to TEN and determine which levels of the psychological and/or physiological response it may represent.

4.6. TEN Improved Heart Rate Variability in ASD

We found that HRV significantly increased (i.e., improved) with TEN treatment, although this change was not progressive over days. This suggests that TEN positively impacted sympathetic regulation and that HRV may be a promising outcome measure for future studies. HRV has been used as a measure of ANS activity in both adults [82–85] and children [39,86–88] with ASD. Lower HRV has been associated with symptoms of gastrointestinal problems, such as constipation in children with ASD [39]. HRV has also been used as an outcome measures in clinical trials of yoga and repetitive transcranial magnetic stimulation in children with ASD [88–90]. Thus, HRV appears to be a promising biomarker of the ANS in children with ASD.

4.7. Dynamic Changes in Autonomic Nervous System Measures with TEN

Some ANS measures positively peaked only on the first day of TEN and then reverted to baseline. These include EDA during all tasks and HRV during the SST. Although this could be interpreted as the effect of TEN wearing off after the first day, such a notion is counter to the continuing positive effect of TEN on anxiety measurements and task performance. An alternative explanation is that this might demonstrate homeostatic mechanisms adapting to the TEN effect on the ANS and compensating for the effect of TEN on the ANS. This demonstrates some of the difficulties in using ANS measures for proxies of anxiety or other cognitive states, as they are regulated by multiple higher-level and lower-level influences. Furthermore, this return to baseline in ANS measures across days may also indicate that TEN is resetting the brainstem circuitry, and thereby facilitating a calmer and more consistent reaction to anxiety provoking stimuli.

4.8. Further Refinement of TEN Protocol

This study suggests that TEN may be useful for short-term improvement of anxiety, but long-term use of this device for individuals with ASD has not been studied. Extended long-term use is important, particularly with respect to the stimulation protocol. For responders, positive changes in C-SCARED (Figure 7B) and task performance (Figure 4F,H) as well as changes in ANS measures (Figures 5 and 6) were strongest after the first TEN treatment. From our studies it is not clear if consecutive-day treatment is necessary, nor whether it is optimal for stimulation to occur every week or every month to maintain and enhance the effect. Electrical stimulation regiments for other disorders vary considerably. Furthermore, only a single set of stimulation parameters were evaluated. Though the stimulation parameters used in this study are based on studies of healthy adults [41], personalized or group-wise optimization could help increase the portion of responders. Determining the optimal stimulation protocol for long-term use will help maximize benefits and minimize burdens. Once that is established, long-term studies can be designed to determine efficacy. Furthermore, improved biomarkers of the response to treatment will help refine future studies and maximize the effect size of treatment.

4.9. Limitations

This study used subjective measures of anxiety, but subjective measures are standard for clinical care and clinical trials. This weakness was mitigated by obtaining both participant and observer (parent) measures. Individuals with ASD by definition have trouble communicating, so it is important to obtain a measure of their experience. Physiological measures relating to ANS activity were also used as a proxy for anxiety, but such measures are only preliminary in their ability to measure psychological states. Future studies should concentrate on validating reliable outcome measure to provide the most accurate representation of the effectiveness of TEN.

This study was limited to high-functioning individuals with ASD, as communication is necessary to assess anxiety. Interestingly, IQ was related to perceived improvement in anxiety on the parent-rated scales, suggesting that the ability of the individual with ASD to communicate complex emotions may have influenced the rating of anxiety as well as its changes during the study.

A procedural limitation was that the sham day was always on the first day of participation. This was meant as a run-in to check for a placebo effect, but future studies should include a longer treatment period, with sham days dispersed throughout. Participants, as well as the researchers who are scoring the participant, should be blinded to the status of the stimulation.

5. Conclusions

Applying tuned, high-frequency stimulation to the cervical nerves appears to be a promising non-pharmacological, biologically informed, non-invasive and safe neuromodulation for managing anxiety in individuals with ASD. Such a treatment could potentially be particularly impactful for young people transitioning into adulthood, where anxiety and sleep problems can be exacerbated by time-based testing and the increased need to interact socially in order to function independently. With recent interest in TEN treatment for ASD, the expanding use of these devices in many disorders, the increased availability of these devices, and the well-established history of its safety, it would not be surprising if these devices were being recommended 'off-label' without any ASD-specific studies to guide their use. This study provides some insight into the safety and effectiveness of TEN for ASD. While there is preliminary evidence suggesting effectiveness in some of the individuals in our study, further studies are needed to better understand its benefits and develop an optimal protocol for its use.

6. Patents

Existing patents for the stimulation technology are held by Tyler (WO2013192582A1, US8903494B2 and US9002458B2).

Supplementary Materials: The following are available online at https://www.mdpi.com/article/10.3390/jpm11121307/s1, Supplemental Table S1: CONSORT checklist; Supplemental Figure S1: Individual anxiety and sleep measures. Supplemental Figure S2: Individual autonomic measures.

Author Contributions: Conceptualization, S.T.F., S.V., E.F., W.J.T. and R.E.F.; methodology, S.T.F., A.R.J., A.J., S.V., W.J.T. and R.E.F.; software, S.T.F. and A.J.; formal analysis, S.T.F., A.J. and R.E.F.; resources, S.T.F. and W.J.T.; data curation, S.T.F., A.R.J., A.J. and R.E.F.; writing—original draft preparation, S.T.F., A.R.J., E.F., T.L. and R.E.F.; writing—review and editing, all authors; visualization, S.T.F. and R.E.F.; supervision, S.T.F., A.G., D.B. and R.E.F.; funding acquisition, S.T.F. and W.J.T. All authors have read and agreed to the published version of the manuscript.

Funding: This research was funded by an NSF Cooperative Grant I/UCRC for Building Reliable Advances and Innovation in Neurotechnology (1650566).

Institutional Review Board Statement: The study was conducted according to the guidelines of the Declaration of Helsinki and approved by the Institutional Review Board of Phoenix Children's Hospital (Phoenix, AZ), protocol #19.265. Date of approval: 21 May 2019.

Informed Consent Statement: Informed consent and assent was obtained from all participants, and their parents, involved in the study.

Data Availability Statement: Data and protocol are availability upon request.

Conflicts of Interest: Tyler holds patents on TEN technology. The remaining authors declare no conflict of interest. The funders had no role in the design of the study; in the collection, analyses, or interpretation of data; in the writing of the manuscript; or in the decision to publish the results.

References

1. Rossignol, D.A.; Frye, R.E. A review of research trends in physiological abnormalities in autism spectrum disorders: Immune dysregulation, inflammation, oxidative stress, mitochondrial dysfunction and environmental toxicant exposures. *Mol. Psychiatry* **2012**, *17*, 389–401. [CrossRef]
2. Maenner, M.J.; Shaw, K.A.; Baio, J.; Washington, A.; Patrick, M.; DiRienzo, M.; Christensen, D.L.; Wiggins, L.D.; Pettygrove, S.; Andrews, J.G.; et al. Prevalence of Autism Spectrum Disorder Among Children Aged 8 Years—Autism and Developmental Disabilities Monitoring Network, 11 Sites, United States, 2016. Morbidity and Mortality Weekly Report. *Surveill. Summ.* **2020**, *69*, 1–12. [CrossRef]
3. Hyman, S.L.; Levy, S.E.; Myers, S.M.; Council On Children With Disabilities, S.O.D.; Behavioral, P. Identification, Evaluation, and Management of Children With Autism Spectrum Disorder. *Pediatrics* **2020**, *145*, e20193447. [CrossRef] [PubMed]
4. Lai, M.C.; Lombardo, M.V.; Baron-Cohen, S. Autism. *Lancet* **2014**, *383*, 896–910. [CrossRef]
5. Fein, D.; Barton, M.; Eigsti, I.M.; Kelley, E.; Naigles, L.; Schultz, R.T.; Stevens, M.; Helt, M.; Orinstein, A.; Rosenthal, M.; et al. Optimal outcome in individuals with a history of autism. *J. Child Psychol. Psychiatry Allied Discip.* **2013**, *54*, 195–205. [CrossRef] [PubMed]
6. Fountain, C.; Winter, A.S.; Bearman, P.S. Six developmental trajectories characterize children with autism. *Pediatrics* **2012**, *129*, e1112–e1120. [CrossRef]
7. Magiati, I.; Tay, X.W.; Howlin, P. Cognitive, language, social and behavioural outcomes in adults with autism spectrum disorders: A systematic review of longitudinal follow-up studies in adulthood. *Clin. Psychol Rev.* **2014**, *34*, 73–86. [CrossRef]
8. Rogge, N.; Janssen, J. The Economic Costs of Autism Spectrum Disorder: A Literature Review. *J. Autism Dev. Disord.* **2019**. [CrossRef]
9. Cakir, J.; Frye, R.E.; Walker, S.J. The lifetime social cost of autism: 1990–2029. *Res. Autism Spectr. Disord.* **2020**, *72*, 101502. [CrossRef]
10. Brown, C.C.; Tilford, J.M.; Payakachat, N.; Williams, D.K.; Kuhlthau, K.A.; Pyne, J.M.; Hoefman, R.J.; Brouwer, W.B.F. Measuring Health Spillover Effects in Caregivers of Children with Autism Spectrum Disorder: A Comparison of the EQ-5D-3L and SF-6D. *Pharmacoeconomics* **2019**, *37*, 609–620. [CrossRef]
11. Hartley, S.L.; Papp, L.M.; Bolt, D. Spillover of Marital Interactions and Parenting Stress in Families of Children With Autism Spectrum Disorder. *J. Clin. Child Adolesc. Psychol. Off. J. Soc. Clin. Child. Adolesc. Psychol. Am. Psychol. Assoc. Div.* **2018**, *47*, S88–S99. [CrossRef] [PubMed]
12. Tilford, J.M.; Payakachat, N.; Kuhlthau, K.A.; Pyne, J.M.; Kovacs, E.; Bellando, J.; Williams, D.K.; Brouwer, W.B.; Frye, R.E. Treatment for Sleep Problems in Children with Autism and Caregiver Spillover Effects. *J. Autism Dev. Disord.* **2015**, *45*, 3613–3623. [CrossRef] [PubMed]
13. Dunn, K.; Rydzewska, E.; Fleming, M.; Cooper, S.A. Prevalence of mental health conditions, sensory impairments and physical disability in people with co-occurring intellectual disabilities and autism compared with other people: A cross-sectional total population study in Scotland. *BMJ Open* **2020**, *10*, e035280. [CrossRef] [PubMed]
14. Viscidi, E.W.; Triche, E.W.; Pescosolido, M.F.; McLean, R.L.; Joseph, R.M.; Spence, S.J.; Morrow, E.M. Clinical characteristics of children with autism spectrum disorder and co-occurring epilepsy. *PLoS ONE* **2013**, *8*, e67797. [CrossRef]
15. Holingue, C.; Newill, C.; Lee, L.C.; Pasricha, P.J.; Daniele Fallin, M. Gastrointestinal symptoms in autism spectrum disorder: A review of the literature on ascertainment and prevalence. *Autism Res. Off. J. Int. Soc. Autism Res.* **2018**, *11*, 24–36. [CrossRef]
16. Lai, M.C.; Kassee, C.; Besney, R.; Bonato, S.; Hull, L.; Mandy, W.; Szatmari, P.; Ameis, S.H. Prevalence of co-occurring mental health diagnoses in the autism population: A systematic review and meta-analysis. *Lancet Psychiatry* **2019**, *6*, 819–829. [CrossRef]
17. Hollocks, M.J.; Lerh, J.W.; Magiati, I.; Meiser-Stedman, R.; Brugha, T.S. Anxiety and depression in adults with autism spectrum disorder: A systematic review and meta-analysis. *Psychol. Med.* **2019**, *49*, 559–572. [CrossRef]
18. Grondhuis, S.N.; Aman, M.G. Assessment of anxiety in children and adolescents with autism spectrum disorders. *Res. Autism Spectr. Disord.* **2012**, *6*, 1345–1365. [CrossRef]
19. van Steensel, F.J.A.; Heeman, E.J. Anxiety Levels in Children with Autism Spectrum Disorder: A Meta-Analysis. *J. Child. Fam Stud.* **2017**, *26*, 1753–1767. [CrossRef]
20. Baker, E.K.; Richdale, A.L.; Hazi, A. Employment status is related to sleep problems in adults with autism spectrum disorder and no comorbid intellectual impairment. *Autism Int. J. Res. Pract.* **2019**, *23*, 531–536. [CrossRef]
21. Deliens, G.; Peigneux, P. Sleep-behaviour relationship in children with autism spectrum disorder: Methodological pitfalls and insights from cognition and sensory processing. *Dev. Med. Child Neurol.* **2019**, *61*, 1368–1376. [CrossRef]
22. Kuusikko, S.; Pollock-Wurman, R.; Jussila, K.; Carter, A.S.; Mattila, M.L.; Ebeling, H.; Pauls, D.L.; Moilanen, I. Social anxiety in high-functioning children and adolescents with Autism and Asperger syndrome. *J. Autism Dev. Disord.* **2008**, *38*, 1697–1709. [CrossRef] [PubMed]
23. Park, J.H.; Kim, Y.-S.; Koh, Y.-J.; Song, J.; Leventhal, B.L. A contrast of comorbid condition and adaptive function between children with Autism Spectrum Disorder from clinical and non-clinical populations. *Res. Autism Spectr. Disord.* **2014**, *8*, 1471–1481. [CrossRef]
24. Myles, B.S.; Barnhill, G.P.; Hagiwara, T.; Griswold, D.E.; Simpson, R.L. A Synthesis of Studies on the Intellectual, Academic, Social/ Emotional and Sensory Characteristics of Children and Youth with Asperger Syndrome. *Educ. Train. Ment. Retard. Dev. Disabil.* **2001**, *36*, 304–311.

25. Ader, R.; Cohen, N.; Felten, D. Psychoneuroimmunology: Interactions between the nervous system and the immune system. *Lancet* **1995**, *345*, 99–103. [CrossRef]
26. Padgett, D.A.; Glaser, R. How stress influences the immune response. *Trends Immunol.* **2003**, *24*, 444–448. [CrossRef]
27. Brotman, D.J.; Golden, S.H.; Wittstein, I.S. The cardiovascular toll of stress. *Lancet* **2007**, *370*, 1089–1100. [CrossRef]
28. Hodge, D.; Carollo, T.M.; Lewin, M.; Hoffman, C.D.; Sweeney, D.P. Sleep patterns in children with and without autism spectrum disorders: Developmental comparisons. *Res. Dev. Disabil.* **2014**, *35*, 1631–1638. [CrossRef]
29. Dewrang, P.; Sandberg, A.D. Parental retrospective assessment of development and behavior in Asperger syndrome during the first 2 years of life. *Res. Autism Spectr. Disord.* **2010**, *4*, 461–473. [CrossRef]
30. Barnevik Olsson, M.; Carlsson, L.H.; Westerlund, J.; Gillberg, C.; Fernell, E. Autism before diagnosis: Crying, feeding and sleeping problems in the first two years of life. *Acta Paediatr.* **2013**, *102*, 635–639. [CrossRef]
31. Deliens, G.; Leproult, R.; Schmitz, R.; Destrebecqz, A.; Peigneux, P. Sleep Disturbances in Autism Spectrum Disorders. *Rev. J. Autism Dev. Disord.* **2015**, *2*, 343–356. [CrossRef]
32. Rossignol, D.A.; Frye, R.E. Psychotropic Medications for Sleep Disorders in Autism Spectrum Disorders. In *Handbook of Autism and Pervasive Developmental Disorders*; John Wiley & Sons, Inc.: Hoboken, NJ, USA, 2021.
33. Williams, K.; Brignell, A.; Randall, M.; Silove, N.; Hazell, P. Selective serotonin reuptake inhibitors (SSRIs) for autism spectrum disorders (ASD). *Cochrane Database Syst. Rev.* **2013**, *8*, Cd004677. [CrossRef] [PubMed]
34. Carmody, J.; Baer, R.A. Relationships between mindfulness practice and levels of mindfulness, medical and psychological symptoms and well-being in a mindfulness-based stress reduction program. *J. Behav. Med.* **2008**, *31*, 23–33. [CrossRef] [PubMed]
35. Scully, D.; Kremer, J.; Meade, M.M.; Graham, R.; Dudgeon, K. Physical exercise and psychological well being: A critical review. *Br. J. Sports Med.* **1998**, *32*, 111–120. [CrossRef] [PubMed]
36. Williams Buckley, A.; Hirtz, D.; Oskoui, M.; Armstrong, M.J.; Batra, A.; Bridgemohan, C.; Coury, D.; Dawson, G.; Donley, D.; Findling, R.L.; et al. Practice guideline: Treatment for insomnia and disrupted sleep behavior in children and adolescents with autism spectrum disorder: Report of the Guideline Development, Dissemination, and Implementation Subcommittee of the American Academy of Neurology. *Neurology* **2020**, *94*, 392–404. [CrossRef]
37. Panju, S.; Brian, J.; Dupuis, A.; Anagnostou, E.; Kushki, A. Atypical sympathetic arousal in children with autism spectrum disorder and its association with anxiety symptomatology. *Mol. Autism* **2015**, *6*, 64. [CrossRef]
38. Kushki, A.; Drumm, E.; Pla Mobarak, M.; Tanel, N.; Dupuis, A.; Chau, T.; Anagnostou, E. Investigating the autonomic nervous system response to anxiety in children with autism spectrum disorders. *PLoS ONE* **2013**, *8*, e59730. [CrossRef]
39. Ferguson, B.J.; Marler, S.; Altstein, L.L.; Lee, E.B.; Akers, J.; Sohl, K.; McLaughlin, A.; Hartnett, K.; Kille, B.; Mazurek, M.; et al. Psychophysiological Associations with Gastrointestinal Symptomatology in Autism Spectrum Disorder. *Autism Res. Off. J. Int. Soc. Autism Res.* **2017**, *10*, 276–288. [CrossRef] [PubMed]
40. Daluwatte, C.; Miles, J.H.; Sun, J.; Yao, G. Association between pupillary light reflex and sensory behaviors in children with autism spectrum disorders. *Res. Dev. Disabil.* **2015**, *37*, 209–215. [CrossRef]
41. Tyler, W.J.; Boasso, A.M.; Mortimore, H.M.; Silva, R.S.; Charlesworth, J.D.; Marlin, M.A.; Aebersold, K.; Aven, L.; Wetmore, D.Z.; Pal, S.K. Transdermal neuromodulation of noradrenergic activity suppresses psychophysiological and biochemical stress responses in humans. *Sci. Rep.* **2015**, *5*, 13865. [CrossRef] [PubMed]
42. Cook, I.A.; Schrader, L.M.; Degiorgio, C.M.; Miller, P.R.; Maremont, E.R.; Leuchter, A.F. Trigeminal nerve stimulation in major depressive disorder: Acute outcomes in an open pilot study. *Epilepsy Behav.* **2013**, *28*, 221–226. [CrossRef]
43. Couto, L.B.; Moroni, C.R.; dos Reis Ferreira, C.M.; Elias-Filho, D.H.; Parada, C.A.; Pela, I.R.; Coimbra, N.C. Descriptive and functional neuroanatomy of locus coeruleus-noradrenaline-containing neurons involvement in bradykinin-induced antinociception on principal sensory trigeminal nucleus. *J. Chem. Neuroanat.* **2006**, *32*, 28–45. [CrossRef] [PubMed]
44. Aston-Jones, G.; Shipley, M.T.; Chouvet, G.; Ennis, M.; van Bockstaele, E.; Pieribone, V.; Shiekhattar, R.; Akaoka, H.; Drolet, G.; Astier, B.; et al. Afferent regulation of locus coeruleus neurons: Anatomy, physiology and pharmacology. *Prog. Brain Res.* **1991**, *88*, 47–75. [CrossRef] [PubMed]
45. Berridge, C.W.; Waterhouse, B.D. The locus coeruleus-noradrenergic system: Modulation of behavioral state and state-dependent cognitive processes. *Brain Res. Brain Res. Rev.* **2003**, *42*, 33–84. [CrossRef]
46. McGough, J.J.; Sturm, A.; Cowen, J.; Tung, K.; Salgari, G.C.; Leuchter, A.F.; Cook, I.A.; Sugar, C.A.; Loo, S.K. Double-Blind, Sham-Controlled, Pilot Study of Trigeminal Nerve Stimulation for Attention-Deficit/Hyperactivity Disorder. *J. Am. Acad. Child. Adolesc. Psychiatry* **2019**, *58*, 403–411 e403. [CrossRef]
47. Blech, B.; Starling, A.J. Noninvasive Neuromodulation in Migraine. *Curr. Pain Headache Rep.* **2020**, *24*, 78. [CrossRef]
48. Trevizol, A.P.; Shiozawa, P.; Albuquerque Sato, I.; da Silva, M.E.; de Barros Calfat, E.L.; Alberto, R.L.; Cook, I.A.; Cordeiro, Q. Trigeminal Nerve Stimulation (TNS) for Post-traumatic Stress Disorder: A Case Study. *Brain Stimul.* **2015**, *8*, 676–678. [CrossRef]
49. Trevizol, A.P.; Shiozawa, P.; Sato, I.A.; Calfat, E.L.; Alberto, R.L.; Cook, I.A.; Medeiros, H.H.; Cordeiro, Q. Trigeminal Nerve Stimulation (TNS) for Generalized Anxiety Disorder: A Case Study. *Brain Stimul.* **2015**, *8*, 659–660. [CrossRef]
50. Zhang, R.; Jia, M.X.; Zhang, J.S.; Xu, X.J.; Shou, X.J.; Zhang, X.T.; Li, L.; Li, N.; Han, S.P.; Han, J.S. Transcutaneous electrical acupoint stimulation in children with autism and its impact on plasma levels of arginine-vasopressin and oxytocin: A prospective single-blinded controlled study. *Res. Dev. Disabil.* **2012**, *33*, 1136–1146. [CrossRef]
51. Zhang, J.S.; Zhang, X.T.; Zou, L.P.; Zhang, R.; Han, S.P.; Han, J.S. [A Preliminary Study on Effect of Transcutaneous Electrical Acupoint Stimulation for Children with Autism]. *Zhen Ci Yan Jiu* **2017**, *42*, 249–253.

52. Wang, X.; Ding, R.; Song, Y.; Wang, J.; Zhang, C.; Han, S.; Han, J.; Zhang, R. Transcutaneous Electrical Acupoint Stimulation in Early Life Changes Synaptic Plasticity and Improves Symptoms in a Valproic Acid-Induced Rat Model of Autism. *Neural Plast.* **2020**, *2020*, 8832694. [CrossRef]
53. Jin, Y.; Kong, J. Transcutaneous Vagus Nerve Stimulation: A Promising Method for Treatment of Autism Spectrum Disorders. *Front. Neurosci.* **2016**, *10*, 609. [CrossRef]
54. Eldridge, S.M.; Chan, C.L.; Campbell, M.J.; Bond, C.M.; Hopewell, S.; Thabane, L.; Lancaster, G.A. CONSORT 2010 statement: Extension to randomised pilot and feasibility trials. *BMJ* **2016**, *355*, i5239. [CrossRef]
55. Birmaher, B.; Khetarpal, S.; Brent, D.; Cully, M.; Balach, L.; Kaufman, J.; Neer, S.M. The Screen for Child Anxiety Related Emotional Disorders (SCARED): Scale construction and psychometric characteristics. *J. Am. Acad. Child. Adolesc. Psychiatry* **1997**, *36*, 545–553. [CrossRef]
56. Blakeley-Smith, A.; Reaven, J.; Ridge, K.; Hepburn, S. Parent–child agreement of anxiety symptoms in youth with autism spectrum disorders. *Res. Autism Spectr. Disord.* **2012**, *6*, 707–716. [CrossRef]
57. Stern, J.A.; Gadgil, M.S.; Blakeley-Smith, A.; Reaven, J.A.; Hepburn, S.L. Psychometric Properties of the SCARED in Youth with Autism Spectrum Disorder. *Res. Autism Spectr. Disord.* **2014**, *8*, 1225–1234. [CrossRef]
58. Behrens, B.; Swetlitz, C.; Pine, D.S.; Pagliaccio, D. The Screen for Child Anxiety Related Emotional Disorders (SCARED): Informant Discrepancy, Measurement Invariance, and Test-Retest Reliability. *Child. Psychiatry Hum. Dev.* **2019**, *50*, 473–482. [CrossRef] [PubMed]
59. Scahill, L.; Lecavalier, L.; Schultz, R.T.; Evans, A.N.; Maddox, B.; Pritchett, J.; Herrington, J.; Gillespie, S.; Miller, J.; Amoss, R.T.; et al. Development of the Parent-Rated Anxiety Scale for Youth With Autism Spectrum Disorder. *J. Am. Acad. Child. Adolesc. Psychiatry* **2019**, *58*, 887–896.e882. [CrossRef]
60. Moore, M.; Evans, V.; Hanvey, G.; Johnson, C. Assessment of Sleep in Children with Autism Spectrum Disorder. *Children* **2017**, *4*, 72. [CrossRef] [PubMed]
61. Tombaugh, T.N. A comprehensive review of the Paced Auditory Serial Addition Test (PASAT). *Arch. Clin. Neuropsychol.* **2006**, *21*, 53–76. [CrossRef]
62. Parsons, T.D.; Courtney, C.G. An initial validation of the Virtual Reality Paced Auditory Serial Addition Test in a college sample. *J. Neurosci. Methods* **2014**, *222*, 15–23. [CrossRef] [PubMed]
63. Johnson, S.K.; Lange, G.; DeLuca, J.; Korn, L.R.; Natelson, B. The effects of fatigue on neuropsychological performance in patients with chronic fatigue syndrome, multiple sclerosis, and depression. *Appl. Neuropsychol.* **1997**, *4*, 145–153. [CrossRef] [PubMed]
64. Habib, A.; Harris, L.; Pollick, F.; Melville, C. A meta-analysis of working memory in individuals with autism spectrum disorders. *PLoS ONE* **2019**, *14*, e0216198. [CrossRef]
65. Peirce, J.; Gray, J.R.; Simpson, S.; MacAskill, M.; Höchenberger, R.; Sogo, H.; Kastman, E.; Lindeløv, J.K. PsychoPy2: Experiments in behavior made easy. *Behav. Res. Methods* **2019**, *51*, 195–203. [CrossRef]
66. Speer, K.E.; Semple, S.; Naumovski, N.; McKune, A.J. Measuring Heart Rate Variability Using Commercially Available Devices in Healthy Children: A Validity and Reliability Study. *Eur. J. Investig. Health Psychol. Educ.* **2020**, *10*, 390–404. [CrossRef] [PubMed]
67. Chalmers, J.A.; Quintana, D.S.; Abbott, M.J.; Kemp, A.H. Anxiety Disorders are Associated with Reduced Heart Rate Variability: A Meta-Analysis. *Front. Psychiatry* **2014**, *5*, 80. [CrossRef]
68. Benedek, M.; Kaernbach, C. A continuous measure of phasic electrodermal activity. *J. Neurosci. Methods* **2010**, *190*, 80–91. [CrossRef]
69. Caporino, N.E.; Sakolsky, D.; Brodman, D.M.; McGuire, J.F.; Piacentini, J.; Peris, T.S.; Ginsburg, G.S.; Walkup, J.T.; Iyengar, S.; Kendall, P.C.; et al. Establishing Clinical Cutoffs for Response and Remission on the Screen for Child Anxiety Related Emotional Disorders (SCARED). *J. Am. Acad. Child Adolesc. Psychiatry* **2017**, *56*, 696–702. [CrossRef]
70. Schiltz, H.K.; Magnus, B.E. Differential Item Functioning Based on Autism Features, IQ, and Age on the Screen for Child Anxiety Related Disorders (SCARED) Among Youth on the Autism Spectrum. *Autism Res. Off. J. Int. Soc. Autism Res.* **2021**, *14*, 1220–1236. [CrossRef]
71. Qiu, J.; Kong, X.; Li, J.; Yang, J.; Huang, Y.; Huang, M.; Sun, B.; Su, J.; Chen, H.; Wan, G.; et al. Transcranial Direct Current Stimulation (tDCS) over the Left Dorsal Lateral Prefrontal Cortex in Children with Autism Spectrum Disorder (ASD). *Neural Plast.* **2021**, *2021*, 6627507. [CrossRef]
72. Keogh, S.; Bridle, C.; Siriwardena, N.A.; Nadkarni, A.; Laparidou, D.; Durrant, S.J.; Kargas, N.; Law, G.R.; Curtis, F. Effectiveness of non-pharmacological interventions for insomnia in children with Autism Spectrum Disorder: A systematic review and meta-analysis. *PLoS ONE* **2019**, *14*, e0221428. [CrossRef]
73. Giannotti, F.; Cortesi, F.; Cerquiglini, A.; Bernabei, P. An open-label study of controlled-release melatonin in treatment of sleep disorders in children with autism. *J. Autism Dev. Disord.* **2006**, *36*, 741–752. [CrossRef]
74. Pardo, G.; Coates, S.; Okuda, D.T. Outcome measures assisting treatment optimization in multiple sclerosis. *J. Neurol.* **2021**. Available online: https://link.springer.com/article/10.1007/s00415-021-10674-8 (accessed on 31 August 2021). [CrossRef]
75. Corbett, B.A.; Muscatello, R.A.; Kim, A.; Patel, K.; Vandekar, S. Developmental effects in physiological stress in early adolescents with and without autism spectrum disorder. *Psychoneuroendocrinology* **2021**, *125*, 105115. [CrossRef]
76. Levine, T.P.; Sheinkopf, S.J.; Pescosolido, M.; Rodino, A.; Elia, G.; Lester, B. Physiologic Arousal to Social Stress in Children with Autism Spectrum Disorders: A Pilot Study. *Res. Autism Spectr. Disord.* **2012**, *6*, 177–183. [CrossRef]

77. Taylor, J.L.; Corbett, B.A. A review of rhythm and responsiveness of cortisol in individuals with autism spectrum disorders. *Psychoneuroendocrinology* **2014**, *49*, 207–228. [CrossRef]
78. Hollocks, M.J.; Pickles, A.; Howlin, P.; Simonoff, E. Dual Cognitive and Biological Correlates of Anxiety in Autism Spectrum Disorders. *J. Autism Dev. Disord.* **2016**, *46*, 3295–3307. [CrossRef]
79. Corbett, B.A.; Mendoza, S.; Abdullah, M.; Wegelin, J.A.; Levine, S. Cortisol circadian rhythms and response to stress in children with autism. *Psychoneuroendocrinology* **2006**, *31*, 59–68. [CrossRef] [PubMed]
80. Corbett, B.A.; Mendoza, S.; Wegelin, J.A.; Carmean, V.; Levine, S. Variable cortisol circadian rhythms in children with autism and anticipatory stress. *J. Psychiatry Neurosci.* **2008**, *33*, 227–234. [PubMed]
81. Corbett, B.A.; Schupp, C.W.; Levine, S.; Mendoza, S. Comparing cortisol, stress, and sensory sensitivity in children with autism. *Autism Res. Off. J. Int. Soc. Autism Res.* **2009**, *2*, 39–49. [CrossRef] [PubMed]
82. Kuiper, M.W.M.; Verhoeven, E.W.M.; Geurts, H.M. Heart rate variability predicts inhibitory control in adults with autism spectrum disorders. *Biol. Psychol.* **2017**, *128*, 141–152. [CrossRef] [PubMed]
83. Thapa, R.; Alvares, G.A.; Zaidi, T.A.; Thomas, E.E.; Hickie, I.B.; Park, S.H.; Guastella, A.J. Reduced heart rate variability in adults with autism spectrum disorder. *Autism Res. Off. J. Int. Soc. Autism Res.* **2019**, *12*, 922–930. [CrossRef]
84. Dijkhuis, R.R.; Ziermans, T.; van Rijn, S.; Staal, W.; Swaab, H. Emotional Arousal During Social Stress in Young Adults With Autism: Insights From Heart Rate, Heart Rate Variability and Self-Report. *J. Autism Dev. Disord.* **2019**, *49*, 2524–2535. [CrossRef]
85. Cai, R.Y.; Richdale, A.L.; Dissanayake, C.; Uljarevic, M. Resting heart rate variability, emotion regulation, psychological wellbeing and autism symptomatology in adults with and without autism. *Int. J. Psychophysiol. Off. J. Int. Organ. Psychophysiol.* **2019**, *137*, 54–62. [CrossRef] [PubMed]
86. Bujnakova, I.; Ondrejka, I.; Mestanik, M.; Visnovcova, Z.; Mestanikova, A.; Hrtanek, I.; Fleskova, D.; Calkovska, A.; Tonhajzerova, I. Autism spectrum disorder is associated with autonomic underarousal. *Physiol. Res.* **2016**, *65*, S673–S682. [CrossRef]
87. Harder, R.; Malow, B.A.; Goodpaster, R.L.; Iqbal, F.; Halbower, A.; Goldman, S.E.; Fawkes, D.B.; Wang, L.; Shi, Y.; Baudenbacher, F.; et al. Heart rate variability during sleep in children with autism spectrum disorder. *Clin. Auton. Res. Off. J. Clin. Auton. Res. Soc.* **2016**, *26*, 423–432. [CrossRef] [PubMed]
88. Wang, Y.; Hensley, M.K.; Tasman, A.; Sears, L.; Casanova, M.F.; Sokhadze, E.M. Heart Rate Variability and Skin Conductance During Repetitive TMS Course in Children with Autism. *Appl. Psychophysiol. Biofeedback* **2016**, *41*, 47–60. [CrossRef] [PubMed]
89. Vidyashree, H.M.; Maheshkumar, K.; Sundareswaran, L.; Sakthivel, G.; Partheeban, P.K.; Rajan, R. Effect of Yoga Intervention on Short-Term Heart Rate Variability in Children with Autism Spectrum Disorder. *Int. J. Yoga* **2019**, *12*, 73–77. [CrossRef]
90. Casanova, M.F.; Hensley, M.K.; Sokhadze, E.M.; El-Baz, A.S.; Wang, Y.; Li, X.; Sears, L. Effects of weekly low-frequency rTMS on autonomic measures in children with autism spectrum disorder. *Front. Hum. Neurosci.* **2014**, *8*, 851. [CrossRef]

Journal of *Personalized Medicine*

MDPI

Review

Parental Quality of Life and Involvement in Intervention for Children or Adolescents with Autism Spectrum Disorders: A Systematic Review

Alessandro Musetti [1,*], Tommaso Manari [1], Barbara Dioni [1,2], Cinzia Raffin [2], Giulia Bravo [2], Rachele Mariani [3], Gianluca Esposito [4,5,6], Dagmara Dimitriou [7,8], Giuseppe Plazzi [9,10], Christian Franceschini [11] and Paola Corsano [1]

1 Department of Humanities, Social Sciences and Cultural Industries, University of Parma, Borgo Carissimi 10, 43121 Parma, Italy; tommaso.manari@unipr.it (T.M.); barbara.dioni@unipr.it (B.D.); paola.corsano@unipr.it (P.C.)
2 Fondazione Bambini e Autismo Onlus, 33170 Pordenone, Italy; c.raffin@bambinieautismo.org (C.R.); g.bravo@bambinieautismo.org (G.B.)
3 Department of Dynamic and Clinical Psychology, Sapienza University of Rome, 00185 Rome, Italy; rachele.mariani@uniroma1.it
4 Social and Affective Neuroscience Lab, Psychology Program-SSS, Nanyang Technological University, Singapore 639818, Singapore; gianluca.esposito@unitn.it
5 Lee Kong Chian School of Medicine, Nanyang Technological University, Singapore 636921, Singapore
6 Affiliative Behaviour and Physiology Lab, Department of Psychology and Cognitive Science, University Trento, 38068 Rovereto, Italy
7 Sleep Education and Research Laboratory, Department of Psychology and Human Development, UCL-Institute of Education, London WC1H 0AA, UK; d.dimitriou@ucl.ac.uk
8 The National Institute for Stress, Anxiety, Depression and Behavioural Change (NISAD), 252 21 Helsingborg, Sweden
9 Department of Biomedical, Metabolic and Neural Sciences, University of Modena and Reggio Emilia, 41125 Modena, Italy; giuseppe.plazzi@unimore.it
10 IRCCS Institute of Neurological Sciences of Bologna (ISNB), 40139 Bologna, Italy
11 Department of Medicine and Surgery, University of Parma, 43121 Parma, Italy; Christian.franceschini@unipr.it
* Correspondence: alessandro.musetti@unipr.it; Tel.: +39-0521-034820

Citation: Musetti, A.; Manari, T.; Dioni, B.; Raffin, C.; Bravo, G.; Mariani, R.; Esposito, G.; Dimitriou, D.; Plazzi, G.; Franceschini, C.; et al. Parental Quality of Life and Involvement in Intervention for Children or Adolescents with Autism Spectrum Disorders: A Systematic Review. *J. Pers. Med.* **2021**, *11*, 894. https://doi.org/10.3390/jpm11090894

Academic Editors: Richard E. Frye, Richard Boles, Shannon Rose and Daniel Rossignol

Received: 4 August 2021
Accepted: 6 September 2021
Published: 8 September 2021

Publisher's Note: MDPI stays neutral with regard to jurisdictional claims in published maps and institutional affiliations.

Copyright: © 2021 by the authors. Licensee MDPI, Basel, Switzerland. This article is an open access article distributed under the terms and conditions of the Creative Commons Attribution (CC BY) license (https://creativecommons.org/licenses/by/4.0/).

Abstract: Previous research has examined several parental, child-related, and contextual factors associated with parental quality of life (QoL) among parents with a child or an adolescent with autism spectrum disorders (ASD); however, no systematic review has examined the relationship between parental QoL and parental involvement in intervention. To fill this gap, a systematic review was conducted using four electronic databases and checked reference lists of retrieved studies. Records were included in the systematic review if they presented original data, assessed parental QoL, and involvement in intervention for children or adolescents with ASD, were published in peer-reviewed journals between 2000 and 2020, and were written in English. Among the 96 screened full-texts, 17 articles met the eligibility criteria. The selected studies included over 2000 parents of children or adolescents with ASD. Three categories of parental involvement (i.e., none, indirect, direct) were identified, which varied across studies, although most had direct parental involvement. The results from this review show that increased parental involvement in the intervention for children or adolescents with ASD may be one way to promote their QoL. However, further research specifically focused on parental involvement during the intervention for children and adolescents with ASD is warranted.

Keywords: autism spectrum disorder; quality of life; parents; intervention; systematic review

1. Introduction

Autism spectrum disorder (ASD) is a pervasive neurodevelopmental disorder characterised by persistent atypicalities in social communication and social interactions across different domains, together with restricted, repetitive, stereotyped patterns of behaviour, interest, or activities [1]. Although there is large variability in the expression of ASD symptoms, many individuals with ASD need lifelong assistance in daily life that is usually provided by family members, especially parents [2]. Therefore, the presence of a family member with ASD features such as challenging behaviours [3,4] or sleep problems [5,6] can significantly affect and challenge the entire family system [7], with a mostly negative impact on the quality of life (QoL) and on the relationship quality of closer family members such as siblings [8,9] and parents [10,11].

Although a lot of research has been conducted to examine the relationship between the characteristics of offspring with ASD, distress and psychological difficulties of family members [12,13], less attention has been paid to the impact of the characteristics of the intervention on family functioning [14,15]. Moreover, most of the research on interventions for ASD has so far been focused on child outcomes, disregarding the impact on parents [14]. This is surprising, given the increasing parental involvement in activities of children and adolescents with ASD [16,17] including the intervention process [18]. In many cases, parental involvement in intervention covers a broad range of activities, from parent training and homework routines, even participation in intervention design and implementation [19]. Therefore, taking into account the family outcomes, it would be possible to gain a more comprehensive view of the effectiveness of an intervention and, in turn, better shape intervention design and implementation [14,20,21]. Most early research in this field unilaterally focused on the negative outcomes (e.g., parental stress) of having a child with ASD [22]. However, a growing number of studies have investigated parental QoL in an endeavour to attempt to capture the variability of parental adaptation and to more deeply comprehend difficulties faced by these parents [23,24]. This interesting broadening of perspective highlights how some parents can cope with the stress resulting from caring for their children with ASD, and in turn, learn and improve their competencies in the process [25,26]. For example, when mothers are able to gain emotional resolution on their child's diagnosis of ASD, they tend to develop a more supportive parenting style [27]. QoL is a multidimensional and wide-ranging construct, characterized by the individual's emotional, physical, and financial well-being, interpersonal relationships, goals, expectations and concerns, and their interactions with salient features of the environment [28,29]. According to the World Health Organization (WHO) Quality of Life Assessment Group [30], QoL is defined as an "individual's perception of their position in life in the context of the culture and value systems in which they live, and in relation to their goals, expectations, standards, and concerns" (p. 11). Up to date, only one study [24] has systematically reviewed published literature about the parental QoL of children and adolescents with ASD. Thus far, several variables have been found to be associated with lower QoL among parents of children and adolescents with ASD including parental characteristics (e.g., being a mother, parental mental health problems, maladaptive parental coping strategies, and low parental self-efficacy), child characteristics (e.g., child behavioural problems, child emotional problems, ASD severity, and child's age), and contextual factors (e.g., low employment status, low household income, low availability of social and professional support, and lack of participation in health promoting activities). However, no systematic review exists that summarizes the currently available evidence on the relationship between parental QoL and parental involvement in intervention for their children or adolescents with ASD. This constitutes a relevant gap in the literature considering the recent increased emphasis on family-focused versus professional-driven interventions [14,31], which the present study intends to fill. Specifically, a previous systematic review on parental QoL of children of ASD by Vasilopoulou et al. [24] revealed a need for greater focus on parents to provide tailored intervention for this population. The current review aimed to identify and discuss the role of parental involvement in intervention in relation to QoL among the parents of children or adolescents with ASD.

2. Methods

2.1. Protocol and Registration

The present systematic review adhered to the Preferred Reporting Items for Systematic Reviews and Meta-Analyses (PRISMA) statement [32]. The protocol was registered at the International Prospective Register of Systematic Reviews (PROSPERO) data repository in February 2021 (registration code: CRD42021230103).

2.2. Study Selection

The selection process identified the following eligibility criteria. Inclusion criteria (IC): (IC1) studies had to be focused on parents of children and adolescents (i.e., <21 years old) with a formal diagnosis of ASD; (IC2) they had to contain quantitative, qualitative, or mixed methods approaches; and (IC3) be published between 2000 and 2020 in (IC4) peer-reviewed journals and written in English. We rejected articles that met one of the following excluding criteria (EX): (EX1) case reports, commentaries, editorials, meeting abstracts were not considered; (EX2) other review articles were consulted but not included finally and to narrow our search procedure, and we excluded (EX3) studies that dealt with the quality of life of parents of children with disabilities different from ASD.

A systematic search was carried out in January 2021, in four online databases: Scopus, Web of Science, PubMed, and PsycINFO. To reduce the risk of methodological biases, no filters were applied in the preliminary searches. We combined the selected keywords with the Boolean operators AND/OR in the following order: ("parent*") AND ("ASD") OR ("autis*") AND ("quality") AND ("life") AND ("intervent*"), in Titles, Abstracts, and Keywords.

All references collected through database searches were exported to the systematic reviews web application Rayyan (https://rayyan.qcri.org/ (accessed on 1 August 2021)). Duplicate records were ruled out, then the titles and abstracts of all remaining articles were independently screened. The use of multiple reviewers may reduce the risk of rejecting relevant reports, as noted by Edwards and colleagues [33]. Results were then compared and in the case of disagreement, the conflicting choices were inspected and discussed further until a consensus was reached. The second step included the screening of the full-texts of the chosen studies, in order to select those where the quality of life was a specified outcome. Reference lists of relevant studies and reviews were examined for additional pertinent records. The articles deemed eligible by all reviewers and that met all the inclusion criteria were included for the final screening, and those that met at least one exclusion criteria were formally excluded with reasons.

2.3. Quality Assessment

The critical assessment of each paper was conducted with AXIS, a quality assessment tool for observational and cross-sectional studies [34]. It comprises a checklist of 20 items to evaluate the overall study design as well as the risk of bias. The items were scored as follows: Yes = 1, No and Don't know = 0, and resulted in a final score that ranged from 0 to 20, with higher scores indicating a higher assessed quality. Adopting the classification used in other literature reviews (e.g., [35]), we further distinguished three quality ratings: low quality (0–7 points), moderate quality (8–14 points), and high quality (15–20 points). The qualitative assessment outcome is discussed in the Results section.

3. Results

3.1. Study Selection

The systematic search was first performed in four online databases: Scopus, Web of Science, PubMed, and PsycINFO, and yielded a total of 1217 records. Duplicate articles were removed with the reference manager Mendeley desktop (https://www.mendeley.com/ (accessed on 1 August 2021)) and resulted in 808 unique references, which were imported to the systematic reviews web application Rayyan (https://rayyan.qcri.org/ (accessed on 1 August 2021)). Titles and abstracts were then independently screened for potentially relevant papers, resulting in 96 eligible references and 712 excluded because they did not meet the predefined inclusion criteria. As the last step, 79 full-texts were excluded with reasons (e.g., non-pertinent, non-pertinent outcome, no empirical data, or without intervention for children with ASD) and 17 articles were found to be appropriate for the qualitative synthesis. The four steps defined in the PRISMA procedure (i.e., Identification, Screening, Eligibility, and Inclusion) are represented in Figure 1 and the excluded articles are listed in Supplementary Table S1.

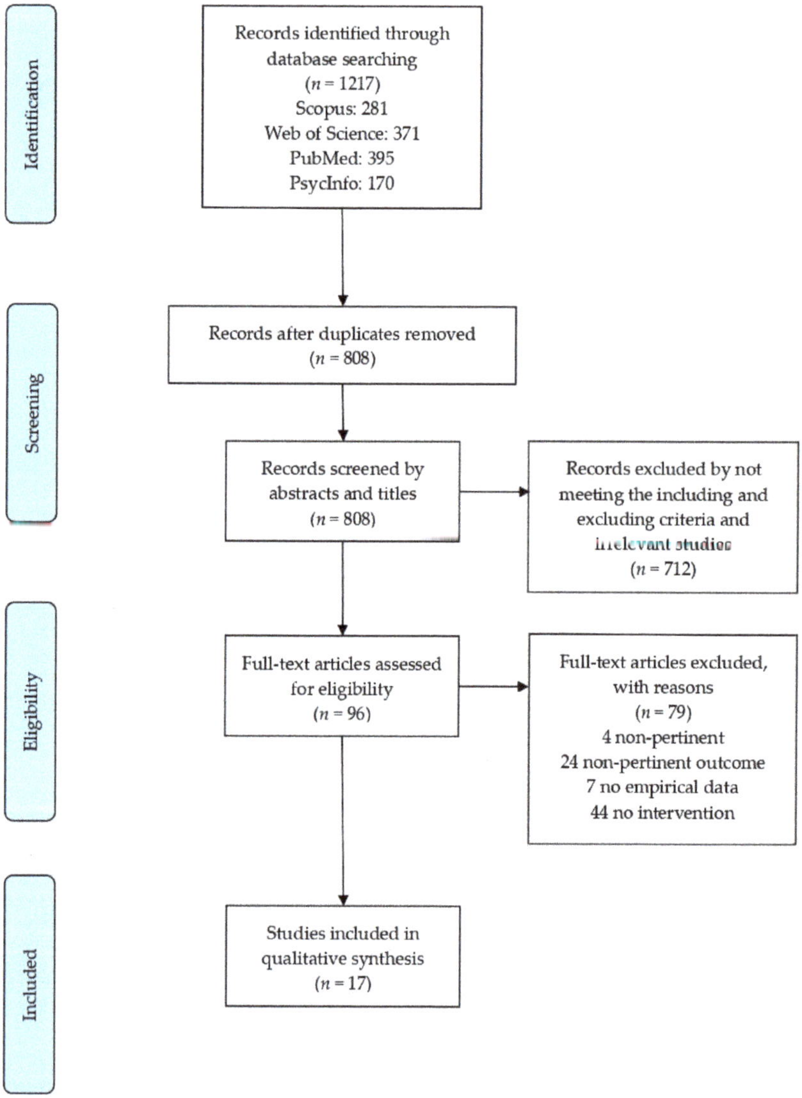

Figure 1. Flow diagram of the search strategy. Modified from the Preferred Reporting Items for Systematic reviews and Meta-Analyses statement flow diagram [32].

3.2. Study Characteristics

A summary of the information extracted from each study is presented in Table 1. The present systematic review examined 17 studies that were published between 2011 and

2020 in peer-reviewed journals that focused on the intrafamilial QoL of parents with a child or an adolescent affected by ASD. The adopted methodological designs were mixed and included cross-sectional designs, qualitative and observational studies, randomized controlled trials, and a validation study.

The reviewed studies involved a total of 1965 children and adolescents and 2040 parents or primary caregivers (partial information was available from three studies). The age of the offspring ranged from 2 to 20 years old ($M = 7.43$, $SD = 3.22$), and 74.48% of the involved participants were female (mothers or female caregivers; partial information was available from three studies).

In relation to the geographical distribution (i.e., where the study was conducted and the data was collected), the 17 studies were carried out in Europe ($n = 8$, United Kingdom, France, Sweden), North America ($n = 2$, United States, Canada), Asia ($n = 2$, China, Taiwan), and Australia ($n = 5$).

The present systematic review was focused on parenting education programmes and interventions. Similarly to previous studies (e.g., [36]), we distinguished between three levels of parental involvement: none (i.e., parents are not involved in intervention design and implementation), indirect (i.e., parents are involved in secondary forms of interventions such as parent training or homework routines), and direct (i.e., parents are actively involved in primary intervention development and implementation).

Accordingly, we identified a heterogeneous number of studies that included no ($n = 2$), indirect ($n = 3$), or direct ($n = 12$) levels of parental involvement. The interventions were performed in clinical settings ($n = 7$), at home ($n = 4$), or a combination of the two (i.e., mixed settings, n = 3; information not available for three records).

The construct dimensions related to the parental QoL were assessed with multiple instruments (see Table 2) including the Family Quality of Life Scale [37], the Parenting Stress Index [38], and the WHOQOL-BREF [28]. Since different studies implemented qualitative and observational approaches, semi-structured interviews, questionnaires, and ad-hoc rating scales were also used.

Table 1. Characteristics of the reviewed studies ($n = 17$).

Authors (Year)	Location	Study Design	Sample Characteristics *N* Age = *M* (*SD*)	Parental Involvement	Intervention	Setting	Length/Frequency	Instruments	Relevant Findings
Aandersson et al. (2017) [39]	Sweden	Qualitative study	56 Parents of Children with ASD ($n = 56$ Children; $M_{age} \approx 9$ Years, Female = 23.21%)	Indirect	Early Intervention, ABA	Clinics	2 Years/25 h/Week	Semi-Structured Questionnaire	Thematic Content Analysis Too much responsivity and lack of knowledge about intervention methods. Perceived support as unequal, uncoordinated, and with variations. Unequal treatments depending on socioeconomic status. lack of individualization of interventions.
Baghdadli et al. (2014) [10]	France	Cross-Sectional	152 Mothers (92.12%) and 13 Fathers of Adolescents with ASD ($n = 152$ Adolescents; $M_{age} = 15$ Years; $SD = 1.6$, Female = 17.8%)	None	Mixed	Clinics	NA/31.3 5 h/week	Par-DD-QoL	Polytomic Logistic Regression Analysis A higher number of hours of specialized intervention is associated with lower parental emotional QoL (ORa = 2.69, 95% CI = 1.1–5.9, $p = 0.04$).
Derguy et al. (2018) [40]	France	Cross-Sectional	115 Parents (Female = 63.5%) of Children with ASD ($n = 78$ Children; $M_{age} = 6.3$, $SD = 2.3$, Female = 23.1%)	None	Psycho-Educational Intervention (74% of the Sample)	NA	NA	WHOQOL-BREF	Hierarchical Regression Analyses Parents showed better QoL whether their child received psychoeducation intervention ($\beta = 0.25$, $p = 0.010$).
Due et al. (2018) [41]	Australia	Mixed-Method Study	27 Parents (Female = 48.14%) of Children with ASD ($n = 27$ Children; $M_{age} = 5$, $SD = 2.0$, Female = 18.52%)	Direct	Early Intervention	Clinics	NA	Quality of Life in Autism Questionnaire; Semi-Structured Interviews	Thematic Content Analysis Parental direct involvement in the intervention increased several aspects of their QoL (e.g., sense of competence and confidence as parents, community participation).
Hwang et al. (2015) [42]	Taiwan	Pre-Post Design	6 Mother-Child dyads (Children with ASD; Age Range = 8–15 Years, Female = 20%)	Direct	Parent-Mediated Home-Based Training	Home	12 Months	Family Quality of Life (FQoL)	Paired Sample Wilcoxon Signed Rank Test The parent-mediated home-based training was associated with marginally significant increase in family quality of life.
Ji et al. (2014) [43]	China	Quasi-Experimental Design	22 Caregivers (Female = 90.9%) of Children with ASD (Intervention Group, $n = 22$ Children with ADS; $M_{age} = 4.93$, $SD = 2.03$, Female = 18.2%) and 20 Caregivers (Female = 90.0%) of Children with ASD (control group, $n = 20$ Children with ASD, $M_{age} = 5.65$, $SD = 1.74$, Female = 15%)	Direct	Parent Education Program	Clinics	8 Weeks	Caregiver Burden Index (CBI)	Independent-Samples *t*-test Parents' mental HRQOL significantly improved after the intervention ($t = -2.138$; $p = 0.039$). Parents' physical HRQOL did not improve after the intervention ($t = -1463$; $p = 0.151$).

Table 1. *Cont.*

Authors (Year)	Location	Study Design	Sample Characteristics *N* Age = *M* (*SD*)	Parental Involvement	Intervention	Setting	Length/Frequency	Instruments	Relevant Findings
Jones et al. (2017) [44]	Canada	Cross-Sectional	151 Caregivers (Female = 78.95%) of children with ASD (n = 151 Children with ASD; M_{age} = 7.3, SD = 3.9, Female = 23.84%)	Indirect	None/Intensive Behavioural Intervention, Intervention from a Speech and Language Pathologist, Occupational Therapy, Physiotherapy Services	NA	NA	Family Quality of Life Survey (FQOLS)	Correlation Analyses Time on waiting list was not significatively associated with family QoL.
Leadbitter et al. (2018) [45]	United King-dom	Pre-Trial Research Design	152 Parents of Children with ASD (n = 152 Children with ASD, M_{age} = 45 Months, Female = 9.21%)	Direct	Parent-Mediated Video-Aided Pre-School Communication-Focused Intervention	Clinics	13 Months	Autism Family Experience Questionnaire (AFEQ)	Effect Estimation Analysis AFEQ total score improved significantly after the treatment and at the 6-year follow-up.
Leadbitter et al. (2020) [46]	United King-dom	Qualitative Study	18 Parents (Female = 66.67%) of Children with ASD (n = 12 Children with ASD, M_{age} = 44.42 Months, SD = 7.04, Female = 8.33%)	Direct	Paediatric Autism Communication Therapy	NA	12 Months	Semi-Structured Interview	Thematic Content Analysis Post-intervention improved family wellbeing.
Mathew et al. (2019) [47]	Australia	Cross-Sectional	161 Parents (Female = 90.7%) of Children with ASD (n = 117 Children with ASD, M_{age} = 4.13, SD = 0.53, Female = 17.9%)	Direct	Early Intervention using the Early Start Denver Model	Clinics	NA	Parenting Sense of Competence Scale (PSOC)	Independent-Samples t-test Significantly greater levels of depression symptoms, anxiety, and stress among mothers (who have the primary caregiver role) than among fathers of children with ASD.
McConkey (2020) [48]	United King-dom	Validation Study	449 Parents (Female = 92.6%) of Children with ASD or with Suspected ASD (n = 449 Children with ASD, Age Range = 2–11 years, Female = 25.6%)	Direct	Family-Centred Intervention	Home	Median = 8 Weeks	Eight Items Questionnaire	Step-Wise, Linear Regression Parental with adequate or poor engagement in intervention showed significantly lower parental well-being than those with good engagement in intervention (β = 4.72; SE 1.54; $p < 0.002$).
McConkey et al. (2020) [49]	United King-dom	Observational Study	92 Families with Children with ASD (n = 96 Children, M_{age} = 7.7, Female = 20.8%)	Direct	Post-Diagnostic Support	Home	12 Months	Two Rating Scales	Thematic Content Analysis Parents reported higher self-confidence and reduced stress within the family after the intervention.
McPhilemy & Dillen-burger (2013) [50]	United King-dom	Observational Study	15 Families with Children or Adolescents with ASD (n = 17 Children or Adolescents with ASD, M_{age}= 38 Months, Age Range = 2–20 Years, Female = 11.76%)	Direct	ABA-based Home Program	Home	M = 48 Months	Questionnaire	Thematic Content Analysis ABA-based home program had significant positive impact on family quality of life.

Table 1. *Cont.*

Authors (Year)	Location	Study Design	Sample Characteristics N Age = M (SD)	Parental Involvement	Intervention	Setting	Length/Frequency	Instruments	Relevant Findings
Milbourn et al. (2017) [51]	Australia/ Sweden	Observational/ Qualitative Study	521 Caregivers (Female = 81%) with Children with ASD (n = 400 Children with ASD (76.78%), M_{age} = 9.92, SD = 4.17, Female = 17%)	Direct	Mixed	NA	NA	Multidimensional Questionnaire	Thematic Content Analysis Respondents indicated that early interventions improved their family life (71.3% answered "somewhat" or "definitely"). Respondents agreed that earlier access to intervention would have led to improved child's quality of life (78.4% answered "somewhat" or "definitely").
Moody et al. (2019) [52]	United States	Randomised Controlled Trial	67 Parents (Active Group, Female = 91.0%; Waitlist, Female = 88.2%) of Children with ASD (n = 33 Intervention Group, Female = 18.2%) (n = 67 Children with ASD, Range age 2–8 Years, Female = 14.7%)	Direct	Colorado Parent Mentoring (CPM) Program	Mixed	Six Months	Family Quality of Life Survey (FQOLS)	Mixed Modelling CPM program positively impacted several areas of family quality of life, regardless the amount of formal intervention received.
Paynter et al. (2018) [53]	Australia	Mixed Methods	26 Fathers of Children with ASD (n = 26 Children with ASD, Age Range 2.5–6 Years, Female = 26.4%)	Indirect	Early Intervention	Clinics	NA	Parenting Stress Index (PSI)	Thematic Content Analysis According to some fathers' family adaptation was negatively affected by inaccessible and/or gender-biased formal supports.
Roberts et al. (2011) [54]	Australia	Randomised Controlled Trial	84 Children with ASD (n = 27 Home-Based Group, n = 29 Centre-Based Group, n = 28 Control, M_{age} = 3.5, SD = 0.61, Female = 9.5%)	Direct and Indirect	Early Intervention (Home-based Intervention vs. Centre-Based Intervention)	Home vs. Clinical Centres	1 Year (40 Weeks)	Family Quality of Life Survey (FQOLS), Parenting Stress Index (PSI)	Analysis of Covariance Parents of children who followed the centre-based intervention showed significant improvements in family QoL. Parents of children who followed the home-based intervention showed the least improvement in family QoL over all groups.

Table 2. Measurement instruments and construct dimensions listed in the included studies (n = 17).

	Measures of QoL	Construct Dimensions	Studies	No. of Studies
Family Quality of Life	Caregiver Burden Index (CBI) [55]	Time Burden, Burden of Personal Development Limitations, Physical Burden, Social Burden, Emotional Burden	Ji et al. (2014) [43]	1
	Family Quality of Life (FQOL) [37]	Emotional Wellbeing, Family Wellbeing, Parenting Wellbeing, Physical/Material Wellbeing, Disability-Related Wellbeing	Hwang et al. (2015) [42]; Moody et al. (2019) [52]; Roberts et al. (2011) [54]	3
	Family Quality of Life Survey (FQOLS) [56]	About Your Family, Health of the Family, Support from Disability-Related Services, Leisure and Recreation, Community Interaction, Overall Family Quality of Life	Jones et al. (2017) [44]	1
	Par-DD-QoL (from Par-ENT-QoL) [57]	Emotional Score, Daily Disturbances Score, Global Score	Baghdadli et al. (2014) [10]	1
	Parenting Sense of Competence Scale (PSOC) [58]	Satisfaction, Interest, Efficacy	Mathew et al. (2019) [47]	1
	Parenting Stress Index (PSI) [38]	Parental Distress, Parent-Child Dysfunctional Interaction, Difficult Child	Paynter et al. (2018) [53]; Roberts et al. (2011) [54]	2
	WHOQOL-BREF [38]	Four Domains (Physical, Psychological, Social Relationships, Environment)	Derguy et al. (2018) [40]	1
	Quality of Life in Autism questionnaire (QoLA) [59]	Subscale A (Quality of Life), Subscale B (Impact of ASD Symptoms)	Due et al. (2018) [41]	1

3.3. Quality Assessment

We implemented the AXIS tool [34] to evaluate each of the 17 included papers. The average quality score was 13.18 out of a total of 20 points (min = 7, max = 19, SD = 3.68), indicating a moderate quality among studies, with two low, eight moderate, and seven high quality ratings (Table 3). Globally, the aims and the objectives were clearly indicated (question number one) and the design was appropriate for the stated aims (question number two). Only three papers [40,43,54], however, reported a specific calculation of the effect size (question number three) to justify the chosen sample. Since the selected interventions were specifically aimed at children with ASD and their parents, the target population was clearly defined in 12 studies (question number four), and the selection process was found to be adequate for most of the studies (questions number five and six). Non-responders were infrequent in the reviewed samples, nevertheless, only one study [43] explicitly reported the measures undertaken to address them (question number seven). The outcome variables were appropriately estimated with suitable instruments in approximately half of the included studies (question number eight, negative scores n = 7; question number nine, negative scores n = 7), and the statistical methods and data were globally specified in sufficient detail (questions from 10 to 12). Overall, the discussions and authors' conclusions were justified by the achieved results, and the inherent limitations of the study designs were correctly presented (question number 18, negative scores n = 4).

Table 3. Quality assessments and total scores using the Appraisal Tool for Cross-Sectional Studies (AXIS).

Author (Year)	Q1	Q2	Q3	Q4	Q5	Q6	Q7	Q8	Q9	Q10	Q11	Q12	Q13 *	Q14	Q15	Q16	Q17	Q18	Q19 *	Q20	Quality Score/20	Quality Rating
Aandersson et al. (2017) [39]	Y	Y	N	N	Y	N	N	N	N	N	N	Y	N	N	Y	Y	Y	Y	N	Y	11	Moderate
Baghdadli et al. (2014) [10]	Y	N	N	Y	Y	Y	N	N	N	Y	N	Y	N	N	Y	Y	Y	Y	N	Y	13	Moderate
Derguy et al. (2018) [40]	Y	Y	Y	Y	Y	Y	N	Y	Y	Y	N	Y	N	N	Y	Y	Y	Y	N	Y	17	High
Due et al. (2018) [41]	Y	Y	N	N	Y	N	N	N	N	N	N	N	N	N	N	Y	Y	Y	N	Y	10	Moderate
Hwang et al. (2015) [42]	Y	Y	N	Y	Y	N	N	Y	Y	N	Y	Y	N	N	Y	Y	Y	Y	na	Y	14	Moderate
Ji et al. (2014) [43]	N	Y	Y	Y	Y	Y	Y	Y	Y	Y	Y	Y	N	Y	Y	Y	Y	Y	N	Y	19	High
Jones et al. (2017) [44]	Y	Y	N	Y	Y	Y	N	Y	Y	N	N	Y	N	N	Y	Y	Y	Y	N	Y	15	High
Leadbitter et al. (2018) [45]	Y	Y	N	N	Y	N	N	N	Y	N	N	Y	N	N	Y	Y	Y	N	N	Y	11	Moderate
Leadbitter et al. (2020) [46]	Y	Y	N	Y	Y	Y	N	Y	N	N	N	Y	N	N	Y	Y	Y	Y	N	Y	14	Moderate
Mathew et al. (2019) [47]	Y	Y	N	Y	Y	Y	N	Y	Y	Y	N	Y	N	N	Y	Y	Y	Y	N	Y	16	High
McConkey (2020) [48]	N	N	N	N	Y	Y	N	N	N	N	Y	Y	N	N	Y	Y	N	N	N	Y	9	Moderate
McConkey et al. (2020) [49]	N	Y	N	Y	N	N	N	N	N	N	N	Y	N	N	Y	N	N	N	N	Y	7	Low
McPhilemy & Dillenburger (2013) [50]	N	N	N	N	Y	N	N	N	N	N	N	Y	N	N	Y	Y	Y	N	na	Y	7	Low
Milbourn et al. (2017) [51]	Y	Y	N	Y	N	N	N	na	na	N	N	N	N	N	Y	Y	Y	Y	N	Y	10	Moderate
Moody et al. (2019) [52]	Y	Y	N	Y	Y	Y	N	Y	Y	Y	Y	Y	N	N	Y	Y	Y	Y	N	Y	17	High
Paynter et al. (2018) [53]	Y	Y	N	Y	Y	Y	na	Y	Y	N	Y	Y	N	N	Y	Y	Y	Y	N	Y	16	High
Roberts et al. (2011) [54]	Y	Y	Y	Y	Y	Y	N	Y	Y	Y	Y	Y	N	N	Y	Y	Y	Y	N	Y	18	High
Mean																					**13.18**	
Standard Deviation																					**3.68**	

Note: Yes = Y; No = N; Don't know = na; Items 13 and 19 are score reversed (see [60]).

3.4. Main Findings

3.4.1. No Parental Involvement

In two studies, interventions were conducted entirely by professionals without any form of parental involvement [10,40]. Derguy et al. [40] found that access to child-focused psycho-educational intervention was positively associated with parental QoL. Baghdadli et al. [10] found that the number of hours of specialized intervention focused on externalizing difficulties of adolescents with ASD was negatively associated with parental QoL.

3.4.2. Indirect Parental Involvement

Four studies used indirect strategies (e.g., parent training and support groups) to involve parents in the interventions [39,44,53,54]. In these cases, the main part of the intervention is centred on the child or the adolescent with ASD and is conducted in a clinical setting.

The results indicated an overall low level of QoL among parents who have been indirectly involved in an intervention for their child or adolescent with ASD. Specifically, Paynter et al. [53] found low levels of family adaptation (e.g., individual mental health, relationship quality, and family well-being) among fathers of children with ASD who participated to the centre-based early intervention. Interventions based on applied behaviour analysis (ABA) were associated with overall negative parent experiences because of the poor quality of the support received at home and the scarce coordination and guidance from the professionals [39]. In addition, findings by Jones et al. [44] showed that time on a waitlist for the ABA treatment was not associated with parental QoL. In contrast, Roberts et al.'s [54] randomised control trial revealed an increase in parent QoL after centre-based early interventions focused on functional impairments of children and on improving the parents' knowledge of ASD.

3.4.3. Direct Parental Involvement

Twelve studies used direct methods (e.g., parent-mediated home-based training, family-centred intervention, parent mentoring program) to involve parents in the interventions [41–43,45,47–52].

The majority of studies found that parental QoL improved after the intervention and, crucially, two studies found that parental direct involvement in the intervention was associated with greater parental QoL [41,43]. Specifically, parents of children with ASD showed significantly improved QoL after they participated in a parent-mediated communication-focused intervention [45,46], a family-centred intervention [49], an ABA-based home program [50], and the Colorado parent mentoring (CPM) program [52]. Moreover, parents of children with ASD who participated in a multidisciplinary parent education program reported increased mental, but not physical, QoL [43,48]. Consistently, Milbourn et al. [51] found that parents of children and adolescents with ASD reported that early access to intervention improved their QoL, especially in terms of fostering their involvement in their child's daily life. However, three studies reported inconsistent results. Roberts et al. [48] found no significant changes in the QoL of parents of children with ASD after a home-based early intervention program. Similarly, Hwang et al. [42] found that mothers of children and adolescents with ASD did not report a significant increase in their QoL after they received a mindfulness parent-mediated home-based training. In addition, parents, especially mothers of children with ASD, who received an early intervention using the Early Start Denver Model showed lower parental well-being compared to the normative population [47].

4. Discussion

To our knowledge, this is the first review to examine the relationship between QoL and involvement in intervention among parents of children and adolescents with ASD. The 17 reviewed studies involved a total of 18 interventions targeting children and adolescents with ASD. Two studies reported no parental involvement in the intervention, three studies reported indirect parental involvement, and 11 studies reported direct parental involvement. One study [54] included both direct and indirect parental involvement in intervention.

The reviewed studies used heterogeneous designs and data collection methods and the majority of the studies had relatively small sample sizes [39,41–43,46,49,50,52–54], which limits our ability to draw firm conclusions about the association between parental QoL and involvement in interventions for youth with ASD.

From the limited data of the reviewed studies, the overall QoL of parents of children and adolescents with ASD appears to be shaped by the way they have been involved in the intervention. In line with a previous systematic review [24], our results showed that access to ASD services is a relevant protective factor not only for children, but also for parents [40]. Children with ASD can be expected to gain significant improvements when diagnosed early and when engaged in structured, intensive, evidence-based programs [61–63]. In contrast, difficulties in meeting the service needs of children with ASDs, ranging from general medical services to supportive services [64], can generate a vicious cycle of worsening symptoms and an overload of responsibility on parents who come to feel exhausted and ineffective [39]. However, the fact that one's child with ASD receives treatment does not in itself guarantee an improvement in parental QoL. In fact, results showed that interventions based on the external difficulties of people with ASD, which do not involve parents in the intervention or involve them only indirectly, do not improve or even worsen parental QoL [10,39,44]. For example, interventions based on ABA are recognised as valid methods used for educating individuals with ASD [65,66], which are characterised by a strong asymmetry of roles of participants in the intervention. Qualified behaviour analysts design, develop, conduct, and directly oversee the ABA-programme that is focused on the child or the adolescent with ASD, while parents receive training to support their offspring in skill practice throughout the day. Behavioural child-focused interventions (e.g., ABA-based interventions), no matter how clinically effective, may be not sufficiently adapted to the broad family needs or may be unsuitable for a family situation. In contrast, when ABA-based interventions are implemented in a home setting and actively involved the whole family, parents report an overall better QoL [50]. In fact, interventions explicitly targeting children's daily living skills in addition to the hallmark symptoms of ASD (i.e., social-communication deficits and repetitive, restrictive behaviours) may enhance parental QoL [54,67].

The majority of the studies examined in this review directly involved parents in the intervention. This may be a sign in the shift in perspective that is occurring in interventions for individuals with ASD and an increased awareness by professionals of the role of parents to implement effective interventions [46]. Parents who were directly involved in the intervention tended to report a higher QoL [43,45,46,49–52]. For example, in one study [43], 22 caregivers of children with ASD participated in an 8-week multidisciplinary education programme, with the intent to learn adaptive strategies and manage the problem behaviours of their child, and consequently to improve the intrafamilial QoL. Results indicated a significant improvement in family functioning, self-efficacy, and coping styles. Another study [49] provided post-diagnostic support to nearly 100 families and children, over a 12-month period. The project implemented a family-centred plan that showed improvements in children's social and communication skills and overall stress reduction in parents. Yet another study [42] described an 8-week training program that comprised six mother–child dyads, aimed at teaching mindfulness strategies to better cope with problem behaviours of their children. At the end of the program, the participants reported positive effects in the targeted areas including parenting stress, intrafamilial QoL, and problematic behaviours. These results can be attributable to various reasons. When parents are actively involved by professionals, the intervention is more personalised and ecological [40]. This is also a way of empowering parents by recognising their expertise and contributions [68,69] and to develop constructive collaboration between different actors involved in the intervention [70]. Based on these findings, clinicians should assess and counsel parents, and identify potential barriers (e.g., lack of resolution of diagnosis) that may prevent them from actively participating in the intervention for their child or adolescent with ASD.

5. Limitations

The present systematic review comes with a number of limitations. Some depend on the relative novelty of the topic and on the absence of shared guidelines in the treatment of children and adolescents with ASD. The selected studies adopted a variety of methods and approaches (e.g., observational studies vs. randomised controlled trials), which limit the possibility to compare their findings. Another limitation regards our search and selection procedure. The construct of parental QoL is very broad and thus some studies may have evaluated some specific dimensions not included in our search keywords. Additionally, we only included articles published in English sources, which may have contributed to a selection bias by overlooking relevant articles published in other languages. In addition, we did not investigate the QoL of family as a whole (e.g., including siblings of children with ASD). However, parents are more generally actively involved in the care and intervention for their children. Furthermore, geographical coverage was dominated by Europe and Australia, therefore further research is needed in Asiatic cultural contexts [71]. Finally, the included studies recruited relatively small samples of self-selected participants who may not be necessarily representative of the general population.

6. Conclusions and Future Directions

Parental involvement in intervention for children or adolescents with ASD is a topic that is attracting increasing attention, as evidenced by the fact that parents were directly involved in interventions in most of the studies selected in this systematic review. The findings suggest that increasing parental involvement in the intervention for children or adolescents with ASD may be one way to promote their QoL. More precisely, this systematic review highlights that a constructive collaboration between professionals and parents in planning and executing interventions may promote more ecological results and better satisfaction among parents. This finding is consistent with the literature on parental QoL [24] and supports the relevance of an ecological and holistic approach in the research on QoL in parents of children with ASD [40]. This could help clinicians to better identify and address parental needs and enhance parenting resources that have a positive impact on the intervention.

Suggestions for future research put forward here include the use of longitudinal studies conducted with wider and demographically diverse samples that would include families from diverse geographical locations who have children with ASD of different ages (e.g., adults).

Supplementary Materials: The following are available online at https://www.mdpi.com/article/10.3390/jpm11090894/s1, Table S1: Full-text articles excluded, with reasons ($n = 79$).

Author Contributions: Conceptualization, A.M. and T.M.; Methodology, A.M. and T.M.; Writing—original draft preparation, A.M. and T.M.; Writing—review and editing, B.D., C.R., G.B., R.M., G.E. and D.D.; Supervision, G.P., C.F. and P.C. All authors have read and agreed to the published version of the manuscript.

Funding: The APC was funded by Fondazione Bambini e Autismo Onlus.

Institutional Review Board Statement: Not applicable.

Informed Consent Statement: Informed consent was obtained from all subjects involved in the study.

Data Availability Statement: Not applicable.

Conflicts of Interest: The authors declare no conflict of interest.

References

1. American Psychiatric Association. *Diagnostic and Statistical Manual of Mental Disorders*, 5th ed.; American Psychiatric Association: Washington, DC, USA, 2013; ISBN 0-89042-555-8.
2. Volkmar, F.R.; Pauls, D. Autism. *Lancet* **2003**, *362*, 1133–1141. [CrossRef]
3. Giovagnoli, G.; Postorino, V.; Fatta, L.M.; Sanges, V.; De Peppo, L.; Vassena, L.; De Rose, P.; Vicari, S.; Mazzone, L. Behavioral and emotional profile and parental stress in preschool children with autism spectrum disorder. *Res. Dev. Disabil.* **2015**, *45–46*, 411–421. [CrossRef]
4. Militerni, R.; Bravaccio, C.; Falco, C.; Fico, C.; Palermo, M.T. Repetitive behaviors in autistic disorder. *Eur. Child Adolesc. Psychiatry* **2002**, *11*, 210–218. [CrossRef] [PubMed]
5. Tudor, M.E.; Hoffman, C.D.; Sweeney, D.P. Children with autism: Sleep problems and symptom severity. *Focus Autism Other Dev. Disabl.* **2012**, *27*, 254–262. [CrossRef]
6. Shaw, A.; Do, T.N.T.; Harrison, L.; Marczak, M.; Dimitriou, D.; Joyce, A. Sleep and cognition in people with autism spectrum condition: A systematic literature review. *Rev. J. Autism Dev. Disord.* **2021**. [CrossRef]
7. Pozo, P.; Sarriá, E.; Brioso, A. Family quality of life and psychological well-being in parents of children with autism spectrum disorders: A double ABCX model. *J. Intellect. Disabil. Res.* **2014**, *58*, 442–458. [CrossRef]
8. Corsano, P.; Musetti, A.; Guidotti, L.; Capelli, F. Typically developing adolescents' experience of growing up with a brother with an autism spectrum disorder. *J. Intellect. Dev. Disabil.* **2017**, *42*, 151–161. [CrossRef]
9. Guidotti, L.; Musetti, A.; Barbieri, G.L.; Ballocchi, I.; Corsano, P. Conflicting and harmonious sibling relationships of children and adolescent siblings of children with autism spectrum disorder. *Child Care Health Dev.* **2021**, *47*, 163–173. [CrossRef] [PubMed]
10. Baghdadli, A.; Pry, R.; Michelon, C.; Rattaz, C. Impact of autism in adolescents on parental quality of life. *Qual. Life Res.* **2014**, *23*, 1859–1868. [CrossRef] [PubMed]
11. Hayes, S.A.; Watson, S.L. The impact of parenting stress: A meta-analysis of studies comparing the experience of parenting stress in parents of children with and without autism spectrum disorder. *J. Autism Dev. Disord.* **2013**, *43*, 629–642. [CrossRef] [PubMed]
12. Bonis, S. Stress and parents of children with autism: A review of literature. *Issues Ment. Health Nurs.* **2016**, *37*, 153–163. [CrossRef] [PubMed]
13. Davis, N.O.; Carter, A.S. Parenting stress in mothers and fathers of toddlers with autism spectrum disorders: Associations with child characteristics. *J. Autism Dev. Disord.* **2008**, *38*, 1278–1291. [CrossRef]
14. Factor, R.S.; Ollendick, T.H.; Cooper, L.D.; Dunsmore, J.C.; Rea, H.M.; Scarpa, A. All in the family: A systematic review of the effect of caregiver administered autism spectrum disorder interventions on family functioning and relationships. *Clin. Child Fam. Psychol. Rev.* **2019**, *22*, 433–457. [CrossRef] [PubMed]
15. McConachie, H.; Diggle, T. Parent implemented early intervention for young children with autism spectrum disorder: A systematic review. *J. Eval. Clin. Pract.* **2007**, *13*, 120–129. [CrossRef]
16. Yan, T.; Hou, Y.; Deng, M. Direct, indirect, and buffering effect of social support on parental involvement among Chinese parents of children with autism spectrum disorders. *J. Autism Dev. Disord.* **2021**. [CrossRef]
17. Đorđević, M.; Glumbić, N.; Memisevic, H.; Brojčin, B.; Krstov, A. Parent-teacher interactions, family stress, well-being, and parental depression as contributing factors to parental involvement mechanisms in education of children with autism. *Int. J. Dev. Disabil.* **2021**, 1–12. [CrossRef]
18. Schertz, H.H.; Baker, C.; Hurwitz, S.; Benner, L. Principles of early intervention reflected in toddler research in autism spectrum disorders. *Top. Early Child. Spec. Educ.* **2011**, *31*, 4–21. [CrossRef]
19. Liu, Q.; Hsieh, W.Y.; Chen, G. A systematic review and meta-analysis of parent-mediated intervention for children and adolescents with autism spectrum disorder in mainland China, Hong Kong, and Taiwan. *Autism* **2020**, *24*, 1960–1979. [CrossRef]
20. Karst, J.S.; van Hecke, A.V. Parent and family impact of autism spectrum disorders: A review and proposed model for intervention evaluation. *Clin. Child Fam. Psychol. Rev.* **2012**, *15*, 247–277. [CrossRef]
21. Payakachat, N.; Tilford, J.M.; Kovacs, E.; Kuhlthau, K. Autism spectrum disorders: A review of measures for clinical, health services and cost-effectiveness applications. *Expert Rev. Pharmacoecon. Outcomes Res.* **2012**, *12*, 485–503. [CrossRef]
22. Hastings, R.P.; Taunt, H.M. Positive perceptions in families of children with developmental disabilities. *Am. J. Ment. Retard.* **2002**, *107*, 116. [CrossRef]
23. Cappe, E.; Wolff, M.; Bobet, R.; Adrien, J.L. Quality of life: A key variable to consider in the evaluation of adjustment in parents of children with autism spectrum disorders and in the development of relevant support and assistance programmes. *Qual. Life Res.* **2011**, *20*, 1279–1294. [CrossRef] [PubMed]
24. Vasilopoulou, E.; Nisbet, J. The quality of life of parents of children with autism spectrum disorder: A systematic review. *Res. Autism Spectr. Disord.* **2016**, *23*, 36–49. [CrossRef]
25. Hastings, R.P.; Kovshoff, H.; Ward, N.J.; Degli Espinosa, F.; Brown, T.; Remington, B. Systems analysis of stress and positive perceptions in mothers and fathers of pre-school children with autism. *J. Autism Dev. Disord.* **2005**, *35*, 635–644. [CrossRef] [PubMed]
26. Lickenbrock, D.M.; Ekas, N.V.; Whitman, T.L. Feeling good, feeling bad: Influences of maternal perceptions of the child and marital adjustment on well-being in mothers of children with an autism spectrum disorder. *J. Autism Dev. Disord.* **2011**, *41*, 848–858. [CrossRef]

27. Wachtel, K.; Carter, A.S. Reaction to diagnosis and parenting styles among mothers of young children with ASDs. *Autism* **2008**, *12*, 575–594. [CrossRef]
28. Dardas, L.A.; Ahmad, M.M. Validation of the World Health Organization's quality of life questionnaire with parents of children with autistic disorder. *J. Autism Dev. Disord.* **2014**, *44*, 2257–2263. [CrossRef] [PubMed]
29. Mello, C.; Rivard, M.; Terroux, A.; Mercier, C. Quality of life in families of young children with autism spectrum disorder. *Am. J. Intellect. Dev. Disabil.* **2019**, *124*, 535–548. [CrossRef]
30. WHO Quality of Life Assessment Group. The World Health Organization quality of life assessment (WHOQOL): Development and general psychometric properties. *Soc. Sci. Med.* **1998**, *46*, 1569–1585. [CrossRef]
31. Dixon, L.; Lucksted, A.; Stewart, B.; Burland, J.; Brown, C.H.; Postrado, L.; McGuire, C.; Hoffman, M. Outcomes of the peer-taught 12-week family-to-family education program for severe mental illness. *Acta Psychiatr. Scand.* **2004**, *109*, 207–215. [CrossRef]
32. Liberati, A.; Altman, D.G.; Tetzlaff, J.; Mulrow, C.; Gøtzsche, P.C.; Ioannidis, J.P.A.; Clarke, M.; Devereaux, P.J.; Kleijnen, J.; Moher, D. The PRISMA statement for reporting systematic reviews and meta-analyses of studies that evaluate health care interventions: Explanation and elaboration. *J. Clin. Epidemiol.* **2009**, *62*, e1–e34. [CrossRef]
33. Edwards, P.; Clarke, M.; DiGuiseppi, C.; Pratap, S.; Roberts, I.; Wentz, R. Identification of randomized controlled trials in systematic reviews: Accuracy and reliability of screening records. *Stat. Med.* **2002**, *21*, 1635–1640. [CrossRef] [PubMed]
34. Downes, M.J.; Brennan, M.L.; Williams, H.C.; Dean, R.S. Development of a critical appraisal tool to assess the quality of cross-sectional studies (AXIS). *BMJ Open* **2016**, *6*, 1–7. [CrossRef]
35. Moor, L.; Anderson, J.R. A systematic literature review of the relationship between dark personality traits and antisocial online behaviours. *Pers. Individ. Dif.* **2019**, *144*, 40–55. [CrossRef]
36. Raber, M.; Swartz, M.C.; Santa Maria, D.; O'Connor, T.; Baranowski, T.; Li, R.; Chandra, J. Parental involvement in exercise and diet interventions for childhood cancer survivors: A systematic review. *Pediatr. Res.* **2016**, *80*, 338–346. [CrossRef] [PubMed]
37. Hoffman, L.; Marquis, J.; Poston, D.; Summers, J.A.; Turnbull, A. Assessing family outcomes: Psychometric evaluation of the beach center family quality of life scale. *J. Marriage Fam.* **2006**, *68*, 1069–1083. [CrossRef]
38. Abidin, R.R. *Parenting Stress Index—Short Form*; Psychological Assessment Resources: Lutz, FL, USA, 1995.
39. Aandersson, G.W.; Miniscalco, C.; Ggillberg, N. A 6-year follow-up of children assessed for suspected autism spectrum disorder: Parents' experiences of society's support. *Neuropsychiatr. Dis. Treat.* **2017**, *13*, 1783–1796. [CrossRef] [PubMed]
40. Derguy, C.; Roux, S.; Portex, M.; M'bailara, K. An ecological exploration of individual, family, and environmental contributions to parental quality of life in autism. *Psychiatry Res.* **2018**, *268*, 87–93. [CrossRef] [PubMed]
41. Due, C.; Goodwin Smith, I.; Allen, P.; Button, E.; Cheek, C.; Quarmby, L.; Stephens, M.; Paku, S.; Ferguson, S.; Fordyce, K. A pilot study of social inclusion and quality of life for parents of children with autism spectrum disorder. *J. Intellect. Dev. Disabil.* **2018**, *43*, 73–82. [CrossRef]
42. Hwang, Y.S.; Kearney, P.; Klieve, H.; Lang, W.; Roberts, J. Cultivating mind: Mindfulness interventions for children with autism spectrum disorder and problem behaviours, and their mothers. *J. Child Fam. Stud.* **2015**, *24*, 3093–3106. [CrossRef]
43. Ji, B.; Sun, M.; Yi, R.; Tang, S. Multidisciplinary parent education for caregivers of children with autism spectrum disorders. *Arch. Psychiatr. Nurs.* **2014**, *28*, 319–326. [CrossRef] [PubMed]
44. Jones, S.; Bremer, E.; Lloyd, M. Autism spectrum disorder: Family quality of life while waiting for intervention services. *Qual. Life Res.* **2017**, *26*, 331–342. [CrossRef]
45. Leadbitter, K.; Aldred, C.; McConachie, H.; Le Couteur, A.; Kapadia, D.; Charman, T.; Macdonald, W.; Salomone, E.; Emsley, R.; Green, J.; et al. The Autism Family Experience Questionnaire (AFEQ): An ecologically-valid, parent-nominated measure of family experience, quality of life and prioritised outcomes for early intervention. *J. Autism Dev. Disord.* **2018**, *48*, 1052–1062. [CrossRef]
46. Leadbitter, K.; Macdonald, W.; Taylor, C.; Buckle, K.L.; Aldred, C.; Barrett, B.; Barron, S.; Beggs, K.; Blazey, L.; Bourne, K.; et al. Parent perceptions of participation in a parent-mediated communication-focussed intervention with their young child with autism spectrum disorder. *Autism* **2020**, *24*, 2129–2141. [CrossRef]
47. Mathew, N.E.; Burton, K.L.O.; Schierbeek, A.; Črnčec, R.; Walter, A.; Eapen, V. Parenting preschoolers with autism: Socioeconomic influences on wellbeing and sense of competence. *World J. Psychiatry* **2019**, *9*, 30–46. [CrossRef] [PubMed]
48. McConkey, R. A brief measure of parental wellbeing for use in evaluations of family-centred interventions for children with developmental disabilities. *Children* **2020**, *7*, 120. [CrossRef]
49. McConkey, R.; Cassin, M.T.; McNaughton, R. Promoting the social inclusion of children with ASD: A family-centred intervention. *Brain Sci.* **2020**, *10*, 318. [CrossRef] [PubMed]
50. Mcphilemy, C.; Dillenburger, K. Parents' experiences of applied behaviour analysis (ABA)-based interventions for children diagnosed with autistic spectrum disorder. *Br. J. Spec. Educ.* **2013**, *40*, 154–161. [CrossRef]
51. Milbourn, B.; Falkmer, M.; Black, M.H.; Girdler, S.; Falkmer, T.; Horlin, C. An exploration of the experience of parents with children with autism spectrum disorder after diagnosis and intervention. *Scand. J. Child Adolesc. Psychiatry Psychol.* **2017**, *5*, 104–110. [CrossRef]
52. Moody, E.J.; Kaiser, K.; Sharp, D.; Kubicek, L.F.; Rigles, B.; Davis, J.; McSwegin, S.; D'Abreu, L.C.; Rosenberg, C.R. Improving family functioning following diagnosis of ASD: A randomized trial of a parent mentorship program. *J. Child Fam. Stud.* **2019**, *28*, 424–435. [CrossRef]
53. Paynter, J.; Davies, M.; Beamish, W. Recognising the "forgotten man": Fathers' experiences in caring for a young child with autism spectrum disorder. *J. Intellect. Dev. Disabil.* **2017**, *43*, 112–124. [CrossRef]

54. Roberts, J.; Williams, K.; Carter, M.; Evans, D.; Parmenter, T.; Silove, N.; Clark, T.; Warren, A. A randomised controlled trial of two early intervention programs for young children with autism: Centre-based with parent program and home-based. *Res. Autism Spectr. Disord.* **2011**, *5*, 1553–1566. [CrossRef]
55. Novak, M.; Guest, C. Application of a multidimensional caregiver. *Gerontologist* **1989**, *29*, 798–803. [CrossRef] [PubMed]
56. Brown, I.; Brown, R.; Baum, N.; Isaacs, B.; Myerscough, T.; Neikrug, S.; Roth, D.; Shearer, J.; Wang, M. *Family Quality of Life Survey: Main Caregivers of People with Intellectual or Developmental Disabilities*; Surrey Place Centre: Toronto, ON, Canada, 2006.
57. Berdeaux, G.; Hervié, C.; Smajda, C.; Marquis, P. Parental quality of life and recurrent ENT infections in their children: Development of a questionnaire. *Qual. Life Res.* **1998**, *7*, 501–512. [CrossRef] [PubMed]
58. Johnston, C.; Mash, E.J. A measure of parenting satisfaction and efficacy. *J. Clin. Child Psychol.* **1989**, *18*, 167–175. [CrossRef]
59. Eapen, V.; Črnčec, R.; Walter, A.; Tay, K.P. Conceptualisation and development of a quality of life measure for parents of children with autism spectrum disorder. *Autism Res. Treat.* **2014**, *2014*, 160783. [CrossRef]
60. Harst, L.; Lantzsch, H.; Scheibe, M. Theories predicting end-user acceptance of telemedicine use: Systematic review. *J. Med. Internet Res.* **2019**, *21*, e13117. [CrossRef] [PubMed]
61. Lake, J.K.; Tablon Modica, P.; Chan, V.; Weiss, J.A. Considering efficacy and effectiveness trials of cognitive behavioral therapy among youth with autism: A systematic review. *Autism* **2020**, *24*, 1590–1606. [CrossRef] [PubMed]
62. Eisenhower, A.; Martinez Pedraza, F.; Sheldrick, R.C.; Frenette, E.; Hoch, N.; Brunt, S.; Carter, A.S. Multi-stage screening in early intervention: A critical strategy for improving ASD identification and addressing disparities. *J. Autism Dev. Disord.* **2021**, *51*, 868–883. [CrossRef]
63. Magán-Maganto, M.; Bejarano-Martín, Á.; Fernández-Alvarez, C.; Narzisi, A.; García-Primo, P.; Kawa, R.; Posada, M.; Canal-Bedia, R. Early detection and intervention of ASD: A European overview. *Brain Sci.* **2017**, *7*, 159. [CrossRef]
64. Bishop-Fitzpatrick, L.; Smith DaWalt, L.; Greenberg, J.S.; Mailick, M.R. Participation in recreational activities buffers the impact of perceived stress on quality of life in adults with autism spectrum disorder. *Autism Res.* **2017**, *10*, 973–982. [CrossRef] [PubMed]
65. Anderson, S.R.; Romanczyk, R.G. Early intervention for young children with autism: Continuum-based behavioral models. *J. Assoc. Pers. Sev. Handicap.* **1999**, *24*, 162–173. [CrossRef]
66. Peters-Scheffer, N.; Didden, R.; Korzilius, H.; Sturmey, P. A meta-analytic study on the effectiveness of comprehensive ABA-based early intervention programs for children with autism spectrum disorders. *Res. Autism Spectr. Disord.* **2011**, *5*, 60–69. [CrossRef]
67. Gardiner, E.; Iarocci, G. Family quality of life and asd: The role of child adaptive functioning and behavior problems. *Autism Res.* **2015**, *8*, 199–213. [CrossRef]
68. Hou, Y.; Kim, S.Y.; Hazen, N.; Benner, A.D. Parents' perceived discrimination and adolescent adjustment in Chinese American families: Mediating family processes. *Child Dev.* **2017**, *88*, 317–331. [CrossRef] [PubMed]
69. Robert, M.; Leblanc, L.; Boyer, T. When satisfaction is not directly related to the support services received: Understanding parents' varied experiences with specialised services for children with developmental disabilities. *Br. J. Learn. Disabil.* **2015**, *43*, 168–177. [CrossRef]
70. Moh, T.A.; Magiati, I. Factors associated with parental stress and satisfaction during the process of diagnosis of children with autism spectrum disorders. *Res. Autism Spectr. Disord.* **2012**, *6*, 293–303. [CrossRef]
71. Wang, H.; Hu, X.; Han, Z.R. Parental stress, involvement, and family quality of life in mothers and fathers of children with autism spectrum disorder in mainland China: A dyadic analysis. *Res. Dev. Disabil.* **2020**, *107*, 103791. [CrossRef]

MDPI
St. Alban-Anlage 66
4052 Basel
Switzerland
Tel. +41 61 683 77 34
Fax +41 61 302 89 18
www.mdpi.com

Journal of Personalized Medicine Editorial Office
E-mail: jpm@mdpi.com
www.mdpi.com/journal/jpm

www.ingramcontent.com/pod-product-compliance
Lightning Source LLC
LaVergne TN
LVHW070251100526
838202LV00015B/2207
* 9 7 8 3 0 3 6 5 3 2 2 1 9 *